The Epidemiology of Eye Disease

Third Edition

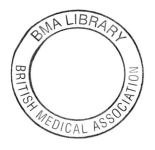

THE EPIDEMIOLOGY OF EYE DISEASE

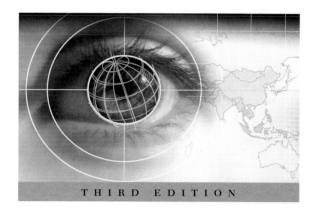

THIRD EDITION

Edited by

Gordon J Johnson
MA MD FRCS(C) FRCOphth
Honorary Professor, London School of Hygiene and Tropical Medicine, UK

Darwin C Minassian
MB BS FRCS MSc(Epidemiol) FRCOphth
Emeritus Reader, University College London, UK

Robert A Weale
MSc MPhil PhD DSc
Institute of Gerontology, King's College London, UK

Sheila K West
PhD
El-Maghraby Professor of Preventive Ophthalmology
The Johns Hopkins University School of Medicine, Baltimore, MD, USA

Associate Editors

Emily W Gower
PhD
Associate Professor, Wilmer Eye Institute, The Johns Hopkins University School of Medicine, Baltimore, MD, USA

Hannah Kuper
ScD
Senior Lecturer, London School of Hygiene and Tropical Medicine, UK

Robert Lindfield
MB ChB MSc MRCOphth MFPH
Clinical Lecturer in International Ophthalmic Public Health, London School of Hygiene and Tropical Medicine, UK

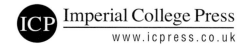

Imperial College Press
www.icpress.co.uk

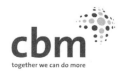

Published by

Imperial College Press
57 Shelton Street
Covent Garden
London WC2H 9HE

Distributed by

World Scientific Publishing Co. Pte. Ltd.
5 Toh Tuck Link, Singapore 596224
USA office: 27 Warren Street, Suite 401-402, Hackensack, NJ 07601
UK office: 57 Shelton Street, Covent Garden, London WC2H 9HE

British Library Cataloguing-in-Publication Data
A catalogue record for this book is available from the British Library.

THE EPIDEMIOLOGY OF EYE DISEASE
Third Edition

ISBN-13 978-1-84816-625-7
ISBN-10 1-84816-625-7

Typeset by Stallion Press
Email: enquiries@stallionpress.com

Printed by FuIsland Offset Printing (S) Pte Ltd Singapore

Contents

List of Contributors ix
Foreword to the first edition xiii
Foreword to the second edition xv
Foreword to the third edition xvii
Acknowledgements xix

SECTION 1: INTRODUCTION

1   **Prevalence, incidence and distribution of visual impairment** 3
GVS Murthy and Gordon Johnson

SECTION 2: METHODOLOGY

2   **Epidemiological research methods: an outline** 65
Darwin Minassian and Hannah Kuper

3   **Cross-sectional studies** 79
Darwin Minassian and Hannah Kuper

4   **Case-control studies** 95
Astrid Fletcher

5   **Cohort studies** 109
Emily Herrett and Hannah Kuper

6   **Genetic epidemiology** 117
Christopher Hammond

7   **Clinical trials** 131
Maureen Maguire

8   **Screening in ophthalmology** 147
Richard Wormald and Robert Lindfield

9   Research synthesis   **169**
Jennifer Evans and Richard Wormald

SECTION 3: SPECIFIC ENTITIES   **175**

10   Age-related cataract   **177**
Emily Gower and Sheila West

11   Epidemiology of refractive errors and presbyopia   **197**
Leslie Hyman and Ilesh Patel

12   The epidemiology of low vision   **227**
Gary Rubin

13   Glaucoma   **241**
Paul Foster and Harry Quigley

14   Visual impairment and blindness in children   **267**
   14a   Magnitude and causes   269
         Clare Gilbert and Jugnoo Rahi
   14b   Vitamin A deficiency disorders   291
         Keith West Jr and Alfred Sommer
   14c   Ophthalmia neonatorum   317
         Volker Klauss and Ulrich Schaller
   14d   Corneal disease in children   323
         Clare Gilbert
   14e   Cataract in children   331
         Edward Wilson and Rupal Trivedi
   14f   Glaucoma in children   341
         Maria Papadopoulos and Peng Tee Khaw
   14g   Retinopathy of prematurity   353
         Subhadra Jalali and Graham Quinn

15   Dry eye disease   **369**
Debra Schaumberg and Giulio Ferrari

16   Corneal and external diseases   **391**
   16a   Microbial keratitis   393
         John Whitcher, Mathua Srinivasan and Madan Upadhyay
   16b   Viral infectious keratoconjunctivitis   403
         Stephen Tuft and Bita Manzouri
   16c   Acanthamoeba keratitis   409
         Stephanie Watson and John Dart
   16d   Ocular manifestations of leprosy   419
         Paul Courtright and Susan Lewallen
   16e   Vernal keratoconjunctivitis   429
         Stephen Tuft and Bita Manzouri
   16f   Mooren's ulcer   435
         Stephen Tuft and Bita Manzouri

16g Climatic droplet keratopathy   439
     Gordon Johnson
16h Pterygium   447
     Gordon Johnson

17   **Epidemiology of trachoma**   455
     Sheila West and Robin Bailey

18   **Onchocerciasis**   487
     Adrian Hopkins

19   **The epidemiology of uveitis**   509
     Jennifer Thorne and Douglas Jabs

20   **Ocular complications of human immunodeficiency virus infection** 517
     John Kempen

21   **Diabetic retinopathy**   547
     Barbara Klein and Ronald Klein

22   **Age-related macular degeneration**   571
     Jennifer Evans and Tien Wong

SECTION 4: PREVENTION STRATEGIES   585

23   **From epidemiology to programme**   587
     Robert Lindfield, Hans Limburg and Allen Foster

24   **Global initiative for the elimination of avoidable blindness** 601
     Robert Lindfield, Ivo Kocur, Hans Limburg and Allen Foster

Glossary   607

Index   617

List of Contributors

Robin Bailey
Professor of Tropical Medicine, Department of Infectious and Tropical Diseases, London School of Hygiene and Tropical Medicine, London; and Consultant, Hospital for Tropical Diseases, London, UK

Paul Courtright
Co-Director, Kilimanjaro Centre for Community Ophthalmology, Tumaini University, Moshi, Tanzania and University of British Columbia, Vancouver, Canada

John KG Dart
Consultant Ophthalmologist, Moorfields Eye Hospital, London; and Reader in Ophthalmology, Institute of Ophthalmology, University College London, UK

Jennifer Evans
Lecturer in Epidemiology, London School of Hygiene and Tropical Medicine, London, UK

Giulio Ferrari
Schepens Eye Research Institute, Harvard Medical School, Boston, MA, USA; and G B Bietti Eye Foundation, IRCCS, Rome, Italy

Astrid Fletcher
Professor of Epidemiology of Ageing, Department of Epidemiology and Population Health, London School of Hygiene and Tropical Medicine, London, UK

Allen Foster
President, CBM International; and Professor of International Eye Health, London School of Hygiene and Tropical Medicine, London, UK

Paul J Foster
Reader in Epidemiology, Division of Genetics, Institute of Ophthalmology, University College London; and Consultant, Glaucoma Service, Moorfields Eye Hospital, London, UK

Clare Gilbert
Professor of International Eye Health, London School of Hygiene and Tropical Medicine, London, UK

Emily W Gower
Associate Professor, Wilmer Eye Institute, The Johns Hopkins University School of Medicine, Baltimore, MD, USA

Christopher Hammond
Frost Professor of Ophthalmology, Departments of Ophthalmology and Twin Research and Genetic Epidemiology, King's College London, St Thomas' Hospital, London, UK

Emily Herrett
Research Student, Department of Epidemiology and Population Health, London School of Hygiene and Tropical Medicine, UK

Adrian D Hopkins
Director, Mectizan Donation Program (MDP) Secretariat, Task Force for Global Health, Emory University, Atlanta, GA, USA

Leslie Hyman
Professor of Epidemiology, Department of Preventive Medicine, Stony Brook University Medical Center, Stony Brook, NY, USA

Douglas A Jabs
Professor and Chair, Department of Ophthalmology; Professor of Medicine; and Dean for Clinical Affairs, Mount Sinai School of Medicine, New York, NY; Adjunct Professor of Epidemiology, Johns Hopkins Bloomberg School of Public Health, Baltimore, MD, USA

Subhadra Jalali
Consultant Ophthalmologist, Jasti Ramanamma Children's Eye Centre, L V Prasad Eye Institute, Hyderabad, Andhra Pradesh, India

Gordon J Johnson
Honorary Professor, London School of Hygiene and Tropical Medicine, London, UK

John H Kempen
Associate Professor of Ophthalmology, Departments of Ophthalmology and Biostatistics and Epidemiology, Center for Clinical Epidemiology and Biostatistics, University of Pennsylvania, Philadelphia, PA, USA

Peng T Khaw
Professor of Glaucoma and Ocular Healing, Institute of Ophthalmology, University College London; and Consultant Ophthalmic Surgeon, Moorfields Eye Hospital, London, UK

Volker Klauss
Professor of Ophthalmology, Department of Tropical Ophthalmology, University Eye Hospital, Ludwig-Maximilians-Universität, Munich, Germany

Barbara E K Klein
Professor, Department of Ophthalmology and Visual Sciences, University of Wisconsin School of Medicine and Public Health, Madison, WI, USA

Ronald Klein
Professor, Department of Ophthalmology and Visual Sciences, University of Wisconsin School of Medicine and Public Health, Madison, WI, USA

Ivo Kocur
Team Leader, Prevention of Blindness and Deafness, World Health Organization, Geneva, Switzerland

Hannah Kuper
Senior Lecturer, London School of Hygiene and Tropical Medicine, London, UK

Susan Lewallen
Co-Director, Kilimanjaro Centre for Community Ophthalmology, Tumaini University, Moshi, Tanzania and University of British Columbia, Vancouver, Canada

Hans Limburg
Senior Research Fellow, International Centre for Eye Health, London School of Hygiene and Tropical Medicine, UK; and Consultant in Community Eye Health, Health Information Services, Grootebroek, Netherlands

Robert Lindfield
Lecturer, London School of Hygiene and Tropical Medicine, London, UK

Maureen G Maguire
Carolyn F Jones Professor of Ophthalmology, and Director, Center for Preventive Ophthalmology and Biostatistics, Department of Ophthalmology, University of Pennsylvania, Philadelphia, PA USA

Bita Manzouri
Clinical Fellow, Moorfields Eye Hospital, London, UK

Darwin C Minassian
Emeritus Reader in Ophthalmic Epidemiology, Institute of Ophthalmology, University College London, UK

GVS Murthy
Director, Indian Institute of Public Health, Hyderabad; Director, PHFI South Asia Centre for Disability, Development and Inclusive Research, Hyderabad, Andhra Pradesh, India; and Senior

Lecturer, London School of Hygiene and Tropical Medicine, London, UK

Ilesh Patel
Research Fellow, Dana Center for Preventative Ophthalmology, Wilmer Eye Institute, Johns Hopkins University, Baltimore, MD, USA

Maria Papadopoulos
Consultant Ophthalmic Surgeon, Moorfields Eye Hospital, London, UK

Harry Quigley
Professor of Ophthalmology, and Director, Glaucoma Service, Dana Center for Preventative Ophthalmology, Wilmer Eye Institute, Johns Hopkins University, Baltimore, MD, USA

Graham E Quinn
Professor of Ophthalmology, The Children's Hospital of Philadelphia, University of Pennsylvania, Philadelphia, PA, USA

Jugnoo S Rahi
Professor of Ophthalmic Epidemiology; Director, Ulverscroft Vision Research Group, Institute of Child Health and Institute of Ophthalmology, University College London; and Honorary Consultant Ophthalmologist, Great Ormond Street Hospital NHS Trust, London, UK

Gary S Rubin
Hellen Keller Professor of Visual Rehabilitation, Institute of Ophthalmology, University College London, UK

Ulrich C Schaller
Department of Ophthalmology, Klinikum Augsburg Teaching Hospital of the Ludwig-Maximilians-Universität, Munich, Germany

Debra A Schaumberg
Associate Professor of Epidemiology, Harvard Medical School, Boston; Associate Professor in the Department of Epidemiology, Harvard School of Public Health, Boston; and Director of Ophthalmic Epidemiology, Division of Preventative Medicine, Brigham and Women's Hospital, Boston, MA, USA

Alfred Sommer
Dean Emeritus; Professor of Epidemiology, Ophthalmology and International Health, Johns Hopkins Bloomberg School of Public Health, Baltimore, MD, USA

Muthiah Srinivasan
Aravind Eye Hospitals and Postgraduate Institute of Ophthalmology, Madurai, Tamil Nadu, India

Hugh R Taylor
Harold Mitchell Chair of Indigenous Eye Health, School of Population Health, University of Melbourne, Victoria, Australia

Jennifer E Thorne
Associate Professor of Ophthalmology and Epidemiology, and Director, Division of Ocular Immunology, Wilmer Eye Institute, Johns Hopkins School of Medicine, Baltimore, MD, USA

Rupal H Trivedi
Research Associate Professor of Ophthalmology, Albert Florens Storm Eye Institute, Medical University of South Carolina, Charleston, SC, USA

Stephen Tuft
Director, Corneal Service, Moorfields Eye Hospital, London; Honorary Senior Lecturer, University College London, UK

Madan P Upadhyay
B.P. Koirala Lions Center for Ophthalmic Studies, Tribhuvan University Institute of Medicine and Teaching Hospital, Maharajgunj, Kathmandu, Nepal

Stephanie Watson
Consultant Ophthalmologist, Sydney Eye Hospital, Prince of Wales Hospital and Sydney Children's Hospital; Associate, Save Sight Institute, University of Sydney; and Conjoint Senior Lecturer, University of New South Wales, Australia

Keith P West Jr
George G. Graham Professor of Infant and Child Nutrition, International Health and Ophthalmology, Johns Hopkins Bloomsberg School of Public Health, Baltimore, MD, USA

Sheila K West
El-Maghraby Professor of Preventive Ophthalmology, Dana Center for Preventative Ophthalmology, Wilmer Eye Institute, the Johns Hopkins University School of Medicine, Baltimore, MD, USA

John P Whitcher
Emeritus Professor of Ophthalmology, Epidemiology and Biostatistics, Francis I Proctor Foundation, University of California, San Francisco, CA, USA

M Edward Wilson
Pierre G. Jenkins Professor of Ophthalmology and Pediatrics, Albert Florens Storm Eye Institute, Medical University of South Carolina, Charleston, SC, USA

Wong Tien Y
Professor and Director, Singapore Eye Research Institute, National University of Singapore, Singapore

Richard Wormald
Honorary Senior Lecturer, London School of Hygiene and Tropical Medicine and University College London; Consultant Ophthalmologist, Moorfields Eye Hospital, London, UK; and Coordinating Editor of Cochrane Eyes and Vision Group

Foreword to the first edition

During the 1970s, I faced the challenge of conceptualizing and establishing an International Centre for Eye Health that could provide academic leadership and manpower to address the worldwide challenges of avoidable blindness. This movement was being promulgated by Sir John Wilson and others, through the World Health Organization, but urgently needed trained workers. The fundamental requirement was to foster epidemiology within ophthalmology, along with an in-depth understanding of the main blinding diseases and the principles of public health and management. An additional requirement was to attract established mainstream epidemiologists to work on priorities in the prevention of blindness.

We were greatly encouraged by Professors Geoffrey Rose and Peter Smith and helped by the flow of epidemiologists from their MSc Course in Epidemiology at the London School of Hygiene and Tropical Medicine. Increasingly, this has included ophthalmologists trained through Wellcome Fellowships in Clinical Epidemiology.

Ophthalmic epidemiology is most importantly about the application of mathematics to the understanding of causation and control of blindness. Unfortunately, many workers in medicine are weak in mathematics and are afraid of it. In trying to awaken enthusiasm for epidemiology, through our courses at ICEH, Darwin Minassian and I felt strongly that wherever possible we needed to teach through eye examples, leading our students gently but firmly through mathematics into epidemiological understandings, constantly keeping in mind the relevance to blindness and its prevention. A main obstacle was the lack of examples of well worked out ophthalmic problems.

The subject has now developed to the point where the present landmark volume provides many ophthalmic examples and should stimulate more work in this area. Within a rounded coverage, Part One gives an excellent account of methodology. Part Two discusses all the main blinding diseases and gives perspectives for public health. Discussions of trachoma, glaucoma, childhood blindness, vitamin A deficiency, onchocerciasis, eye injuries and age-related macular degeneration are outstanding. As a guide to action, Part Three outlines planning and management of prevention of blindness programmes and the roles of WHO and the international non-governmental organizations. I warmly welcome this book which should stimulate focused research.

Professor Barrie Jones
1998

Foreword to the second edition

Epidemiology is, at its heart, mere counting — but 'counting' of a practical and insightful sort. By establishing the magnitude and distribution of disease, it is fundamental to designing effective intervention strategies. By establishing statistical associations and relationships between a disease and patient characteristics, it can reveal critical causal pathways.

Other than Ida Mann's *Culture, Race, Climate, and Eye Disease: An Introduction to the Study of Geographical Ophthalmology*, few publications before 1980 drew together epidemiologic information spanning more than a single disease or population. Few individuals and fewer institutions were interested in its academic pursuit.

This has changed dramatically during the past two decades. Early population-based studies, like the Framingham Eye Study, and randomized clinical trials like the Diabetic Retinopathy Study, proved the importance of moving clinical science beyond clinical case series. The International Agency for Prevention of Blindness, founded in 1978, gave voice to the need for informed, effective blindness prevention activities, particularly for poor people in the developing world. Through its advocacy, IAPB gave birth to WHO's Prevention of Blindness Programme, which helped establish a global network of 'collaborating centres'. These 'centres', mostly academic institutions, conducted critical ophthalmic epidemiologic research and trained future scientists and programme leaders.

The editors and authors of The Epidemiology of Eye Disease were very much leaders of the eye-epidemiology revolution. The fact that a second edition follows the first after a mere five years speaks of the continuing pace at which new information is being gathered and the new premium being placed on such knowledge by Vision 2020, the global effort to reverse the tide of unnecessary visual impairment and blindness.

As with all second editions, the scope, depth, and 'heft' of this new volume considerably exceed the first (which was by no means insubstantial!). Its four sections provide focused, critical treatises on interrelated aspects critical to understanding the magnitude and nature of ocular disease and visual impairment, and global plans for their control: an introduction to the epidemiology of visual impairment and blindness around the world; a description of epidemiologic methods; an exposition of the epidemiology of each of the major visually disabling entities, and a discussion of Vision 2020 and its rationale and motivation.

This new edition of an 'instant classic' provides a ready reference and study guide for those interested in advancing ophthalmic knowledge, in better understanding the nature, extent, and causal pathways of the world's major blinding diseases, and in appreciating (and perhaps participating in) a uniquely collective global enterprise to improve the human condition.

Alfred Sommer MD MHS
2003

Foreword to the third edition

A book that sells enough of its first edition to warrant a second edition is a huge success. One that goes into a third edition is well on its way to become an established classic. This is one reason I am delighted to be asked to contribute a foreword to this important book.

The second reason for my delight in accepting the invitation is the opportunity to pay tribute to the outstanding editors, each of whom has made tremendous contributions in their own right. They have provided great leadership to both ophthalmology and epidemiology through their research and teaching. However, when they work together they form a truly formidable team and when this team is combined with the world class authors who have contributed chapters, the book they have produced is a real tour de force.

Thirdly, I am delighted to write this foreword because I believe the field of ophthalmic epidemiology is of great importance and this outstanding book provides an excellent foundation and resource for those interested in this field.

One of my mentors used to say that epidemiology was "only organised common sense". The trick was to learn how to do that organisation: how to make sense out of what, at times, can be masses of complex data; how to distil the important findings and key messages. Another mentor told me "Taylor, all you need to do is to learn how to count (properly)", emphasising the importance of careful numeration whether of the numerator or, even more importantly, the denominator. But

also built into the apparently simple statement about counting was the need, for example, to be mindful of all the potential biases in the inclusion or exclusion of those data to be counted; a point Professor Alfred Sommer emphasises in his foreword to the second edition of this book. The reader will find these basic skills of epidemiology are beautifully extolled and explained. The clearly written and constructed chapters show the honing that comes from experienced teachers who have presented their material over time and worked out all the bugs.

Epidemiology is important to ophthalmology because it gives us clear indications as to how to better manage the problems we encounter in delivering eye care as well as in managing individual patients. Epidemiology guides the way we provide eye care and treatment, whether this is by generating information about the frequency and distribution of disease, its aetiology and risk factors, or the efficacy of various forms of prevention or treatment. The epidemiologic aspects of a wide range of ophthalmic diseases and conditions are beautifully presented and each chapter is completed with a list of issues for further research. In addition, this work provides the wider framework for fashioning eye health care policy and practice that eventually leads us to the noble goal of Vision 2020 and the Right to Sight for All.

This magnificent third edition builds on both the scholarship and the inspiration of the late

Professor Barrie Jones who was a founding giant in this field and who wrote the foreword to the first edition. Although significantly expanded this new, third edition presents a crisp, authoritative and up-to-date account of the very broad field of ophthalmic epidemiology, or rather "organised common sense about vision".

Professor Hugh R. Taylor AC MD
2011

Acknowledgements

The preparation of this book has been sponsored by CBM.

The Editors are indebted to Jenni Sandford for her work in the compilation of this third edition.

The assistance of Sarah Polack with maps of disease distribution, Pak Sang Lee, Jyoti Shah and Michael Geraghty with technical assistance, and Astrid Leck and Stephen Tuft with their comments on specific questions, are gratefully acknowledged. We thank all those who have contributed the colour illustrations.

SECTION 1

INTRODUCTION

1

Prevalence, incidence and distribution of visual impairment

GVS MURTHY AND GORDON JOHNSON

1.1	Introduction: the scope of ophthalmic epidemiology	3
1.2	The magnitude of global blindness	4
1.3	Sources of data for blindness and visual impairment	5
1.5	Prevalence data derived from surveys	11
1.6	Limitations of prevalence surveys	13
1.7	Trends of prevalence with time	14
1.8	Incidence of blindness	15
1.9	Causes of blindness	16
1.10	Patterns of distribution of blindness	18
1.11	Conclusions	21

1.12	Future research needs	21
	EPIDEMIOLOGICAL DATA	23
	Commentary on Table 1.7	
	Table 1.7: Population-based surveys of blindness prevalence	31
	Commentary on Table 1.8	
	Table 1.8: Causes of blindness from comprehensive studies	43
	Commentary on Table 1.9	
	Table 1.9: Causes of blindness from RACSS and RAAB	50
	References	53

1.1 INTRODUCTION: THE SCOPE OF OPHTHALMIC EPIDEMIOLOGY

Why are ophthalmic conditions important? Surveys consistently reveal that loss of sight ranks second or third in people's perceptions after the most feared conditions of cognitive loss or cancer. Although a good quality of life is usually achieved by people without high quality vision, normal vision nevertheless enables individuals to participate more fully in the myriad of activities that make up daily living and opportunities for recreation. Prevention of visual loss, or restoration of vision loss, has become an important priority for public health; it requires a multidisciplinary approach engaging as stake-holders researchers, eye care workers, the designers and managers of programmes of prevention and funders.

Why is epidemiology important? Epidemiology, in its broadest sense, is the study of the distribution and determinants of disease. First, epidemiological research contributes to the body of scientific knowledge about diseases of the eye and provides clues to their likely aetiological pathways, which may not emerge from laboratory research or observation in the clinic.

Second, it contributes to the public health approach to blindness prevention by identifying the magnitude of the problem, and describing the main causes and distribution of eye diseases that result in impairment and disability. It also identifies differences between populations that may be modifiable.

Third, epidemiological research also contributes to blindness prevention through understanding the determinants of disease in human populations. Establishing an association between exposure to a risk factor or causative agent, and the presence or absence of disease, requires an analytical study design. This may be either a case-control study (Chapter 4), or a longitudinal (cohort) study (Chapter 5), which may, in turn, be retrospective or prospective.

Finally, epidemiology evaluates preventive measures, treatments or other intervention to reduce the impact of vision loss, by conducting clinical trials that require randomization of populations or persons, together with standardized assessments of outcomes (Chapter 7).

Thus the epidemiology of eye disease has made, and continues to make, critical contributions to both scientific knowledge and blindness prevention. In this book, we review these contributions, and suggest new avenues for research that will further enhance eye health. In this first chapter we begin by describing the research that documents the magnitude of the problem of visual loss in the world, and its main causes.

1.2   THE MAGNITUDE OF GLOBAL BLINDNESS

1.2.1   Summary of global blindness

The most recent global estimates by the Global Databank of the World Health Organization Programme for the Prevention of Blindness and Deafness were published in 2004, based on the data available to 2002. The number of **visually impaired people** (best corrected vision <6/18, 20/60, 0.33) **was 161 million**, of whom **37 million were blind** (<3/60, 20/400, 0.05). The history of the sequence of estimates by the World Health Organization (WHO) of the burden of global blindness is outlined in Section 1.5.1 below, and summarized in Fig. 1.1.

In the lists of figures for prevalence and causes of blindness by country in Tables 1.7, 1.8 and 1.9, we have added those surveys published since 2002 which meet the criteria described in the text. In the past there have been few firm data on the prevalence of blindness, and even now the results of individual surveys must be interpreted with care if extrapolated to a region.

No. Blind (Millions)

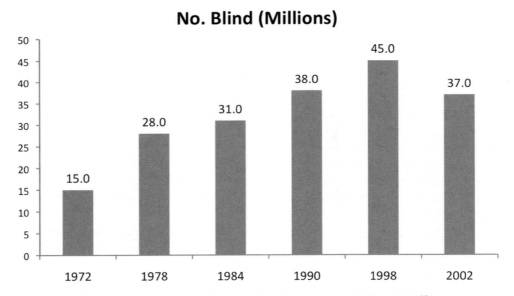

Figure 1.1 *Estimated global magnitude of blindness by date (best corrected VA < 3/60)*[18]

1.2.2 Summary of global causes

The most recent estimates from the WHO on the causes of blindness need to be examined in two ways because the proportions vary depending on the definition of blindness used. When the estimates were first published in 2004, the conventional definition of best corrected vision was used.[1] With this definition, **cataract** was responsible for nearly half the global blindness (**47.8%**); and **glaucoma** (**12.3%**) became the second most important cause. However, if presenting vision were to be considered (as in the revised WHO definition described below),[2,3] **uncorrected refractive errors** would be the second commonest cause (**18%**). The comparison between the causes based on presenting and best corrected vision is shown in Figs. 1.2 and 1.3.

1.3 SOURCES OF DATA FOR BLINDNESS AND VISUAL IMPAIRMENT

A proper epidemiological study requires considerable planning (see Section 1.3.4), which may be helped by advance information. It is often possible to obtain, from existing sources, a rough idea of the magnitude of visual impairment, to identify geographical areas of high prevalence and to suggest the major causes of visual loss. The gathering of this initial information has been referred to as a 'Preliminary Assessment'.[4,5]

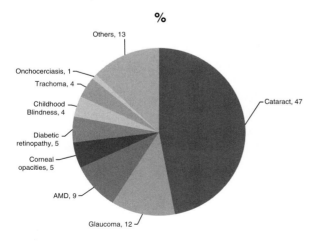

Figure 1.2 *Global causes of blindness (best corrected vision <3/60, excluding refractive errors)*[18]

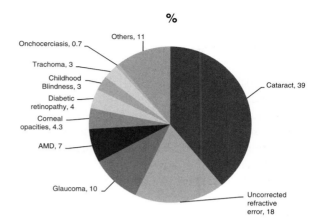

Figure 1.3 *Global causes of blindness (presenting vision <3/60, including uncorrected refractive errors)*[196]

1.3.1 Possible sources of preliminary data

➢ Hospital and clinic statistics of both outpatients and inpatients, and eye camp records; these may allow ethnic, geographical and seasonal variations in the distribution of the main eye conditions to be recognized.

➢ Health and social insurance records. An example was the ascertainment of known cases of glaucoma in Iceland, from the records of anti-glaucoma medications dispensed throughout the country plus records of surgically treated cases of glaucoma.[6] However, we know from population-based glaucoma surveys that much glaucoma is not diagnosed, and also that some of the treatment will have been for ocular hypertension.

➢ Health surveys undertaken for other purposes.

➢ Censuses; some national censuses have included questions about disabilities, including blindness.

1.3.2 Blindness registration statistics

Blindness registration in most countries[7,8] is incomplete. This is largely because the main purpose of registration is not for medical information, but to enable the patient to receive social benefits. Observations in the UK and other countries suggest that only about half of those eligible are in fact registered,[7] and under-certification could be as high as 64% for blind people and 77% for the partially sighted.[8] Registration of all individuals with visual impairment according to WHO definitions has become compulsory in Norway and Finland, and this is being extended to other Nordic countries. In some well-documented, small populations, the number of known blind people may approximate closely to the true number of blind persons, for example in Iceland and Greenland.[9]

Some blind people do not wish to be 'registered blind' because of what they perceive to be the stigma of blindness, or for fear that their employment may be jeopardized. What is required, therefore, if more reliable figures are to be obtained in industrialized countries, is a system of 'notification of irreversible blindness' to an appropriate independent authority, in the same way that cases of cancer or some infectious diseases must be notified. Perhaps the use of the term 'visual impairment' implying different levels of severity, rather than 'blindness' or 'partial sight', would find broader acceptance. Chapter 12 emphasizes that there are other measures of the burden of visual impairment besides conventional visual acuity.

Where additional information about a registered or notified person may become available at a later date, some mechanism must exist by which the entry can be updated. This is particularly important when evidence of genetic aetiology becomes available, as was illustrated in a study of all the registered blind people in the Canadian province of Newfoundland and Labrador.[10] The percentage attributable to hereditary disease was doubled when extensive pedigrees had been explored and further examinations carried out.[10]

1.3.3 Schools and institutions for the blind

The limitations of data drawn from examination of children in schools for the blind are considered in Chapter 14. In some countries children from rural areas, from lower socio-economic strata and girls, are likely to be seriously under-represented. Nevertheless, examinations of children in as many schools for the blind in a country as possible may give an idea of the relative proportions of different causes in that country, and with proper caveats may be used to identify changes over time as well as the emergence of new problems.

1.3.4 Population-based sample surveys

The only secure sources of prevalence data are population-based prevalence surveys conducted according to strict criteria. The principles and some practical aspects are described in Chapter 3.

While still being population-based, rapid assessment techniques have also been improved over the last 15 years. Employed initially for assessment of cataract blindness (**Rapid Assessment of Cataract Surgical Services — RACSS**), these methods are now being increasingly used for gathering evidence of other causes of visual impairments, both at local and national level (**Rapid Assessment of Avoidable Blindness — RAAB**).

Because data are now available from a large number of surveys, it becomes important to identify those which can stand the test of scientific rigour. In this chapter we have required some basic criteria, as follows, before including the results in the Tables 1.7, 1.8 and 1.9.

1. The survey must have identified the population to which it refers and selected a sample using random sampling methods, so that the results can be generalized to the wider population in that area.
2. If it is to be generalizable, the survey should include a representative population and not be limited only to specific groups in, for example, areas endemic for onchocerciasis, leprosy villages or trachoma-endemic populations. This will allow the findings to be extrapolated to a wider population.
3. A sample large enough to provide **confidence intervals (95%)** on the prevalence measures. If blindness is relatively rare, the estimate will be un-interpretable unless the sample size is large.

4. Clear-cut descriptions should be provided of the sampling process, definitions used, enumeration procedures adopted, clinical examination protocol followed and methods of data analysis.

We have included the most recent data available for a country and have arbitrarily taken 1990 as the cut-off year. Most earlier surveys were reported in the second edition of this book. With increased access to services, older figures may no longer be valid for a particular country or region today. Only if no studies since 1989 were available from a particular country have we retained the older data, so that the readers can understand at least the extent of the problem in the past.

1.4   Definitions

1.4.1   Definition: magnitude

Magnitude is the size of the problem of a condition or disease. The two measures used are **prevalence** and **incidence** (which will be described in more detail in Chapter 2 under 2.2.1). Prevalence is a static measure that provides a snapshot of the disease in the population at a particular point in time, and includes all cases of disease regardless of duration.

Prevalence is a proportion and relates to a defined population.

$$\text{prevalence} = \frac{\text{number of cases of disease at a particular time}}{\text{total number of the population}}$$

This crude prevalence measure can be made more specific by giving the prevalence in a particular age group; for example, the number of people with blindness aged 50–59 years as a proportion of the total defined population aged 50–59 years. This is called the age-specific prevalence. For meaningful comparison between studies in different populations, or in the same population at different times, prevalence can be adjusted to a reference population with a known age and sex structure.

Incidence is a more dynamic measure of the magnitude of the problem, and measures the

(Continued)

(Continued)

number of new cases of disease in the population at risk (that is, the population that does not already have the disease) over a defined period of time. Incidence can be expressed in two main ways: either as a proportion or as a rate (**the incidence rate**, explained further in Chapter 2 under 2.2.2). Incidence expressed in the simplest way, as a proportion, is known as **cumulative incidence (CI)**.

$$CI = \frac{\text{number of new cases occurring in a given time}}{\text{total number of population at risk at the beginning of the period}}$$

1.4.2   Definition: blindness, low vision and visual impairment

Blindness and low vision are conventionally measured and defined in terms of **visual acuity (VA)** and of reduction of visual field. The equivalence between the different notations used in different countries for visual acuity is given in Table 1.1.

Each country has its own definition of blindness for legal and social purposes. Because there are wide variations in these requirements, and so that global comparisons could be made, a WHO study group in 1972 recommended a standardized method of testing and a uniform definition of blindness and visual impairment.[4] This was incorporated into the **International Statistical Classification of Diseases and Related Health Problems, 10th revision (ICD-10)**[11] (Table 1.2).

Blindness was defined internationally as a VA of less than 3/60 (20/400, 0.05) in the better eye with best possible correction, or a visual field loss in each eye to less than 10° from fixation. This corresponded to categories of visual impairment 3, 4 and 5 in ICD-10.

Low vision was defined as VA of less than 6/18 (20/60, 0.3) but equal to or better than 3/60 in the better eye with best possible correction (corresponding to visual impairment categories 1 and 2 in ICD-10). Category 1 was visual impairment less than 6/18 to 6/60, and category 2 was severe visual impairment less than 6/60 to 3/60.

(Continued)

Table 1.1 *Conversions between the notations for recording visual acuity*

LogMAR	Snellen (6 m)	Snellen (20 ft)	Decimal
1.8	1/60*	20/1200	0.02
1.3	3/60*	20/400	0.05
1.0	6/60*	20/200	0.10
0.9	6/48	20/160	0.26
0.8	6/38	20/125	0.16
0.7	6/30	20/100	0.20
0.6	6/24	20/80	0.25
0.5	6/19	20/63	0.32
0.48	6/18*	20/60	0.33
0.4	6/15	20/50	0.40
0.3	6/12	20/40	0.50
0.2	6/9.5	20/32	0.63
0.1	6/7.5	20/25	0.80
0.0	6/6	20/20	1.00
−0.1	6/4.8	20/16	1.25
−0.2	6/3.8	20/12.5	1.60
−0.3	6/3	20/10	2.00

*WHO blindness categories

Table 1.2 *Original WHO categorization of blindness and visual impairment*

	Distance visual acuity with best possible correction	
Category	Worse than	Equal to or better than
1 (Low Vision)	6/18	6/60
2 (Low Vision)	6/60	3/60
3 (Blindness)	3/60	1/60 (finger counting at 1 metre)
4 (Blindness)	1/60 (finger counting at 1 metre)	Light perception
5 (Blindness)	No light perception	
9	Undetermined or unspecified	

(Continued)

At the time of the Technical Group Meeting in 1972, four major causes of blindness were identified as the most common worldwide, and it was recommended that information should be collected with respect to these four conditions. They were trachoma, onchocerciasis, xerophthalmia and cataract. At that time, there was no consideration of refractive error as a cause of blindness or visual impairment. It is now widely recognized that collected evidence should help in formulating

(Continued)

(Continued)

effective strategies for action to prevent visual impairment as well as blindness. To the extent that the absence of corrective glasses is an impediment to normal functioning of an individual, in areas/countries where refraction services are not well developed the lack of access calls for an international response. Evidence on the extent of the problem and the magnitude of refractive errors can only be collected if the definition of blindness and visual impairment includes uncorrected and

(Continued)

Table 1.3 *Revised WHO categorization of blindness and visual impairment*

Category	Presenting distance visual acuity with available correction	
	Worse than	Equal to or better than
0 (Mild or No Visual Impairment)		6/18 (0.3) 20/70
1 (Moderate Visual Impairment)	6/18 (0.3) 20/70	6/60 (0.1) 20/200
2 (Severe Visual Impairment)	6/60 (0.1) 20/200	3/60 (0.05) 20/400
3 (Blindness)	3/60 (0.05) 20/400	1/60 (0.02) 20/1200 (Finger counting at 1 metre)
4 (Blindness)	1/60 (0.02) 20/1200 (Finger counting at 1 metre)	Light perception
5 (Blindness)	No light perception	
9	Undetermined or unspecified	

(Continued)

under-corrected refractive errors. Most surveys in the late 1990s and the first decade of the 21st century have therefore used presenting or habitual vision to define blindness. This trend has accelerated further in the last ten years with the introduction and widespread use of rapid methods for assessment of blindness, where it is usually only practical to collect presenting vision.

Recently, therefore, the WHO has recommended that instead of best corrected vision, presenting vision should be used to define blindness.[2]

Other reasons why the WHO believed that changes were necessary to the prevailing definition of blindness were that:

1. The nomenclature did not distinguish between 'visual loss' and 'low vision'; and that
2. Inconsistencies existed within the H54 sub categories in ICD-10, which did not distinguish between those who had irreversible blindness (no perception of light) from those with vision <3/60 but who could perceive light.

In addition, the International Council of Ophthalmology (ICO) had resolved that ICD-10 should be revised.

(Continued)

(Continued)

Based on these observations, the WHO made two major recommendations to ICD-10:

1. Replace 'best corrected' by 'presenting vision' in defining blindness.
2. Delete the term 'Low Vision' from the previous ICD-10 terminology to collectively refer to visual impairment categories 1 and 2.

The revised categorization is shown in Table 1.3.

If the extent of the visual field was taken into account, patients with a field no greater than 10° but greater than 5° around central fixation had been placed in category 3, and patients with a field no greater than 5° around central fixation had been placed in category 4, even if the central acuity was not impaired.

In the revised categorization, it has been recommended that subjects with a visual field of the better eye, no greater than 10° in radius around central fixation, should all be placed in category 3, so that the old categories 3 and 4 on the basis of field are now clumped together.

(Continued)

(Continued)

1.4.3 Methods and definitions: measuring visual acuity

In visual acuity testing the test object should be adequately illuminated, but the illumination has not been specified and the degree of contrast not defined for use under field conditions. Each eye is tested separately. Vision of 3/60 means that the eye can recognise correctly only at 3 metres a target which a normal eye could recognise at 60 metres. Vision of 3/60 may be regarded as approximately equivalent to the ability to count clearly separated, extended fingers against a contrasting background at a distance of three metres. The ability to count fingers at one metre is roughly equivalent to vision of 1/60. This may be useful if it is suspected that the examinee does not understand a test using letters or an illiterate 'E' chart or a Landholt 'C' card.

A vision chart and notation has been designed aimed at improving the consistency of VA measurement so that the only chart feature that would influence the visual acuity score would be the letter size.[12] The notation is the **logMAR**, which stands for 'the logarithm of the Minimal Angle of Resolution', that is, the widths of the strokes of the letters viewed from six metres. The principles are as follows: there should be a constant ratio between letter size and spacing; there should be a logarithmic progression of letter size; letters should be of equal legibility; and there should be the same number (five) of letters on each row. The point of equal legibility is not being met at present if all the letter sizes are presented in full black rather than with variable contrast depending on size. Previous acuity charts had irregular progression of letter size. A ratio or multiplier between rows of 0.1 log unit means that the new chart can be used accurately at non-standard distances. The conversions between logMAR and earlier notations for visual acuity are shown in Table 1.1. A reduced logMAR has recently been introduced to simplify and speed up this type of acuity

(Continued)

(Continued)

testing.[13] This reduced logMAR chart was validated[14] and has been extensively used in the surveys in Bangladesh, Pakistan and Nigeria.[15–17]

A definition based on visual field constriction was originally included to allow for surveys in geographical areas where onchocerciasis was present. Confrontational testing was regarded as the only practical method under field conditions.[5] Now that there is more interest in the prevalence of different types of glaucoma, and portable perimeters are available, routine visual field testing is regarded as essential in a survey if the true prevalence of glaucoma and of glaucoma blindness is to be estimated. Unfortunately, when the definition of blindness based on visual field constriction was formalized, the size of the test target to be used for field testing was not stipulated. This aspect of visual fields testing needs to be resolved. In practice, many population surveys do not include visual field testing because of the time and cost involved, so that VA alone is used when deciding who is blind.

1.4.4 Definitions in recent surveys

In the past few years, most people conducting population-based sample surveys have in practice departed from the WHO guidelines and definitions in two respects. First, they have recorded presenting vision (habitual vision), i.e. the visual acuity of the patients as they come to the examination site.

Second, the cut-off level of acuity for visual impairment has been moved to less than 6/12 in recognition of the increasing visual demands in all countries, for example, for driving and use of computers. In these surveys the best corrected visual acuity (or pin-hole visual acuity), and also vision less than 6/18, are usually recorded as well so that comparisons with earlier surveys and other countries can still be made.

In addition, near vision is now being recorded in some surveys.

1.5 PREVALENCE DATA DERIVED FROM SURVEYS

1.5.1 The Global Data Bank of WHO/PBD

The **WHO Programme for the Prevention of Blindness (WHO/PBL)**, now the **Programme for the Prevention of Blindness and Deafness (PBD)**, was established in 1978. It has sought to collate the data on prevalence (Figure 1.1) and causes of blindness as they became available (Figures 1.2 and 1.3), and it established the WHO Global Data Bank on Blindness.

The first estimate of global blindness was made in 1972, compiled from information supplied by member states. The figure of 10–15 million was already recognized by the Study Group on the Prevention of Blindness as an underestimate. The first epidemiological estimate drawn up by WHO/PBL was based on data up to and including 1978, and suggested that the total number of blind people was 28 million, using the visual acuity criterion of less than 3/60. If those with a visual acuity of less than 6/60 were added, the total with blindness and severe visual impairment was 42 million.

The first nationwide survey of the prevalence and causes of blindness was conducted in Nepal from December 1980 to April 1981.[18] The population sample included all age groups, and the WHO definition of blindness was used.

A revision and update based on the 1984 global population was 31 million blind people. A complete and epidemiologically sound new estimate of 38 million was made in 1994, based on information held by the WHO Global Data Bank on Blindness up to 1990.[19] This 1994 report provided the global estimates that were used as the evidence base for launching the Global Initiative for the Elimination of Avoidable Blindness. The surveys, which were included by the Global Data Bank, were selected on such criteria as being population-based and representative of the country or region.

In 1998 the figure was 44.8 million blind (WHO World Health Report 1998, Geneva, WHO 1998:53).

The next estimate of global blindness was made by the WHO in 2004, based on available data up to 2002 and using the 17 sub-regions employed at that time by the Global Burden of Disease Commission.[20] Surveys from 55 countries were used,[1] and the list of surveys has also been published.[3] The number of visually impaired people worldwide was 161 million, of whom 37 million were blind. Over 30 million (30.3 million) of the 37 million blind were thought to be aged 50+ years, indicating a shift from the early 1980s when childhood blindness, and the sequelae of past infections like measles, small pox and onchocerciasis, affected the younger population in much larger numbers than is seen today. Among the 37 million projected blind, 12.5 million were in the South East Asia region of WHO and another 7.2 million in Africa. Owing to increased recognition of refractive errors as an important cause of blindness and visual impairment when presenting vision is used to define visual impairment, the WHO compiled estimates for refractive errors. It estimated that 153 million people (range of uncertainty: 123 million to 184 million) were visually impaired from uncorrected refractive errors, of whom eight million were blind (2004).[21] Combined with the 161 million people visually impaired estimated in 2002 according to best corrected vision, the WHO has stated that 314 million people are visually impaired from all causes based on the 2002 and 2004 revised estimates.

Recently there has been a recognition that near vision is important for ensuring quality of life. Studies on near-vision impairment have been conducted in Kenya,[22] Zanzibar,[23] India[24] and Tanzania.[25] Available data have also been used to project the global burden on near-vision impairment and presbyopia. It is estimated that globally there are 1.04 billion people with presbyopia (2005) and that 517 million of them have no, or only inadequate, spectacles.[26] If quality of life is to be improved, then adequate attention needs to be paid to near correction as well as distance visual acuity.

1.5.2 Trends in global blindness with time

Although the earliest estimate in 1972 lacked the accuracy of later studies, which were based on different methodologies, there has clearly been an increase in the number of blind people (Fig. 1.1). Applying age-specific prevalence to the world population Thylefors *et al.* had projected that the expected number of blind, considering only the age group of 60 years and over, would be around 54 million by 2020. Of these, 50 million would be in developing countries.[27] This assumed that there would be no change in age-specific prevalence rates. In the interim, however, it was thought that there were already 50 million totally blind by 2000,[28] and projections by the authors suggested that there would be 76 million blind by 2020 if there were no additional interventions.

Why should the numbers be increasing at this rate? First, there is, of course, an overall increase in world population. Second, there is a relative increase in the proportion of older people in the population, and this is expected to accelerate with time. However, the WHO global estimates of 2004 indicated that the extent of visual impairment in 2002 was in fact lower than what had been projected earlier.[1] The recent global initiative for elimination of avoidable blindness, and the action plans charted for all countries, have led to augmentation of eye care services through technical cooperation between developed and developing countries, training, infrastructure support and increased funding.[29] Together with earlier intervention, this intervention seems to have reversed the trend of increasing global blindness observed until 2000, and may actually indicate some progress towards the goal of elimination of avoidable blindness in most countries by 2020.

1.5.3 Prevalence of blindness by health region

The publication by the WHO in 1994 arranged countries according to the grouping used by the World Bank's Development Report of 1993.[30] This is based largely on the types of economy and on stages of economic development. However, as noted above, the subsequent global estimates in 2004 grouped the WHO Member States into 17 sub-regions according to the classification adopted by the Global Burden of Disease working group.[20]

Table 1.4 presents the combined prevalence of blindness, for three age groups and all ages in the

Table 1.4 *Global prevalence of blindness*

WHO Region	Sub-Region	Prevalence of Blindness (%)			
		< 15 years	15–49 years	≥ 50 years	All ages
Africa	Afr-D	0.124	0.2	9	1.0
	Afr-E	0.124	0.2	9	1.0
America	Amr-A	0.03	0.1	0.4	0.2
	Amr-B	0.062	0.15	1.3	0.3
	Amr-D	0.062	0.2	2.6	0.5
Eastern Mediterranean	Emr-B	0.08	0.15	5.6	0.8
	Emr-D	0.08	0.2	7	0.97
Europe	Eur-A	0.03	0.1	0.5	0.2
	Eur-B1	0.051	0.15	1.2	0.4
	Eur-B2	0.051	0.15	1.3	0.3
	Eur-C	0.051	0.15	1.2	0.4
South East Asia	Sear-B	0.083	0.15	6.3	1.0
	Sear-D	0.08	0.2	3.4	0.6
Western Pacific	Wpr-A	0.03	0.1	0.6	0.3
	Wpr-B1	0.05	0.15	2.3	0.6
	Wpr-B2	0.083	0.15	5.6	0.8
	Wpr-B3	0.083	0.15	2.2	0.3

Source: Bulletin World Health Organ 2004; 82: 844–851.

countries of each sub-region according to this grouping.

This working group is now called the Global Burden of Diseases, Injuries and Risk Factors Study Group (GBD), and has recommended the use of 21 distinct geographical regions[21] (shown alphabetically in Table 1.5). The objective of this re-organization was to define regions that were as epidemiologically homogenous as possible so that extrapolations could be made to other countries of the region.[31] We have used this classification for the presentation of evidence in Tables 1.7, 1.8 and 1.9, in the Epidemiological Data. However, because of their size, complexity and the large number of surveys performed, we have listed India and China as separate entities within their stipulated regions.

Some of the information used by the WHO came from unpublished sources. The data presented in Tables 1.7, 1.8 and 1.9 are, however, confined to published surveys, or to reports that can be readily obtained from the government or agency that conducted them. The aim is to present

Table 1.5 *Revised arrangement of countries recommended by the Global Burden of Disease, Injuries and Risk Factors Study Group (CBD)*[31]

1. Asia Pacific — High Income
2. Asia — Central
3. Asia — East including China
4. Asia — South including India
5. Asia — South East
6. Australasia
7. Caribbean
8. Europe — Central
9. Europe — Eastern
10. Europe — Western
11. Latin America — Andean
12. Latin America — Central
13. Latin America — Southern
14. Latin America — Tropical
15. North Africa/ Middle East
16. North America — High Income
17. Oceania
18. Sub-Saharan Africa — Central
19. Sub-Saharan Africa — East
20. Sub-Saharan Africa — Southern
21. Sub-Saharan Africa — West

surveys published since the 2004 report as well as those available up to 2002.

1.6 LIMITATIONS OF PREVALENCE SURVEYS

A glance at the studies displayed in Table 1.7 will show that many are not representative countrywide surveys, but that provinces or districts have been chosen for convenience or because of a particular interest. Results from countries such as Nigeria, Pakistan, Chad, Togo and India demonstrate that major differences can exist between regions of a country. These variations could partly result from sampling variations, as well as from real differences in prevalence between areas. In extrapolating the results of a local survey to a whole country, assumptions are made that may not be valid without further information. Similarly, results from one country cannot always be extrapolated to a whole region.

The published surveys have tended to favour rural areas. This is partly because the burden of avoidable blindness in developing countries has been thought to be higher in rural than urban parts of the country. It is perhaps also because it is easier to carry out a census and to identify the participants in rural villages than in multi-storied apartment buildings in a town, and because the response rate is usually better. Some of the recent surveys, such as India,[32–35] the Gambia,[36] Bangladesh,[15] Pakistan,[16] Nigeria[17] and Ethiopia have, however, specifically sampled from urban as well as rural areas.

Ascertainment of prevalence of blindness in children presents special problems, which are discussed in Chapter 14. With an average prevalence of less than one blind child per 1,000 children aged 15 years or under in developing countries, it is possible to examine several thousand children without finding a single case of blindness. Blindness is strongly age-related. For this reason, many prevalence surveys restrict the age group examined to 30 or 40 years and above, in order to give a better yield and make optimal use of limited resources. Some studies use the age structure of a country to extrapolate the measured prevalence to an all-age population. However, even with a good knowledge of the age structure of the population of the country, only an estimated figure can be given, since firm data are not available for blindness in the younger age groups.

The results of many published surveys are expressed as single figures. The prevalence is, however, an estimate, the accuracy of which depends on total numbers examined and on the sampling method, as explained in Chapter 3. A simple random sample is usually impractical for a national or even district population. Most surveys are therefore based on cluster sampling, the population often having first been stratified. Precision is expected to be less than with a simple random sample and, if there is a complex survey design, it may be difficult to calculate. Prevalence should be expressed with **95% confidence intervals (95% CI)**, as has been done for some of the more recent surveys. The meaning of 95% CI is that there is a 95% probability that the range of values indicated by the CI contains the true value of the population parameter (see also Chapter 3 and Glossary). Even then there is a 1 in 20 chance that the reported confidence interval does not include the true prevalence.

In a given community, there may be a right month or season of the year, and even a best time in a working day, when a survey should be done in order that the subjects examined are truly representative. For example, the survey in the Wenchi district of Ghana was conducted just before the planting season so that most adults would be at home.[37] These practical aspects of survey planning are important if a valid result is to be obtained.

Finally, it must be appreciated that many surveys of blindness that have been conducted have not been published in scientific journals. There may be a variety of reasons for this, but the consequence is that the methodology cannot be examined and the results are not available for use in global comparisons or in the effort to eliminate blindness.

1.7 TRENDS OF PREVALENCE WITH TIME

Trends in estimates of global prevalence have been presented in Fig. 1.1 and Section 1.5.1 above.

There is limited information on the change of prevalence in a particular country or region over time, but this is clearly essential in the planning, evaluation and further planning of intervention programmes. A decline in prevalence is illustrated by data for the Eastern Region of Saudi Arabia, where a high prevalence of over 3% in 1984[38] appears to have been reduced by concerted action to 1.5% in 1990[39] (Table 1.7).

In two countries, the Gambia and India, repeat surveys have been conducted to assess the impact of national eye care programmes.

In the Gambia the crude prevalence of blindness fell from 0.70% to 0.42%[40] after an interval of ten years.[36] During the same period the population increased from 775,000 to 1,169,000. When the prevalence for the whole country in 1996 was age-standardized to the 1986 sample, it became 0.55%, not a statistically significant difference from 1986. However, the programme had been phased in across the three health regions from west to east. Where the eye care programme had been introduced first in 1986 in the western region, the prevalence of blindness had halved, and there was a significant gradient of risk factors across the three regions, suggesting a causal relationship between the intervention and the reduction in risk of blindness.

Some interesting data are available from India. A series of surveys, covering the population aged 50+ years, have been conducted over the period 1998–2007. Though they have used different protocols of examination (RACSS, comprehensive or RAAB), the data can be compared in respect of presenting visual acuity. In 15 states, in 16 selected districts where RACSS or comprehensive surveys were carried out during the period 1998–2002, a repeat survey was done in 2007 (by RAAB) (Table 1.6). In three districts where a comprehensive survey had been carried out in 2001–2002, the 2007 RAAB recorded an increase; in one of these a very small increase. The other 13 districts showed a decrease in prevalence over time, usually substantial, in one case even over the short term of three years. Unfortunately the 95% confidence limits were not available for the data; hence it is not possible to say whether the difference observed was a true difference. Despite all the limitations of the comparisons, it is evident that there has been an appreciable change during the period 1998–2007.

This was the period in India when the benefits of concerted efforts for control of cataract blindness were becoming apparent and it strongly suggests that such organized interventions can play a significant role in blindness alleviation. However, it has to be remembered that this period in Indian history was also coupled with improvements in the socio-economic fabric of society owing to the adoption of a market economy and the subsequent steep increase in industrial growth in the country, as well as a sudden improvement in life expectancy. It therefore becomes difficult to attribute the success or failure of such a programme directly to the programme itself if other important relevant changes are occurring in the country at the same time.

Surveys done during this time, including the Andhra Pradesh Eye Study, showed very high prevalence. Some of these sources of data, including the Andhra Pradesh Eye Study, were used to extrapolate the prevalence to the whole country, and a steep increase in the number of blind was predicted. It was felt that the number of blind persons would increase to 24 million by the year 2010 and 31.6 million in 2020.[41] Current indications are that this may not be the case, particularly if the gains made in the recent past are consolidated.

1.8 INCIDENCE OF BLINDNESS

Because of the paucity of data, Podgor, Leske and Ederer developed a formula, based originally on the Framingham results, to calculate incidence from age-specific prevalence for the major conditions causing blindness.[43] Until recently, there was virtually no direct measurement of the incidence of blindness, that is, the number of new cases of blindness in a defined population in one year. An exception was for the incidence of childhood blindness in the Nordic population for

Table 1.6 Changes in prevalence of blindness and severe visual impairment in India (Presenting VA < 6/60 in better eye, age 50+ years, 1998–2007)[42]

| State | District | Blindness prevalence (%) | | |
		1998–1999 RACSS	2001–2002 comprehensive	2007 RAAB
Himachal Pradesh	Solan		5.4	3.2
Punjab	Bhatinda		7.8	4.4
Uttar Pradesh	Deoria	19.3		12.4
Uttar Pradesh	Jhansi	23.8		10.6
Rajasthan	Nagaur	24.9		8.7
Bihar	Vaishali		6.0	9.4
West Bengal	Malda		9.2	6.7
Orissa	Ganjam	19.9		10.0
Chattisgarh	Rajnandgaon		12.4	13.2
Madhya Pradesh	Shadol	21.0		5.3
Gujarat	Surendranagar		8.1	5.7
Maharashtra	Parbhani		7.9	11.3
Andhra Pradesh	Prakasam	21.8	10.9	8.5
Karnataka	Gulbarga		13.7	7.9
Kerala	Palakkad		4.2	3.7
Tamilnadu	Cuddalore		15.3 (RACSS)	7.3
India	Pooled Data	18.4	8.5	8.0

the year 1993.[44] The annual incidence varied between 5.7 and 11.1 per 100,000 children in the five countries.

Two longitudinal follow-up studies in industrialized countries were completed in the 1990s. The surviving persons in the original population-based cohort in Beaver Dam, WI, USA, who were aged 43–86 years at the baseline in 1988–1990, were re-examined after five years and after ten years.[45] The ten-year cumulative incidence of bilateral severe visual impairment (≥ 6/60) was 0.8%, and 5.9% of the population at risk had developed some degree of visual impairment (< 6/12). People who were 75 years of age or older at baseline were 19.8 times more likely to develop severe visual impairment than people younger than 75 years of age at baseline. Similarly, in the Blue Mountains Eye Study, 2,335 persons were available for follow-up at five years.[46] Based on their presenting VA in the better eye, there were 8.4% with incident visual impairment worse than 6/12, 2.5% worse than 6/21 (20/70) and 0.1% (two persons) worse than 6/60. Both the latter cases were a result of age-related maculopathy. There were, however, 21 persons with incident unilateral impairment worse than 6/60, the majority resulting from age-related maculopathy.

The cumulative incidence of visual impairment among the African-Caribbean population of Barbados has been published.[47] Using best corrected vision <3/60, the overall four-year incidence of blindness was 3.6% among those aged 40–84 years at baseline. Nearly 50% of this visual loss was attributed to cataract. The nine-year incidence of blindness has recently become available and it was 1.0% (95% CI: 0.7–1.4) among the surviving cohort of this African-Caribbean population.[48]

In a follow-up of the national Nigeria blindness survey, the people aged 40+ years in Bauchi state who were examined in 2005 were re-examined in 2007. The three-year cumulative incidence of blindness was 5.5% (95% CI: 2.34–8.66). Of those who had normal vision at baseline, 1.19% (two cases) became blind over the three year period.[49] A study is currently underway in India where the subjects examined at baseline in the Andhra Pradesh Eye Disease Study will be re-examined to document changes in visual status over a ten-year period.

1.9   CAUSES OF BLINDNESS

The proportions of blindness caused by different disease entities, available from published population surveys, are given in the Epidemiological Data. Because of the widely different methods of ascertaining causes of blindness, data are being presented separately for the comprehensive surveys (Table 1.8) and rapid surveys (RACSS/RAAB) (Table 1.9). Estimates of the proportion of blindness attributed to the main causes in the global population were summarized in Section 1.2.2 and Figs. 1.2 and 1.3.

1.9.1   Problems of nomenclature

There are discrepancies between surveys in the way causes are measured and how they are recorded; for example, the complications of cataract surgery are sometimes included with 'cataract' and sometimes listed separately. Similarly, blindness resulting from uncorrected aphakia is sometimes recorded under 'cataract' and sometimes under the heading 'refractive errors'. Causes of corneal opacity other than trachoma may be distinguished from trachoma as 'corneal scar', 'corneal ulcers' or 'corneal opacities'; in other reports trachoma and other causes are combined together as 'corneal opacities', 'corneal lesions', 'corneal scarring', 'corneal diseases', including, on occasion, cases of xerophthalmia. Similarly many studies report on macular degeneration based on a clinical picture without specifying whether it is AMD or not, while some studies report on AMD and DR based on photographic evidence only. Even more problematic is that few surveys attempt to determine blindness caused by glaucoma, which is often undercounted or attributed to other causes.

1.9.2   The problem of multiple causes and of different causes in the two eyes

A common problem is that there may appear to be more than one cause of blindness in the same eye. Examples might include cataract and optic atrophy, or cataract and severe glaucoma. In these cases a clinical judgment is often made as to which disease process is contributing most to the visual impairment. In the first example, the judgment might be made that the degree of optic atrophy is so severe that the eye would still be blind, even if the incomplete cataract were to be removed. Other studies permit primary and secondary causes to be listed, so that both are counted.

A more difficult problem is when each eye is assigned to a different cause of blindness. What is the cause in the individual? The convention adopted by the WHO simplified methodology for the assessment of blindness and its main causes was that the cause in the individual should be the one 'most easily preventable or curable'. An alternative approach would be to give the cause for the individual as the cause in the second eye to become blind: this is the condition which actually rendered the individual bilaterally blind. However, much valuable information is lost by either of these approaches. The condition that was less preventable or curable, or was the first to occur, is still making an equal contribution to the present state of blindness. Even using the logic of 'most preventable', there could be an argument on the temporal status of the cause. Is it preventable or curable at the time of the survey or was it preventable or curable in the past? For example, if it occurred in childhood, is it no longer preventable or curable? Therefore, even with the benefit of WHO guidelines, the examining clinicians may take different views in recording the final cause of visual loss. With this background, care has to be taken in comparing causes of blindness across different studies, with different methods adopted and different interpretations by examining clinicians.

An extension of this approach, in reporting the results of a survey, is to enumerate those individuals with the same cause in both eyes, and then to list those with different causes in the two eyes, specifying the combinations. The data can then be re-arranged for comparison with other surveys. A good example of this method of presentation is in the report of the survey by Cook and colleagues in northern KwaZulu.[50] Dandona and colleagues adopted a further variation for the Andhra Pradesh survey.[32] If the two eyes of a subject were blind from two different causes, both were given 50% weight, rather than 'arbitrarily choosing one or the other as the cause for that participant'. For the Shunyi[51,52] and Doumen County[33] surveys in China and the Tirunelvelli survey[53] in India, the authors reported the causes of blindness for eyes, not for individual subjects. In this case it was not possible to rearrange the data to give causes for individual people. While these different approaches make use of all the data, these surveys are difficult to compare with those that follow the WHO guidelines.

1.9.3   Trends in causes with time

In the earlier estimates of 1990, there was an uncertainty regarding the proportion caused by two conditions, trachoma and glaucoma: the estimates worked out by Thylefors and Négrel were 16% and 15% respectively, that is, 5.6 million for trachoma in 1990 and 5.2 million for glaucoma.[19] At that time it was widely believed that the incidence of blindness from trachoma had been declining for some time in certain populations, under the influence both of control programmes and improving living conditions. (In the 1986–1989 India survey it constituted less than 1% of blindness.)[54] For glaucoma, the 1984 estimate of 3 million blind was revised in 1990 to 5.2 million.[55] Independently, Quigley analyzed the available data for glaucoma and projected a figure of 6.7 million blind from glaucoma by the year 2000.[56] Quigley recently estimated that there would be 60.5 million people with glaucoma in 2010 and 79.6 million by 2020, among whom 74% would have open-angle glaucoma.[57] In the latest estimates the global picture has been revised based on the present situation in previously trachoma-endemic populations and the recent appreciation of the importance of glaucoma.

1.9.4   Numbers for particular causes

There are some important causes of blindness for which reasonably confident estimates have now been reached. An Expert Committee on onchocerciasis reported a figure of 268,000 for world blindness from the parasite *Onchocerca volvulus* (see Chapter 18). The current working figure for planning purposes is 400,000. The figure for blindness from leprosy arrived at by a WHO workshop in 1988 was 250,000 (although there were dissenting opinions). If leprosy patients who have age-related cataract are also included, the current figure may be up to 300,000 (see Chapter 16d). A workshop on childhood blindness in 1990* concluded that an estimate of 1.5 million children under the age of 16 years were blind, of whom 70% would be as a result of vitamin A deficiency (see Chapter 14b). This cause is now thought to have decreased as a proportion of childhood blindness. In most surveys blindness caused by eye injuries is included in the categories of 'other causes' or 'other corneal opacities'. It therefore remains difficult to obtain a correct estimate of trauma-related blindness. In 1997, it was estimated that 1.6 million people were blind because of eye injuries.[†] However, this figure may be an overestimate, and has not been updated. Thylefors *et al.* found in 1994 that the lack of epidemiological data for diabetic retinopathy and age-related maculopathy made it impossible to arrive at precise estimates for these causes.[19] However, the WHO does now include estimates for these conditions.

1.10   PATTERNS OF DISTRIBUTION OF BLINDNESS

1.10.1   Demography

The overall prevalence of blindness is a function of age, affecting mainly the older section of any population. This is illustrated in individual countries, such as the Gambia (Fig. 1.4), and also for the global population (Fig. 1.5).

Over the previous 12–18 years, the estimated prevalence of global blindness has risen more or less in step with the increase in world population. However, the number of people in the group aged

* WHO. Report of the WHO meeting on the Prevention of Childhood Blindness. London, 29 May–1 June 1990. Geneva. WHO/PBL/90.19.

† Négrel AD, in Johnson GJ, Minassian DC, Weale R, eds. *The Epidemiology of Eye Disease*, 1st Edition, 1998. London: Chapman and Hall.

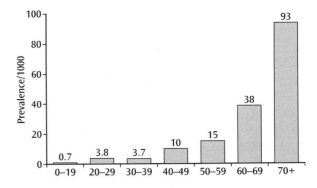

Figure 1.4 *Prevalence of blindness by age in the national survey of the Gambia (1986)[40]*

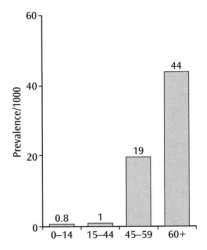

Figure 1.5 *Global estimated prevalence of blindness by age (From Thylefors B, Négrel AD, Pararajasegaram R, Dadzie KY. Global data on blindness: an updated. WHO/PBL/94.40. Geneva: WHO)*

25–40 years has been larger than in earlier age strata. As this works its way into the older age bands in around 20 years' time, the prevalence of blindness would be expected to rise at a faster rate than the total population, if appropriate interventions are not put in place.

A meta-analysis has been completed to show the influence of gender on blindness.[58] Published population-based studies were collected and analyzed. Globally, women have an excess of blindness, so that women account for 64.5% of all blind people. The overall ratio of blind women to men was 1.43%, ranging from 1.39% in Africa and 1.41% in Asia, to 1.63% in industrialized countries.

The prevalence of blindness by gender varies according to the cause; for example, blindness as a result of trachoma is higher in women because of a cycle of re-infection from young children. Males are more likely to become blind from onchocerciasis, because they may be working beside or on water from an early age as fishermen or ferry operators, close to the breeding sites of the *Simulium* vector. The Barbados survey is unusual in that, in each age group, blindness is around twice as common in men as in women and this was associated with the high rate of glaucoma.[59] Conversely blindness as a result of cataract may be higher in females compared with males, not just because of epidemiological factors but also because women in many developing countries, especially in South Asia, have poorer access to surgical services as compared with men.

The influence of ethnicity on prevalence of blindness is uncertain. It is often very difficult to disentangle environmental influences from ethnic ones. The Baltimore survey showed that the rate of blindness in the black African-American population was almost twice that in white population living in the same city district, when examined using identical methods.[60,61] This survey is now almost 30 years old, and the findings may have changed, although the SEE study also examined African-Americans and Caucasians, and found a higher rate of blindness in African-Americans. Certainly anatomical characteristics appear to account for the high level of blindness from angle-closure glaucoma in central Asian populations.[62] There was a striking contrast in the proportion of blindness attributable to glaucoma in the two studies in Singapore. Among the Chinese, 60% of all blindness was due to glaucoma[63] while among the Malays, glaucoma was responsible for only 5% of blindness.[64] It is possible, however, that there could have been confounding factors as the studies were conducted six years apart and the numbers of blind individuals were low.

1.10.2 Geography

Local variations

According to the surveys from Africa there is wide causal variation between countries. This is partly because of the occurrence of onchocerciasis in West and Central Africa, so that in Kaduna State in Nigeria, in the late 1980s, onchocerciasis caused 43% of cases of blindness, and cataract only 6%.[65] Within a given country, the prevalence depends on the geography; for example, in Togo the

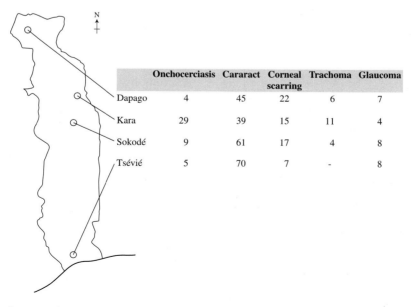

	Onchocerciasis	Cararact	Corneal scarring	Trachoma	Glaucoma
Dapago	4	45	22	6	7
Kara	29	39	15	11	4
Sokodé	9	61	17	4	8
Tsévié	5	70	7	-	8

Figure 1.6 *Map of Togo, showing the proportion of the different causes of blindness in different geographical regions (Note that some of the variation may be a result of sampling variation).*

prevalence of blindness as a result of onchocerciasis, and hence the proportions attributable to other causes, varies widely from region to region (Fig. 1.6). In the non-onchocercal areas of Africa, the main causes are generally cataract, corneal opacities and glaucoma, in that order. In the recently completed national survey in Nigeria, the prevalence of trachoma-related severe visual impairment and blindness was 1% or more in the northern part of Nigeria (the north-east, north-west and north-central geopolitical zones) compared with 0.1–0.4% in the geopolitical zones in southern Nigeria. Even the cases in the south are unlikely to be caused by local transmission as the environmental characteristics of the south are not conducive to Chlamydial growth and transmission.

In Italy there is a striking gradient in prevalence of blindness, increasing from the north to the south of the country, based on three different methods for ascertaining prevalence: a national household health survey; the national registry of the blind; and the welfare list of the Ministry of the Interior.[66]

As noted, Mongolia (central Asian region) and Barbados (Caribbean region) are unusual among all the countries surveyed in that glaucoma accounts for 28–35% of blindness, the same as for cataract.[59,67] Most of these cases are of angle-closure glaucoma in Mongolia, but open-angle glaucoma in Barbados.

Variations between regions

Current estimates of prevalences of blindness throughout the world are presented in Plate 1.1. In the analysis by Thylefors *et al.* published in 1995,[27] the overall prevalence of blindness in the world using World Bank regions was 0.7%. This varied from 0.3% in the Established Market Economies (EME), to 1.4% in Sub-Saharan Africa, with regions such as Latin America and China intermediate at 0.5–0.6%. Other authors would put the level for the EME slightly lower at 0.1–0.2%. The update of the global figures in 2002 also showed stark differences between regions.[1] Global prevalence was estimated to be 0.57%, with the highest estimate of 1.0% for the WHO Africa Region and the South Asian countries of the WHO

South East Asia Region. Prevalence in the European region was estimated at 0.2–0.4%, the same as for the North American region. Other regions were intermediate. Within each WHO region there was also a variation among the countries.

1.10.3   Socio-economic factors

Socio-economic status can be measured in a number of ways. Obtaining information on monthly family incomes, especially in the rural areas of most developing countries is usually very difficult. Many studies have therefore used literacy as a proxy indicator for socio-economic status. This is a sensitive indicator. Data from studies in India,[32,33] Pakistan,[16] Nigeria[17] and from many other countries have shown that literacy is one of the most important determinants of prevalence of blindness.

The association of poverty with blindness has been studied extensively. The national survey in Pakistan showed that the prevalence of blindness caused by cataract, glaucoma and corneal opacity was lower in affluent clusters and households.[68] It has been stated that a combination of factors like poverty, lack of education and inadequate health services were responsible to a great extent for the burden of blindness in Africa.[69]

The importance of access to services is generally borne out by studies where there is a rural/urban differential in blindness prevalence. Rural areas have significantly more blindness than urban ones, not only in the developing countries, but even in Victoria, Australia.[121]

1.10.4   The concept of 'avoidable blindness'

A term frequently used is **avoidable blindness**. This is defined as blindness that could 'reasonably be prevented or cured within the limits of resources likely to be made available'. Figures of 75% or 85% are often quoted. With the adoption of VISION2020: The Right to Sight initiative and the advent of RAAB methodology, more and more studies are reporting on avoidable blindness. In Nigeria, the recent national survey found that 84% of blindness was avoidable (if glaucoma was included),[70] while in Rwanda, it was 87.2% (excluding glaucoma).[71] The RAABs in India found that avoidable blindness was responsible for 88.2% (excluding glaucoma).[34] The variations depend in part on whether glaucoma is considered to come within this definition of 'avoidable'. The proportion of avoidable blindness also varies greatly from region to region, being much higher in those areas of the world where cataract blindness and ocular infections predominate. Despite some inconsistencies, the concept is considered valuable because it focuses attention on the proportion of visual impairment, and on those causes, for which an effective programme of intervention is likely to make a difference.

1.11 CONCLUSIONS

Population-based sample surveys are the most reliable sources of data from which to analyze the magnitude and causes of blindness and visual impairment, so that priorities for intervention can be determined and resources used most effectively. The recent change in the definition of blindness will mean that new global estimates of the prevalence and magnitude based on the models developed by WHO will need to be generated. For some countries this will not be a problem as surveys are already reporting presenting vision, but for the countries in Europe, Australia, America and the rich countries in the Asia Pacific region, which have always reported results based on best corrected vision, some mathematical assumptions will need to be made to arrive at estimates comparable with presenting vision.

The causes of blindness vary widely from region to region, within regions and even within countries. Globally, uncorrected cataract is the leading cause of blindness. The estimate for trachoma is now lower than for glaucoma. The populations affected are quite different, and it is likely that cases of glaucoma will continue to increase in the future, whereas trachoma cases are expected to decrease further. We await more reliable data on the prevalence of blindness caused by corneal opacities

(other than trachoma), diabetic retinopathy and age-related maculopathy.

Based on the surveys collated by the Global Databank of WHO/PBD, it is clear that the total number of people suffering from blindness and visual impairment in the world has been steadily increasing. As mentioned before, this is partly a result of the increase in world population, but is more particularly attributable to the relatively greater increase in the numbers of elderly people in the population. Nevertheless, the most recent estimate for global blindness based on surveys until 2002, suggests that, for the first time, a reversal of this remorseless increase may have been observed. It is possible that this can be attributed, at least in part, to the co-ordinated worldwide intervention embodied in the Vision 2020: The Right to Sight initiative. It is therefore important that accurate population-based prevalence figures continue to be collected in order to monitor the progress of the international effort to prevent blindness.

1.12 FUTURE RESEARCH NEEDS

1. More population-based data are required, using standardized survey methodology. Information is lacking particularly from Eastern and Central Europe (former socialist republics), Indonesia and Thailand in South East Asia, and the Caribbean. For many countries in North and South Africa, the available data are nearly two decades old and need to be updated. Standardized methodologies will include the use of the ICD-10 definition of blindness and low vision, but will also include 'presenting vision' as well as corrected vision; testing of visual fields on all patients over a certain age to detect blindness on the basis of visual field constriction; expressing the results of prevalence with confidence intervals for the estimate; and making age-specific and sex-specific prevalence data available.
2. Longitudinal studies, or repeat surveys in the same population, especially in the developing countries, are necessary toss give estimates of incidence.

3. Accurate figures for the prevalence of blindness resulting from causes of corneal opacities (other than trachoma), diabetic retinsssopathy and age-related maculopathy in different regions and geographical locations are needed.

4. The estimates of prevalence, incidence and causes of blindness and visual impairment for each demographic region should continue to be regularly collected, and as far as possible be subjected to meta-analysis, in order to guide and monitor the policies of eye care and blindness prevention programmes.

5. More research is indicated into standardizing the methods of measuring visual acuity in the field, including the effects of contrast and colour of the targets, type of target, and degree of illumination. If more surveys are going to include assessment of near vision, this testing also needs to be standardized.

6. The ICD-10 criterion for blindness based on visual field could be reconsidered, so that, as more surveys of glaucoma prevalence are conducted, guidelines are available for size and intensity of stimulus to be used with perimeters, and a definition be developed for the density of field defect to qualify as blindness. In view of vision requirements for driving, should the binocular visual field now be included in the definition of visual impairment?

7. RAAB Methodology has been evolving over the last ten years. Due to world-wide resource constraints, there will be increasing interest in RAAB as a cost-effective tool to provide timely data for planning of need-based services. Supplementing the protocol to facilitate a rapid diagnosis of glaucoma and diabetic retinopathy would be very desirable.

EPIDEMIOLOGICAL DATA

COMMENTARY ON TABLE 1.7: POPULATION-BASED SURVEYS OF BLINDNESS PREVALENCE

Overview of Global Prevalence

The global prevalence of blindness was estimated as 0.57%, with the highest prevalence being reported for countries in Africa and South East Asia.[1]

In adults aged 15–49 years, blindness prevalence (Table 1.5) was estimated for each WHO region (arranged alphabetically). The sub-regions have been defined using the mortality stratum of each country, as indicated: A –0.1%; B or C –0.15% and D or E –0.2% mortality per annum.

Asia pacific — high income

In this sub-region of four countries, which includes South Korea and Brunei, surveys are available from Japan and Singapore.[63,64,72,73] Four comprehensive studies were restricted to populations > 40 years of age and were localized, not national in coverage. The study in Nagoya, Japan, had the very low response rate of 29%.[72] Response rates below 70% may make it difficult to generalize the findings to a larger population as the blindness profile among those not examined may be completely different from those who were examined. However, it has been retained here since information from the rich nations in the Asia Pacific region is sparse. Based on the four studies from the sub-region, the prevalence of blindness was low (ranging from 0.05 to 0.6% in those over 40).

Central Asia

There are nine countries in this region: the five 'stan' states of Central Asia, plus Armenia, Azerbaijan, Georgia and Mongolia. Data are available from only two of these. The survey in Turkmenistan[74] was a Rapid Assessment of Cataract Surgical Services (RACSS) among those aged 50+ years, and the sample included the entire country. As in most of the rapid assessments, presenting vision was recorded. The 1992 study in Mongolia[67] was conducted in three provinces; the second in 1995 in a fourth province with the primary objective of assessing glaucoma among those aged 40+ years.[29] The prevalence of blindness in the sub-region is likely to be over 1% in those aged 40+, based on the available data.

East Asia

Four countries comprise this sub-region, of which China is predominant. Therefore we have provided separate estimates for China and for the other countries — North Korea, Hong Kong and Taiwan.

China

Recently there has been much attention paid to the blindness situation in China, and many population-based studies were undertaken from 1995 to 2007. Unlike the earlier surveys in the 1980s, recent surveys tended to be more localized.[51,52,75-85] The prevalence of blindness (best corrected vision) ranged from 0.4–2.59%, with the higher figures being reported from Tibet, where people of all ages were examined,[82] and from Guangdong (among those aged 50+ years).[52] The only RAAB in China, in Yunan Province, also revealed a high prevalence (3.7%) among those aged 50+ years.[84] Apparently, there is a wide variation in the prevalence of blindness across the country. This is to be expected owing to its size, geographical and cultural diversity, and differential access to services. In general, prevalence appears to be inversely related to the degree of economic development. One of the difficulties of assessing the present situation is the rapid urbanization that has taken place in the country over the past two decades, from 20% to more than 50% of the population today. The overall prevalence of blindness considering all ages appears to be low (0.3–0.5%) in China, and in Beijing it is even lower, where the prevalence among those aged 40+ years was only 0.4%.[80]

The surveys in Shunyi[51] and Doumen[52] counties used a standardized methodology developed by the WHO. (This protocol was also used in surveys in Nepal, India, Hong Kong and also Chile.)

Other East Asia

Surveys have been undertaken in Hong Kong[86] and Taiwan.[87,88] These covered only elderly populations. The prevalence of blindness in those over 60 was similar across these populations (0.46–0.6%), probably lower than in most areas of China. We have no survey from North Korea, the fourth member of this subgroup.

South Asia

South Asia is the most populous region of the world as it includes Bangladesh, India and Pakistan, as well as Afghanistan, Bhutan and Nepal. The magnitude of blindness in this sub-region is a major determinant of the global magnitude of blindness. The sub-region is also unique in that some of the population-based studies have been rigorously conducted using standardized protocols that allow international comparisons to be made with relative ease. There have been national surveys in India, Nepal and Pakistan in the 1980s and more recently in Bangladesh and Pakistan.

Because of the size of its population, data for India are being presented separately.

India

It has been a particularly difficult problem to determine the magnitude of blindness in India because of the size of the country and the great variety of populations and socio-economic development in different regions. It should be noted that the accepted definition of blindness in India is 'economic blindness' (presenting vision less than 6/60 in the better eye). Figures for 'social blindness' (presenting vision less than 3/60 in the better eye, as in the WHO definition) are usually also recorded for international comparison.

India was one of the first countries to have a national programme for the prevention and control of blindness (now the **National Programme for the Control of Blindness, NPCB**). In 1971–1974 the **Indian Council of Medical Research (ICMR)** conducted a survey in seven selected areas in which a total of 395,788 persons of all ages were examined.[89] It is questionable whether the sampling procedure was representative, as the urban population was over-represented. The authors arrived at a pooled prevalence of blindness of 0.54% at the <3/60 level.

Between 1986 and 1989 a national survey (all ages) was conducted for the NPCB by the Dr Rajendra Prasad Centre of the All India Institute of Medical Sciences. This included samples from all the states and union territories of India.[54] In different states the prevalences ranged from 0.18% in Delhi (similar to Europe and other market economies) to 1.69% in Jammu and Kashmir. Seven states accounted for two-thirds of the blindness in the country: Uttar Pradesh, Rajasthan, Madhya Pradesh, Maharashtra, Orissa, Andhra Pradesh and Tamilnadu. These states were selected in 1994 for the World Bank assisted Cataract Blindness Control Project.

The data from the 1970s and 1980s are presented here because of their historical significance. India has been an example where the National Programme activities were based on evidence generated from periodic population-based surveys. The initial focus of the National Programme was on Trachoma and Vitamin A deficiency, before the evidence from the nationwide and state surveys provided evidence of cataract as an important cause of blindness. There has been a sudden up-scaling of services, especially cataract surgical services, in the country, and the access to services has increased tremendously. The tradition of evidence from population-based surveys has continued well into the 21st century and improved access has led to a 25% reduction in the prevalence of blindness in the country, at the same time as life expectancy has increased.[42]

The first survey to include a detailed examination of each visually impaired eye, including dilation of the pupils and visual field examination, was conducted in Hyderabad and three rural areas in Andhra Pradesh by Dandona and colleagues from the LV Prasad Eye Institute.[32] The urban part of the survey included all age groups, but no blindness was found in any person below the age of 30. At around the same time, another WHO collaborating centre located in India (the Aravind Eye Care System) undertook a population survey with detailed examination, including dilation if vision was < 6/18, in three rural districts in Tamilnadu in the south of India.[91] This survey included those aged 40+ years.

Further information about the 50+ age group comes from rapid assessments of blindness in the seven states assisted by the World Bank,[92] as a mid-term appraisal, and also in the rural and urban areas of Gujarat.[93,94] In the World Bank study, visual acuity was measured with E-optotypes, rotated at six metres and, if necessary, three metres. The lenses were examined for cataract with a torch in a semi-dark area. This study of over 28,000 people could be completed within eight weeks from planning to implementation, and results were available for the Government of India within six weeks of data collection. This methodology was widely adopted in the RACSS which followed this study. Since then, most surveys in India have been undertaken only among those aged 50+ years on the assumption that the prevalence of blindness was very low at younger ages and programmatic inputs needed to target the older population.

In the late 1990s two surveys, conducted in Bharatpur District, Rajasthan[54] and Sivaganga District, in Tamilnadu,[96] used sound sampling methods and a comprehensive examination, but the age group was restricted to 50 years and over. Using the same standard protocol, the Government of India conducted similar studies in 13 other districts (one district randomly selected in each state).[33,97] The data were presented for all the 13 states plus the two states of Rajasthan and Tamilnadu, where comprehensive surveys had been done a year earlier.[95,96] Though the sampling was done at district level, the data were pooled to arrive at a national estimate. There was wide variation across the different districts in the country, and it was generally observed that in states that had a better socio-economic profile the prevalence of blindness at the district level was lower compared with the sampled districts in the states with a poorer socio-economic profile.[97]

Most of the recent surveys have sampled at the district level, and results from one district may not be representative of an entire state, because of considerable variation between districts. But when a series of studies done at the same time are pooled together, they can provide meaningful insights into the national situation provided the series is spread across the geographical span of the country.

RACSS was also undertaken in all other states that were not covered by the comprehensive survey in 1999–2001, including the north-eastern states.[98,101–103] The government of India developed a method for rapid assessment of avoidable blindness (RAAB), and undertook surveys in 16 districts spread across 15 states.[34] RAAB surveys were done in those districts where either a RACSS or a comprehensive survey had been done in the previous 5–7 years to track changes over time (Table 1.6).

Looking at the data from the different surveys in India from 1989 onwards, there is a distinct reduction in the prevalence of blindness among those aged 50+ years across the country, especially after 2000. The overall estimate for India based on extrapolation of these data is 1.2% (presenting vision <6/60).

South Asia — Other countries

The benchmark survey in Nepal was the first comprehensive national survey of blindness in the world.[18] Later surveys in Nepal were done on populations aged 45+ years in specified locations.[104,105] For the first time the survey in 1995 also looked at qualitative analysis of barriers and visual functioning.[104]

In Pakistan, two RACCS and two comprehensive surveys were undertaken recently, all covering older age populations.[16,106–108] The prevalence ranged from 1.9 to 3.8% when presenting vision was considered. Over the past decade, the International Centre for Eye Health developed a protocol for comprehensive national surveys which was used first in Bangladesh[15] and later in Pakistan.[16] The two surveys provided national level estimates for populations aged 30+ years. The same protocol was later used in the Nigeria national survey. This development, along with the WHO protocol developed and used in Nepal, China, Chile, Hong Kong and India, has helped to compare data across countries with more scientific rigour. The Pakistan national survey, which examined 16,507 persons aged 30+ years over the period 2003–2005, showed a prevalence of 2.7%.[16] It also documented that there were wide variations among the different provinces in the country,[16] and that level of blindness was closely related to poverty.[68]

Two studies are available from Bangladesh, one comprehensive and one RACSS.[15,109] The comprehensive national survey covered those aged 30+ years, and showed a prevalence for presenting vision of 1.52%, lower than for the comparable survey in Pakistan. The RACSS covered those aged 50+ in one district, giving a result intermediate between the two equivalent RACSS in districts of Pakistan.

The studies from India and South Asia show that blindness prevalence is similar across the countries of the region but that there are variations both between and within the countries, which seems to be related to poverty and access to services.

South East Asia

This sub-region includes Cambodia, Laos, Malaysia, Myanmar, Sri Lanka, Thailand and Vietnam, as well as the large populations of Indonesia and the Philippines. In addition there are small island communities: Maldives, Mauritius, Mayotte, Seychelles and Timor-Leste. A mix of RACSS, RAAB and comprehensive surveys is available from seven of these countries,[110–116] showing a wide variation in blindness prevalence. The all-age prevalence of blindness in Malaysia (0.29%)[111] is similar to that reported from most of the economically developed nations in the world. The highest prevalence in the region (8.1% presenting vision and 5.3%, best corrected) was in Myanmar where a representative rural population aged 40+ was surveyed.[114] The situation in the poorer countries is similar to that seen in South Asia.

Indonesia is the most populated country in this sub-region, and also the country that has the maximum disparity in access to services because of the complexity of providing services in the different island communities. Surveys have so far been restricted to Sumatra, and lack of data from elsewhere in Indonesia hampers needs-based planning.

Australasia

This sub-region consists of Australia and New Zealand, and data are only available for Australia. No national level estimate is available. An early survey in Australia, confined to the Aborigine population, showed that the prevalence of blindness (1.4%) was much higher than could be expected in the white population.[117] This survey is more than three decades old. More recently a small survey among indigenous adults aged 40+ years in two communities found that the prevalence of blindness (2%) was 40 times higher than in the urban population in Australia, after adjusting for age differences.[118] However, this study examined only 260 individuals and cannot be generalized.

A survey was conducted on a geographically representative population aged 50+ years in South Australia. The prevalence of blindness in this age range, and based on a definition of less than 6/60, was 0.66% although the response rate of 41% was disappointing.[119] Results have been published of large, comprehensive blindness prevalence surveys in predominantly Caucasian populations in New South Wales (Blue Mountains Eye Study)[120] and in urban and rural areas of Victoria.[121] The prevalence of blindness ranged between 0.16% and 0.66% in Australia among older people, a little lower than in the similar age groups in Western Europe. The most recent study in Victoria among people aged 40+ included visual field restriction in the definition.

The prevalence for the white population of Australia may be presumed to apply equally to the European population of New Zealand, but with its large Maori population and recent immigration from Polynesia, New Zealand warrants its own surveys.

Caribbean

This sub-region of 27 countries includes all the islands of the Caribbean, Bermuda, and four countries on the mainland: Belize, French Guiana, Guyana and Surinam. Data are only available for Barbados (comprehensive)[59] and Cuba (RACSS).[122] The Barbados study covered the predominantly black population aged 40–84 years, and showed that the prevalence of blindness was higher among the African-Caribbean population and those of mixed ancestry compared with the white population. In Cuba, the RACSS was done in the capital region. The prevalence of blindness was similar in the two countries, 1.6% and 1.8% in those aged 40 or 50 and over.

Europe — Central

The countries of the Europe Central sub-region are erstwhile socialist market economies: Albania, Bulgaria, Czech Republic, Hungary, Poland, Romania, Slovakia, and the republics of former Yugoslavia. The only population-based survey is from Bulgaria, carried out in the Sofia district and Sofia city in 1996, where the prevalence of blindness in those aged 40 and over was 0.49%,[123] similar to Western Europe.

Europe — East

The seven countries that comprise this sub-region are Russia, Ukraine, Belarus, Estonia, Latvia, Lithuania and Moldova. There is no population-based datum from this region. A RAAB was recently completed in Russia: the results are awaited.

Europe — Western

This region includes 29 developed economies of Europe, plus Israel, Greenland, and Saint Pierre and Miquelon. Population-based data are available from only nine. The one survey in Europe that considered all age groups was in the Bouche du Rhône Department of France, which includes the city of Marseille.[124] The all-age blindness prevalence was 0.2%. The Copenhagen City Eye Study (60–80 years), Denmark,[125] the Roscommon Study in Ireland (50+),[126] the Rotterdam Eye Study, Netherlands (55+),[127] Iceland (50+)[131] and two studies in Italy, Sicily[128] and Ponza (both 40+),[132] all found prevalences ranging between 0.47 and 0.6%. This indicates a relative homogeneity in these countries with similar health systems. The two studies in the UK[129,130] covered older populations aged 65+ and 75+ years respectively and found higher prevalences. Small surveys in Finland[133] and Spain,[134] which covered populations aged 70+ and 64+ years respectively, found results similar to an early study in the UK.[135] However, whether these West European studies can be extrapolated to the population of Israel is unknown. A comprehensive review of all the information on blindness and visual impairment in Germany was prepared, but this did not include a population-based survey. This information is more than two decades old and it may not be representative of present-day Germany.

Latin America — Andean

Until recently little evidence was available from Latin America. With the increased use of RAAB/RACSS many studies have now been undertaken in the Latin American region, all in those aged 50+ years, and there was one comprehensive survey in Brazil, also in those aged 50+.

The small Andean sub-region is composed of three countries, Bolivia, Ecuador and Peru. In Peru the prevalence of blindness was 2.6% among those aged 50+ years.[136]

Latin America — Central

There are nine countries in this sub-region, and RACSS/RAAB have been completed in three: Guatemala,[137] Mexico and Venezuela.[122] Guatemala had a significantly higher prevalence among those aged 50+ years than the other two countries –3.5% compared with 1.3% and 2.0% respectively (no overlap in the confidence intervals). The countries without data are Colombia, Costa Rica, El Salvador, Honduras, Nicaragua and Panama.

Latin America — Southern

RACSS/RAAB have been done in Argentina and Chile.[122] The prevalence of blindness among those aged 50+ years was very similar in the two countries — 1.0% and 1.2%. There are no equivalent data for Uruguay or the Falkland Islands.

Latin America — Tropical

Brazil and Paraguay comprise the sub-region. All three population-based surveys in the region were among those aged 50+ years and included one RACSS each in Paraguay[139] and Brazil[140] and one comprehensive survey in Sao Paulo, Brazil.[108] The prevalence was higher in Paraguay (2.6% compared with 1.4% and 1.07%) but the survey was done five years before those in Brazil.

North Africa/Middle East

The region is made up of Turkey, Iran and 18 predominantly Arab-speaking countries of North Africa, the Eastern Mediterranean and Arabian Peninsula. A survey in two provinces of Turkey in 1989 revealed a prevalence of blindness of 0.4% (all ages).[141] The original nationwide survey of Saudi Arabia in 1984 showed a surprisingly high prevalence of 1.5%, with a figure for the eastern province of 3%.[38] It should be noted that this survey represented not only affluent town-dwellers, but also the semi-nomadic tribes, who had received little direct medical intervention up to that time. Energetic programmes of eye care followed, so that when the eastern region was surveyed again in 1990 the prevalence was down to 1.5%.[39] A corresponding figure in the south west of the country for 1991 was 0.66%.[142] There has been no further survey. The figures for Morocco (0.76%),[143,144] Tunisia (0.8%)[145] and Lebanon (0.6%)[146] suggest an estimated prevalence (for all ages) for North Africa and the eastern end of the Mediterranean of around 0.7%.

A national survey (all ages) was conducted in Oman where the prevalence, based on presenting vision, was 1.1%.[147] Two recent studies in Iran showed prevalences from 0.28% (urban) to 0.79% (rural).[148,149]

North America

While there are as yet no population-based data from Canada, some of the most representative population-based surveys have been done in the USA. However, none of them have looked at younger populations as they have been restricted to ages 40+ years or higher. The legal definition of blindness in USA and Canada is 6/60 (20/200) or less. The well-known survey in Framingham, a white suburb of Boston in Massachusetts in the age band 52–85 years,[150] is now only of historical interest, as there has been a significant change in the USA over the past three decades.

One of the earlier studies in the USA was the **Beaver Dam Eye Study** (**BDES**).[151] Prevalence of blindness in 1990 was 0.5% among those aged 43–86. The Baltimore survey has been particularly valuable because it was conducted in the inner city, and directly compared the black and white populations aged 40+ years living side-by-side in the same neighbourhood.[60] The examination included visual field testing by the Humphrey Field Analyser on all subjects, as careful attention was being paid to the detection of cases of glaucoma. The prevalence of blindness in the black population (1.65%) was more than three times than that in the white population (0.5%) of the same age. A two-fold difference was found between African-Caribbeans (0.9%) and Caucasians (0.5%) in Salisbury.[152] These studies emphasize the importance of surveying different social and racial groups in North America, Europe and Australia, if measures for eye care and the prevention of blindness are to be appropriately focused. The pattern of blindness in minority groups may be quite different from that in larger background populations.

A small survey in an under-served rural population in Kentucky in the early 1990s gave a similar prevalence for a white population aged 40+ years of 0.44%.[153]

A study of native Americans in Oklahoma in the 1990s found a relatively low prevalence of blindness among those aged 40+ years,[154] as did a survey of Mexican Americans in Arizona.[155] However, a recent report of a prevalence of 3.13% among Latinos in Los Angeles[156] seems excessively high as compared with the Arizona result.

Oceania

This sub-region consists of Papua New Guinea and 21 small island states of the Pacific. There have been surveys in Vanuatu[157] and Tonga,[158] which gave, for the first time, an idea of the prevalence and causes of blindness in the Pacific Islands. In Vanuatu the prevalence was 0.4%. The Tonga survey examined only people aged 20 years or over, and all the cases of blindness occurred in people aged 50 years and over, while those aged under 20 years made up 54% of the population. The prevalence of blindness, if all ages had been included, was estimated to be 0.26%.

A RACSS was done in Papua New Guinea in 2005 across the whole country among those aged

50+ years, and revealed a prevalence of 3.9% which was similar to that in South East Asia.[159]

Sub-Saharan Africa — Central

There is no recent survey from this sub-region of six countries, which includes Angola, Democratic Republic of the Congo and Gabon. Surveys covering all ages were conducted in Congo,[160] Central African Republic[161] and Equatorial Guinea[162] more than 15 years ago. The Central African Republic and Equatorial Guinea had high blindness prevalences of 2.2% (best corrected) and 3.2% (presenting) respectively. The low prevalence (0.3%) in the Republic of Congo requires some explanation.[160] This country (capital Brazzaville), with a population of only 2.3 million people, had a relatively high standard of living at the time, and trachoma and other infectious diseases were not prominent.

Sub-Saharan Africa — East

This sub-region is comprised of 13 nations in mainland East Africa, extending from Sudan and Eritrea in the north to Mozambique in the south, plus two island states — Madagascar and the Comoros. Survey data are available from eight countries.[50,71,163–174] The surveys in Zambia[163] and Tanzania[164] were conducted around 1985 and may not reflect the present situation, but are being mentioned here as there has been no later survey in these two countries. All the other surveys were conducted in local/regional pockets and generally had an age restriction, except for the national survey in Ethiopia. This was undertaken in 2005 and the prevalence of blindness was recorded as 1.6% in all age groups.[171] Though a national survey was conducted in Kenya in the 1980s, subsequent surveys have been conducted only in localized population groups, in Nakuru[174] and in Nairobi slums,[173] where the lowest prevalence in the sub-region was recorded (0.6%).

Sub-Saharan Africa — Southern

Of the six countries that form this sub-region, data are available from two, South Africa[50] and Botswana.[176] (The other four countries are Lesotho, Namibia, Swaziland and Zimbabwe.) The study from South Africa is nearly 20 years old and included all ages in Kwazulu, finding a prevalence of 1.0%. In Botswana, the population aged 50+ was covered in the whole country through a randomly selected sample, where the prevalence of blindness was 3.69% (presenting vision). With only two results it is difficult to make comparisons, but the prevalence in this sub-region appears to be similar to that in comparable age groups in South Asia.

Sub-Saharan Africa — West

This sub-region consists of 16 countries of mainland West Africa, south of Algeria and Libya, and the islands of Cape Verde, Sao Tome and Principe, and Saint Helena. Ten of these countries have undertaken population-based surveys either locally or nationally. The first nationwide surveys on the African continent were in Chad in 1985[177] and the Gambia in 1986.[40]

In Benin (0.6%)[178] and Mali (1.7%)[179] surveys were done in 1990. In Ghana, two regional surveys done ten years apart among those aged 30+ and 40+ years respectively found similar prevalences (1.7–2.0%).[37,180] Surveys from the early 1990s in Sierra Leone[181] and Cameroon,[182,183] among all age populations, found a prevalence of 1.2–1.4%. Recently RAABs were done in Cameroon among those aged 40+ years in two regions of the country, in the north and south.[184,185] Both found a prevalence above 1% using the revised WHO classification of blindness.

Two national surveys were conducted in the Gambia, ten years apart.[36,40] The most recent survey was in 1996, which showed that the prevalence was 0.42%, which was lower than that reported a decade earlier.[36] A similar low prevalence was observed in Cape Verde islands[187] while the prevalence in Togo was high.[186]

A series of local surveys and one national survey have been undertaken in Nigeria over the past two decades.[17,188–197] There was a wide variation in the results from localized surveys. The most recent piece of evidence from Nigeria is the national survey, which covered a **population proportionate to size** (pps) sample from the entire country.[17] This survey revealed a national prevalence of blindness of 3.4% for the population aged 40+ years, with the north east geopolitical zone having the highest prevalence and the south west having the lowest prevalence, mirroring the access to services in Nigeria.

The available data from the 46 states which make up the whole region shows that Sub-Saharan Africa has, in general, the widest coverage by well-conducted and published prevalence surveys of any region. The impression is of an overall prevalence in the all-age population of between 1.0% and 1.3% for the whole of Sub-Saharan Africa, higher than in any other region. A review of 22 surveys by Lewallen and Courtright arrived at a figure of approximately 1% of Africa's population regarded as blind at the <3/60 level.[198] However, there is considerable variation across the continent, from Equatorial Guinea (3.2% presenting vision), Chad (2.31% best corrected vision) and the Central African Republic (2.2% best corrected vision) to the Gambia (0.42% best corrected vision) and the Republic of Congo (0.3% best corrected vision). Within individual countries there may also be considerable regional variations, for instance in Nigeria, Chad and Togo. The highest rates reflect foci of high prevalence of onchocerciasis and sometimes of trachoma in the past.

Table 1.7 Prevalence of blindness in different regions/countries of the world

Country	Year of survey	Population covered	Restriction of age; age range or definition	Type of survey	Number examined	Prevalence of blindness (%; 95% CI) Presenting	Prevalence of Blindness (%; 95% CI) best corrected/pin hole	Reference
Asia Pacific High Income Countries								
Japan	1997–2000	Nagoya	40–79; < 3/60	Comprehensive	2263	Response rate: 29%	0.09	72
Japan	2000–2001	Tajimi City	40+; < 3/60	Comprehensive	2977		0.14 (0.06–0.32)	73
Singapore	1997–1998	Tanjong Pagar District	40–79; < 3/60 & < 10° central fixation	Comprehensive	1232		0.6 (0.2–1.8)	63
Singapore	2004–2006	Malay population	40–79; < 3/60	Comprehensive	3280	0.12 (0.1–0.14)	0.05 (0.04–0.07)	64
Central Asia								
Turkmenistan	2000–2001	National	50+; < 3/60	RACSS	6011	1.26		74
Mongolia	1992	3 provinces	40+; < 3/60	Comprehensive	4345		1.5 (0.8–2.3)	67
Mongolia	1995	1 province	40+; < 3/60	Comprehensive	942		1.2 (0.36–2.04)	62
East Asia – China								
Yunan Province	1995–1996	Gejiu City	All; < 3/60	Comprehensive	361,214		0.29	75
Shandong Province	1996	Zhangqiu City	All; < 3/60	Comprehensive	11,884		0.31	76
Shunyi County	1996	Beijing Province	50+; < 3/60	Comprehensive	5084	1.9		51
Doumen County	1997	Guangdong Province	50+; < 3/60	Comprehensive	5342	2.67 (2.09–3.24)		52
Guangdong Province	1998–1999	Meixian County	All; < 3/60	Comprehensive	11,327		0.47	77
Tibet Autonomous Region	1999–2000	Lhoka, Nakchu, and Lingzhr prefectures	All; < 6/60	Comprehensive	12,644	1.4 (1.3–1.5)		78
Lasa	2000	Linzhou County	40+; < 3/60	Comprehensive	3153		2.3 (1.8–2.8)	79
Beijing Eye Study	2001	Beijing, North China	40+; < 3/60	Comprehensive	4438		0.4	80
Nantong city	2003	8 communities in Xinchengqiao administrative sub-district	60+; < 3/60	Comprehensive	3040	1.32 (0.94–1.79)	1.35 (0.97–1.83)*	81

(Continued)

Table 1.7 (Continued)

Country	Year of survey	Population covered	Restriction of age; age range or definition	Type of survey	Number examined	Prevalence of blindness (%; 95% CI) Presenting	Prevalence of Blindness (%; 95% CI) best corrected/pin hole	Reference
Motuo County, Tibet	2003	6 villages	All; < 3/60	Comprehensive	735		2.59	82
Chongqing County	2004	Nan'an District,	50+; < 3/60	Comprehensive	5079		1.8	83
Yunan Province	2006	Kunming prefecture	50+; < 3/60	RAAB	2588	3.7 (2.8–4.6)		84
Yongnian County, Handan North China	2006–2007	Han Chinese; rural	30+; < 3/60	Comprehensive	6799	0.6	0.5	85
East Asia – Other Countries								
Hong Kong	1998	Shatin area	60+; < 3/60	Comprehensive	3441	0.71 (0.31–1.1)	0.46 (0.19–0.73)	86
Taiwan	1999–2000	Shihpai	65+; < 3/60	Comprehensive	1361		0.5 (0.25–1.16)	87
Taiwan	2002	National	65+; < 3/60	Comprehensive	3160		0.6	88
South Asia – India								
Karnataka State	1995	19 districts	50+; < 3/60	RACSS	21,950	4.93 (4.52–5.34)		90
Andhra Pradesh State	1996–2000	3 rural; 1 urban area	All; < 3/60 & < 10° central fixation	Comprehensive	10,293	1.34 (1.07–1.61)		32
Tamilnadu State	1995–1997	3 districts Aravind Study	40+; < 3/60	Comprehensive	5150	4.3 (3.8–4.9)		91
World Bank Project States	1997–1998	7 states	50+; < 3/60	RACSS	24,818	5.3 (5.05–5.6)		92
Gujarat State	1997	All districts	50+; < 6/60	RACSS	61,194	7.98		93
Gujarat State #	1998	Ahmedabad Urban	50+; < 3/60	RACSS	1962	2.9		94
Rajasthan State	1998–1999	Bharatpur District	50+; < 3/60	Comprehensive	4284	8.9 (7.2–10.5)	5.1 (3.9–6.3)	95
Tamilnadu State	1998–1999	Sivaganga District	50+; < 3/60	Comprehensive	4642	5.2 (4.3–6.0)	2.8 (2.2–3.5)	96
15 states π	1999–2001	15 districts (pooled data)	50+; < 6/60	Comprehensive	63,337	8.5 (8.1–8.9)		33
Andhra Pradesh		Prakasam			4329	6.5 (5.1–7.9)		97
Chattisgarh		Rajnandgaon			4015	6.5 (5.2–7.7)		97
Madhya Pradesh		Dewas			3738	6.4 (5.4–7.5)		97
Maharashtra		Satara			4618	4.8 (3.8–5.8)		97
Orissa		Dhenkanal			4228	5.9 (5.0–6.8)		97
Uttar Pradesh		Sultanpur			5396	5.0 (4.3–5.6)		97
Bihar		Vaishali			5048	3.8 (3.2–4.5)		97

(Continued)

Table 1.7 (Continued)

Country	Year of survey	Population covered	Restriction of age; age range or definition	Type of survey	Number examined	Prevalence of blindness (%; 95% CI) Presenting	Prevalence of Blindness (%; 95% CI) best corrected/pin hole	Reference
Gujarat		Surendranagar			3736	4.5 [3.6–5.5]		97
Himachal Pradesh		Solan			2856	3.6 [2.9–4.3]		97
Karnataka		Gulbarga			3265	7.3 [6.3–8.3]		97
Kerala		Palakkad			5211	2.1 [1.6–2.7]		97
Punjab		Bhatinda			4688	6.0 [5.0–7.0]		97
West Bengal		Mada			4289	6.0 [5.2–6.8]		97
Tamilnadu State	2000	Tirunelveli District	50+; < 6/60	Comprehensive	5411	11	4.6	53
9 states	2001–2002	12 districts	50+; < 3/60	RACSS	23446	4.67		98
Tamilnadu State	2001–2003	Chennai (rural)	40+; < 3/60 & < 10° central fixation	Comprehensive	3924	19.2	3.37 (2.8–3.93)	99
Karnataka State	2002	Udipi District, rural	50+; < 3/60	Comprehensive	1505	6.6 [5.3–7.8]		100
North East states	2003	8 states	50+; < 3/60	RACSS	7519	4.95		101
6 states	2004	1 district in each state	50+; < 3/60	RACSS	NA			102
Goa		Goa				5.0		102
Haryana		Panipat				6.8		102
Jharkhand		Ranchi				5.2		102
Uttaranchal		Haridwar				2.7		102
Delhi		Delhi				1.7		102
Jammu & Kashmir		Jammu				4.6		102
Gujarat State	2005	Bharuch District	50+; < 3/60	RACSS	3068	5.3		103
15 states (pooled)	2007	16 districts in 15 states	50+; < 3/60	RAAB	40458	3.6 [3.3–3.9]	3.0	34
Gujarat State	2008	Navsari District	50+; < 3/60	Comprehensive	4738	4.3 [3.5–5.1]	2.7 (2.1–3.3)	35
South Asia — Other countries								
Nepal	1995	2 zones	45+; < 3/60	Comprehensive	4602	3.0 [2.05–3.86]		104
Nepal	2002	3 districts, Gandaki Zone	45+; < 6/60	Comprehensive	5002	2.6 [2.2–3.9]		105
Pakistan	1998	Budni, Peshawar, NWFP	40+; < 3/60	Comprehensive	1106	1.9 [1.1–2.7]		106
Pakistan	1999	Chakwal District	50+; < 3/60	RACSS	1505	3.8 [2.6–5.4]	3.1 [2.3–4.1]	107
Pakistan	2003	Dt. Lower Dir, NWFP	50+; < 3/60	RACSS	1076	2.6		108

(Continued)

Table 1.7 (Continued)

Country	Year of survey	Population covered	Restriction of age; age range or definition	Type of survey	Number examined	Prevalence of blindness (%; 95% CI) Presenting	Prevalence of Blindness (%; 95% CI) best corrected/pin hole	Reference
Pakistan	2003–2005	National	30+; < 3/60	Comprehensive	16,507	2.7 (2.4–2.9)		16
Bangladesh	2000–2001	National	30+; < 3/60	Comprehensive	11,624	1.52 (1.31–1.75)		15
Bangladesh	2005	Satkhira District	50+; < 3/60	RACSS	4868	2.9 (2.4–3.5)		109
South East Asia								
Cambodia	1996	Kandal Province	All; < 3/60	Comprehensive	5803	1.1 (0.9–1.4)		110
Malaysia	1996	National	All; < 3/60	Comprehensive	18,027	0.29 (0.19–0.39)		111
Indonesia	2002	Sumatra (5 rural; 1 urban)	21+; < 3/60	Comprehensive	989	2.2 (1.1–3.2)		112
Timor-Leste	2004	National	40+; < 6/60	RACSS	1414	7.4 (6.1–8.8)		113
Myanmar	2005	Rural Meiktila District	40+; < 3/60	Comprehensive	2076	8.1 (6.5–9.9)	5.3 (4.0–6.6)	114
Philippines	2005	Negros Island	50+; < 3/60	RAAB	2774	2.6 (2.0–3.2)		115
Philippines	2006	Antique District	50+; < 3/60	RAAB	3177	3.0 (2.4–3.6)		115
Sri Lanka	2006–2007	Kandy District	40+; < 3/60	Comprehensive	1375		1.1 (0.002–0.02)	116
Australasia								
Australia	1989–1990	South Australia	50+ 6/60	Comprehensive	2115		0.66	119
Australia (Blue Mountains)	1992–1993	New South Wales	49+; ≤ 6/60	Comprehensive	3647		0.27	120
Australia	1992–1996	Victoria	40+; < 3/60 & < 5° central fixation	Comprehensive	4744		0.16 (0.06–0.26)	121
Caribbean								
Barbados	1988–1992	Barbados	40–84; < 3/60	Comprehensive	4631 (Afro-carib: 4314)		Afro-Caribbean– 1.7 (1.3–2.1); Mixed – 1.6 (0.3–4.7)	59
Cuba	2004	Havana City	50+; < 3/60	RACSS	2760	1.9 (1.3–2.5)	1.8 (1.2–2.4)	122

(Continued)

Table 1.7 (Continued)

Country	Year of survey	Population covered	Restriction of age; age range or definition	Type of survey	Number examined	Prevalence of blindness (%; 95% CI) Presenting	Prevalence of Blindness (%; 95% CI) best corrected/pin hole	Reference
Central Europe								
Bulgaria	1993	Sofia district	≥40	Comprehensive	6275		0.49	123
Western Europe								
France	1985	Bouche du Rhone Dept.	All	Comprehensive	69,356		0.2	124
Denmark	1986–1988	Copenhagen	60–80; < 3/60	Comprehensive	969		0.53	125
Ireland	1990	Roscommon	50+	Comprehensive	2186		0.5	126
The Netherlands	1990–1993	Rotterdam	55+;	Comprehensive	6775		0.47	127
Italy	1992	Casteldaccia, Sicily	40+	Comprehensive	1068		0.47	128
UK	1995–1996	North London	65+; < 6/60 worse eye	Comprehensive	1547		5.95	129
UK	1995–1999	England, Scotland, Wales	75+; < 3/60	Nurse examination & records	15,126		2.1 (1.8–2.4)	130
Iceland	1996	Reykjavik	50+; < 3/60 & < 5° central fixation	Comprehensive	1045		0.57 (0.12–1.03)	131
Italy	2000	Ponza	40+; < 3/60 & < 10° central fixation	Comprehensive	847	0.8	0.6 (0.3–1.4)	132
Finland	2000–2001	Oulu County	70+; < 3/60	Comprehensive	500		1.9	1133
Spain	2005	Cuenca	64+; < 3/60	Comprehensive	1155		2 (1.1–2.7)	134
Latin America – Andean								
Peru	2002	Piura and Tumbes	50+; < 3/60	RACSS	4782	4 (3.2–4.8)	2.6 (2.2–3.1)	136
Latin America – Central								
Guatemala	2004	4 provinces	50+; < 3/60	RACSS	4806	4.1 (3.4–4.8)	3.5 (3.0–4.2)	137
Venezuela	2004	National	50+; < 3/60	RACSS	3317	2.3 (1.7–2.8)	2.0 (1.5–2.5)	122
Mexico	2005	Nuevo Leon State	50+; < 3/60	RAAB	3780	1.5 (1.1–1.9)	1.3 (0.9–1.7)	122
Latin America – Southern								
Argentina	2003	Buenos Aires	50+; < 3/60	RACSS	4302	1.3 (0.9–1.6)	1.0 (0.7–1.3)	122
Chile	2006	Bio-Bio Province	50+; < 3/60	RAAB	3000	1.4 (0.8–1.9)	1.2 (0.7–1.7)	122

(Continued)

Table 1.7 (Continued)

Country	Year of survey	Population covered	Restriction of age; age range or definition	Type of survey	Number examined	Prevalence of blindness (%; 95% CI) Presenting	Prevalence of Blindness (%; 95% CI) best corrected/pin hole	Reference
Latin America – Tropical								
Paraguay	1999	National	50+; <3/60	RACSS	2136	3.1 (2.2–4.4)	2.6 (1.6–3.6)	138
Brazil	2003	Campinas	50+; <3/60	RACSS	2224	1.6 (0.9–2.2)	1.4 (0.7–2.1)	139
Brazil	2004–2005	Sao Paulo low–middle income area	50+; <6/60	Comprehensive	3678	1.51 (1.2–1.82)	1.07 (0.79–1.35)	140
North Africa/Middle East								
Turkey	1989	2 provinces South East	All; <3/60	Comprehensive	8571		0.4 (0.3–0.5)	141
Saudi Arabia	1990	Eastern province	All; <3/60	Comprehensive	4340		1.5	39
Saudi Arabia	1991	Risha Region, South West	All; <3/60	Comprehensive	2882		0.66	142
Morocco	1992	Whole country	All; <3/0	Comprehensive	8878		0.76 (0.57–0.94)	143,144
Tunisia#	1992–1993	Whole country	All; <3/60	Comprehensive	3547		0.8	145
Lebanon	1995	Whole country	All ; <3/60	Comprehensive	10,148		0.6	146
Oman	1996–1997	National	All; <3/60	Comprehensive	11,417	1.1 (0.9–1.3)		147
Iran: Tehran Eye Study	2002	Tehran	1+; <3/60	Comprehensive	6497	1.39 (1.07–1.71)	0.28 (0.14–0.42)	148
Iran: Zahedan Eye Study	2004–2005	Sistan-va-Baluchestan Province	10+; <3/60	Comprehensive	5446		0.79 (0.5–1.08)	149
North America – High Income								
USA	1988–1990	Beaver Dam	43–86; ≤6/60	Comprehensive	4897		0.5	151
USA	1990	Baltimore, Maryland	40+; ≤6/60	Comprehensive	5341		White: 0.52; Afro-Carib: 1.65	60
USA	1993	Salisbury, Maryland	65–84; ≤6/60	Comprehensive	2520		0.83 (White: 0.54; Black: 0.92)	152
USA	1995–1998	Oklahoma Indians	48–82; ≤6/60	Comprehensive	1019		0.6	154
USA	1997–1998	Hispanics, Southern Arizona	40+; <3/60	Comprehensive	4774		0.29 (0.16–0.29)	155

(Continued)

Table 1.7 (Continued)

Country	Year of survey	Population covered	Restriction of age; age range or definition	Type of survey	Number examined	Prevalence of blindness (%; 95% CI) Presenting	Prevalence of Blindness (%; 95% CI) best corrected/pin hole	Reference
USA	2000–2003	Latinos, LA, California	40+; ≤6/60	Comprehensive	6122		3.13 (0.3–3.8)	156
Oceania								
Vanuatu	1989	Whole country	6+; <3/60	Comprehensive	3520		0.37 (0.16–0.69)	157
Tonga	1991	Whole country	20+; <3/60	Comprehensive	4056		0.56 (0.1–1.13)	158
Papua New Guinea	2005	Whole country	50+; <3/60	RACSS	1174	3.9 (3.4–6.1)		159
Sub-Saharan Africa – Central								
Congo	1989	Whole country	All; <3/60	Comprehensive	6185		0.3	160
Central African Republic	1994	Bossangoa District	All; <3/60	Comprehensive	6086		2.2 (1.83–2.57)	161
Equatorial Guinea	1999	Bioko (Oncho endemic area)	All; <3/60	Comprehensive	3218	3.2 (2.6–3.9)		162
Sub-Saharan Africa – East								
Zambia	1985	Luapula Valley	6+;	Comprehensive	2503		3.6 (2.9–4.3)	163
Tanzania	1986	Kongwa Area	7+; <3/60	Comprehensive	1827		1.26 (0.8–1.89)	164
Malawi	1998	Nkhoma	40+; <3/60	RACSS	993	3.72		165
Malawi	1999	Chikwawa District	50+; <6/60	Comprehensive	1384	5.39		166
Ethiopia	1995	Jimma Zone	All; <3/60	Comprehensive	7423		0.85 (0.63–1.07)	167
Ethiopia	1995?	Central Ethiopia	40+; <3/60	Comprehensive	60,820?		1.1	168
Ethiopia	2000	Gurage Zone, Central Ethiopia		Comprehensive	2693	7.9 (6.9–8.9)		169
Ethiopia	2005?	Goro District, Central Ethiopia	50+; <3/60	Comprehensive	1497	4.7		170
Ethiopia	2005–06	National	All; <3/60	Comprehensive	25,650	1.6		171
Uganda	1998?	Rural South West Uganda in an HIV sero surveillance cohort	13+; <3/60	Comprehensive; 2 stage	4076	1.6 (1.3–2.1)		172

(Continued)

Table 1.7 (Continued)

Country	Year of survey	Population covered	Restriction of age; age range or definition	Type of survey	Number examined	Prevalence of blindness (%; 95% CI) Presenting	Prevalence of Blindness (%; 95% CI) best corrected/pin hole	Reference
Kenya	2002–2003	Kibera slums, Nairobi	2+; <3/60	Comprehensive	1438	0.6 (0.21–1.0)		173
Kenya	2005	Nakuru District	50+; <3/60	RAAB	3784	2.0 (1.5–2.4)		174
Sudan	2005	Mankien District, Southern Sudan	5+; <3/60	Comprehensive	2499	4.1 (3.4–4.8)		175
Rwanda	2006	Western Province	50+; <3/60	RAAB	2206	1.8 (1.2–2.4)		71
Sub Saharan Africa – Southern								
South Africa	1991	Northern Kwazulu	All; <3/60	Comprehensive	6090		1.0 (0.7–1.2)	50
Botswana	2006	National	50+; <3/60	Comprehensive	2127	3.69 (2.38–5.0)		176
Sub Saharan Africa – West								
Chad	1985	Whole country	All; <3/60	Comprehensive	5002		2.31 (1.5–3.1)	177
Benin	1990	Whole country	All; <3/60	Comprehensive	7047		0.6	178
Mali	1990	Ségou Region	All; <3/60	Comprehensive	5871		1.7	179
Ghana	1991	Wenchi District:	30+; <3/60	Comprehensive	962		1.7 (1.1–2.5)	37
Ghana	2001	Volta Region (3 districts)	40+; <6/60	Comprehensive	2298	2.8	2.0	180
Sierra Leone	1992	Tabe River Valley, hyperendemic onchocerciasis	1+; <3/60	Comprehensive	1625		1.3 (0.7–1.9)	181
Cameroon	1992	Extreme North Province	All; <3/60	Comprehensive	10647		1.2	182
Cameroon	1992	Rural forest area	6+; <3/60	Comprehensive	5066	1.4 (0.9–2.0)	1.4 (1.0–1.8)	183
Cameroon	2004	Muyuka district (rural)	40+; <3/60	RAAB	1787			184
Cameroon	2006	Limbe urban area, South West province	40+; <3/60	RAAB	2215	1.1 (0.7–1.5)		185
Gambia	1996	Whole country	All; <3/60	Comprehensive	13046		0.42	36
Togo	1998	Rural area in south	5+; <3/60	Comprehensive	1738		2.47	186

(Continued)

Table 1.7 (Continued)

Country	Year of survey	Population covered	Restriction of age; age range or definition	Type of survey	Number examined	Prevalence of blindness (%; 95% CI) Presenting	Prevalence of Blindness (%; 95% CI) best corrected/pin hole	Reference
Cape Verde Islands	1998	National	All; <3/60	Comprehensive	3374	0.8 (0.5–1.1)		187
Nigeria	1991	Ife North LGA, Osun State	All ; <3/60	Comprehensive	2921		0.9	188
Nigeria	1995	Dambatta LGA, Kano State	All; <3/60	Comprehensive	3596	1.14 (0.8–1.48)		189
Nigeria	1999	Rural Katsina	40+; <3/60	RACSS	1461	8.2 (5.8–10.5)		190
Nigeria	2001	Ughelli North LGA, Delta State	50+; <3/60	RACSS	684	9.9		191
Nigeria	2001?	Egbedore LGA, Osun State, SW Zone	All; <3/60	Comprehensive	3204	1.18		192
Nigeria	2003?	Ozoro Town, Delta State, SW Zone	40+; <3/60	Comprehensive	815	6.3 (4.6–8.0)		193
Nigeria	2004	Atakunmosa West LGA, SW Nigeria	5+; <3/60	Comprehensive	1248	1.1		194
Nigeria	2005–2007	Whole country	40+; <3/60	Comprehensive	15,027	4.2 (3.8–4.6)	3.4 (3.0–3.8)	17
Nigeria	2005?	Sabon Birni LGA, Sokoto State	All; <3/60	Trachoma Survey	?2760	2 (1.4–2.6)		195
Nigeria	2006	Kaduna State	All; <3/60	Comprehensive	8400	0.6 (0.4–0.8)		196
Nigeria	2006	Birnin-Kebbi LGA, Kebbi State	50+; <3/60	RACSS	2424	4.5 (3.7–5.3)		197

Age/gender adjusted.
π This includes the two surveys in Rajasthan (Bharatpur) and Sivaganga (Tamilnadu), which have been reported separately and not included again.

COMMENTARY ON TABLE 1.8: CAUSES OF BLINDNESS FROM COMPREHENSIVE STUDIES

Asia Pacific — High income countries

In the Singapore Tanjong Pagar study of people predominantly of Chinese origin and aged 60–79, 60% of vision <6/60 was due to glaucoma,[63] while among the Malays glaucoma was the cause to which only 5% of blindness was attributed.[64] On the other hand, cataract was responsible for 65.2% and refractive errors for 18.0% of blindness.[64] So a wide variation was observed in Singapore according to ethnic background. In Japan, cataract (28.6%) and glaucoma, AMD and optic atrophy (14.3% each) were the predominant causes of visual impairment when vision < 6/18 was considered.[73] All three studies from the sub-region used different visual acuity cut-offs in reporting results, which can affect the assignment of major causes.

Central Asia

The studies from Mongolia among those aged 40+ years found that a third of all blindness was due to glaucoma while the proportion due to cataract differed between the two studies.[62,67] The result from Mongolia differed from those from almost all other developing countries, except perhaps Barbados, in that glaucoma was as frequent a cause of blindness as cataract.

East Asia — China

In two surveys in China, in the mid 1980s, the three leading causes were cataract, corneal opacities (with or without trachoma) and glaucoma. In several locations the corneal opacities resulting from other causes were judged more numerous than those attributable to trachoma. In most of the recent studies, whether using best corrected vision or presenting vision, cataract was the predominant cause of blindness (31.6%–71%).[51,52,75–85] Corneal opacities and glaucoma were the other major causes of blindness. The studies in Shunyi and Doumen depended on counting causes in eyes and therefore cannot be compared with data based on persons.[51,52]

East Asia — Others

In Hong Kong[86] cataract was responsible for more than half of blindness and severe visual impairment (< 6/60) while in the Shihpai study in Taiwan retinal causes including AMD predominated, but cataract did not figure at all.[87]

South Asia — India

Comprehensive eye examinations since 1995 in India have documented cataract as the single largest cause of blindness (45.5–85.6%).[32,33,35,55,91,95,96,99,100] Two of these studies reported on vision <6/60.[95,96] All except the Andhra Pradesh Eye Diseases survey[32] were done on older adults. Only two of these studies — in Andhra Pradesh[32] and Chennai[99] — additionally included the constriction of visual fields when diagnosing glaucoma. Nevertheless, these reported a high proportion of blindness to be cataract-related. In Table 1.8, in classification of the causes, surgical complications following cataract surgery have been clubbed together with cataract; it does not mean that this high proportion of cataract directly translates into a backlog of operable cases. The proportion attributable to glaucoma, even where visual fields were included in the diagnosis, was much lower in India than that reported from other regions.

Recent evidence on refractive errors as a cause of blindness is also available since presenting vision has been used to define blindness. The proportion of refractive error as a cause of blindness is directly related to the proportion of uncorrected/undercorrected aphakia as this has been grouped with refractive errors in the earlier surveys, where a significant proportion of surgery was intracapsular extraction. In Gujarat, using a strict definition of refractive errors, coupled with the fact that an overwhelming proportion of the surgery used an IOL implant, the proportion attributable to refractive errors as a cause of blindness was very low.

When the first survey was undertaken in India by the ICMR, trachoma was an important cause of blindness.[89] None of the recent studies except the survey in Rajasthan have flagged up trachoma or corneal causes as significant.

South Asia — Other countries

National surveys have been conducted in Bangladesh[15] and Pakistan[16] covering all areas of these countries. All the studies in this sub-region document cataract as the predominant cause of blindness, ranging from 55.1% to 79.6%. Only one study in Nepal showed that trachoma was an important cause of blindness. The proportion attributable to glaucoma ranged from 0.4% to 7.1%.

The available evidence from all the countries in South Asia, including India, show that the proportion of blindness due to cataract is much higher than that reported from any other region in the world. This is despite the scaling up of cataract surgical services in the region. It is also well known that life expectancies are increasing at a rapid pace in the whole region and this may be one of the causes for surgical services not being able to keep pace with new incident cases of cataract blindness. The reasons for high cataract-related blindness, in this sub-region, merits further epidemiological investigation.

South East Asia

The few studies available from this sub-region mirrored the situation in South Asia, except in Malaysia, where cataract accounted for a smaller proportion, 39%.[111] Glaucoma did not appear as a significant cause of blindness in these countries, except in Myanmar (10.5%),[114] but the results for glaucoma would depend on how specifically it was looked for.

Australasia

Age-related macular degeneration (AMD) emerged clearly as the most common cause of blindness in Australia, 50% in Victoria and up to 88% in the Blue Mountains, which were primarily Caucasian populations.[120,121]

Caribbean

In Barbados, cataract and glaucoma were almost equally important as causes of blindness.[59] Here all glaucoma blindness was open-angle, except for one case of secondary glaucoma. Because this study was done in an area with a known high rate of glaucoma, it is not clear that these results can be extrapolated to other Caribbean countries.

Europe — Central

In Bulgaria, cataract and glaucoma were responsible for a fifth of blindness each.[123] A similar picture was seen in Herzegovina.[200]

Europe — Western

In these older, primarily white Caucasian populations, AMD was clearly the single largest cause of blindness, followed by cataract and glaucoma in most countries. In Rotterdam AMD was responsible for 58% of blindness,[127] while in Iceland AMD reached 83.4%.[131]

Latin America — Tropical

The only comprehensive study in this sub-region is from Sao Paulo in Brazil, where cataract was found to be responsible for 40% of blindness while glaucoma, AMD and diabetic retinopathy were the other significant causes,[140] reflecting a pattern intermediate between the developing countries of South Asia and the established market economies of Western Europe.

North Africa — Middle East

Except in Tehran, cataract accounted for a quarter to two thirds of all blindness. Trachoma was still responsible for blindness in this region, up to nearly a quarter of all blindness in Oman.[147] Glaucoma, refractive errors and corneal opacities were other important causes.

North America — High Income

AMD and other posterior segment diseases were the common causes of blindness in America. However, there was no case of AMD among the African-Caribbean population in Baltimore[60] and similarly a much lower proportion among the black population segment than among the white in Salisbury.[152] The proportion of blindness due to

AMD was also low among the Hispanic population.[155] In most studies in the USA, cataract did not figure as a major cause of blindness, and in the Salisbury (White) population[152] and the Latino study[202] in California blindness due to cataract did not occur. In the USA most cataract surgeries are done while visual acuity is still reasonably good. However, in Arizona the complications of cataract surgery were an issue.[155]

Oceania

The two comprehensive surveys in this sub-region showed that cataract was responsible for 68% and 85% of the blindness. However, both these studies[157,158] were undertaken two decades ago and may not accurately estimate the current situation in these countries.

Sub-Saharan Africa — Central

Throughout Sub-Saharan Africa, cataract was in general the predominant cause of blindness, as in the Republic of Congo[160] and Equatorial Guinea.[162] In the Central African Republic, however, onchocerciasis was responsible for three-quarters of blindness.[161] All these surveys were done in the 1990s, and it is likely that the situation in the Central African Republic may be different today due to the Ivermectin distribution programme.

Sub-Saharan Africa — East

Most surveys showed cataract as the predominant cause of blindness, but in this sub-region trachoma and other corneal opacities emerged as major causes. The most recent survey in this region was in Ethiopia where 50% of the blindness was due to cataract, with another fifth due to trachoma and other causes of corneal scarring.[171]

Sub-Saharan Africa — Southern

The only study was from an area in South Africa where 60% of blindness was due to cataract and another quarter was attributable to glaucoma.[50]

Sub-Saharan Africa — West

Again, in almost all the surveys in this sub-region, cataract was the predominant cause of blindness. The situation was different in an onchocercal endemic area in Sierra Leone, where nearly half the blindness was due to onchocerciasis. Glaucoma, trachoma and other causes of corneal scarring were also important causes. The most recent survey in this sub-region was the national survey in Nigeria, where 43% of blindness was due to cataract, 16.7% to glaucoma, 9.8% to refractive errors, 4.2% to trachoma and 1.1% to onchocerciasis.[70] Trachoma and onchocerciasis were seen in the north and south respectively, but not across the whole country.

Table 1.8 Causes of blindness from comprehensive studies

Region/country	Year	Age	VA	Cataract & complications	Refractive error & aphakia	Trachoma	Other cornea	Glaucoma	AMD/MD	DR	Chorio retinal	OA	Other post seg	All post segment	Oncho	Other	Ref
								%									
Asia Pacific – High Income Countries																	
Singapore: Tanjong Pagar	1997–1998	60–79	BC	20.0				60.0	20.0								63
Singapore: Malay ✳	2004–2006	40–79	PV	65.2	18.0			5.0	5.0	5.0						1.8	64
Japan: Tajmi City β	2000–2001	40+	BC	28.6			7.1	14.3	14.3			14.3	14.3			7.1	73
Central Asia																	
Mongolia: 3 provinces	1992	40+	BC	36.2			8.7	34.8	2.9			5.8				11.5	67
Mongolia: 1 province	1995	40+	PV	16.7	16.7		8.3	33.3	8.3							16.7	62
East Asia-China																	
Gejiu; Yunan	1995–1996	All	BC	51.98			16.0	10.0								21.99	75
Zhangqiu, Shandong	1996	All	BC	45.95			5.41	24.32				5.41		13.5		5.41	76
Shunyi County; Beijing Ω	1996	50+	PV	32.9	11.1		13.8	9.4					13.0			19.9	51
Doumen County; Guangdong Ω	1997	50+	PV	53.7	15.2		15.1	3.9						6.5		5.6	52
Meixian, Guangdong	1998–1999	All	BC	71.0	3.8	3.8	5.7	9.4						1.9		4.4	77
Linzhou, Lasa	2000	40+	PV	52.9	9.2		5.6	4.8								27.5	79
Beijing Eye Study	2001	40+	BC	38.5			15.4	7.7	7.7	7.7		7.7	15.4				80
Nantong	2003	60+	PV	63.4	9.76		2.44							21.95		2.44	81
Tibet: Motuo County	2003	All	BC	42.1			21.1	15.8								21.0	82
Nan'an; Chongqing β	2004	50+	PV	31.6	17.0		9.3	7.8						20.1		14.2	83
Yongnian County, Handan	2007	30+	PV	36.6	9.8		7.3	7.3	2.4	2.4		21.9				12.2	85

(Continued)

Table 1.8 (Continued)

Region/country	Year	Age	VA	Cataract & complications	Refractive error & aphakia	Trachoma	Other cornea	Glaucoma	AMD/ MD	DR	Chorio retinal	OA	Other post seg	All post segment	Oncho	Other	Ref
East Asia – Other																	
Hong Kong ¥	1998	60+	BC	51.7			9.2	7.7	27.1			2.1	14.3			9.6	86
Taiwan: Shihpai	1999	65+	BC					12.5	25.0	12.5	37.5					12.5	87
South Asia – India																	
Tamilnadu: ACES	1995–1997	40+	BC	77.5			2.0	10.2	2.0			8.2					91
Andhra Pradesh: APED	1996–2000	All	PV	45.5	11.2		9.0	9.0				4.5	12.7			8.2	32
Rajasthan: Bharatpur ¥	1998–1999	50+	PV	52.8	11.5		8.4	3.0		0.5		1.5	4.6			11.4	95
Tamilnadu: Sivaganga ¥	1998–1999	50+	PV	57.36	20.93		3.18	4.39				2.43		0.37		11.08	96
15 states	1999–2001	50+	PV	64.45	19.65		0.89	5.83				0.9		4.72		4.47	33
Tamilnadu: Tirunelveli Ω	2000	50+	PV	64.9	23.3		1.6	2.3	2.9				0.5			3.7	53
Tamilnadu: Chennai	2001–2003	40+	BC	75.38			6.06	3.79#	1.89	0.38		3.79	7.97			0.76	99
Karnataka: Udipi	2002	50+	PV	80.7	12.0							1.0	2.0			4.0	100
Gujarat: Navsari	2008	50+	PV	72.7	1.5		5.4	3.4	3.4	0.5		1.9	2.9			8.3	35
South Asia – Other																	
Pakistan: Budni	1998	40+	PV	66.6	14.3		4.7	4.8				9.5					106
Pakistan: National	2003–2005	30+	PV	55.1	11.3		11.8	7.1	2.1	0.2		0.9				11.6	16
Bangladesh: National	2000–2001	30+	PV	79.6	7.4			1.23	3.09		0.62	2.47	2.47			3.09	15
Nepal: 2 provinces Ω¥	1995	45+	BC	71.4	10.8	4.6	3.7	2.1								7.4	104
Nepal: Gandaki Ω	2002	45+	PV	66.1	13.2		3.1	0.4			0.4	0.8	11.7			4.3	105
South East Asia																	
Cambodia: Kandal	1996	All	PV	67.4	9.1	3.0	5.3					3.0				12.2	110

(Continued)

Table 1.8 (Continued)

Region/country	Year	Age	VA	Cataract & complications	Refractive error & aphakia	Trachoma	Other cornea	Glaucoma	AMD/MD	DR	Chorio retinal	OA	Other post seg	All post segment	Oncho	Other	Ref
Malaysia: National	1996	All	PV	39.1	4.7		3.1	1.6	4.7	1.6		1.6	16.6			27.0	111
Indonesia: Sumatra	2002	21+	PV	62.5					12.5							25.0	112
Indonesia: Purwakarta West Java ≠	2006	40+	PV	62.5	20.7											16.6	199
Myanmar: Meiktila	2005	40+	PV	71.8		4.7	1.2	14.1	1.2				1.2			5.9	114
Sri Lanka: Kandy β	2006–2007	40+	BC	79.0			3.0		15.0							3.0	116
Australasia																	
Australia: S. Australia	1989–1990	50+	BC	28.6					50	7.1		14.2					119
Australia: Blue Mountains New South Wales α	1992–1993	49+	BC	4					88		4					4	120
Australia: Victoria	1992–1996	40+	PV					25	50				12.5			12.5	121
Caribbean																	
Barbados	1988–1992	40–84	BC	32				28	5.0		15.0	11.0				8.0	59
Central Europe																	
Bulgaria: Sofia	1993	≥40	BC	20.0			3.0	20.0	20.0	7.0	10.0					20.0	123
Herzegovina: Srpska ¥	2005	All	BC	17.0	13.0			22.0		12.0						36.0	200
Western Europe																	
Denmark: Copenhagen2	1986–1988	60–80	BC	40.0				40.0#					20.0				125
Denmark: Copenhagen3	1999–2000	20–84	BC					14.0	43.0	7.0			32.0			4.0	201
The Netherlands: Rotterdam	1990–1993	55+	BC	6.0				9.0	58.0		9.0	6.0				12.0	127
UK: MRC Trial β	1995–1999	75+	BC	35.9				11.6	52.9	3.4			4.2				130

(Continued)

Table 1.8 (Continued)

Region/country	Year	Age	VA	Cataract & complications	Refractive error & aphakia	Trachoma	Other cornea	Glaucoma	AMD/MD	DR	Chorio retinal	OA	Other post seg	All post segment	Oncho	Other	Ref
Iceland: Reykjavik	1996	50+	BC					#	83.4		16.7						131
Italy: Ponza	2000	40+	BC	47.7				21.7#	13.0				17.3				132
β Finland:Oulu County ++	2000–2001	70+	BC	75.4				21.1	68.4								133
Latin America – Tropical																	
Brazil: Sao Paulo ++	2004–2005	50+	PV	40.0	5.5			20.0	16.4	16.4		1.8	14.5			16.4	140
North Africa/Middle East																	
Turkey: 2 provinces	1989	All age	BC	38.0	12.0	3.0	12.0	12.0				6.0				17.0	141
Saudi Arabia: East Province	1990	All age	BC	37.5	15.7	9.4	7.9	9.4								20.5	39
Saudi Arabia: Risha Region	1991	All age	BC	52.6	21.0			5.3						5.3		15.8	142
Morocco: Whole country	1992	All age	BC	45.5	10.4	3.9	6.5	14.3	3.9	1.3		2.6				10.3	143 144
Tunisia: Whole country	1992–1993	All age	BC	66.0	6.4	2.1	2.1	6.4	2.1	2.1						10.7	145
Lebanon: Whole country	1995	All age	BC	41.3	12.6		7.5	2.5	3.8	2.5		7.5				22.3	146
Oman: National	1996–1997	All age	PV	30.5	2.3	23.7	7.9	11.5	2.9			5.0	3.1			11.0	147
Iran: Tehran β	2002	1+	PV	25.4	33.6		3.7	2.2	12.7			2.2	2.2			17.9	148
Iran: Sistan ¥	2004–2005	10+	BC	37.7	5.34		14.95	5.69				1.07	12.81			22.43	149
North America – High Income																	
USA: Beaver Dam β	198–1990	43–86	BC	44.4					22.2	18.5	14.8						151
USA: Baltimore: White	1990	40+	BC	13			7	12	37	6	11	5				25	60
USA: Baltimore: Black	1990	40+	BC	27			4	26		5		5				22	60

(Continued)

Table 1.8 (Continued)

Region/country	Year	Age	VA	Cataract & complications	Refractive error & aphakia	Trachoma	Other cornea	Glaucoma	AMD/MD	DR	Chorio retinal	OA	Other post seg	All post segment	Oncho	Other	Ref
USA: Salisbury: White	1993	65–84	BC					10	70		10	10					152
USA: Salisbury: Black	1993	40+	BC	9				9	18	18	9	18				18	152
USA: Hispanics, Arizona	1997–1998	40+	BC	14.3				28.6	14.3	14.3			14.3			14.3	155
USA: Oklahoma Indians α; # ++	1995–1998	48–82	BC	50.0				33.3	33.3				50.0				154
USA: Latinos; California	2000–2003	40+	BC				8.3		25.0	8.3			25.0			33.3	202
Oceania																	
Vanatu: National	1989	6+	BC	84.6					7.7							7.7	157
Tonga: National	1991	20+	BC	68.4		5.3	5.3			5.3						15.8	158
Sub Saharan Africa – Central																	
Congo: National	1989	All age	BC	76.0	5.0			9.0			5.0					5.0	160
Central African Republic: Bossangoa	1994	All age	BC	16.4		4.5	0.7	2.2				1.5			73.1	1.4	161
Equatorial Guinea: Bioko Oncho Area ++	1999	All	PV	61.3			2.1π	10.7				16.0		25.3		8.6	162
Sub Saharan Africa – East																	
Tanzania: Kongwa	1986	7+	BC	21.7		26.1	17.4	17.4			4.4					13.2	164
Malawi: Chikwawa	1999	50+	PV	61.5	4.6		9.2									24.6	166
Uganda: South West	1998	13+	PV	23.1	7.7		7.7	38.5			7.7	15.4					172
Ethiopia: Gurage	2000	40+	PV	50.4	6.8	19.5	7.8	7.7								15.5	169
Ethiopia: National	2005–2006	All	PV	49.9	7.8	11.5	7.8	5.2								13.0	171
Sudan: Mankien	2005	5+	PV	41.2		35.3	18.6		4.8							4.9	175

(Continued)

Table 1.8 (Continued)

Region/country	Year	Age	VA	Cataract & complications	Refractive error & aphakia	Trachoma	Other cornea	Glaucoma	AMD/MD	DR	Chorio retinal	OA	Other post seg	All post segment	Oncho	Other	Ref
Sub Saharan Africa – Southern																	
South Africa: Kwazulu	1991	All age	BC	59.0			1.6	24.6	1.6		3.3		1.6			8.2	50
Sub Saharan Africa – West																	
Chad: National	1985	All	BC	48.0		23.0	14.0	15.0									177
Benin: National	1990	All age	BC	47.5	6.5		11.0	15.0				7.0				13.0	178
Mali: Segou	1990	All age	BC	68.7		12.1	7.1	8.1				1.0		2.0		1.0	179
Sierra Leone:	1992	1+	BC	19.0			14.3	9.5							47.6	9.5	181
Oncho Area																	
Nigeria: Osun	1991	All	PV	48.1			7.4	11.1	3.7			7.4	7.4		14.8		188
Nigeria: Katsina	1999	40+	PV	55.9	0.8		15.8	5.8								21.7	190
Nigeria:Osun	2001	40+	PV	47.4	20.7			15.8	2.6			2.6	5.2			5.3	192
Nigeria:	2004	5+	PV	57.1	8.1		7.1π	14.3							7.1	14.3	194
Atakunmosa																	
Nigeria: Kaduna	2006	All	PV	37.8	9.8		7.9	21.6								32.7	196
Nigeria: National	2005–2007	40+	PV	43	9.7	4.2	3.3	16.7	1.8	0.5		3.7	3.0		1.1	8.2	70
Cameroon:	1992	All age	BC	55.0		7.4	3.3	12.0						4.1		8.5	182
Extreme North																	
Cameroon:	1992	6+	BC	85.0			8.0									7.0	183
Rural Forest																	
Ghana: Wenchi	1991	30+	BC	62.5	4.2		8.2					4.2		4.2	12.5	4.2	37
Ghana: Volta ¥ ++	2001	40+	PV	53.9	16.7			20.6				8.8		8.8		3.9	180
Cape Verde Islands	1998	All	PV	57.7	3.8		7.7	15.4				3.8		7.7		3.8	187
Togo: South rural	1998	5+	BC	86.0			4.7	4.7								4.7	186
Gambia: National	1996	All age	PV	45.0	24.0	5.0	16.0	9.0									36

π Includes trachoma
Visual fields included
++ % >100% as causes not mutually exclusive
β Includes both low vision & blindness
Ω Eyes of bilaterally blind persons
* VA < 6/60
α ≤6/60
PV Presenting Vision
BC Best Corrected Vision

COMMENTARY ON TABLE 1.9: CAUSES OF BLINDNESS FROM RACSS AND RAAB

In every sub-region and country in which RACSS or RAAB have been conducted, with one exception, cataract has been the predominant cause of blindness. The 19 reports of RACSS show a range for the proportion of cataract from 41% to 83%, and the 12 RAAB listed have a range for cataract from 45% to 75%, with an outlier of 25% for an area of Cameroon.[185]

In the RACSS, where the examination of the eye is basically by a torch and external evaluation, the impact of cataract is probably over-emphasized. This is because the pupil is constricted in a routine examination carried out in natural daylight and the lens opacity becomes very obvious unless there is corneal scarring. To improve on this, RAAB now incorporates a dilated eye examination if the visual acuity is <6/18. An additional feature of the RAAB is the inclusion of the ophthalmologist as an integral part of the team, which allows a better diagnosis of causes as compared with an allocation by an ophthalmic assistant or an ophthalmic nurse.

The introduction of pin-hole vision testing also allows an estimate of refractive errors.

Because of differences in locality, timing, and the age ranges included, it is difficult to make direct comparisons of causation conducted by RACSS/RAAB with figures by comprehensive examination. But a comparison of Table 1.9 with Table 1.8 suggests some general correspondence by the two approaches for the proportions of blindness due to cataract in a sub-region. Where results are available for close or overlapping locations, the results for proportion due to cataract may appear to be more congruent. For example, in Bangladesh cataract was 79.6% in the national survey (age 30+, 2000–2001)[15] and 80.4% by RACSS in a district (age 50+, 2005);[109] or in Malawi the proportion of cataract in Nkhoma was 62.0% by RACSS (age 40+, 1998)[165] compared with 61.5% in Chikwawa by comprehensive examination (age 50+, 1999).[166] RACSS/RAAB can be regarded as adding valuable information for those countries, or districts of a country, where comprehensive national or area surveys have not been carried out. They will also be valuable for monitoring the progress achieved by programmes for control of blindness.

Table 1.9 Causes of blindness from RACSS and RAAB

Region/ Country	Year	Age	VA	Cataract & complications	Refractive error & aphakia	Trachoma	Other cornea	% Glaucoma	AMD/ MD	DR	Chorio retinal	OA	Other post seg	All post segment	Oncho	Other	Ref
Central Asia																	
Turkmenistan *	2000–2001	50+	PV	42.0												58.0	74
East Asia – China																	
Kunming, Yunan ≠	2006	50+	PV	64.3	2.1		14.7	7.4					5.2			6.3	84
South Asia – India																	
Karnataka: 20 districts *	1995	50+	PV	71.9												28.1	90
Gujarat: 19 districts *	1997	50+	PV	48.4												51.6	93
7 states: World Bank *	1997–1998	50+	PV	82.1	9.6											8.2	92
Gujarat: Ahmedabad *	1998	50+	PV	41.3												58.7	94
Gujarat: Bharuch ≠	2005	50+	PV	60.7	14.8		6.9						6.2			11.4	103
15 states ≠	2007	50+	PV	75.2	6.3	0.6	5.9	4.4	0.7	0.1			2.2			4.5	34
South Asia – Other																	
Pakistan: Chakwal *	1999	50+	PV	46.5												53.5	107
Bangladesh: Satkhira *	2005	50+	PV	80.4	2.1		3.5						13.3			0.7	109
South East Asia																	
Timor-Leste: National * ¥	2004	40+	PV	82.5	5.5		4.6						6.4			0.9	113

(Continued)

Table 1.9 (Continued)

Region/Country	Year	Age	VA	Cataract & complications	Refractive error & aphakia	Trachoma	Other cornea %	Glaucoma	AMD/MD	DR	Chorio retinal	OA	Other post seg	All post segment	Oncho	Other	Ref
Philippines: Negros ≠	2005	50+	PV	55.0	5.0		6.0							31.0		3.0	115
Philippines: Antique ≠	2006	40+	PV	64.0			18.0							16.0		2.0	115
Caribbean																	
Cuba: Havana City *	2005	50+	PV	51.0	1.0		5.0							43.0			122
Latin America – Andean																	
Peru *	2002	50+	PV	53.3												46.7	136
Latin America – Central																	
Guatemala: 4 regions *	2004	50+	BC	68.0												32.0	137
Venezuela: National *	2004	50+	PV	68.0	4.0		3.0							25.0		1.0	122
Mexico: Nuevo Leon ≠	2005	50+	PV	70.0										30.0			122
Latin America – Southern																	
Argentina: Buenos Aires *	2003	50+	PV	47.0	6.0									44.0		2.0	122
Chile: Bio Bio ≠	2006	50+	PV	57.0	2.0	4.0								34.0		2.0	122
Latin America – Tropical																	
Paraguay: National *	1999	50+	PV	59.0	2.3		2.3									41.0	138
Brazil: Campinas *	2003	50+	PV	47.7	2.3		2.3	11.4	15.9				20.5				139
Oceania																	
Papua New Guinea *	2005	50+	PV	75.0	10.7		3.6	1.8		1.8			5.4			1.8	159

(*Continued*)

Table 1.9 (Continued)

Region/ Country	Year	Age	VA	Cataract & complications	Refractive error & aphakia	Trachoma	Other cornea	% Glaucoma	AMD/ MD	DR	Chorio retinal	OA	Other post seg	All post segment	Oncho	Other	Ref
Sub-Saharan Africa – East																	
Malawi: Nkhoma *	1998	40+	PV	62.0												37.8	165
Kenya: Nakuru ≠	2005	50+	PV	44.9	10.1	5.8	5.8							30.4		2.9	174
Rwanda: West province≠	2006	50+	PV	65.0		2.5	12.5							20.0			71
Sub-Saharan Africa – Southern																	
Botswana ≠	2006	50+	PV	46.9		6.2	13.1			20.0						13.8	176
Sub-Saharan Africa – West																	
Nigeria: Delta *	2001	50+	PV	41.2	23.5	2.7	5.5									35.3	191
Nigeria: Kebbi *	2006	50+	PV	66.0	4.5	2.7	5.5	11.8	2.7				1.8			3.6	197
Cameroon: Muyuka ≠	2004	40+	PV	62.1										13.8	13.8	10.4	184
Cameroon: Limbe ≠	2006	40+	PV	25.0	4.0							21.0		29.0	17.0	4.0	185

* RACSS
≠ RAAB
¥ VA < 6/60

REFERENCES

1. Resnikoff S, Pascolini D, Etya'ale D, *et al.* Global data on visual impairment in the year 2002. *Bull World Health Organ* 2004; 82:844–851. Epub 2004 Dec 14.

2. WHO. Change the definition of blindness. Accessed 1st September 2009. http://www.who.int/blindness/Change%20the%20Definition%20of%20Blindness.pdf.

3. Pascolini D, Mariotti SP, Pokharel GP, *et al.* 2002 Global update of available data on visual impairment: a compilation of population-based prevalence studies. *Ophthalmic Epidemiol* 2004;11(2):67–115.

4. WHO Study Group on the Prevention of Blindness. *WHO Technical Report Series No.* 518. WHO, Geneva, 1973.

5. Methods of Assessment of Avoidable Blindness. *WHO Offset Publication No.* 54. Geneva: WHO 1980.

6. Viggosson G, Björnsson G, Ingvason JG. The prevalence of open-angle glaucoma in Iceland. *Acta Ophthalmol* 1986; 64:138–141.

7. Brennan ME, Knox EG. An investigation into the purposes, accuracy, and effective uses of the Blind Register in England. *Br J Prev Soc Med* 1973; 27:154–159.

8. Evans JR, Wormald RPL. Epidemiological functions of BD8 certification. *Eye* 1993; 7:172–179.

9. Rosenberg T. Prevalence and causes of blindness in Greenland. *Arct Med Res* 1987; 46:13–17.

10. Green JS, Bear JC, Johnson GJ. The burden of genetically determined eye disease. *Br J Ophthalmol* 1986; 70:696–699.

11. International Statistical Classification of Diseases and Related Health Problems, 10th Revision. Geneva: WHO 1992. pp. 456–457.

12. Bailey IL, Lovie JE. New design principles for visual acuity letter charts. *Am J Optom Phys Optics* 1976; 53:740–745.

13. Rosser DA, Laidlaw DAH, Murdoch IE. The development of a 'reduced logMAR' visual acuity chart for use in routine clinical practice. *Br J Ophthalmol* 2001; 85:432–436.

14. Bourne RR, Rosser DA, Sukudom P, *et al.* Evaluating a new logMAR chart designed to improve visual acuity assessment in population based surveys. *Eye* 2003; 17:754–758.

15. Dineen BP, Bourne RR, Ali SM, *et al.* Prevalence and causes of blindness and visual impairment in Bangladeshi adults: results of the National Blindness and Low Vision Survey of Bangladesh. *Br J Ophthalmol* 2003; 87(7):820–828.

16. Jadoon MZ, Dineen B, Bourne RR, *et al.* Prevalence of blindness and visual impairment in Pakistan: the Pakistan National Blindness and Visual Impairment Survey. *Invest Ophthalmol Vis Sci* 2006; 47(11):4749–4755.

17. Kyari F, Gudlavalleti MV, Sivsubramaniam S, *et al.* Nigeria National Blindness and Visual Impairment Study Group. Prevalence of blindness and visual impairment in Nigeria: the National Blindness and Visual Impairment Study. *Invest Ophthalmol Vis Sci* 2009; 50(5):2033–2039. Epub 2008 Dec 30.

18. Brilliant LB, Pokhrel RP, Grasset NC, *et al.* Epidemiology of blindness in Nepal. *Bull World Health Organ* 1985; 63:375–386.

19. Thylefors B, Négrel AD, Pararajasegaram R, *et al.* Available data on blindness (update 1994). WHO/PBL/94.38, WHO, Geneva. (This is also published in *Ophthalmic Epidemiol* 1995; 2:5–39.)

20. Murray CJL, Lopez AD, Mathers CD, *et al.* The Global Burden of Disease 2000 Project: aims, methods and data sources. Geneva: World Health Organization 2001; Global Programme on Evidence for Health Policy Discussion paper No. 36. http:/www.who.int/entity/en.

21. Resnikoff S, Pascolini D, Mariotti SP, *et al.* Global magnitude of visual impairment caused by uncorrected refractive errors in 2004. *Bull World Health Organ* 2008; 86(1):63–70.

22. Sherwin JC, Keeffe JE, Kuper H, *et al.* Functional presbyopia in a rural Kenyan population: the unmet presbyopic need. *Clin Exp Ophthalmol* 2008; 36(3):245–251.

23. Laviers H. The prevalence of presbyopia and the feasibility of community distribution of near spectacles in adults in Zanzibar, East Africa. *Community Eye Health J* 2007; 20(64):73.

24. Nirmalan PK, Krishnaiah S, Shamanna BR, *et al.* A population-based assessment of presbyopia in the state of Andhra Pradesh, south India: the Andhra Pradesh Eye Disease Study. *Invest Ophthalmol Vis Sci* 2006; 47(6):2324–2328.

25. Burke AG, Patel I, Munoz B, et al. Population-based study of presbyopia in rural Tanzania. *Ophthalmology* 2006; 113(5):723–727.

26. Holden BA, Fricke TR, Ho SM, et al. Global vision impairment due to uncorrected presbyopia. *Arch Ophthalmol* 2008; 126(12):1731–1739.

27. Thylefors B, Négrel AD, Pararajasegaram R, et al. Global data on blindness. *Bull World Health Organ* 1995; 73:115–121.

28. Dandona L, Foster A. Patterns of blindness. In: Tasman W, Jaeger EA, eds. *Duanes Clinical Ophthalmology*. Philadelphia: Lippincott-Raven; 2001. Chapter 53.

29. WHO. VISION 2020: The Right to Sight. Global initiative for the elimination of avoidable blindness. Action Plan 2006–2011. WHO, Geneva, 2008. pp. 1–97.

30. World Development Report 1993. Oxford: The International Bank for Reconstruction and Development/The World Bank; 1993. p. 52.

31. The Global Burden of Diseases, Injuries, and Risk Factors Study. Operations Manual Final Draft January 2008; 1–15:25–31.

32. Dandona L, Dandona K, Srinivas M, et al. Blindness in the Indian State of Andhra Pradesh. *Invest Ophthalmol Vis Sci* 2001; 42:908–916.

33. Murthy GV, Gupta SK, Bachani D, et al. Current estimates of blindness in India. *Br J Ophthalmol* 2005; 89(3):257–260.

34. Neena J, Rachel J, Praveen V, et al. Rapid Assessment of Avoidable Blindness India Study Group. Rapid Assessment of Avoidable Blindness in India. *PLoS One* 2008; 3(8):e2867.

35. Dept. of Community Ophthalmology, AIIMS, New Delhi, India. Prevalence and Causes of Visual Impairment & Blindness in Adults in Navsari district, Gujarat, India: A Report. 2008:1–53.

36. Faal H, Minassian DC, Dolin PJ, et al. Evaluation of a national eye care programme: re-survey after 10 years. *Br J Ophthalmol* 2000; 84:948–951.

37. Moll AC, van der Linden AJH, Hogeweg M, et al. Prevalence of blindness and low vision of people over 30 years in the Wenchi district, Ghana, in relation to eye care programmes. *Br J Ophthalmol* 1994; 78:275–279.

38. Tabbara KF, Ross-Degnan D. Blindness in Saudi Arabia. *J Am Med Ass* 1986; 255:3378–3384.

39. Badr IA, Al-Saif AM, Al-Rajhi AA, et al. Changing pattern of visual loss in the Eastern province of Kingdom of Saudi Arabia. *Saudi J Ophthalmol* 1992; 6:59–68.

40. Faal H, Minassian D, Sowa S, et al. National survey of blindness and low vision in The Gambia: results. *Br J Ophthalmol* 1989; 73:82–87.

41. Dandona L, Dandona R, John RK. Estimation of blindness in India from 2000 through 2020: implications for the blindness control policy. *Natl Med J India* 2001; 14:327–333.

42. NPCB. Rapid Assessment of Avoidable Blindness-India: A Report. 2006–07. Ophthalmology Section, Directorate General of Health Services, Ministry of Health & Family Welfare, Govt. of India. pp. 1–56.

43. Podgor MJ, Leske MC, Ederer F. Incidence estimates for lens changes, macular changes, open-angle glaucoma, and diabetic retinopathy. *Am J Epidemiol* 1983, 118:206–212.

44. Rosenberg T, Flage T, Hansen E, et al. Incidence of registered visual impairment in the Nordic child population. *Br J Ophthalmol* 1996; 80:49–53.

45. Klein R, Klein BEK, Lee KE, et al. Changes in visual acuity in a population over a 10-year period. The Beaver Dam Study. *Ophthalmology* 2001; 108:1757–1766.

46. Foran S, Wang JJ, Mitchell P. Causes of incident visual impairment. The Blue Mountains Eye Study. *Arch Ophthalmol* 2002; 120:613–619.

47. Leske MC, Wu SY, Hyman L, et al. Four-year incidence of visual impairment: Barbados Incidence Study of Eye Diseases. *Ophthalmology* 2004; 111:118–124.

48. Hennis AJ, Wu SY, Nemesure B, et al. Nine-year incidence of visual impairment in the Barbados Eye Studies. *Ophthalmology* 2009; 6(8):1461–1468. Epub 2009 Jun 4.

49. Abdull M. Incidence of blindness and low vision in Bauchi State, Nigeria. *Community Eye Health J* 2008; 21(68):66.

50. Cook CD, Knight SE, Crofton-Briggs I. Prevalence and causes of low vision and blindness in northern KwaZulu. *S Afr Med J* 1993; 83:590–593.

51. Zhao J, Jia L, Sui R, et al. A survey of blindness and cataract surgery in Shunyi County, China. *Am J Ophthalmol* 1998; 126:506–574.

52. Li S, Xu J, He M, *et al*. A survey of blindness and cataract surgery in Doumen County, China. *Ophthalmology* 1999; 106:1602–1608.

53. Nirmalan PK, Thulasiraj RD, Maneksha V, *et al*. A population based eye survey of older adults in Tirunelveli district of south India: blindness, cataract surgery, and visual outcomes. *Br J Ophthalmol* 2002; 86(5):505–512.

54. Mohan M. National Survey of Blindness, India. NPCB-WHO Report. Government of India, New Delhi: Ministry of Health and Family Welfare; 1989.

55. Thylefors B, Négrel AD. The global impact of glaucoma. *Bull World Health Organ* 1994; 72:323–326.

56. Quigley HA. Number of people with glaucoma worldwide. *Br J Ophthalmol* 1996; 80:389–393.

57. Quigley HA, Broman AT. The number of people with glaucoma worldwide in 2010 and 2020. *Br J Ophthalmology* 2006; 90:262–267.

58. Abou-Gareeb I, Lewallen S, Barrett K, *et al*. Gender and blindness: a meta-analysis of population-based prevalence surveys. *Ophthalmic Epidemiol* 2001; 8:39–56.

59. Hyman L, Wu SY, Connell AM, *et al*. Prevalence and causes of visual impairment in The Barbados Eye Study. *Ophthalmology* 2001;108(10): 1751–1756.

60. Tielsch JM, Sommer A, Witt K, *et al*. Blindness and visual impairment in an American urban population. *Arch Ophthalmol* 1990; 108:286–290.

61. Sommer A, Tielsch JM, Katz J, *et al*. Racial differences in the cause-specific prevalence of blindness in east Baltimore. *N Engl J Med* 1991; 325:1414–1417.

62. Foster P, Baasanhu J, Alsbirk PH, *et al*. Glaucoma in Mongolia. A population based survey in Hovsgol province, Northern Mongolia. *Arch Ophthalmol* 1996; 114:1235–1241.

63. Saw SM, Foster PJ, Gazzard G, *et al*. Causes of blindness, low vision, and questionnaire-assessed poor visual function in Singaporean Chinese adults: The Tanjong Pagar Survey. *Ophthalmology* 2004; 111(6):1161–1168.

64. Wong TY, Chong EW, Wong WL, *et al*. Singapore Malay Eye Study Team. Prevalence and causes of low vision and blindness in an urban Malay population: the Singapore Malay Eye Study. *Arch Ophthalmol* 2008; 126(8):1091–1099.

65. Abiose A, Murdoch I, Babalola O, *et al*. Distribution and aetiology of blindness and visual impairment in mesoendemic onchocercal communities, Kaduna State, Nigeria. *Br J Ophthalmol* 1994; 78:8–13.

66. Nicolosi A, Marighi PE, Rizzardi P, *et al*. Prevalence and causes of visual impairment in Italy. *Int J Epidemiol* 1994; 23:359–364.

67. Baasanhu J, Johnson GJ, Burendei G, *et al*. Prevalence and causes of blindness and visual impairment in Mongolia: a survey of populations aged 40 years and older. *Bull World Health Organ* 1994; 72: 771–776.

68. Gilbert CE, Shah SP, Jadoon MZ, *et al*. Poverty and blindness in Pakistan: results from the Pakistan national blindness and visual impairment survey. *Br Med J* 2008; 336(7634):29–32.

69. Naidoo K. Poverty and blindness in Africa. *Clin Exp Optom* 2007; 90(6):415–421.

70. Abdull MM, Sivasubramaniam S, Murthy GV, *et al*. Causes of blindness and visual impairment in Nigeria: The Nigeria National Blindness and Visual Impairment Survey. *Invest Ophthalmol Vis Sci* 2009; Apr 22; Epub ahead of print.

71. Mathenge W, Nkurikiye J, Limburg H, *et al*. Rapid assessment of avoidable blindness in Western Rwanda: blindness in a post-conflict setting. *PLoS Med* 2007; 4(7):e217.

72. Iwano M, Nomura H, Ando F, *et al*. Visual acuity in a community-dwelling Japanese population and factors associated with visual impairment. *Jpn J Ophthalmol* 2004; 48(1):37–43.

73. Iwase A, Araie M, Tomidokoro A, *et al*; Tajimi Study Group. Prevalence and causes of low vision and blindness in a Japanese adult population: the Tajimi Study. *Ophthalmology* 2006; 113(8): 1354–1362.

74. Amansakhatov S, Volokhovskaya ZP, Afanasyeva AN, *et al*. Cataract blindness in Turkmenistan: results of a national survey. *Br J Ophthalmol* 2002; 86(11):1207–1210.

75. Li N, Wang C, Wang C. A survey and treatment of blindness in Gejiu City of Yunnan Province [Article in Chinese]. *Zhonghua Yan Ke Za Zhi* 2001; 37(3):218–221.

76. Dang G, Zheng X, Yang Z, *et al*. An epidemiological survey and treatment of blindness in Zhangqiu city of Shandong province [Article in

Chinese]. *Zhonghua Yan Ke Za Zhi* 1999; 35(5):352–354.

77. Liang X, Li F, Qiu W. An epidemiological survey of blindness and low vision in Meixian County [Article in Chinese]. *Zhonghua Yan Ke Za Zhi* 2001; 37(1):12–15.

78. Dunzhu S, Wang FS, Courtright P, *et al.* Blindness and eye diseases in Tibet: findings from a randomized, population based survey. *Br J Ophthalmol* 2003; 87(12):1443–1448.

79. Hou B, De J, Wu H, *et al.* Prevalence of blindness among adults aged 40 years or above in Linzhou county of Lasa [Article in Chinese]. *Zhonghua Yan Ke Za Zhi* 2002; 38(10):589–593.

80. Xu L, Cui T, Yang H, *et al.* Prevalence of visual impairment among adults in China: the Beijing Eye Study. *Am J Ophthalmol* 2006;141(3):591–593.

81. Li L, Guan H, Xun P, *et al.* Prevalence and causes of visual impairment among the elderly in Nantong, China. *Eye* 2008; 22(8):1069–1075. Epub 2008 May 9.

82. Luobuciren, Li JF. A survey of blindness and low vision in Motuo county of Tibet [Article in Chinese]. *Zhonghua Yan Ke Za Zhi* 2007; 43(9):803–805.

83. Liu S, Chen L, Ouyang L, *et al.* The survey of prevalence of blindness in Nan'an District of Chongqing [Article in Chinese]. *Zhonghua Yan Ke Za Zhi* 2007; 43(8):722–725.

84. Wu M, Yip JL, Kuper H. Rapid assessment of avoidable blindness in Kunming, china. *Ophthalmology* 2008; 115(6):969–974. Epub 2007 Oct 22.

85. Liang YB, Friedman DS, Wong TY, *et al.* Handan Eye Study Group. Prevalence and causes of low vision and blindness in a rural Chinese adult population: the Handan Eye Study. *Ophthalmology* 2008; 115(11):1965–1972. Epub 2008 Aug 5.

86. Michon JJ, Lau J, Chan WS, *et al.* Prevalence of visual impairment, blindness, and cataract surgery in the Hong Kong elderly. *Br J Ophthalmol* 2002; 86(2):133–139.

87. Hsu WM, Cheng CY, Liu JH, *et al.* Prevalence and causes of visual impairment in an elderly Chinese population in Taiwan: the Shihpai Eye Study. *Ophthalmology* 2004; 111(1):62–69.

88. Tsai CY, Woung LC, Chou P, *et al.* The current status of visual disability in the elderly population of Taiwan. *Jpn J Ophthalmol* 2005; 49(2):166–172.

89. National Programme for Control of Blindness, India. A Report. DGHS 2/86. Government of India, New Delhi: Directorate General of Health Services (Ophthalmic Section), Ministry of Health and Family Welfare; 1985.

90. Limburg H, Kumar R. Follow-up study of blindness attributed to cataract in Karnataka State, India. *Ophthalmic Epidemiol* 1998; 5:211–223.

91. Thulasiraj RD, Nirmalan PK, Ramakrishnan R, *et al.* Blindness and vision impairment in a rural south Indian population: the Aravind Comprehensive Eye Survey. *Ophthalmology* 2003; 110(8):1491–1498.

92. Bachani D, Murthy GVS, Gupta KS. Rapid assessment of cataract blindness in India. *Indian J Public Health* 2000; 44:82–89.

93. State Ophthalmic Cell, Commissionerate of Health, Medical Services and Medical Education, Govt. of Gujarat, Gandhinagar, India. Rapid Assessment of Cataract Blindness in Districts of Gujarat: A Report 1998:1–67.

94. Limburg H, Vasadava A, Muzundar G, *et al.* Rapid assessment of cataract blindness in an urban district of Gujarat. *Indian J Ophthalmol* 1999; 47:135–141.

95. Murthy GVS, Gupta S, Ellwein LB *et al.* A population-based eye survey of older adults in a rural district in Rajasthan. I. Central vision impairment, blindness, and cataract surgery. *Ophthalmology* 2001; 108:679–685.

96. Thulasiraj RD, Rahmatullah R, Saraswati A, *et al.* The Sivaganga Eye Survey: 1 Blindness and Cataract Surgery. *Ophthalmic Epidemiol* 2002; 9(5):299–312.

97. National Programme for Control of Blindness: National Survey on Blindness and Visual Outcomes after Cataract Surgery, Directorate General Health Service, Govt. of India, 2002: A Report. pp. 1–79.

98. Ophthalmology Section, Directorate General Health Services, Ministry of Health & Family Welfare, Govt. of India, New Delhi. Rapid Assessment of Blindness: A Report 2001–2002: 1–48.

99. Vijaya L, George R, Arvind H, *et al.* Prevalence and causes of blindness in the rural population of the Chennai Glaucoma Study. *Br J Ophthalmol* 2006; 90(4):407–410.

100. Chandrashekhar TS, Bhat HV, Pai RP, *et al*. Prevalence of blindness and its causes among those aged 50 years and above in rural Karnataka, South India. *Trop Doct* 2007; 37(1):18–21.

101. Ophthalmology Section, Directorate General Health Services, Ministry of Health & Family Welfare, Govt. of India, New Delhi, India. Rapid Assessment of Blindness in North Eastern States of India 2003: A Report. 2003:1–48.

102. Rapid Assessment of Blindness in Selected States of India: 2002–2004. *NPCB India* 2003; 2(3):6–8.

103. Ophthalmology Section, Directorate General Health Services, Ministry of Health & Family Welfare, Govt. of India, New Delhi, India. Rapid Assessment of Blindness in 50+ population (Bharuch, Gujarat): A Report, 2006: 31–51.

104. Pokharel GP, Regmi G, Shrestha SK, *et al*. Prevalence of blindness and cataract surgery in Nepal. *Br J Ophthalmol* 1998; 82:600–605.

105. Sapkota YD, Pokharel GP, Nirmalan PK, *et al*. Prevalence of blindness and cataract surgery in Gandaki Zone, Nepal. *Br J Ophthalmol* 2006; 90(4):411–416.

106. Ahmad K, Khan MD, Qureshi MB, *et al*. Prevalence and causes of blindness and low vision in a rural setting in Pakistan. *Ophthalmic Epidemiol* 2005; 12(1):19–23.

107. Haider S, Hussain A, Limburg H. Cataract blindness in Chakwal District, Pakistan: results of a survey. *Ophthalmic Epidemiol* 2003; 10(4):249–258.

108. Shaikh SP, Aziz TM. Rapid assessment of cataract surgical services in age group 50 years and above in Lower Dir District Malakand, Pakistan. *J Coll Physicians Surg Pak* 2005; 15(3):145–148.

109. Wadud Z, Kuper H, Polack S, *et al*. Rapid assessment of avoidable blindness and needs assessment of cataract surgical services in Satkhira District, Bangladesh. *Br J Ophthalmol* 2006; 90(10): 1225–1229. Epub 2006 Jul 26.

110. Rutzen AR, Ellish NJ, Schwab L, *et al*. Cambodia Eye Survey Group. Blindness and eye disease in Cambodia. *Ophthalmic Epidemiol* 2007; 14(6):360–366.

111. Zainal M, Ismail SM, Ropilah AR, *et al*. Prevalence of blindness and low vision in Malaysian population: results from the National Eye Survey 1996. *Br J Ophthalmol* 2002; 86(9):951–956.

112. Saw SM, Husain R, Gazzard GM, *et al*. Causes of low vision and blindness in rural Indonesia. *Br J Ophthalmol* 2003; 87(9):1075–1078.

113. Ramke J, Palagyi A, Naduvilath T, *et al*. Prevalence and causes of blindness and low vision in Timor-Leste. *Br J Ophthalmol* 2007; 91(9):1117–1121.

114. Casson RJ, Newland HS, Muecke J, *et al*. Prevalence and causes of visual impairment in rural Myanmar: the Meiktila Eye Study. *Ophthalmology* 2007; 114(12):2302–2308. Epub 2007 Apr 19.

115. Eusebio C, Kuper H, Polack S, *et al*. Rapid assessment of avoidable blindness in Negros Island and Antique District, Philippines. *Br J Ophthalmol* 2007; 91(12):1588–1592. Epub 2007 Jun 13.

116. Edussuriya K, Sennanayake S, Senaratne T, *et al*. The prevalence and causes of visual impairment in central Sri Lanka the Kandy Eye study. *Ophthalmology* 2009; 116(1):52–56. Epub 2008 Nov 17.

117. Taylor HR. Prevalence and causes of blindness in Australian aborigines. *Med J Aust* 1980; 6:71–76.

118. Wright HR, Keeffe JE, Taylor HR. Trachoma, cataracts and uncorrected refractive errors are still important contributors to visual morbidity in two remote indigenous communities of the Northern Territory, Australia. *Clin Exp Ophthalmol* 2009; 37(6):550–557.

119. Newland HS, Hiller JE, Casson RJ, *et al*. Prevalence and causes of blindness in the South Australian population aged 50 and over. *Ophthalmic Epidemiol* 1996; 3:97–107.

120. Attebo K, Mitchell P, Smith W. Visual acuity and causes of visual loss in Australia. The Blue Mountains Eye Study. *Ophthalmology* 1996; 103:357–364.

121. Van Newkirk MR, Weik L, McCarty CA, *et al*. Cause-specific prevalence of bilateral visual impairment in Victoria, Australia. *Ophthalmology* 2001; 108:960–967.

122. Limburg H, Barria von Bischhoffshausen F, Gomez P, *et al*. Review of recent surveys on blindness and visual impairment in Latin America. *Br J Ophthalmol* 2008; 92(3):315–319. Epub 2008 Jan 22.

123. Vassileva P, Gieser SC, Vitale S, *et al.* Blindness and visual impairment in Western Bulgaria. *Ophthalmic Epidemiol* 1996; 3:143–149.

124. Queguiner P, Guillaumat L, Gattef C. Epidemiology of blindness in Bouches-du-Rhône: Methodology [Article in French]. *Bull Soc Ophthalmol Fr* 1988; 93:23–26.

125. Buch H, Vinding T, La Cour M, *et al.* The prevalence and causes of bilateral and unilateral blindness in an elderly urban Danish population. The Copenhagen City Eye Study. *Acta Ophthalmol Scand* 2001; 79(5):441–449.

126. Coffey M, Reidy A, Wormald R *et al.* Prevalence of glaucoma in the west of Ireland. *Br J Ophthalmol* 1993; 77:17–21.

127. Klaver CC, Wolfs RCW, Vingerling JR, *et al.* Age-specific prevalence and causes of blindness and visual impairment in an older population. The Rotterdam Study. *Arch Ophthalmol* 1998; 116:653–658.

128. Ponte F, Giuffr'e G, Giammanco R. Prevalence and causes of blindness in the Casteldaccia Eye Study. *Graefes Arch Clin Exp Ophthalmol* 1994; 232:469–472.

129. Reidy A, Minassian DC, Vafidis G, *et al.* Prevalence of serious eye disease and visual impairment in a north London population: population based, cross sectional study. *Br Med J* 1998; 316:1643–1646.

130. Evans JR, Fletcher AE, Wormald RPL, *et al.* Prevalence of visual impairment in people aged 75 years and older in Britain: results from the MRC Trial of assessment and management of older people in the community. *Br J Ophthalmol* 2002; 86:795–800.

131. Gunnlaugsdottir E, Arnarsson A, Jonasson F. Prevalence and causes of visual impairment and blindness in Icelanders aged 50 years and older: the Reykjavik Eye Study. *Acta Ophthalmol* 2008 ; 86(7):778–785. Epub 2008 May 30.

132. Cedrone C, Nucci C, Scuderi G, *et al.* Prevalence of blindness and low vision in an Italian population: a comparison with other European studies. *Eye* 2006; 20(6):661–667. Epub 2005 May 27.

133. Hirvelä H, Laatikainen L. Visual acuity in a population aged 70 years or older; prevalence and causes of visual impairment. *Acta Ophthalmol Scand* 1995; 73(2):99–104.

134. Esteban JJ, Martínez MS, Navalón PG, *et al.* Visual impairment and quality of life: gender differences in the elderly in Cuenca, Spain. *Qual Life Res* 2008; 17(1):37–45. Epub 2007 Nov 17.

135. Gibson JM, Lavery JR, Rosenthal AR. Blindness and partial sight in an elderly population. *Br J Ophthalmol* 1986; 70:700–705.

136. Pongo Aguila L, Carrión R, Luna W, *et al.* Cataract blindness in people 50 years old or older in a semirural area of northern Peru [Article in Spanish]. *Rev Panam Salud Publica* 2005; 17(5–6):387–393.

137. Beltranena F, Casasola K, Silva JC, *et al.* Cataract blindness in 4 regions of Guatemala: Results of a population based survey. *Ophthalmology* 2007; 114:1558–1563.

138. Duerksen R, Limburg H, Carron JE, *et al.* Cataract blindness in Paraguay — results of a national survey. *Ophthalmic Epidemiol* 2003; 10(5):349–357.

139. Arieta CE, de Oliveira DF, Lupinacci AP, *et al.* Cataract remains an important cause of blindness in Campinas, Brazil. *Ophthalmic Epidemiol* 2009; 16(1):58–63.

140. Salomao SR, Cinoto RW, Berezovsky A, *et al.* Prevalence and causes of vision impairment and blindness in older adults in Brazil: the Sao Paulo Eye Study. *Ophthalmic Epidemiol* 2008; 15(3):167–175.

141. Negrel AD, Minassian DC, Sayek F. Blindness and low vision in south east Turkey. *Ophthalmic Epidemiol* 1996; 3:127–134.

142. Al Fran MF, Al-Rajhi AA, Al-Omar OM, *et al.* Prevalence and causes of visual impairment and blindness in the south western region of Saudi Arabia. *Int Ophthalmol* 1993; 17:161–165.

143. World Health Organization Prevention of Blindness. Prevalence and causes of blindness and low vision in Morocco. *Wkly Epidemiol Rec* 1994; 69:129–131.

144. Chami-Khazaraji Y, Akalay O, Negrel AD. Prevalence and causes of blindness and low vision in the Kingdom of Morocco [Article in French]. Ministère de la Santé Publique.

145. Ayed S, Negrel AD, Nabli M *et al.* Prevalence and causes of blindness in the Republic of Tunisia. Results of a national survey conducted in 1993 [Article in French]. *Cahiers Santé* 1998; 8:275–282.

146. Mansour AM, Kassak K, Chaya M *et al.* National survey of blindness and low vision in Lebanon. *Br J Ophthalmol* 1997; 81:905–906.

147. Khandekar R, Mohammed AJ, Negrel AD, *et al.* The prevalence and causes of blindness in the Sultanate of Oman: the Oman Eye Study (OES). *Br J Ophthalmol* 2002; 86(9):957–962.

148. Fotouhi A, Hashemi H, Mohammad K, *et al.* Tehran Eye Study. The prevalence and causes of visual impairment in Tehran: the Tehran Eye Study. *Br J Ophthalmol* 2004; 88(6):740–745.

149. Shahriari HA, Izadi S, Rouhani MR, *et al.* Prevalence and causes of visual impairment and blindness in Sistan-va-Baluchestan Province, Iran: Zahedan Eye Study. *Br J Ophthalmol* 2007; 91(5):579–84. Epub 2006 Nov 23.

150. Leibowitz HM, Krueger DE, Maunder LR, *et al.* The Framingham eye study monograph. *Surv Ophthalmol* 1980; 24(suppl.):335–608.

151. Klein R, Klein BEK, Linton KLP, *et al.* The Beaver Dam Eye Study: visual acuity. *Ophthalmology* 1991; 98:1310–1315.

152. Munoz B, West SK, Rubin GS, *et al.* Causes of blindness and visual impairment in a population of older Americans. The Salisbury Eye Evaluation Study. *Arch Ophthalmol* 2000; 118:819–825.

153. Dana MR, Tielsch JM, Enger C, *et al.* Visual impairment in a rural Appalachian community: prevalences and causes. *JAMA* 1990; 264:2400–2405.

154. Lee TE, Russel D, Morris T, *et al.* Visual Impairment and Eye abnormalities in Oklahoma Indians. *Arch Ophthalmol* 2005; 123:1699–1704.

155. Rodriguez J, Sanchez R, Munoz B, *et al.* Causes of blindness and visual impairment in a population-based sample of U.S. Hispanics. *Ophthalmology* 2002; 109(4):737–743.

156. Varma R, Ying-Lai M, Klein R, *et al.* Los Angeles Latino Eye Study Group. Prevalence and risk indicators of visual impairment and blindness in Latinos: the Los Angeles Latino Eye Study. *Ophthalmology* 2004; 111(6):1132–1140.

157. Newland HS, Harris MF, Walland M, *et al.* Epidemiology of blindness and visual impairment in Vanuatu. *Bull World Health Organ* 1992; 70:369–372.

158. Newland HS, Woodward AJ, Taumoepeau LA, *et al.* Epidemiology of blindness and visual impairment in the kingdom of Tonga. *Br J Ophthalmol* 1994; 78:344–348.

159. Garap JN, Sheeladevi S, Shamanna BR, *et al.* Blindness and vision impairment in the elderly of Papua New Guinea. *Clin Exp Ophthalmol* 2006; 34(4):335–341.

160. Négrel AD, Massembo-Yako B, Botaka E, *et al.* Prevalence and causes of blindness in the Congo. *Bull World Health Organ* 1990; 68:237–243.

161. Schwartz EC, Huss R, Hopkins A, *et al.* Blindness and visual impairment in a region endemic for onchocerciasis in the Central African Republic. *Br J Ophthalmol* 1997; 81:443–447.

162. Moser CL, Martín-Baranera M, Vega F, *et al.* Survey of blindness and visual impairment in Bioko, Equatorial Guinea. *Br J Ophthalmol* 2002; 86(3):257–260.

163. Sukwa TY, Mwandu DH, Ngalande TC, *et al.* Prevalence of blindness and visual impairment in the Luapula Valley, Zambia. *Trop Geogr Med* 1988; 40:237–240.

164. Rapoza PA, West SK, Katala SJ, *et al.* Prevalence and causes of vision loss in central Tanzania. *Int Ophthalmol* 1990; 15:123–129.

165. Eloff J, Foster A. Cataract surgical coverage: results of a population-based survey at Nkhoma, Malawi. *Ophthalmic Epidemiol* 2000; 7(3): 219–221.

166. Courtright P, Hoechsmann A, Metcalfe N, *et al.* Chikwawa Survey Team. Changes in blindness prevalence over 16 years in Malawi: reduced prevalence but increased numbers of blind. *Br J Ophthalmol* 2003; 87(9):1079–1082.

167. Zerihun N, Mabey D. Blindness and low vision in Jimma Zone, Ethiopia; results of a population-based survey. *Ophthalmic Epidemiol* 1997; 4:19–26.

168. Alemayehu W, Tekle-Haimanot R, Forsgren L, *et al.* Causes of visual impairment in central Ethiopia. *Ethiop Med J* 1995; 33(3):163–174.

169. Melese M, Alemayehu W, Bayu S, *et al.* Low vision and blindness in adults in Gurage Zone, central Ethiopia. *Br J Ophthalmol* 2003; 87(6):677–680.

170. Bejiga A, Tadesse S. Cataract surgical coverage and outcome in Goro District, Central Ethiopia. *Ethiop Med J* 2008; 46(3):205–210.

171. Berhane Y, Worku A, Bejiga A, *et al.* Prevalence and causes of blindness and low vision in Ethiopia. *Ethiopian J Health Dev* 2007; 21(3):204–210.

172. Mbulaiteye SM, Reeves BC, Karabalinde A, *et al.* Evaluation of E-optotypes as a screening test and the prevalence and causes of visual loss in a rural population in SW Uganda. *Ophthalmic Epidemiol* 2002; 9(4):251–262.

173. Ndegwa LK, Karimurio J, Okelo RO, *et al.* Prevalence of visual impairment and blindness in a Nairobi urban population. *East Afr J Med* 2006; 83(4):69–72.

174. Mathenge W, Kuper H, Limburg H, *et al.* Rapid assessment of avoidable blindness in Nakuru district, Kenya. *Ophthalmology* 2007; 114(3): 599–605. Epub 2006 Nov 30.

175. Ngondi J, Ole-Sempele F, Onsarigo A, *et al.* Prevalence and causes of blindness and low vision in southern Sudan. *PLoS Med* 2006; 3(12):e477.

176. Nkomazana O. Disparity in access to cataract surgical services leads to higher prevalence of blindness in women as compared with men: results of a national survey of visual impairment. *Health Care Women Int* 2009; 30(3):228–229.

177. World Health Organization. Prevention of Blindness. Chad. *Wkly Epidemiol Rec* 1987; 43:322–323.

178. Négrel AD, Avognon Z, Minassian DC, *et al.* Blindness in Benin [Article in French]. *Trop Med* 1995; 55:409–414.

179. Kortlang C, Koster JCA, Coulibalys, *et al.* Prevalence of blindness and visual impairment in the region of Ségou, Mali. A baseline survey for a primary eye care programme. *Trop Med Int Health* 1996; 1:314–319.

180. Guzek JP, Anyomi FK, Fiadoyor S, *et al.* Prevalence of blindness in people over 40 years in the volta region of Ghana. *Ghana Med J* 2005; 39(2):55–62.

181. Whitworth JAG, Gilbert CE, Mabey DM, *et al.* Visual loss in an onchocerciasis endemic community in Sierra Leone. *Br J Ophthalmol* 1993; 77:30–32.

182. Wilson MR, Mansour M, Ross-Degnan D, *et al.* Prevalence and causes of low vision and blindness in the Extreme North Province of Cameroon, West Africa. *Ophthalmic Epidemiol* 1996; 3:23–33.

183. Migliani R, Louis J-P, Anduge A, *et al.* Evaluation of visual impairment and blindness in Cameroon [Article in French]. *Cahiers Santé* 1993; 3:17–23.

184. Oye JE, Kuper H, Dineen B, *et al.* Prevalence and causes of blindness and visual impairment in Muyuka: a rural health district in South West

185. Province, Cameroon. *Br J Ophthalmol* 2006; 90(5):538–542.

185. Oye JE, Kuper H. Prevalence and causes of blindness and visual impairment in Limbe urban area, South West Province, Cameroon. *Br J Ophthalmol* 2007; 91(11):1435–1439. Epub 2007 Mar 27.

186. Balo PK, Wabagira J, Banla M, *et al.* Specific causes of blindness and visual deficiency in an area of southern Togo [Article in French]. *J Fr Ophthalmol* 2000; 23:459–464.

187. Schémann JF, Inocencio F, de Lourdes Monteiro M, *et al.* Blindness and low vision in Cape Verde Islands: results of a national eye survey. *Ophthalmic Epidemiol* 2006; 13(4):219–226.

188. Adeoye A. Survey of blindness in rural communities of south-western Nigeria. *Trop Med Int Health* 1996; 1(5):672–676.

189. Abdu L. Prevalence and causes of blindness and low vision in Dambatta local government area, Kano State, Nigeria. *Niger J Med* 2002; 11(3):108–112.

190. Rabiu MM. Cataract blindness and barriers to uptake of cataract surgery in a rural community of northern Nigeria. *Br J Ophthalmol* 2001; 85(7):776–780.

191. Patrick-Ferife G, Ashaye AO, Osuntokun OO. Rapid assessment of cataract blindness among Ughelli clan in urban/rural district of Delta State, Nigeria. *Annals African Med* 2005; 4:52–57.

192. Adeoti CO. Prevalence and causes of blindness in a tropical African population. *West Afr J Med* 2004; 23(3):249–252.

193. Patrick-Ferife G, Ashaye AO, Qureshi BM. Blindness and low vision in adults in Ozoro, a rural community in Delta State, Nigeria. *Niger J Med* 2005; 14(4):390–395.

194. Onakpoya OH, Adeoye AO, Akinsola FB, *et al.* Prevalence of blindness and visual impairment in Atakunmosa West Local Government area of southwestern Nigeria. *Tanzan J Health Res* 2007 May; 9(2):126–131.

195. Mansur R, Muhammad N, Liman IR. Prevalence and magnitude of trachoma in a local government area of Sokoto State, north western Nigeria. *Niger J Med* 2007; 16(4):348–353.

196. Rabiu MM. Prevalence of blindness and low vision in north central, Nigeria. *West Afr J Med* 2008; 27(4):238–244.

197. Rabiu MM, Muhammed N. Rapid assessment of cataract surgical services in Birnin-Kebbi local

government area of Kebbi State, Nigeria. *Ophthalmic Epidemiol* 2008; 15(6):359–365.

198. Lewallen S, Courtright P. Blindness in Africa: present situation and future needs. *Br J Ophthalmol* 2001; 85:897–903.

199. Ratnaningsh N. Prevalence of blindness and low vision in Sawah Kulon village, Purwakarta district, West Java, Indonesia. *Community Eye Health J* 2007; 20:9.

200. Ceklić L, Latinović S, Aleksić P. Leading causes of blindness and visual impairment in the region of Eastern Herzegovina [Article in Serbian]. *Med Pregl* 2006; 59(1–2):15–18.

201. Buch H, Vinding T, Morten La Cour, *et al.* Prevalence and causes of Visual Impairment and Blindness among 9980 Scandinavian adults. *Ophthalmology* 2004; 111:53–61.

202. Cotter SA, Varma R, Ying-Lai M, *et al.* Los Angeles Latino Eye Study Group. Causes of low vision and blindness in adult Latinos: the Los Angeles Latino Eye Study. *Ophthalmology* 2006; 113(9):1574–1582.

SECTION 2

METHODOLOGY

2

Epidemiological research methods: an outline

DARWIN MINASSIAN AND HANNAH KUPER

2.1	Introduction	65		2.5	Types and objectives of	71
2.2	Basic measures of occurrence	65			epidemiological research	
	in epidemiological research			2.6	Future direction of ophthalmic	76
2.3	Measures of effect	69			epidemiology: concluding notes	
2.4	Notes on estimation of effect measures	71			References	76
	and hypothesis testing					

2.1 INTRODUCTION

Epidemiology is the scientific discipline that studies health and disease in populations, as distinct from individuals. Epidemiological research aims to describe the health of a population, detect patterns and causes of ill health, and identify effective means of controlling disease. It addresses questions such as 'How common is the disease?'; 'Who is most affected?'; 'What are the underlying causes?' and 'What can be done to prevent or treat it?'. Epidemiological research, therefore, addresses both scientific and administrative problems in virtually all areas of medicine, ranging from clinical practice through to health service management and health protection. The focus on populations distinguishes epidemiology from clinical practice, which centres on individual cases.

Epidemiology began with studies of the epidemics of communicable diseases. Principles and methods that were developed to relate the disease occurrence rates to possible determinants and suspected causal factors were subsequently used to study the endemic occurrence of communicable diseases. The work of John Snow on cholera is a famous example of the application of classic epidemiological principles and methods.[1] The same methodological principles for studying infectious disease could also apply to non-infectious diseases, both chronic and acute. This led to a major expansion of epidemiology, mainly concerning chronic 'degenerative' diseases.

For readers interested in a more profound understanding of the principles of epidemiological research, Olli Miettinen provides an elegant and intellectual discussion of the 'principles of occurrence research in medicine' in his book on Theoretical Epidemiology.[2]

2.2 BASIC MEASURES OF OCCURRENCE IN EPIDEMIOLOGICAL RESEARCH

Case definition

The first step in epidemiological research is the definition of the disease or condition of interest. That is, epidemiologists first ask the question 'When is a case a case?' To give an ophthalmic example, in order to count the number of people in a population with glaucoma, the definition of who is eligible to be included as a case must be clearly defined, and this would typically be in terms of visual field, and features of the optic disc. Changing the definition of glaucoma, perhaps by changing the cut-off for severity of the visual field loss, will change the number of people counted as cases of glaucoma in a population. The need for a clear 'case' definition need not necessarily be limited to an adverse event such as occurrence of disease, but applies equally well to favourable outcomes such as 'cure', occurrence of other types of event or a health-related state. For simplicity's sake we will introduce the epidemiological concepts in terms of measurements of magnitude and causes of disease, rather than another health state.

Measures of occurrence

The hallmark of epidemiological investigations is the measurement of the frequency of occurrence of an event (e.g. disease) in a defined population. It is generally not feasible to measure the occurrence of disease in the entire population and so it is usual in epidemiological research to assess disease occurrence in a sample of the population and then extrapolate these findings to the entire population. A 'population' can mean the whole population of a country or region, or a group defined by a common characteristic (e.g. people with diabetes or smokers).

The two basic occurrence measures are **prevalence** and **incidence**. Prevalence assesses the occurrence of existing disease in a population, while incidence focuses on the occurrence of new cases of a disease. These will be explained in detail below. An important purpose of measuring the occurrence of disease, whether through prevalence or incidence, is to assess the magnitude of disease in a population, in order to uncover epidemics, and plan and monitor health services. Measurement of disease frequency also allows us to compare the occurrence of disease in different groups (e.g. compare the occurrence of cataract in people with diabetes to those without diabetes) in order to

identify predictors of disease. In the comparison of two populations or sub-groups, the ratio of the incidences or of the prevalences gives a relative measure of effect (such as **relative risk**, **RR**), and the difference in incidence or in prevalence gives an absolute measure of effect (such as **attributable risk**, **AR**). The following sections describe these measures briefly, and also consider the concept of risk in epidemiology and how it relates to incidence.

Readers interested in more detailed consideration and advanced statistical analysis of aspects of occurrence and effect measures should refer to general texts in epidemiology such as those by Kleinbaum et al.[3] and Rothman et al.[4]

2.2.1   Prevalence

The **prevalence** of a disease in a population is the proportion of individuals in that population who have the disease at a given time. Prevalence (P) is a proportion which can have values 0 to 1 (often expressed as a percentage), and is said to be dimensionless.

> Prevalence of a disease in a defined population (**P**) = **D/N**
> where:
> **D** is the number of cases with the disease in the defined population at a point in time, and
> **N** is the total number of individuals in the defined population at that time.

For instance, the National Blindness and Visual Impairment Survey conducted in Nigeria during 2005–2007 examined 13,599 people aged 40 years and above.[5] Among those examined, 569 were 'cases' of blindness (case definition: presenting visual acuity <20/400 or 3/60 in the better eye). This gives a prevalence of 569 divided by 13,599, which is 0.042 or 4.2%. Prevalence is thus a population measure, concerning the magnitude of disease at a given time. It is important to state the 'point' in time when the prevalence was estimated. Moreover, the population examined must also be described in terms of demographic or geographical features — the prevalence of blindness in the whole population would be lower than the prevalence in those aged 40 years and above. Therefore, the correct description for the Nigeria survey is that prevalence of blindness in the sample was 4.2% among people aged 40 years and above, examined in 2005–2007.

Prevalence (P) for a large population is usually estimated by an examination of a sample drawn from it and extrapolating back to the large population. Although the estimated 'case' pool gives a static view of the magnitude of the health problem at a point in time, the pool itself has a dynamic nature. The number of 'cases' in the population pool changes with time as new (i.e. incident) 'cases' enter it and others leave it through death or cure (e.g. by successful treatment). The dynamics of prevalence over time are therefore determined by the occurrence of new cases, and the duration of disease (determined by the death rate among cases and/or the cure rate). Assessment of the population need for health services requires knowledge and consideration of the measures that determine the pool, as well as a static view of the pool at the start of a time period through which the population need is to be projected. Prevalence is determined by incidence: incidence of new cases entering the pool per unit time, and the incidence of death and of reversal, removing cases from the pool per unit time. Epidemiological models have been developed to simulate the dynamics of disease in large populations, projecting the changes in the 'case' pool over time, under various scenarios of service provision, level of intervention, and of changes in demography and risk factor status. Examples include models for onchocerciasis control[6] (see Chapter 18) and for cataract.[7] Simplistic approaches to needs assessment tend to be focused on prevalence (backlog) without taking proper account of the time dimension, the incidence and their root determinants (demographic and risk factors). Such approaches may be misleading, and have no place in epidemiology.

In addition to its utility in planning, provision and monitoring of health services and needs assessment, prevalence data from cross-sectional studies (see Chapter 3) have also been used to compare various sub-groups of the population, defined by level of exposure to a suspect determinant of the disease. Examples include comparison of cataract prevalence in sub-groups with various levels of exposure to nutritional factors or comparing the prevalence among men and women. If the suspected exposure definitely preceded the onset of the disease, such as for genes, gender, ethnicity, or blood group, then these comparisons can give insights into the development and predictors of the disease. However, this is more difficult for potential exposures that change over time, such as ageing, weight or blood pressure, because both exposure and disease are measured at the same point in time and so it cannot be determined if either is the causal agent. This latter point also holds true for potential **confounders** of the association between exposure and disease (e.g. smoking confounding the association between ethnicity and cataract), which need to be taken into account during the analyses. Such comparative analyses, however, have been helpful in generating new aetiological hypotheses (concerning possible determinants of disease), which could then be tested through more appropriate studies (such as case-control or cohort studies, discussed in Chapters 4 and 5 respectively), designed to generate comparative measures of occurrence based on incidence.

2.2.2 Incidence

Incidence refers to the occurrence of new cases in the population at risk, as opposed to prevalence, which measures the frequency of existing cases in the total population of cases and non-cases. There are two main measures of incidence described in detail below: **cumulative incidence** (which is the proportion of the population that is disease free at baseline that develops a disease over a given time period) and **incidence density** or **incidence rate** (which is the number of cases that occur in the population per unit of person-time at risk and is a rate as it has a time dimension). Both measures concern a change of status in individuals who are candidates for such change; e.g. occurrence of primary open-angle glaucoma in individuals who do not have the disorder and who have at least one eye intact which may develop the disorder, that is, who are 'at risk' or susceptible. As described for prevalence, incidence figures are meaningful when a clear 'case' definition is specified, together with the population 'at risk', and the time interval or unit.

Cumulative Incidence (CI)

The **cumulative incidence** (**CI**) of a disease in a population is the number of new 'cases' that occur in a population that is disease free at baseline (i.e. excluding prevalent cases) over a specified period of time. Cumulative incidence, like prevalence, is a proportion which can have values 0 to 1 (often expressed as a percentage) and is said to be dimensionless. The CI is directly interpretable as the risk of the event in the period t because it is the probability of the event occurring in that time period.

> CI in time t, in a defined population = D_{new}/N_{free}
>
> where:
>
> t is the time period
>
> D_{new} is the number of new cases occurring in time t, in the defined population
>
> N_{free} is the number of individuals free of the disease at baseline in the defined population, (i.e. individuals at risk)

For instance, in the Wisconsin Epidemiologic Study of Diabetic Retinopathy (see Chapter 21), 610 people with young onset insulin-taking diabetes and 652 with older onset diabetes but no macular oedema were followed for four years.[8] During the follow-up there were 50 new cases of macular oedema among the younger onset diabetics and 34 among the older onset diabetics. The cumulative incidence of macular oedema is therefore 50 divided by 610 in the young onset group, which is 0.082 or 8.2%, and 34 divided by 652 in the older onset group, which is 0.052 or 5.2% over a four-year period.

CI gives important information for planning and provision of services, and needs assessment, as it can be used to derive the number of new cases that are expected in a given time period in a given population. The main utility of CI, however, is in an aetiological study where the objective is to compare risk between groups that have various levels of exposure to potential risk factors, such as comparing risk of disease in smokers to that in non-smokers. CI is also a simple and highly interpretable measure of the risk of cure (better termed as the probability of cure) for the treatment groups in a clinical trial.

The main problem with CI is that, in most circumstances, disease occurrence is a rare event and so long follow-up is often required to assess CI meaningfully. Long follow-up (one year or more) means that some members of the cohort are bound to be lost to follow-up. Such loss, if non-trivial, may introduce an unknown amount of bias into the CI estimate as loss to follow-up may be related to their risk of becoming a case.

Incidence Rate or Density (IR)

The **incidence rate** (**IR**) uses person-time at risk as the denominator rather than the number of people at risk. Imagine we are following a group of 1,000 people who are disease free at baseline for a given period of time to assess the incidence of cataract blindness. During the follow-up people may: (a) develop a cataract, (b) be lost to follow-up, (c) die or develop another condition so that they are no longer at risk of cataract (e.g. have eyes removed) or (d) remain disease free until the end of follow-up. Person-time of follow-up across the 1,000 people is accrued from the start of follow-up until one of the four events occurs. The total person-time at risk is the sum of the person-time at risk for each subject in the study. The incidence rate calculates the number of new cases that occur during follow-up divided by the total amount of person-time of follow-up of the participants. Note that once a person becomes a case, he/she is no longer at risk of the disease and moves out of the denominator. Incidence rate is expressed as cases per unit of person-time (e.g. 5 per 100,000 person-years).

> Incidence Rate (IR) = Number of new cases/Total person-time at risk

As an example, 297,756 people from 2,315 villages in 11 countries were followed up during 1971–2001 to assess the incidence of blindness as part of the Onchocerciasis Control Programme in western Africa.[9] In total, 367,788 person-years of follow-up were accumulated and 200 people became blind as a result of onchocerciasis. The incidence rate of onchocerciasis in this population was 200 divided by 367,788 person-years, which is 0.00054 cases per person-year of follow up, or 5.4 cases per 10,000 person-years of follow-up.

Note that IR has a time dimension and is a measure of speed of occurrence or rate. It is an instantaneous rate of occurrence and in practice is difficult to conceptualize and interpret. The IR, however, can be estimated from longitudinal studies that have variable follow-up periods and losses as people only contribute person-time during the period that they are actually at risk of being recorded as a case in the study. It forms a valid and useful comparative measure in aetiological studies and trials, in spite of the fact that it has no direct interpretation as risk. In the example given, the incidence rate was 5.4 per 10,000 person-years at risk, and although it is tempting to interpret this to mean 54 new cases per 100,000 persons per year, in fact the '100,000 person-years' cannot be meaningfully segregated into units of persons and of years.

Prevalence and incidence are distinct, but related, concepts. If the prevalence is relatively low (<10%) then prevalence approximates the incidence multiplied by the average duration of the disease.[4]

2.3   MEASURES OF EFFECT

The strength of the association between risk of disease and a potential causative factor can be evaluated by comparing the occurrence measure (e.g. incidence or prevalence) for a group that is exposed to a possible causative factor to that of a group that is unexposed (or less exposed). The main effect measures are discussed in Chapters 3–5, under the appropriate study methods. Here, an outline description is given to familiarize the reader with the basic concepts.

2.3.1   Difference (absolute) measure

Consider the comparison of two risks R_0 and R_1, where R_0 is a baseline risk in those not exposed

(or least exposed) to the factor of interest, and R_1 is the risk in those exposed. For instance, in the Blue Mountains Eye Study, a cohort of people were followed for ten years, and the risk of nuclear cataract among non-diabetics (R_0) was 35% while the risk of nuclear cataract among diabetics (R_1) was 54%.[10] To compare the risk among the exposed and unexposed we can simply calculate the difference $R_1 - R_0$, which is an absolute measure of effect, commonly called **attributable risk** (**AR**). For the Blue Mountains Eye Study the attributable risk of nuclear cataract related to diabetes was 54%–35% = 19%. From a public health perspective, the magnitude of AR indicates the amount of risk in the exposed group that could be avoided if the group became unexposed, assuming the putative factor is responsible for the difference. A large AR, however, may simply reflect a large R_0 and R_1. Similarly, a small AR may arise when R_0 and R_1 are small, even when R_1 is several times larger than R_0. Thus the AR is not a good measure of the strength of association between an exposure and a disease in the context of aetiological research.

2.3.2   Relative measures

Relative risk (RR)

The natural solution to estimating the association between an exposure and a disease is to calculate a relative measure that is independent of the magnitude of R_0. In epidemiological studies the most common relative measure is the **relative risk**, or R_1/R_0. This can also be called the **risk ratio, rate ratio, odds ratio** or **incidence rate ratio** (when R_0 and R_1 are incidence density measures). Relative risk is a good indicator of the strength of association; for example, a value of 1.0 (or close to unity) indicates no association, 2.0 suggests doubling of risk in the exposed, and 0.5 may indicate halving of the risk in the exposed. For the above example, the relative risk for the association between diabetes and nuclear cataract is 54%/35% = 1.5. This means that the risk of nuclear cataract was 50% higher (1.5 times higher) among people with diabetes compared with people without diabetes during ten years of follow-up. It is also possible to calculate the prevalence ratio, by dividing the prevalence of disease in the exposed group by the prevalence in the unexposed group.

Population attributable risk percent (PAR%)

A population is made up of people who are exposed and those who are unexposed, and these people may have a different risk of disease. The risk in the total population is therefore determined by the risk in those who are exposed and those who are unexposed, as well as the proportion of subjects who are exposed (i.e. the prevalence of exposure). Although a large relative risk may indicate that the exposure is of aetiological importance, this does not necessarily mean that the exposure is of public health concern; for example, when the disease or the exposure is extremely rare. For a holistic appreciation of the importance of an exposure (detrimental or beneficial) at the population level, it is necessary to quantify both relative risk and one of its derivatives. **Population attributable risk percent (PAR%)** gives the proportion of all 'cases' (occurring in a general population) that is attributable to the exposure, by subtracting the risk in the unexposed groups from the risk in the total population. That is:

Population attributable risk percent PAR% = $100 (R_{total} - R_0)/R_{total}$

In terms of the diabetes and nuclear cataract example, if the risk of nuclear cataract in the total population was 36% then the PAR% = (36%–35%)/36% = 0.03 or 3%, suggesting that 3% of nuclear cataract could be avoided if diabetes were eliminated from the population. This has meaning only when a causal relationship is assumed between a detrimental exposure (diabetes) and the 'case' status (nuclear cataract). Another form of the equation (which is mathematically the same as the above), provided by Miettinen,[11] shows the relation between PAR% and RR:

PAR% = P(RR–1)/RR

where P is the prevalence (%) of exposure among the 'cases'.

The utility of PAR% is clear in so far as it gives an impression of the amount of the disease problem that might 'disappear' if exposure to the risk factor at issue is removed. This could be valuable in the planning of a preventive intervention.

Odds ratio (OR)

When separate estimates for R_1 and R_0 cannot be made (e.g. in case-control studies, see Chapter 4), the risk ratio or rate ratio cannot be estimated directly. Usually in such situations, the study design ordains that a sample of 'cases' (individuals with the disease or condition of interest) are obtained and compared with a contemporaneous sample of non-cases. In the simplest form, the data from such studies may be summarized in a 2 by 2 contingency table (Table 2.1).

Table 2.1 *Summary of data (in the simplest form) from a case-control or a cross-sectional study. Individuals are classified according to disease status (cases and non-cases) and also by status of exposure to the factor of interest. The cell frequencies are denoted by the letters a, b, c and d*

	Exposed	Not exposed
Cases	a	b
Non-cases	c	d

The odds of being 'exposed' can be computed for the 'cases' and the 'non-cases' as a/b and c/d, respectively. The exposure **Odds Ratio (OR)** is expressed as:

OR = (a/b)/(c/d) = ad/bc

From the diabetes and nuclear cataract example, the odds of exposure to diabetes among the cases of cataract was 37/415 and among the people without cataract was 32/775. This gave an OR of (37/415)/(32/775) = 0.090/0.041 = 2.2. This indicates that the odds of exposure to diabetes is 2.2 times higher among cases with cataract than among people without cataract.

The OR obtained from well-designed case-control studies is generally believed to give a good indirect estimate of **incidence rate ratio (IRR)**, particularly when the incidence of the 'case' status is low (e.g. for rare diseases). Regardless of its validity as an indirect measure of IRR, the OR remains a valid measure of the strength of association between exposure and 'case' status. Like IRR, greater deviations from unity indicate stronger associations. The OR has become a very popular choice, even when direct estimation of IRR may be possible, due to the ready availability of robust statistical procedures for OR analysis, such as the logistic regression model. Thus the OR is frequently used in the analysis of data that come not only from case-control studies, but also from clinical trials, and from cross-sectional studies (prevalence data).

2.4 NOTES ON ESTIMATION OF EFFECT MEASURES AND HYPOTHESIS TESTING

Most published reports of epidemiological studies include estimation of the risk ratio, rate ratio or odds ratio after adjustment for other factors besides the exposure of interest that may influence the association (these are called **confounders**). For such an approach, multiple regression analysis is undertaken using statistical tools such as the logistic regression model. These models are used to test hypotheses and to estimate the pertinent effect measure, with adjustments for the effect of other (extraneous) exposure factors (possible confounders). The analyses also quantify the level of precision for the estimate, usually reported as **confidence limits**. Estimation of the effect measure in practice is thus considerably more complex than the above-mentioned equations would suggest. The objectives and the type of epidemiological study that generates the data largely determine the choice of effect measure and the analysis tool. The following section outlines the commonly used study designs and related objectives.

2.5 TYPES AND OBJECTIVES OF EPIDEMIOLOGICAL RESEARCH

The diversity of methods used in epidemiological research may be grouped into two primary types.

The first is **experimental studies**, where the researcher assigns the exposure to the factor of interest to participants, and this includes randomized clinical trials, randomized screening trials, field trials and community intervention trials. The second type is **observational studies**, where the exposure is not under the control of the investigator (i.e. exposure is 'observed' rather than assigned by the investigator). Observational studies include cross-sectional studies, case-control studies, longitudinal cohort studies, and their variants.

2.5.1 Randomized experimental studies

The gold standard of randomized experimental studies is the **randomized controlled trial** (**RCT**) (see Chapter 7). In this type of study, the researchers randomly allocate participants to 'exposure' (therapeutic or preventive intervention) or not (control). The 'unexposed' or control group may receive nothing, a placebo or the standard treatment. Allocation is random so that if the groups are sufficiently large they should be similar with respect to all extraneous factors, known and unknown, which might influence the outcome. For instance, they will be similar in terms of age structure, health conditions and body size. This means that any difference in outcome between the comparison groups could be attributed to the exposure to 'treatment' under study rather than any other difference between the two groups. The intervention and control groups are then followed over time to assess disease incidence; the incidence in the intervention group is compared with that in the control group to assess the effect of the intervention on the disease risk. Participants and researchers are typically masked to the exposure status of the participants, meaning that they do not know to which group the participant has been assigned, and this is done in order to reduce bias in reporting and assessment of disease.

As an example, a randomized clinical trial was undertaken to assess whether beta carotene supplementation reduced the incidence of age-related maculopathy (ARM).[12] The investigators randomly allocated 22,071 male doctors to receive beta carotene or placebo. They were treated and followed up for 12 years and neither the investigators nor the participants knew to which treatment arm they had been assigned. At the end of follow-up there were 162 cases of ARM in the beta carotene group and 170 cases in the placebo group to give a relative risk of 0.96 (95% CI 0.78–1.20) showing no protective effect of supplementation on the development of ARM.

(For explanation of **95% CI** (**95% confidence intervals**) please see box in Chapter 1).

Variants on the randomized clinical trial model exist, such as the **randomized screening trial** (see Chapter 8). Another variant is the **field trial**, where individuals in a population are randomized to a preventive intervention (e.g. a vaccine) or no intervention (or placebo), and the incidence of disease compared in the two groups. Such trials have been used for diseases that are of great public health concern. Some of the largest experimental studies have been of this type; for example, the Salk vaccine trial for poliomyelitis, involving more than one million children. **Community intervention trials** are similar to field trials but in this design convenient clusters of people (communities) rather than individuals are randomized to the preventive intervention. An example is the first community-based vitamin A trial[13] (see Chapter 14b).

The main limitations of randomized experimental studies arise from two sources. First, for practical reasons, strict eligibility criteria have to be used in selection of subjects, so that the observations are often made on a highly selected sample. Consequently the inferences may be limited to small, and sometimes peculiar, populations rather than to a large population of general interest. Second, randomization may be unethical if one of the interventions or treatments is regarded to be more beneficial by clinicians or by the patients. Moreover, it may not be feasible to randomize exposure to certain biological, behavioural or other psychosocial factors (e.g. smoking, stress or alcoholism). The high cost of experimental studies in some situations is an additional disadvantage; for example, in the UK, the cost of a major ophthalmic clinical trial has been in excess of £2,000 per randomized individual. Much higher costs have been incurred in the USA. Such studies require

considerable justification. In view of these limitations, most epidemiological investigations of aetiological factors are observational in design.

2.5.2   Observational studies — basic designs

In observational studies the investigators observe the events as they unfold naturally. There are three main basic types of observational study: cross-sectional studies or surveys (see Chapter 3), case-control studies (see Chapter 4) and cohort (longitudinal, follow-up) studies (see Chapter 5).

Cross-sectional studies

In a cross-sectional study the investigators carefully sample people from the population. They then examine and/or interview the participants to assess whether or not they have the disease and exposure(s) of interest. This allows assessment of the prevalence of disease (and exposure), so that the magnitude of disease in the population can be estimated. The prevalence can also be compared in different groups (e.g. those exposed and those unexposed) to explore whether there may be an association between the exposure and the disease. As an example, in the national survey of blindness conducted in Nigeria described above, the overall prevalence of blindness was 4.2% (95% confidence intervals: 3.8 to 4.6%).[5] The prevalence of blindness was higher among people who were illiterate (5.8%) compared with those who could read and write easily (1.5%) to give a prevalence ratio of 3.9, suggesting that socio-economic status may play a role in the incidence or persistence (duration) of blindness. However, with cross-sectional surveys we must emphasize the adage that 'association does not equal causation'. We do not know whether the exposure or disease came first, or if both are caused by a third factor.

Cohort studies

Cohort studies allow us to measure disease incidence, rather than focusing on prevalence as in the cross-sectional studies. To conduct a cohort study, a group of people free from the disease of interest are selected (i.e. prevalent cases are excluded). The participants are then examined or interviewed and are categorized as 'exposed' or 'unexposed' with respect to the risk factor of interest. The participants are then followed over time and the number of incident cases of disease that arise are assessed. This allows the investigators to calculate the incidence of disease (whether cumulative incidence or incidence rate). The incidence can be calculated separately in the exposed and unexposed group so that the relative risk (CIR or IRR) can be estimated.

The Copenhagen City Eye Study is a long-running cohort study.[14] During 1986–1988, 946 volunteers aged 60–80 living in Copenhagen were examined and participated in the study. The cohort was re-examined 14 years later and 359 (97% of survivors) were re-examined and 301 included in the analyses (81%). At follow-up 163 of the subjects had ARM to give a risk (cumulative incidence) or ARM of $163/301 = 0.54 = 54\%$. Risk of ARM was higher among people who had a family history of ARM ($24/30 = 80\%$) compared with the risk in people without a family history ($139/271 = 51\%$) to give a risk ratio of 1.56 (confidence intervals 1.26–1.93). These results indicate that having a family history of ARM may increase the risk of developing ARM by 56%.

This example illustrates the problem of loss to follow-up, which is often encountered by cohort studies. Not all of the initial cohort were included in the final analyses, and it is not known what happened to those lost to follow-up in terms of ARM. Although the majority were lost through death, it is not known whether or not they developed ARM before they died. This means that the risk measured may not be the 'true' risk in that study population. Another problem with cohort studies is that they usually either require a large sample or long follow-up to accumulate enough incident cases of disease to have sufficient **power** to make meaningful inferences, (for further discussion of 'power' see also Chapter 7). This makes cohort studies expensive and time consuming, which is why they are rare in the ophthalmic literature. The strengths of cohort studies are that incidence can be estimated and that the

researchers are relatively confident that the exposure preceded the disease.

Case-control studies

The third type of observational study that is frequently used is the case-control study, which is used to study the aetiology of disease. Case-control studies are conducted by recruiting people who have the disease of interest (cases) as well as people without the disease (controls) to allow comparison. The cases and controls are then interviewed or examined to assess whether they have the exposure of interest. The odds of being exposed are then compared for cases and controls to see if there is an association between exposure and being a case. Ideally, cases are 'incident cases', so that they are newly diagnosed and have not had time to change their exposure status as a result of their diagnosis. The controls are selected from the same population that gave rise to the cases and represent the exposure distribution in the source population. Case-control cannot be used to estimate the burden of disease, since the ratio of cases to controls is determined by the investigators.

A case-control study was undertaken to investigate the association between childbearing and risk of cataract in young women.[15] The cases selected were women aged 35–45 attending an eye hospital in central India with bilateral 'senile' cataract. Controls were selected among women of the same age with clear lenses attending the hospital with other complaints. Cases and controls were interviewed about their history of pregnancy and childbirth. The investigators found that the cases had statistically significantly more live births than the control subjects. Compared with women who had had 1–3 children, the odds of a case having 4–6 children was 1.9 times higher (95% CI 1.1–3.1) than for controls, and the odds of a case having 7–11 children was 4.6 times (2.0–10.6) higher than for controls. These results suggest that in central India there is an association between high parity and having a cataract.

There are many advantages to case-control studies. They are relatively quick and cheap to carry out, and can be used to investigate rare diseases. Recall bias is a problem, since cases and controls may report exposure history differently because of their case status. Avoiding bias due to selection of inappropriate controls is also a major challenge.

Nested case-control studies combine some of the advantageous features of case-control and cohort studies. For example, in one common form all disease 'cases' occurring in a given population are identified through a registry. A sample of non-cases (sometimes matched for age etc.) is also drawn from the same population. The past exposure status is then ascertained for both the cases and the sample of non-cases. Here, the number of non-cases that have to be investigated for past exposure is only a small fraction of the numbers in a longitudinal cohort study (particularly when the disease is rare). An important advantage over a case-control study design is that a measure of disease frequency can be estimated for the population.

2.5.3 Variants of the basic observational studies

There are also variants of the basic observational designs that arise from a diversity of design options which are available in observational studies. The more pertinent variants are briefly described below.

Ecological studies

In the ecological study design the exposure status data are not available for individuals but are obtained as an average for groups. The unit of observation is thus the group rather than an individual. The groups are commonly defined geographically (e.g. as a whole country or region) but could be defined by other factors, such as socio-economic, occupational and demographic factors. A proxy measure is often used to describe the exposure status of the group as individual measures are not obtained. For instance, average per capita gross domestic product for the country could be used as the measure of socio-economic status. Comparisons are made between the groups in respect of frequency of disease occurrence. Examples in eye research include older studies of the relationship between ultraviolet radiation from

the sun and frequency of cataract. In one such study in Australia, various geographical zones were defined according to average levels of ambient ultraviolet radiation. The zones were then compared with respect to the population prevalence of cataract.[16] It is now well known that inferences from ecological data may be misleading. The problem, named 'ecologic fallacy', arises because there are often insufficient data on other pertinent exposures to allow control of confounding in the analysis (i.e. third factors that could explain the association between the exposure and the disease). In addition, the exposure and disease status of individuals is not known, and so even if an association between the exposure and disease exists at the population level, it may not exist at the individual level.

Self-controlled case series

A self-controlled case series can be used to assess the effect of a transient exposure on disease risk. A patient who has developed a disease is interviewed about his/her exposure pattern during a specific period of time. This time is divided into 'risk' periods and 'control' periods. For instance, imagine that an investigator wishes to assess the relationship between administration of dilatation drops and the development of acute open angle glaucoma. The investigator would interview cases of acute open angle glaucoma about whether or not they had received dilatation drops during the 24 hours prior to disease onset. The period in the two hours before disease onset could be defined as the 'risk' period, while the previous 22 hours are the 'control' period. The investigator can then assess whether the onset of disease is associated with administration of drops. This study design includes only cases, and the cases act as their own controls, therefore any potential association between the exposure and disease cannot be attributed to differences in age or other risk factors (i.e. confounding is removed).

Space/time cluster studies

Space clustering studies share the features of ecological studies in so far as exposure data are not available for individuals and clusters or groups are compared. In addition, the grouping need not be according to levels of exposure to a particular putative risk factor. The studies are designed to detect clustering in space, that is, a non-uniform distribution of 'cases' over the total study area, beyond the level of clustering that might be expected from the population distribution and chance. The studies have been used to implicate or assess general environmental influences in the disease aetiology. Examples include international comparisons of disease risk or prevalence.

Time clustering studies are designed to detect non-uniform distribution of the occurrence of 'cases' over a time period for a defined population. The main objectives are to identify secular trends in large populations, including cyclic fluctuations, and to explore local epidemics. A study of optic neuritis in Sweden is an example of the method in ophthalmology.[17] The clustering (in time, and separately in space) of incident cases over a six-year period among the population of Stockholm County was investigated. Only a seasonal variation emerged: highest incidence in spring, and lowest in winter.

Time clustering designs are sometimes combined with space clustering designs to detect clustering in time and space. Clustering of 'cases' in both time and space suggests the involvement of infectious agents in causation of the disease.

Genetic studies

There is enormous interest in identifying genetic risk factors for disease (Chapter 6). This can be investigated through cross-sectional surveys, cohort studies or case-control studies by including genotype as the 'exposure' and assessing its role in the aetiology of disease. There are also specific study designs used for genetic studies: twin studies, familial aggregation studies and pedigree studies.

Twin studies are generally very effective in providing evidence for the 'genetic effect' in the aetiology of disease. The sample of twin pairs are grouped according to a two-way classification: (i) as monozygotic ('identical') or dizygotic ('non-identical'), and (ii) as concordant or discordant with respect to the presence or absence of disease (i.e. same or different disease status). Significantly

greater concordance among the monozygotic pairs is regarded as evidence for the genetic role in causation of the disease, because members of a monozygotic pair share all of their genes, whereas members of a dizygotic pair differ in respect of some genes. The measure used to summarize the results is the '**heritability**' proportion,[18] which estimates the percentage of the total variance in disease status attributable to genetic factors (although an environmental component is usually needed for the disease to become manifest). A recent example of a twin study in ophthalmology reports the heritability for cataract.[19,20]

In **familial aggregation studies**, the variability of the trait or disease (prevalent or incident) within families is compared to the variability between families. A large between-family variance (relative to within-family variance) indicates a correspondingly high degree of familial aggregation. A US study (1997) of diabetic retinopathy and nephropathy may serve as an example of the method.[21] The study involved patients from the **Diabetes Control and Complications Trial** (**DCCT**) and their first-degree relatives. The interclass correlation was computed from 'severity-of-retinopathy' scores for all family members. Significant interclass correlation levels were found for parent–offspring, mother–child and father–child relationships, thus providing evidence that the severity of diabetic retinopathy is influenced by familial (possibly genetic) factors.

Pedigree studies involve investigation of disease or traits in large families of at least three generations, in order to classify members according to their genotype and disease status, so that a specific genetic mechanism may be identified in relation to other factors in the development of disease, such as diet. Well-designed studies of this type allow estimation of heritability for the population and also provide a description of the mode of inheritance. The main difficulties are obtaining sufficient data from each pedigree.

2.5.4 Limitations of observational studies

There is a general limitation with all these observational studies. They utilize experiments arising from accidental circumstances. Assessments of outcome are made in a sample of individuals whose exposure status is determined by an interacting mixture of natural, political, economic, cultural, social and behavioural forces. Observational studies can be conducted in populations where these 'natural' forces have created a marked (easily measurable) variation in the level of exposure to the suspect factor(s). These influences, however, do not allocate exposure randomly. In a 'natural' non-experimental setting, a person exposed to the putative harmful agent of interest is often also more likely to have a multitude of other exposures that might enhance the risk of the disease under study; for example, persons 'exposed' to alcohol abuse are more likely to be heavy smokers; and children exposed to poor personal hygiene in a rural trachoma-endemic community tend to be also more exposed to conditions of malnutrition, overcrowding and poverty, with all the associated complex of risk factors. Clearly, in assessing the effect of any particular exposure on risk of disease or disability, the influence of all other pertinent extraneous factors should be taken into account (adjusted for), as fully and as simultaneously as possible. Such adjustment is commonly referred to as the control of 'confounding', which is elaborated upon in Chapter 4. The problem is made more challenging when many of the extraneous factors act in synergy with the study exposure, and/or with one another, to influence the study outcome in a complex way. Many of the recent advances in epidemiology have been made through the development and refinement of study designs and of statistical models to resolve these complex problems, which are often shared by experimental studies.

2.6 FUTURE DIRECTION OF OPHTHALMIC EPIDEMIOLOGY: CONCLUDING NOTES

In this book, many experimental and observational studies are discussed in the context of the epidemiology of the major eye disorders. The structure is traditional insofar as various aetiological factors are considered together, in relation to a particular disease. This disease-oriented approach is in keeping with the process of research in ophthalmic epidemiology, where most studies are initiated or led by disease experts. Recent advances in molecular biology and genetics open new, exciting avenues of research, including the highly challenging study of gene–environment interactions in disease causation, where modern epidemiology and the related advanced statistical methods have a central role. The approach in eye research, however, may become even more profoundly disease-oriented as various genetic and environmental risk factors are considered in relation to a specific disease. The tendency is already apparent in the more recent studies of cataract aetiology.

An alternative or complementary approach would be to consider all disease or health outcomes of exposure to a particular risk factor or protective factor. Such exposure-oriented research should lead to a more holistic appreciation of the importance for public health of the exposure factor. The approach would require the working collaboration of disease experts and exposure experts (e.g. nutritionists), that is, epidemiologists with special interest in public health aspects of a particular exposure or risk factor complex. The methodology would focus on major cohort follow-up studies and large-scale randomized trials with long-term outcome assessment. Potential candidates for this research approach may include nutritional/dietary factors, tobacco use, alcohol consumption and hormone replacement therapy, with a wide spectrum of ocular and other health indicators included as outcomes.

Earlier, mention was made of some work in construction of epidemiological models for cataract and for onchocerciasis, and the utility of such models (see Section 2.2.1). As more information is harvested from future research, epidemiological models could be developed to study the population dynamics of the major eye disorders (specifically and collectively), in relation to their determinants and their management and control.

REFERENCES

1. Snow J. *On the Mode of Communication of Cholera*, 2nd Edition. London: Churchill; 1855. Reproduced in: *Snow on Cholera*. New York: Commonwealth Fund; 1936. New York: Hafner; 1965.
2. Miettinen OS. *Theoretical Epidemiology: Principles of Occurrence Research in Medicine*. New York: John Wiley & Sons; 1985.

3. Kleinbaum DG, Kupper LL, Morgenstern H. *Epidemiologic Research: Principles and Quantitative Methods.* New York: Van Nostrand Reinhold Company Inc; 1982.

4. Rothman KJ, Greenland S, Lash TL. *Modern Epidemiology*, 3rd Edition. Philadelphia: Lippincott Williams & Wilkins; 2008.

5. Kyari F, Gudlavalleti MV, Sivasubramaniam S, *et al.* Prevalence of blindness and visual impairment in Nigeria: the National Blindness and Visual Impairment Study. *Invest Ophthalmol Vis Sci* 2009; 50:2033–2039.

6. Plaisier AP, van Oortmarssen GJ, Habbema JD, *et al.* ONCHOSIM: a model and computer simulation program for the transmission and control of onchocerciasis. *Comput Methods Programs Biomed* 1990; 31:43–56.

7. Minassian DC, Reidy A, Desai P, *et al.* The deficit in cataract surgery in England and Wales and the escalating problem of visual impairment: epidemiological modelling of the population dynamics of cataract. *Br J Ophthalmol* 2000; 84:4–8.

8. Klein R, Moss SE, Klein BE, *et al.* The Wisconsin epidemiologic study of diabetic retinopathy. XI. The incidence of macular edema. *Ophthalmology* 1989; 96:1501–1510.

9. Little MP, Basanez MG, Breitling LP, *et al.* Incidence of blindness during the Onchocerciasis control programme in western Africa, 1971–2002. *J Infect Dis* 2004; 189:1932–1941.

10. Tan JS, Wang JJ, Mitchell P. Influence of diabetes and cardiovascular disease on the long-term incidence of cataract: the Blue Mountains eye study. *Ophthalmic Epidemiol* 2008; 15:317–327.

11. Miettinen OS. Proportion of disease caused or prevented by a given exposure, trait or intervention. *Am J Epidemiol* 1974; 99:325–332.

12. Christen WG, Manson JE, Glynn RJ, *et al.* Beta carotene supplementation and age-related maculopathy in a randomized trial of US physicians. *Arch Ophthalmol* 2007; 125:333–339.

13. Sommer A, Tarwotjo I, Djunaedi E, *et al.* Impact of vitamin A supplementation on childhood mortality. A randomised controlled community trial. *Lancet* 1986; 1:1169–1173.

14. Buch H, Nielsen NV, Vinding T, *et al.* 14-year incidence, progression, and visual morbidity of age-related maculopathy: the Copenhagen City Eye Study. *Ophthalmology* 2005; 112:787–798.

15. Minassian DC, Mehra V, Reidy A. Childbearing and risk of cataract in young women: an epidemiological study in central India. *Br J Ophthalmol* 2002; 86:548–550.

16. Hollows F, Moran D. Cataract — the ultraviolet risk factor. *Lancet* 1981; 2:1249–1250.

17. Jin YP, de Pedro-Cuesta J, Soderstrom M, *et al.* Incidence of optic neuritis in Stockholm, Sweden, 1990–1995: II. Time and space patterns. *Arch Neurol* 1999; 56:975–980.

18. Elston RC, Rao DC. Statistical modeling and analysis in human genetics. *Annu Rev Biophys Bio* 1978; 7:253–286.

19. Hammond CJ, Snieder H, Spector TD, *et al.* Genetic and environmental factors in age-related nuclear cataracts in monozygotic and dizygotic twins. *N Engl J Med* 2000; 342:1786–1790.

20. Hammond CJ, Duncan DD, Snieder H, *et al.* The heritability of age-related cortical cataract: the twin eye study. *Invest Ophthalmol Vis Sci* 2001; 42:601–605.

21. The Diabetes Control and Complications Trial Research Group. Clustering of long-term complications in families with diabetes in the diabetes control and complications trial. *Diabetes* 1997; 46:1829–1839.

3

Cross-sectional studies

DARWIN MINASSIAN AND HANNAH KUPER

3.1	Introduction	79	3.5	Sources of bias	89
3.2	Bias and precision	80	3.6	Sample size for estimating prevalence	90
3.3	Probability sampling	82	3.7	Future directions	91
3.4	Sampling schemes	82		References	92

3.1 INTRODUCTION

In a cross-sectional study a sample is drawn from a defined population, and the findings are then used to make estimates for the population. The study is undertaken in as short a time as practicable, so that the data will reflect the status of the sample members at 'a point in time'. The usual primary objectives are to estimate the prevalence of disease and dysfunction (health states) for the population and for subgroups of particular interest, and to assess the need for health services. Generally, the principal aim is to provide the necessary data for devising improved healthcare services, including improved access and utilization, with the expectation of reducing the population burden of disease and disability. These data include the **prevalence** (magnitude) of conditions, as well as the behaviours of the population that may increase or reduce their risk of disease and may provide understanding about the development of disease and targets for prevention.

Population-based surveys of blindness and eye disease are examples of cross-sectional studies. Many of these have been carried out over the past decade in various countries, some major ones in the USA, Australia and Western Europe, but mostly outside of the Established Market Economies. Information from these surveys, collated and analyzed by the World Health Organization (WHO), has provided global and regional estimates of the prevalence of visual impairment and of the main blinding eye disorders[1,2] (see Chapter 1). Such data are valuable in the continuing advocacy effort within the 'Vision 2020' initiative (see Chapter 24). Individually, many surveys have led to additional funding and improvements in the eye care services, and have helped to establish or strengthen local or national programmes for the prevention of blindness. Some have influenced government health policy in the maintenance or expansion of community-based eye care services and in new initiatives. Notable examples of studies with such influence include: the national surveys of blindness in Nepal,[3] the Gambia,[4] Bangladesh,[5] Pakistan[6] and Nigeria,[7] the Irish Glaucoma Survey,[8] the **North London Eye Study** (**NLES**)[9] and the initial cross-sectional phase of a longitudinal study in the USA — the **Salisbury Eye Evaluation Project** (**SEE**).[10]

Information from cross-sectional studies has often been used to make comparisons between regions or countries (ecological studies; see Chapter 2). In the ophthalmic field it is common practice to use the cross-sectional data to compare prevalence in various subgroups, such as socio-economic, ethnic, age and sex groupings, to elucidate their relationship with the prevalence of particular eye diseases or with visual impairment. For this purpose, the data are often analyzed to estimate the prevalence ratio. Cross-sectional studies can also be repeated in the same place over time to monitor the impact of programmes or other changes on the prevalence of disease. As mentioned in Chapter 2, cross-sectional data can be used as analytical studies of aetiology where we are confident that the exposure clearly preceded the disease, as is the case for gender, genes and other variables. For other potential exposures this is not the case and, since both exposure and disease are assessed at the same point in time, this means that their temporal relationship cannot be ascertained with certainty in many situations. More appropriate methods are described in Chapters 4 and 5.

Some of the recent major population-based cross-sectional studies in ophthalmic epidemiology have progressed (some by prior intent) as longitudinal cohort studies — the cross-sectional data providing the baseline, and the sample becoming the cohort for the follow-up. One example is the NLES sample,[9] which became a cohort for a longitudinal study of mortality and cataract; another is the SEE project,[10] designed as a longitudinal study of risk factors for age-related eye diseases, which has also given valuable cross-sectional data on the prevalence of visual impairment (and on the relationship between various measures of visual function).

This chapter gives an outline of the methodology for cross-sectional studies, focusing on the study designs that are population-based (i.e. drawing a sample from a defined population) with the primary objective of estimating prevalence. Such studies are referred to as **sample surveys** (or simply as surveys) in this chapter. Here it is essential that the sample selection should be unbiased. Sampling principles and methods are, therefore, considered in some detail. The aspects of methodology covered in this chapter pertain to two central issues. The first, and more important, concerns the avoidance or minimization of bias. The second issue is the precision in estimating prevalence. Other aspects of survey methodology concerning mainly operational and administrative issues such as cost, logistics, public

relations and return of benefit to the surveyed communities, are not covered here. Examples from some eye surveys are given to illustrate the methods in study design and implementation.

3.2 BIAS AND PRECISION

Before describing methodology, it may be helpful to consider the concepts of **bias** and of **precision** in estimating an occurrence measure.

Bias is the distortion of the estimated prevalence away from the true population value (see also Chapter 4). Bias may arise because of how subjects are selected into the survey, and this is called **selection bias**. Alternatively bias may arise as a result of how information is collected from the subjects, and this is called **information bias**. Both are discussed below.

As mentioned, in most cross-sectional studies a sample is drawn from the population and examined in detail; this is used to make inferences about the prevalence of disease in the general population. One of the most important concerns in any sampling procedure is therefore the avoidance of bias in selecting the sample so that it is reasonable to extrapolate results to the general population. The easiest and most acceptable way of avoiding such bias is for the sample to be drawn 'at random', using a probability-sampling scheme (see Section 3.3), which gives all eligible members of the population an equal or known probability of being selected. Given that a sample of size n is drawn from a population of N individuals, the value p obtained from the sample (e.g. proportion with a disease) is considered as an estimate of the corresponding true value (P) in the population, with the expectation that some error may have occurred simply because of sampling variation. This type of error, known as **sampling error** (or **random sampling error**), arises entirely because only n members are measured instead of all N individuals. It is expected to occur because of chance differences between the members of the sample (n) and those not included in the sample. If all individuals in the population (N) were examined there would be no sampling and no sampling error. When a probability-sampling scheme has been used, the sampling error can be quantified and is usually presented in the form of '95% confidence limits' (95% CI) for the estimated value; for example, the prevalence of primary open-angle glaucoma (POAG) in a population in Rotterdam[11] was estimated as 1.1% with 95% confidence limits of 1.09–1.11%. This indicates a probability of 0.95 that the reported limits contain the true population prevalence. Sampling error is thus a measure of precision because, other things being equal, the smaller it is the closer the confidence limits and the more precise the estimate.

Investigators also need to decide how many people to sample as well as how to sample the individuals. Sample size is an important determinant of the sampling error. The Rotterdam example gives a prevalence estimate with high precision.

The sample size was 3,062 individuals. The POAG prevalence estimate for an older population in the NLES[9] was 3% with 95% confidence limits of 2.3–3.6%, for a sample size of 1,547. The lower precision (wider confidence limits, higher sampling error) in the NLES is mainly a result of the smaller sample size, and if the sample size were increased the confidence limits would narrow. Other determinants of the amount of sampling error are the type of the probability-sampling scheme used (see Section 3.4.3) and the variation in the population (or the variance of p). Sampling errors tend to increase to a maximum as P approaches 50%. Figure 3.1 demonstrates the relationships.

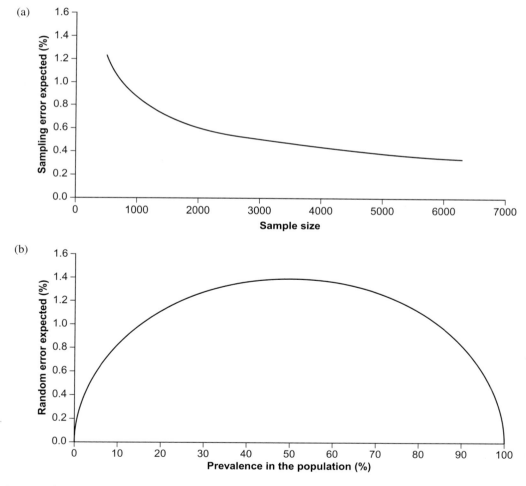

Figure 3.1 *Random sampling error in relation to (a) sample size, and (b) population prevalence. (a) Relationship between sample size and expected sampling error, assuming a population prevalence of 2%, population size 1 million, and simple random sampling. (b) Variation of random sampling error with population prevalence. Simple random sampling, with sample size of 5,000.*

The investigators need to take care to assess accurately the disease status for all individuals to reduce information bias. For example, a tendency to misclassify true cases of POAG in the sample (without a parallel reverse trend) would be expected to result in a biased estimate (i.e. an underestimate) of POAG prevalence.

The concept of bias is further considered in relation to sampling in the following section. Selection and information bias are considered in more detail in Section 3.5.

3.3   PROBABILITY SAMPLING

As mentioned earlier, the hallmark of probability sampling schemes is that the probability of selection is known for every eligible member of the population. For instance, if the investigators have decided to sample 100 people from a total population of 100,000 giving equal probability of selection to all individuals, then the probability of selection for each person is 0.1%. Having decided that a sample of n units is required from a defined population of size N eligible units, then in reality there are a great number of different combinations of n individual units out of the N eligible units that are possible. In practice, probability of selection is specified for the individual units, which are drawn one by one or in clusters, until the desired sample of size n units is obtained.

A great variety of different probability-sampling schemes are possible. Here only the most practicable and commonly used methods are considered, in which each population member has the same probability of being selected, collectively known as **epsem** (equal probability selection methods). **Simple random sampling** (**SRS**) and some forms of **cluster sampling** (**CLS**) are examples of epsem. SRS is the most basic and the easiest to handle statistically. It also provides a basis for the CLS methods where, instead of selecting individuals to examine, clusters of people (e.g. households) are selected, as this is often more practicable and economical to implement.

When a probability-sampling scheme such as an epsem is used, a statistically unbiased estimate (**p**) of the true prevalence in the population (**P**) can be obtained and the sampling error can be calculated. This is because the calculations are based on the **sampling distribution of p,** which in turn will be known, as it can be defined when a probability sampling scheme is employed.

Sampling distribution of p: an explanation

Suppose a sample of size n individuals is to be drawn from a population of size N using an epsem. In most practical situations, there would be a vast number of distinct samples of size n that were candidates for selection. Even for a small population of N = 49 units and a sample of size n = 6 (as in the UK national lottery), there are more than 13.9 million distinct samples of size 6. Each of the distinct samples of size n could theoretically generate an estimate **p**, resulting in a multitude of values for p. The frequency distribution of these values is known as the **sampling distribution of p**. This is a theoretical probability distribution that could be defined for any given (or assumed) value of the true population prevalence. In many instances where an epsem is used, the sampling distribution of p may follow the binomial probability distribution, which is well known.

3.4   SAMPLING SCHEMES

The ideal in designing a survey is to devise a sampling scheme that yields unbiased estimates of prevalence with the highest attainable precision, and that is economical and easy to implement. Usually a compromise is needed in practice. A variety of methodological options available within the broad scheme of SRS and CLS make it possible to devise several distinct sampling methods that provide a statistically unbiased estimate. Some may be devised for maximal precision for a given sample size but may be difficult to operate in the field. Yet others could be easy to manage and be well within the budget but may not give the desired precision for some of the secondary objectives. The task is thus a challenging one and may require the skills of a 'sampling specialist'. The study objectives are central in the decision to adopt a particular scheme, as are the geographical features of the survey location and the socio-economic and demographic features of the population at issue. Budgetary constraints, however, often overrule most other considerations. The design process, which includes a calculation of sample size, may at times force a drastic trimming of the initial objectives. Most eye surveys have used sampling methods that are based on the broad schemes described below.

3.4.1 Simple random sampling (SRS)

In practice, the defined population to be sampled is first enumerated so that a complete numbered list of all eligible members may be constructed. Eligible members are those that should be given a chance of being selected. The list, comprising all of the eligible members (and no ineligible members), is called a **sampling frame**. Each member in the list is called a **sampling unit (SU)**. In simple random sampling the SU is an individual. In some situations a suitable sampling frame may be readily available in the form of a computerized membership list, such as an electoral register. The required number of sampling units is drawn from the frame by reference to a list of random numbers (published tables or random numbers generated by a computer for the purpose), so that each unit is given the same probability of selection. The selected members so identified from the list are then sought in the population.

A popular alternative procedure is **systematic sampling**. The total sampling frame is divided by the number of subjects required, to derive the **sampling interval (y)** (e.g. if 1,000 subjects are required out of 1,000,000 people then the sampling interval is 1,000). The first sampled individual is selected by multiplying the sampling interval with a random number between 0 and 1 (e.g. if the sampling interval is 1,000 and the random number is 0.98 then the first person selected is person number 980). The resulting person is traced in the sampling frame and selected. The resulting individuals are selected by adding the sampling interval (1,000) to the previous number

(980). The sampling scheme is therefore to select the required number of units by taking every yth unit in the sampling frame (in our example the 1,000th unit), with y (the sampling interval) being defined so that the whole frame is covered. For a sample of size n from a population N, the sampling interval is given by:

$$N = (n - 1)y + v$$

where the value of the variable **v** is non-zero and less than or equal to y. The first unit is selected randomly from the first v. Thereafter, every yth unit is taken.

The procedure is attractive not only because of convenience, but also because it seems to give a better apparent coverage of the population. The method, however, is not always equivalent to SRS in so far as not all the SUs are given the same chance of selection. Consequently, estimates of sampling error and confidence limits are problematic. The method is employed in many eye surveys to select units of individuals or clusters as if it were effectively an SRS, and the data are analyzed accordingly.

Simple random sampling is the most basic and straightforward of the sampling schemes and, as such, is the most desirable in many respects. Yet very few eye surveys have employed the scheme. There are, however, two notable examples outlined below.

The first, the Roscommon Glaucoma Survey[8] conducted in the west of Ireland, successfully used an SRS scheme. The primary objective was to measure the prevalence of glaucoma in the older population of the county. The sampling design was made possible because computerized electoral register data were available. The Economic and Social Research Institute in Dublin was able to generate sampling frames and to draw an SRS, giving contact addresses for each member. The selected individuals were invited to attend an eye examination in one of more than 50 clinics held throughout the county at 18 different sites. Those who could not attend the clinics were examined in their homes. Good public relations and advertising helped to produce an excellent response. Of the 2,200 individuals invited, 99.5%

were examined, including 12.8% examined in their own homes.

The other example is the Barbados Eye Study,[12] designed to obtain epidemiological data on glaucoma and other major eye disorders in a predominantly black population. The study report is highly informative with respect to the methodology and the data on prevalence of glaucoma in various age and gender subgroups for the black population. An SRS scheme was employed to select the sample from a frame representing the Barbados-born resident population of the island, aged 40–84 years. The Barbados Statistical Services Department handled the random selection, which was based on their national registration numbers. The 4,709 participants represented about 84% of the eligible members selected from the sampling frame.

Generally, for a given sample size, SRS gives the most precise results with the smallest random sampling error, other things being equal. In many situations, however, SRS may be too difficult and/or uneconomical to perform. It might not be possible to construct the necessary sampling frame, particularly in rural areas of many developing countries. Even if this were possible, the selected individuals might be widely scattered over a large area, with only one or two persons at any one address. Travelling long distances to a particular address to find and examine only a few individuals might present serious logistic and economic problems, as might the setting up of a large number of examination stations. The high likelihood of 'non-response' in such situations is an additional serious concern. An attractive solution is to adopt a cluster sampling scheme.

3.4.2   Cluster sampling (CLS)

In CLS the population members are divided into non-overlapping groups ('clusters') of individuals, and a sample of the clusters is chosen to yield a sample of the population members. Three main varieties of CLS may be defined, as follows.

One-stage cluster sampling

The population is divided into a number of primary clusters (usually 30 or more), either by census, or

enumeration areas, neighbourhoods or villages. Having randomly selected a number of clusters, no further sampling is carried out, and all population members (individuals) within the selected clusters are included in the final sample of individuals. When the clusters have approximately the same number of individuals, SRS is used to draw the sample of clusters in which case the procedure approximates an epsem. When the cluster sizes differ appreciably, the above procedure for selecting a sample of clusters is modified to 'ensure' epsem. This involves allocating a proportionally higher probability of selection to clusters that are larger, an important principle known as **probability-proportional-to-size (pps)**. This is done because most populations are made up of a few large clusters (e.g. towns) and many small clusters (e.g. villages), and if SRS were applied then all clusters would have an equal chance of being selected and the selected sample would over-represent people from small clusters and under-represent people from large clusters, compared with the actual population. As the prevalence of a disease may vary between the small and large clusters (e.g. due to access to treatment) this could bias the prevalence estimate. However, statistical methods are available for obtaining unbiased estimates in such situations. Most eye surveys using cluster sampling employ pps because in most populations it is very difficult to define or identify convenient boundaries that delineate groups of equal size.

Two-stage cluster sampling or sub-sampling

In this procedure a number of clusters are selected randomly from the primary clusters (as above), but within each chosen cluster only a sample of the individuals are included. As in one-stage CLS, pps is usually employed to select the clusters, but a fixed (predefined) number of individuals are drawn from every chosen cluster. Selection of individuals within the clusters can be through SRS of all the eligible participants. In this case, the individuals within each chosen cluster are listed in a sampling frame and a random sample (usually SRS) is drawn from the frame. All the individuals thus selected are included in the final sample. Another frequently used method is the **random walk method**, where a starting point is defined in the cluster and a bottle is spun to select an arbitrary starting direction. A house in the line of the bottle is chosen and the enumerators include individuals door to door until the desired cluster size is achieved. There are also variations of the basic random walk method (e.g. choosing consecutive houses at a set interval). There are a number of limitations to the random walk method. This method does not select households from a sampling frame and so the sample is not selected with a known probability. Furthermore, this method of selection may be open to conscious or unconscious bias of the enumerator in selecting households.

Another method for selecting individuals within clusters is through the **compact segment method**. In this method the cluster is divided into areas so that each area includes approximately the same number of people. One of the areas is chosen at random and either all the participants in that area are included, or else a specified number are included (in which case the method would be more like three-stage cluster sampling), and sampling ceases when the required sample size is obtained.

Multi-stage cluster sampling

When the defined population to be sampled is that of a large region or country, it may be more convenient (logistically and for economy) to group the population members first in large clusters (called **primary sampling units** or **PSU**) that may correspond to, for example, counties or provinces. Within each PSU, the individuals are grouped into a number of smaller convenient clusters (second-stage units). These subunits may be administrative divisions within the PSU (e.g. districts). Yet smaller subgroups of individuals may be defined within each second-stage unit (e.g. enumeration areas), and so on. Selecting first from among PSUs, then from secondary units within selected PSUs, and then within the secondary units and so on generates the sample. Figure 3.2 gives a schema of the process. This method of sampling enables a representative sample to be obtained across provinces so that the sample may be more generalizable.

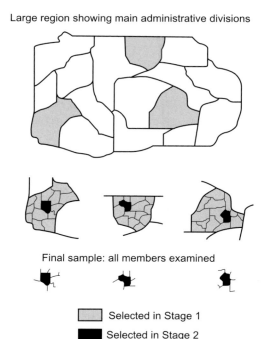

Large region showing main administrative divisions

Final sample: all members examined

▨ Selected in Stage 1
■ Selected in Stage 2

Figure 3.2 *Schematic example of two-stage cluster random sampling*

3.4.3 The design effect (deff)

The sampling error tends to be higher in cluster random sampling than in simple random sampling schemes, but the former are often more attractive operationally. The following numerical example may help to illustrate the issue.

Example

A rural population of 240,000 individuals resides in 800 villages, each containing (for simplicity) approximately 300 persons. A sample of 2,400 individuals is to be drawn from the population. There are various ways in which the total sample may be obtained, as shown in Table 3.1.

Scheme A is an SRS scheme, without stratification. This would be possible if a sampling frame could be constructed, for example, from a suitable complete and up-to-date register and 2,400 individuals are selected at random from the register. Without such a frame it may be impractical. Scheme B does not involve a selection of a sample of villages: all are used. It is thus an SRS with stratification,

Table 3.1 *Possible sampling schemes to select 2,400 persons from 800 villages*

Sampling Scheme	Number of villages to be selected Stage 1	Number of persons to be selected from each selected village Stage 2
A	not applicable	2,400 simple random sampling
B	800	3
C	240	10
D	120	20
E	60	40
F	8	300

whereby a simple random sample is taken from every village (stratum). Schemes C to E are two-stage sampling schemes, and F is a single-stage CLS scheme. In scheme C, each village constitutes a cluster of 10 persons, and there are 240 clusters. In D, there are 120 clusters, each of size 20, and so on. From the logistic convenience and cost point of view, the schemes become more attractive from A to F. Schemes A and B, however, are expected to have the least random sampling error and therefore give the highest precision. There is likely to be more random sampling error when one selects clusters of people rather than individuals. The extent to which this happens will partly depend on how highly clustered conditions are within geographical areas, and as such is likely to be most problematic for infectious conditions.

The random sampling errors in CLS depend not only on the size of the clusters, but also on the sum of the differences between the overall prevalence and the prevalence in each cluster. In general, when such differences are large and numerous, the random sampling error is also large. The **design effect** (**deff**) is a ratio of two variances (measures of random sampling error) V_1/V_2, where V_1 is the variance when a CLS method has been used, and V_2 is calculated assuming an SRS method, and gives a measure of how highly clustered a condition is within communities. The deff is close to 1.0 when the sampling method used is equivalent to SRS insofar as the sampling error is concerned. It is usually (but not invariably) higher than 1.0 when a CLS method has been employed. The following approximate equation demonstrates the main determinants of the magnitude of the design effect.

$$\text{Design Effect} = \frac{\sum m_i^2(p_i - P)^2}{NMPQ}$$

where:
Σ denotes the sum of
m_i is the size of the ith cluster (i.e. number of individuals in the cluster)
p_i is the prevalence in the ith cluster
P is the overall prevalence, and $Q = 1-P$
N is the number of clusters
M is the average cluster size

A number of readily available statistical software packages, such as STATA and Epi-Info, may be used to compute deff from survey data. The design effect is important in calculating the required sample size for a planned survey (see Section 3.6). If the anticipated design effect is underestimated or if no allowance is made for it, then the desired precision may not be attained and the confidence interval for the prevalence estimate may be considerably wider than hoped for.

3.4.4   Cluster sampling in eye surveys: some examples

Population-based sample surveys covering large regions, particularly in developing countries, commonly use a CLS design, whereby geographical area units are selected in two (or more) stages, sometimes with stratification. The 1981 Nepal Blindness Survey[3] is a good example to illustrate some of the methodological issues. The survey was the first phase of the Nepal Prevention of Blindness Programme, initiated in 1979 under the auspices of the government and the World Health Organization, with financial support from many non-governmental organizations and trusts. The study was the first nationwide, population-based sampling survey of blindness and eye disease conducted anywhere.

The population of approximately 14 million people lives in a partially mountainous rectangle

100 by 500 miles. The smallest defined area unit was the ward, which comprised one or more villages. Nine wards made up a panchayat. There were 4,000 panchayats. A collection of 5–108 panchayats made up a district, of which there were 75. Some of the panchayats were rural and some were urban.

The rural population was divided into 12 strata, primarily according to the geographical characteristics of the region and terrain. From these strata, the rural portion of the sample was drawn in two stages. In stage 1, 97 rural panchayats were selected randomly, with the probability of selection being proportional to the estimated number of residents (pps). Adjustments were made within each selected panchayat to link small wards into a single unit of 80–90 households, and to split larger wards accordingly. This helped to generate clusters of approximately equal size. In stage 2, a single ward (or ward-like unit) was drawn randomly from each selected panchayat. These final-stage units were the survey sites, expected to contain 80–90 households and 450–500 persons each. Following an enumeration by an advance team, all residents of the selected survey sites were then examined. In urban areas, eight 'wards' were selected randomly from the 23 town panchayats in the country and all residents were examined. The response rate was good. Of a total of 46,905 persons enumerated, 39,887 (85%) were examined. Locating and obtaining lists and maps of all the panchayats in Nepal was a difficult task and could not have been achieved without the good will and assistance of government offices.

The Baltimore Eye Survey conducted in the USA is another example.[13] This was a population-based prevalence survey, the primary aim being the comparison of the black and white populations with respect to the prevalence of eye disease. A CLS scheme was chosen that employed pps. In view of the main aim, however, the study plan was designed to generate a sample that had approximately equal numbers from each broad ethnic group. The population was stratified accordingly and clusters were classified according to ethnic composition based on the census, and were selected from each ethnic stratum by systematic sampling. The methodology is a useful example of

how the basic sampling schemes may be modified to serve the study objectives. Also of interest are the main reasons given for adopting the CLS scheme: '… to minimize the distance between subjects' homes and our neighbourhood screening centres and to enable the use of community leaders and the media to encourage participation'.[13] These reasons are germane in the elimination of bias arising from non-response (see Section 3.5).

The Melbourne Visual Impairment Project,[14,15] a population-based, cross-sectional, detailed study of eye disease in the Melbourne metropolitan region, has published informative accounts of the methods, particularly of the operational aspects, including the protocol summary for standardized methods of eye examination and assessment of visual function. The survey used a CLS scheme incorporating pps and systematic sampling.

Examples of eye surveys that cover a defined total population without sampling include the Beaver Dam Eye Study[16] (designed to estimate the prevalence and severity of lens opacities in a rural community in the USA), and the Blue Mountains Eye Study[17] (designed to investigate vision and the causes of visual impairment in a defined urban population in Australia). In these cases the estimation of sampling error or confidence limits for occurrence measures such as the overall prevalence is a non-issue, since the entire population was included. Nevertheless, confidence intervals are sometimes reported and inferences made to the larger population of the country, albeit with dubious validity. These studies, however, give valuable information in the form of an effect measure, such as arises in the comparison of subgroups and in the evaluation of associations (e.g. comparing the prevalence of a condition by age, ethnicity or other characteristics). The statistical significance and precision of these effect measures are highly pertinent because, for the effect measure (unlike the occurrence measure), inference is based on an abstract (infinitely large) population. Published reports from the two studies cover important methodological issues that are relevant even when sampling is not involved. The Beaver Dam Eye study employed a private census of the local community using 'total digit dialling by phone'.[18] The Blue Mountains Eye Study carried out a door-to-door census of the area to identify the eligible residents and to invite them to attend a local hospital clinic for a detailed eye examination. In the event of 'no-contact', several call-back visits were made at different times and on different days to ensure good coverage. The survey plan included taking a sample from residents of nursing homes, considered as a separate population for analysis. The response rate was 88%. For most of the non-responders, some basic information could be ascertained concerning vision, gender, age, etc., so that they could be compared with the responders. Such comparisons are useful in evaluating non-response as a source of bias.

Many population-based eye surveys conducted outside of the Established Market Economies in the last decade or so have used multi-stage or CLS of area units. These include surveys in the Gambia,[4,19] southern Turkey,[20] Benin,[21] Congo,[22] Togo,[23] Bangladesh,[5] Pakistan[6] and Nigeria.[7] Useful examples of the sampling method (and of other methodological issues) are to be found in the published accounts of these eye surveys.

The Rapid Assessment of Avoidable Blindness

The **Rapid Assessment of Avoidable Blindness** (**RAAB**) is a survey design using CLS sampling to achieve the desired sample size,[24,25] (see also Chapter 1). It was developed as a simple and rapid survey methodology to provide data on the prevalence and causes of blindness, and is a modified version of the **Rapid Assessment of Cataract Surgical Services** (**RACSS**).[26] A RAAB is ideally carried out at the level of a district or province that has a population size of 0.5 to 5 million people. The sample size required for a RAAB is usually between 2,000 and 5,000 people, but depends on the expected prevalence of blindness and the desired precision of the estimate. Clusters of people to include in the survey are randomly selected from across the survey area through pps. Each day a team visits one population unit (preferably an enumeration area used by the census office, which is a small, clearly demarcated area with a known population often corresponding to a village or suburb of a town).

Individuals within the cluster are selected through a modification of compact segment sampling. The cluster is divided into geographical units each including approximately 50 people aged 50+ and one segment is randomly selected. The team then goes to the selected area and visits the households door-to-door until they have enumerated 50 people aged over 50 years (the cluster). All selected people undergo visual acuity screening with a tumbling E chart and have their lenses examined. The main cause of VA < 6/18 is determined by an ophthalmologist or ophthalmic clinical officer. The information collected in the RAAB is used to estimate the prevalence of blindness in the survey area, taking into account the design effect, and causes of blindness are also estimated. Data from RAAB can also be used to assess outcomes after cataract surgery, barriers to cataract surgery and cataract surgical coverage.

3.4.5   Stratification

Several mentions have already been made of the population being 'stratified' in the context of sampling. Here the topic is considered in a little more detail.

Stratification is the process of defining population subgroups (or strata) that are non-overlapping, and these are often geographically defined (e.g. districts in a province, or urban and rural areas). Samples are then selected from within every stratum rather than across the whole population. A stratified population may offer three main advantages. First, for a given sample size n, it may be logistically more convenient to obtain a random sample from each stratum to make up n, rather than taking n units from the whole population (see scheme B in the example in Section 3.4.3).

Second, the sampling error of the estimate p may be reduced by sampling from each stratum separately, provided that there is more homogeneity within the strata than in the whole population, in respect of the measurement that is being made on the sample members. Consider a simplistic example. In a population that can be divided into two broad ethnic strata A and B, if a visual function score shows less variation within each stratum than in the whole population, then a stratified SRS scheme would estimate the mean visual function score for the population more efficiently (less sampling error for a given sample size and cost) than would a non-stratified SRS.

Third, in the above example the main interest may well be in separate estimates of the visual function score for each ethnic group, perhaps standardized for age, and a comparison of the score between them. These objectives would be best served if an adequate sample were obtained from each ethnic stratum.

Both SRS and CLS could be applied to a stratified population. The requirement is that a sample is taken from each and every defined stratum. Usually, the stratum-specific sample size is made proportional to the population size of the stratum. In the Baltimore Eye Survey[13] (see Section 3.4.4), the sample size from each ethnic stratum was not made proportional to the stratum size because the study objectives required approximately equal numbers of each ethnic group for efficient comparisons, and so clusters were over-sampled from ethnic minority groups. In estimating the overall prevalence in the population in such situations, adjustments are made to allow for the disproportionate representation of the stratum members in the sample.

In eye surveys, stratification often involves identifying geographical areas and/or subpopulations that are similar in respect of the risk of blindness, and so on, and grouping them into a stratum. Examples include grouping all towns into an 'urban' stratum and all villages into two or three strata, according to size. Many of the eye surveys mentioned in Sections 3.4.1 and 3.4.4 have used a stratified sampling scheme.

3.5 SOURCES OF BIAS

As mentioned earlier, non-sampling errors are difficult to quantify and may invalidate the survey findings. Statistical models have been developed to evaluate the possible effect of bias arising from sources such as non-response,[27] but their utility in eye surveys has been limited. The main sources

of such systematic errors in sample surveys are summarized here.

3.5.1 Biased selection

Biased selection of the eligible members of the population can be avoided by strict adherence to a well-devised random sampling scheme. The importance of allocating the predefined probability of selection to each sampling unit has been discussed earlier.

3.5.2 Faulty coverage

The term 'under-coverage' refers to a situation where some of the eligible members of the population (eligible sampling units) are not included in the sampling frame and therefore not given a chance to be selected. 'Over-coverage' indicates the reverse, whereby members that are not eligible, for example those outside the defined population, are included in the sampling frame (e.g. if people seeking eye care approach the survey team and are included in the sample). The problem, therefore, relates to the aptness of the sampling frame. Precise definition of the eligible members of the population (in terms of residence or other characteristics such as age) is a prerequisite.

3.5.3 Non-response

Many of the reports from the eye surveys mentioned earlier indicate that when a selected member cannot be 'examined' because of absence or refusal or another difficulty, then every reasonable effort (with due regard to resources and to the ethics of the situation) is first made to enable an examination to take place. Substituting the next-door neighbour or arbitrary selection of another member may cause bias. If necessary, an additional eligible member may be selected randomly from the sampling frame; however, this is not a substitute for efforts to maximise response since people who respond may be different from those who do not respond in terms of prevalence and risk factors for blindness which could result in bias. Many of the recent eye surveys in developing countries have managed to minimize the non-response, having examined more than 90% of all those who were selected. By contrast, some eye surveys in urban settings, particularly in large metropolitan areas, have examined only about 60% of the selected sample. Surveys that involve house-to-house visits by the team tend to achieve a better response rate. When persons are invited to attend examination in a remote centre, or when postal questionnaires are used, the response generally tends to be poorer. The well-designed eye survey in the west of Ireland managed to examine 99.5% of all those invited to attend clinics at 18 examination sites throughout the county[8] (see Section 4.3 for more detail). The 4,709 participants in the Barbados Eye Study[12] represented about 84% of the eligible members in the sample. The Melbourne Visual Impairment Project achieved a response rate of 83%.[15] The response rate in the North London Eye Study[9] was 84%. These studies have relied on media publicity and public relations to help provide information to the community and to secure the co-operation of community leaders and other key officials.

3.5.4   Other sources of bias

Other sources of information bias include systematic mistakes in measurement, diagnosis and the classification of individuals, mistakes in recording data, and mistakes in data analysis and reporting. These errors could mean that the estimates of prevalence and causes of blindness from the survey do not reflect the true values in the total population. Procedures that may help to eliminate these sources of bias include:

> Preparation of a detailed protocol (manual of operations) for training and reference.
> Training of the members of the survey team in standardized methods of examination, grading and classification, and assessing the level of agreement between the examiners (observers), before and during the survey, using observer agreement studies.

> Making the examinations and assessments as objective and as automated as possible. This may include (when possible) the use of image-capture systems (such as a fundus camera) and subsequent 'reading' of the images by an expert group, or a computerized image-analysis system.
> Data entry (manual or by scanning of the record sheet) using software with range-checks and validity-checks, and double data entry or formal checking of entered data against original records.

3.6   SAMPLE SIZE FOR ESTIMATING PREVALENCE

The sample size will depend upon the desired level of precision for estimating prevalence, the sampling scheme, the population size, and cost and logistic issues. Having devised an efficient sampling scheme (one that would result in minimal sampling error for any given sample size and cost), an approximate minimum sample size, required to give the desired precision, may be calculated using standard statistical tools which are widely available. The equations require the following criteria to be specified:

> The expected prevalence of the condition in the population. This is usually based on the results of surveys conducted in similar settings.
> The desired **precision** (the maximum sampling error that is acceptable) for estimating the prevalence of the disorder(s) deemed as 'most important' in the objectives of the study. Calculations are also made for the secondary objectives. The desired precision will strongly depend upon the 'expected' prevalence in the population: for example, when the prevalence is expected to be in the region of 0.1 (i.e. 10%) a sampling error of ± 0.02 may be acceptable, whereas a much smaller sampling error (e.g. ± 0.005) is required for an expected prevalence of, for example, 0.025. Calculations are usually made for several different assumed values of the prevalence and the corresponding levels of precision.

- The **power** of the study (i.e. the probability that the test will reject the null hypothesis when the alternative hypothesis is true) insofar as it relates to the probability of not exceeding the specified sampling error (see also Chapter 2). This is usually fixed at 0.95 (for 95% confidence limits), in contrast to the flexibility in other types of study such as a clinical trial (see Chapter 7), or a cross-sectional study for estimation of an effect measure (see Chapter 4).
- The population size, because larger sampling fractions (n/N) tend to yield smaller sampling errors. This may have a negligible effect on sample size when N is very large.
- The expected design effect (see Section 3.4.3). It may be difficult to predict a value for this with any level of certainty, but instances of the actual findings in other similar studies may be useful.[28] Unfortunately, very few eye surveys have reported the observed design effect.[21,29-31]

The following equation is intended to help the understanding of the relationship between sample size and its determinants (excluding any stratification).

$$n = \frac{t^2PQW/E^2}{1+(1/N)((t^2PQW/E^2)-1)}$$

where:
n is the minimum sample size required (approximate)
P is the assumed prevalence in the population (a proportion)
Q is 1 − P
E is the maximum random sampling error acceptable
W is the likely design effect
N is the population size
t is the standardized normal deviate, usually fixed at 1.96, to give 95% probability of not exceeding E

When N is very large in relation to n (e.g. N is more than a million and n < 3,000), the denominator (expression under the line) of the equation will have a value very close to 1.0, giving a simpler equation:

$$n = t^2PQW/E^2$$

Alternatively, the expected precision may be calculated for a given sample size.

3.7 FUTURE DIRECTIONS

- Large eye surveys planned primarily for the estimation of the prevalence of visual impairment and eye disease in countries within the Established Market Economies would probably fail to attract major funding. Those planned to form the initial cross-sectional phase of analytical cohort studies should have a higher chance of success. Generally, the approach in the past has been to limit the study scope to matters of vision and eye disease. Future large sample surveys should be multi-disciplinary, aiming to obtain data on the population burden of a broader spectrum of disability (hearing, mobility, etc.) and the causal disorders, so that the 'general functional health' status of the population may be assessed. Health authorities may increasingly tend to base the planning of future levels and type of service on sound epidemiological models of population need. Such models are scarce and the very few that exist are in great need of more diverse, precise and reliable data. Consequently, studies designed specifically to generate such data and to enable the development of new models may become favoured, particularly if they are made germane to the requirements of the owner-users of the intended model, that is, the health provider (public, private or non-governmental organization).
- Surveys may also contribute towards the development of screening programmes. In general medicine several biological measures exist that can herald the coming of a disease, indicate its presence, or quantify the severity of disease or dysfunction. Many of these measures are 'continuous'. Their population mean values (norms) have had to be established, and the cut-offs that

could be taken to indicate abnormality have had to be defined. Discovery and development of such new objective measures for eye disorders is a reasonable expectation in view of the advances in molecular biology and genetics. Population-based, cross-sectional studies should play a central initial role in establishing the 'norms' and critical cut-off values to identify people at high risk of disease. Biological measures that are permanent markers for transient exposures or which quantify cumulative life-time exposure may be developed, and may require initial assessment through cross-sectional studies.

➢ Other developments may also require future cross-sectional studies for the assessment and exploration of relationships and the assessment of impact of interventions. An example of such new advances would be the development of a sensible scoring system for visual function or for vision-related quality of life, applicable across the spectrum of the major eye disorders and in different settings.

➢ In many developing nations of Asia, Latin America and Africa, local eye surveys should continue to generate important data on the population burden of eye disease and blindness, and on the need for basic eye services. These surveys will contribute towards the planning and monitoring of local programmes for the prevention of blindness and will help with advocacy and raising awareness. New methodologies may need to be developed for the assessment of the prevalence of rare conditions.

REFERENCES

1. Pascolini D, Mariotti SP, Pokharel GP, *et al*. 2002 Global update of available data on visual impairment: a compilation of population-based prevalence studies. *Ophthalmic Epidemiol* 2004; 11:67–115.

2. Resnikoff S, Pascolini D, Etya'ale D, *et al*. Global data on visual impairment in the year 2002. *Bull World Health Organ* 2004; 82:844–851.

3. Brilliant GE (ed). *The Epidemiology of Blindness in Nepal: Report of the 1981 Nepal Blindness Survey*. Chelsea, MI: The Seva Foundation; 1988.

4. Faal H, Minassian D, Sowa S, *et al*. National survey of blindness and low vision in The Gambia: results. *Br J Ophthalmol* 1989; 73:82–87.

5. Dineen BP, Bourne RR, Ali SM, *et al*. Prevalence and causes of blindness and visual impairment in Bangladeshi adults: results of the National Blindness and Low Vision Survey of Bangladesh. *Br J Ophthalmol* 2003; 87:820–828.

6. Jadoon MZ, Dineen B, Bourne RR, *et al*. Prevalence of blindness and visual impairment in Pakistan: the Pakistan National Blindness and Visual Impairment Survey. *Invest Ophthalmol Vis Sci* 2006; 47:4749–4755.

7. Kyari F, Gudlavalleti MV, Sivsubramaniam S, *et al*. Prevalence of blindness and visual impairment in Nigeria: the National Blindness and Visual Impairment Study. *Invest Ophthalmol Vis Sci* 2009; 50:2033–2039.

8. Coffey M, Reidy A, Wormald R, *et al*. Prevalence of glaucoma in the west of Ireland. *Br J Ophthalmol* 1993; 77:17–21.

9. Reidy A, Minassian DC, Vafidis G, *et al*. Prevalence of serious eye disease and visual impairment in a north London population: population based, cross sectional study. *Br Med J* 1998; 316:1643–1646.

10. Rubin GS, West SK, Munoz B, *et al*. A comprehensive assessment of visual impairment in a population of older Americans. The SEE Study. Salisbury Eye Evaluation Project. *Invest Ophthalmol Vis Sci* 1997; 38:557–568.

11. Dielemans I, Vingerling JR, Wolfs RC, *et al*. The prevalence of primary open-angle glaucoma in a population-based study in The Netherlands. The Rotterdam Study. *Ophthalmology* 1994; 101:1851–1855.

12. Leske MC, Connell AM, Schachat AP, *et al*. The Barbados Eye Study. Prevalence of open angle glaucoma. *Arch Ophthalmol* 1994; 112:821–829.

13. Tielsch JM, Sommer A, Witt K, *et al*. Blindness and visual impairment in an American urban population. The Baltimore Eye Survey. *Arch Ophthalmol* 1990; 108:286–290.

14. Wensor MD, McCarty CA, Stanislavsky YL, *et al*. The prevalence of glaucoma in the Melbourne Visual Impairment Project. *Ophthalmology* 1998; 105:733–739.

15. Livingston PM, Carson CA, Stanislavsky YL, *et al*. Methods for a population-based study of eye

disease: the Melbourne Visual Impairment Project. *Ophthalmic Epidemiol* 1994; 1:139–148.

16. Klein BE, Klein R, Linton KL. Prevalence of age-related lens opacities in a population. The Beaver Dam Eye Study. *Ophthalmology* 1992; 99:546–552.

17. Attebo K, Mitchell P, Smith W. Visual acuity and the causes of visual loss in Australia. The Blue Mountains Eye Study. *Ophthalmology* 1996; 103:357–364.

18. Campbell JA, Palit CD. Total digital dialing for small area census by phone. *American Statistical Association Proceedings of the Section on Survey Research Methods*. Alexandra, VA: The Association, 1988.

19. Faal H, Minassian DC, Dolin PJ, *et al.* Evaluation of a national eye care programme: re-survey after 10 years. *Br J Ophthalmol* 2000; 84:948–951.

20. Negrel AD, Minassian DC, Sayek F. Blindness and low vision in southeast Turkey. *Ophthalmic Epidemiol* 1996; 3:127–134.

21. Négrel AD, Avognon Z, Minassian DC, *et al.* Blindness in Benin [Article in French]. *Med Trop* 1995; 55:409–414.

22. Negrel AD, Massembo-Yako B, Botaka E, *et al.* Prevalence and causes of blindness in the Congo [Article in French]. *Bull World Health Organ* 1990; 68:237–243.

23. Balo K, Negrel DA. [Causes of blindness in Togo] [Article in French]. *J Fr Ophthalmol* 1989; 12:291–295.

24. Kuper H, Polack S, Limburg H. Rapid assessment of avoidable blindness. *Community Eye Health* 2006; 19:68–69.

25. Mathenge W, Kuper H, Limburg H, *et al.* Rapid assessment of avoidable blindness in Nakuru district, Kenya. *Ophthalmology* 2007; 114:599–605.

26. Limburg H, Kumar R, Indrayan A, *et al.* Rapid assessment of prevalence of cataract blindness at district level. *Int J Epidemiol* 1997; 26:1049–1054.

27. Cochrane WG. *Sampling Techniques.* New York: John Wiley & Sons; 1977.

28. Katz J, Zeger SL. Estimation of design effects in cluster surveys. *Ann Epidemiol* 1994; 4:295–301.

29. Katz J, Zeger SL, Tielsch JM. Village and household clustering of xerophthalmia and trachoma. *Int J Epidemiol* 1988; 17:865–869.

30. West SK, Munoz B, Turner VM, *et al.* The epidemiology of trachoma in central Tanzania. *Int J Epidemiol* 1991; 20:1088–1092.

31. Dandona L, Dandona R, Naduvilath TJ, *et al.* Burden of moderate visual impairment in an urban population in southern India. *Ophthalmology* 1999; 106:497–504.

4

Case-control studies

ASTRID FLETCHER

4.1	Introduction	95	4.7	Nested case-control studies	103
4.2	What is a case-control study?	95	4.8	Analysis of case-control studies	103
4.3	Study hypothesis and sample size	96	4.9	Reporting the results of case-control studies	104
4.4	Selection of cases	97			
4.5	Selection of controls	99	4.10	Future directions	104
4.6	Assessment of exposures	102		References	105

4.1 INTRODUCTION

The case-control study was one of the earliest study designs in the emerging discipline of epidemiology in the first part of the 20th century.[1] This design has made a major contribution to our understanding of risk factors for many diseases and health problems. Case-control studies became widely used in cancer epidemiology in particular, and it was in this field that many of the methodological and statistical advances in their design and analysis were developed. Although case-control studies were used occasionally in ophthalmology, it was not until the 1980s that they became more commonly applied.

4.2 WHAT IS A CASE-CONTROL STUDY?

The key design feature of a case-control study is the comparison of the odds of an exposure[a] ('risk factor') in people with a particular disease or condition ('cases') with the odds of that exposure in people who do not have the disease or condition ('controls'). This comparison is expressed by the **odds ratio (OR)**.

Example 1

In a case-control study of young adults, the researchers investigated whether high social class was a risk factor for myopia.[2] Table 4.1 shows the results and the calculations.

In a case-control study the cases are already known and the exposures of interest must be retrospective, i.e. have occurred in the past before the onset of disease. In contrast, in a cohort study (Chapter 5) the exposures are measured at the start of the study

---

[a] Epidemiologists use the term 'exposure' to refer to any characteristic that is hypothesized to be related to the disease being investigated. Exposures include demographic factors (e.g. age), lifestyle factors (e.g. diet, smoking), environmental (e.g. sunlight exposure), systemic or ocular factors (e.g. systemic blood pressure, intra-ocular pressure), biological variables (e.g. homocysteine) or genetic variables (e.g. allele frequency).

Table 4.1 *Case-control study of young adults investigating whether high social class is a risk factor for myopia*

High Social Class	Cases N = 99	Controls N = 101
Yes	58	17
No	41	84
Odds of exposure[b]	1.41	0.20
Odds Ratio	7.0	

[b] The odds of the exposure in cases is given by $p_1/1 - p_1$ and in controls by $p_0/1 - p_0$ where $p_1 = 58/(58 + 41)$, $1 - p_1 = 41/(41 + 58)$, $p_0 = 17/(17 + 84)$, $1 - p_0 = 84/(17 + 84)$.

and the cases arise over follow-up. Thus the obvious immediate benefit of a case-control study compared to a cohort study is the potential to examine a study hypothesis within a relatively short period of time.

The essential rationale and design is well set out in the abstract of one of the earliest case-control studies in ophthalmology.[3]

Example 2

*'Senile' macular degeneration (now **age-related macular degeneration** or **AMD**), although a leading cause of visual loss in the USA, remains a poorly understood disease. To assess the effects of host and environmental factors on this condition, a study of 228 cases and 237 controls matched by age and sex, who had visited any of 34 Baltimore ophthalmologists between 1 September 1978 and 31 March 1980, was conducted. Study participants were interviewed for past medical, residential, occupational, smoking and family histories, as well as social and demographic factors.*

In this early study there is no specific hypothesis but 'host and environmental factors' are assessed. This illustrates another benefit of case-control studies, which is that different exposures may be investigated in the same study. Note also the short duration of the study, with recruitment of cases and controls, interviews, analysis and publication, completed within five years.

However a word of warning! The apparent simplicity of the case-control design and the obvious advantages in the speed of results does not mean that case-control studies are easy to undertake. A well-designed and executed case-control study requires careful planning and preparation and there are a number of very serious problems that can arise at all stages. We will now consider in detail the steps in undertaking a case-control study.

4.3 STUDY HYPOTHESIS AND SAMPLE SIZE

A study hypothesis is the starting point for any epidemiological study design. It is a formal statement of the presumed relationship (adverse or protective) of a particular exposure in a particular group of people. Case-control studies may be exploratory with a general hypothesis or may investigate a specific hypothesis. In the case-control study of age-related macular degeneration described above, the exposures were loosely described as host or environmental factors. In contrast, in a case-control study in cataract,[4] the authors stated specific hypotheses.

Example 1

To further investigate the possible relationship of cataract formation with indoor smoke exposure, we conducted a cataract case-control study in the area of the Nepal–India border where cooking with solid fuels in unvented indoor stoves is a common practice. The main objectives of this study were to confirm results of earlier studies using clinically confirmed cataract cases; investigate possible confounding of the relationship; and examine whether the risk of cataract is modified by stove type or ventilation.

The numbers of cases and controls required to investigate the study hypotheses must be calculated before any detailed planning of the study is undertaken. First it is necessary to decide on the effect size (i.e. odds ratio) that is being investigated. The presumed odds ratio may be based on previous or pilot studies, or a judgement about the size of effect that the investigators consider is of public health or clinical importance to detect. In addition to the odds ratio, other information is required for sample size calculations: the expected prevalence of the exposure in the control population; the number of controls to each case; the alpha level[c] (usually 0.05); and the study **power**[d]

---

[c] Alpha level is the probability of a type I error, i.e. falsely rejecting the null hypothesis. Usually we consider an alpha level of at least 0.05, i.e. a 1 in 20 chance that we conclude there is an association with an exposure and a disease when there is none.

[d] The power of a study is the probability of correctly rejecting the null hypothesis. It is related to Beta, which is the probability of a type II error, i.e. failing to reject the null hypothesis when the null hypothesis is false. Power = 1 – Beta.

Table 4.2 *Sample sizes needed for different odds ratios and exposure prevalence*

Odds Ratio	Prevalence of exposure in the controls			
	30%	20%	10%	5%
OR = 3	110	128	200	354
OR = 2	306	372	614	1118
OR = 1.5	892	1124	1914	3548

(usually 0.8 or above). Information on the expected prevalence of exposure may be available from previous studies or surveys. In the situation where no prior information is available it will be necessary to carry out a pilot study to obtain this information.

Table 4.2 gives sample sizes needed for different odds ratios and exposure prevalence using an alpha of 0.05 and a power of 0.8. The numbers given are the total sample size with equal numbers of cases and controls.

The calculations show that the smaller the odds ratio to be investigated, the larger the sample size required. The prevalence of exposure is also a key factor and for less common exposures (5% or less) the sample size required to detect a modest (but potentially important effect) is around ten times greater than to detect a large odds ratio.

Example 2

In a case-control study of 175 cases of primary open-angle glaucoma and an equal number of controls, the prevalence of current smoking in controls was 14%.[5] The researchers found an odds ratio of 1.4, which was not significant. As Table 4.2 shows, the researchers would have required a sample size at least three times larger in order to show a significant effect of smoking with exactly the same odds ratio and smoking prevalence. In a smaller case-control study of 122 cases and 190 controls, a family history of glaucoma was obtained in 13% of controls and 30% of cases; analyses adjusted for confounders gave an odds ratio of 3.1.[6] In this example the study sample size had adequate power to detect such a large odds ratio.

Sample size calculations may also be based on the precision of the odds ratio, i.e. by the 95% confidence interval.[c] If the sample size is based only on the odds ratio there may be a wide 95% confidence interval resulting in uncertainty about the relative importance of the result. For example, as shown in Table 4.2, in a study with a 20% prevalence in controls, to detect an odds ratio of 2 at 80% power and 5% alpha requires 372 (186 cases and 186 controls). This would give a 95% confidence interval of 1.3–3.3. If we doubled the sample size we would reduce the width of 95% confidence interval of the odds ratio to 1.4–2.8.

Study power can also be increased by increasing the number of controls per case. This can be considered in situations when it is difficult or expensive to recruit cases. In the example of 186 cases and an equal number of controls described above, we could reduce the case sample size to 120 for the same power if we increased the number of controls to 360, i.e. recruited three controls per case. In general there is little gain in power for increasing the number of controls per case beyond three.[7]

The main advantage of doing the sample size calculations as the first step in planning the study is that the information aids the investigator in key design considerations, such as whether to recruit cases from many centres, the time necessary for recruitment of cases and controls, and the decision concerning the number of controls per case.

4.4 SELECTION OF CASES

4.4.1 Case definition

The study hypothesis must include a clear statement on the disease or condition being investigated, and whether it is being investigated in any particular subgroup of the case population. A case definition is therefore essential and must be supported by the criteria for defining the case. Case definitions may be simple presences or absences of disease, for example retinoblastoma. Many ophthalmological conditions, such as cataract or myopia, exhibit a continuum of 'disease' or abnormality

---

[c] The confidence interval is the probability that the true but unknown odds ratio lies in the range of values in the confidence interval. Usually we calculate a 95% confidence interval.

and the definition of a case is based on a cut-off point of severity. For others, such as glaucoma, the case definition is based on a variety of features (such as visual fields, cup–disc ratio and asymmetry). The development of standard classification systems for many major ophthalmic conditions has greatly facilitated epidemiological research. For example, the international grading system for age-related macular degeneration[8] and the Lens Opacities Classification System (LOCS III)[9] both permit a common understanding of the case criteria and comparability between studies using these systems and definitions. Cataract definitions should also include the type of opacity, i.e. nuclear, cortical and posterior sub-capsular opacity.

4.4.2 Sources of cases

Depending on the condition or disease being investigated, cases may be recruited from hospital clinics, community clinics (e.g. family practitioner clinics) or via population surveys. Hospitals are the best source for serious conditions likely to be referred and managed in the hospital setting. Milder conditions, e.g. dry eye, are likely to be seen in community clinics or by family doctors. If the source of cases is very restrictive, e.g. a tertiary referral clinic, this will limit the extent to which the results can be generalized, but it will not affect the validity, provided (as discussed later) the controls are appropriately selected. The most important consideration in selection of cases is that they must be selected independently of exposure. However, this can sometimes be difficult to ascertain, e.g. self-referral or physician referral, or choice of hospital may be influenced by factors such as socio-economic status, family history or co-morbidity. People with undiagnosed disease may be different from those who are known to have disease. Critically they may be different with respect to the exposure of interest.

Example 1

Over half the cases of primary open glaucoma identified in a recent population-based survey in Thessaloniki, Greece, were unaware of their diagnosis.[10] Men, those without a family history of glaucoma, *those with infrequent visits to ophthalmologists and those with a smaller cup–disc ratio were less likely to have been previously diagnosed. If a case-control study was conducted using the Eye Hospital Clinics as the source of the POAG cases, the prevalence of family history would have been biased with respect to all POAG cases.*

Ascertainment bias occurs when cases are more likely to be identified because of an exposure.

Example 2

In a case-control study of AMD, a history of cataract surgery was more common in cases than controls.[11] It is possible that this result was biased by people undergoing cataract surgery being more likely to be discovered to have signs of age-related macular degeneration.

4.4.3 Incident or prevalent cases

Another consideration in case selection is whether to recruit incident or prevalent cases. Incident cases are new cases of the disease occurring in a defined time period. Prevalent cases are all those with the disease in a defined time period and are a mixture of new cases and old cases. Incident cases are preferred for several reasons. They are less likely to have changed their behaviour because of knowledge of the condition, and may be more likely to recall their behaviour and exposure before the onset of disease, since this is in the recent past. Incident cases are more likely to represent all cases while prevalent cases may represent only those with a better prognosis if the disease is associated with survival (or conversely with a worse prognosis if 'cured' individuals leave the case population). If the exposure of interest is associated with the prognosis, then the prevalent cases may not be representative of the distribution of the exposure in all cases. For very rare diseases with a good prognosis, using only incident cases may not be feasible because of the long period for recruitment. For rare diseases with a poor prognosis, incident cases are preferred both for feasibility reasons and to avoid any bias associated with prognosis.

Example 1

A large case-control study investigated parental occupation at birth as a risk factor for retinoblastoma.[12] Because of the rarity of this condition 1,318 cases were identified over a 37-year period using the population-based Great Britain National Registry of Childhood Tumours (NRCT). Parental occupation in cases and controls was obtained from the description on the birth certificate. In this example, the cases were incident cases and the exposure of interest was collected from the birth record, and therefore not biased by subsequent prognosis.

Example 2

The Eye Disease Case-Control study recruited prevalent cases of neovascular AMD from eye care centres in five different USA cities.[13] Cases were identified by (i) a check of medical records of patients with scheduled appointments, and (ii) direct referral of patients with neovascular AMD from other eye clinics in the centres. Cases had to be diagnosed in the year prior to enrolment. In this example the cases are prevalent cases but by restricting the period of diagnosis the investigators ensured that there was not substantial variation in the period of recruitment and diagnosis.

4.5   SELECTION OF CONTROLS

The source and criteria for selecting controls is one of the most difficult aspects of a case-control study. Understanding the purpose of a control helps identify the criteria for selection of controls. The control group should represent the population from which the cases derive and hence represent the distribution of the exposure in that population. Controls must fulfil the same eligibility criteria defining cases apart from those relating to the disease. Many case-control studies, especially earlier studies, used hospital-based controls because of the ease of identification. Hospital controls are themselves cases of some other condition with its own set of risk factors and therefore they may not be representative of the exposures in the population. In an attempt to

overcome this potential bias, researchers have sometimes excluded potential controls with certain diagnoses considered to have risk factors similar to those of the disease under investigation.

Selection of controls with a variety of different diagnoses is one method to ensure that no particular control diagnostic group dominates.

Example 1

In the Eye Disease Case-Control study five retinal conditions were investigated in separate case-control studies using a common bank of controls attending hospital for other ocular conditions.[13] The most frequent diagnoses were lid disorders (31%), vitreous disorders (18%), cataract (14%) and conjunctivitis (10%).

Hospital controls may also differ from cases in factors related to attendance at hospital such as area of residence and associated socio-economic characteristics, which themselves may be related to exposure. This may be particularly problematic in settings with substantial socio-economic variation in hospital attendance. For example, if cataract cases are identified from outreach eye care services and attend hospital for surgery, controls attending the same hospital for other conditions may come from very different locations and socio-economic backgrounds. The essential criterion that a control should represent the prevalence of exposure in the population that gives rise to the cases will not have been met.

Example 2

A study conducted in the south of India recruited cataract cases and controls from the same outreach eye screening camps, thus avoiding the problem discussed above.[14]

Studies using hospital controls may not necessarily be biased compared with population controls if hospital controls are unbiased with respect to the exposure of interest. Unfortunately many of the early published case-control studies in ophthalmology do not provide adequate information on hospital control selection (method, conditions, exclusions, participation) for the reader to judge the validity of the controls.

4.5.1   Population controls

For the concerns discussed above, population-based controls are preferred to hospital controls. If the cases come from a well-defined area, then controls can be recruited from the same population. In some countries population registers may be available to investigators and controls can be randomly sampled from the register. It may be difficult, however, to be sure that a particular population really does represent the population from which the cases arise, especially in the situation of specialist hospitals where cases may come from a wide range of geographical locations. 'Neighbourhood' controls are often used to overcome this problem. Each control is selected to come from the same location as the case. For example, in the UK a control may be randomly selected from the age/sex register of the same family practitioner as the case. Random digit dialling with the location codes matched to the case is a popular approach in the USA, but less efficient because many calls may need to be made to locate a control who matches the same inclusion criteria as the case (matching is discussed below). In countries with considerable selection biases in hospital attendance, it may be preferable to recruit both cases and controls using population-based surveillance or a specially conducted survey. Population-based cross-sectional studies have become a more commonly used design to investigate risk factors in many middle and low income settings.[15–17]

Spouses or friends of cases have also been used as controls in some studies but are also unlikely to be representative of the population. Spouses and friends in particular may be biased with respect to exposures such as lifestyle which are likely to be shared with cases.[18] Volunteer controls are also likely to be biased.

Example 1

In an early small case-control study of 26 cases of AMD, 15 spouses were used as controls.[19] This study showed no association with smoking probably because most spouse pairs shared smoking habits. In a recent larger case-control study of 435 cases, 280 spouses were available.[20] This study found no significant association with smoking although the ORs were in the direction of an adverse effect. An analysis by pack years of smoking showed that higher consumption of cigarettes was associated with AMD. This suggests that while spouses may to some extent share smoking behaviour, they differed in the amount consumed.

Example 2

*The **AREDS** study recruited participants to a clinical trial of high-dose vitamin supplementation. Participants included those with intermediate or late AMD (grades 3 and 4), and those with no or minimal signs of early AMD (grades 1 and 2). The AREDS case-control study was a comparison at trial baseline of those with grades 2, 3 and 4 (cases) with grade 1 (controls).[21] The recruitment sources showed that most grades 1 and 2 were recruited through public advertisement (53%) and friends and family of participants (13%). The finding that those with higher levels of education were significantly less likely to have late AMD may be attributed to selection bias of volunteers rather than any true association with education level.*

Low participation rates can be a greater problem amongst population-based controls that have little motivation to participate. This will lead to biased results if participation is related to exposure. For example, if smokers are less likely to participate, the prevalence of smoking in controls will be underestimated (with respect to the prevalence of smoking in the source population) and the odds ratio will be biased upwards.

Some studies have used different types of controls to try to take account of selection biases in control specification.[22,23] The difficulty lies in interpreting the study results. If the results differ according to which type of control is used, does this suggest that one type of control is preferable to the other? Since we do not know the 'true' result there could be a danger of preferring the control type that gives a positive result. If results for different types of controls agree, it may be argued that this strengthens the validity of the results.

Example 3

The Risk Factor for Uveal Melanoma Study recruited incident cases of uveal melanoma in the ophthalmic clinic at the University Clinics of Essen, Germany.[23] The investigators used three control groups with a stated rationale for each. Population-based controls were randomly selected from compulsory resident lists covering the total population of Essen, on the assumption that cases were a random sample of cases in Germany. Hospital controls were randomly selected from private ophthalmologists who referred incident uveal melanoma cases to the referral centre on the assumption that some referral biases existed for cases. Controls with diagnoses of work-related conditions or acute keratitis were excluded. Sibling controls of cases were also chosen to assess whether genetic factors might confound or interact with the effect of exposure. The results revealed both consistent results by type of control and some differences. For iris colour there was a strong association with light iris colour in the comparison with population controls, but no association in the comparison with hospital or sibling controls. Significant associations with any history of eye burns were observed only for the analyses by sibling controls and for high numbers of burns in the analyses with population and hospital controls.

4.5.2 Matching

Before discussing matching it is necessary to consider **confounding**. A potential confounder (see Chapter 5, Section 5.3) is a factor that is associated both with the exposure and with being a case. A potential confounder becomes a confounder if the association between the risk factor and the disease changes, when the confounder is introduced into the statistical analysis. At the most extreme, the introduction of the confounder will totally remove the association with the exposure, i.e. the odds ratio will become null (1.0). The confounder is the explanation for the apparent association of the exposure with the disease.

Hypothetical example of confounding

In a case-control study beer drinking is highly associated with age-related macular degeneration (AMD). However, people who drink beer are also smokers. When smoking is adjusted for in the statistical analysis, the association with beer drinking disappears because the 'true' association of AMD is with smoking. In this example, smoking has confounded the association of beer drinking with AMD. Measuring possible confounding variables is essential to be sure that study results are not explained by factors other than the exposure under investigation.

Matching is different from selecting controls to have the same inclusion criteria as the cases. For example, if the inclusion criteria for cases are women aged 60 and over, then controls should be selected using the same criteria. The main purpose of matching is to increase the efficiency of a case-control study with respect to the adjustment for confounding in the statistical analysis.[24]

This can best be explained by a hypothetical example of a case-control study of age-related macular degeneration in which the principal exposure is smoking. In this example age is a potential confounder because older people (aged 70 and over) are more likely to have age-related macular degeneration and older people are also less likely to smoke. Suppose we select our cases and controls to be in the same broad age group, e.g. 50 years and over, but we do not match more closely on age. Because the chance of being selected as a control is higher in the younger age group aged 50–69 years (simply because in the population there are more people aged 50–69 than people aged 70 and over) then we will have proportionately younger controls than cases. When we adjust smoking for age we carry out an analysis which examines the association of smoking in different age groups (stratified analysis). If we have too many younger controls there would be far more controls than cases in the strata of the age group 50–69 but we will also have too few older controls especially in the oldest age group of aged 80 and above, which contains most cases. This will make it more difficult to adequately control for age in the analysis by smoking, and will result in wide confidence intervals for the odds ratio in those strata.

Example

A hospital-based case-control study recruited 1,401 cases of cataract and 549 controls aged 37–62.[25] There was a substantial difference in the age distribution of the cases and controls; 6% of cases and 47%

of controls were aged less than 50 years, and 66% of cases and 17% of controls were aged more than 55 years. In the very oldest age group of 60 and above there were 575 cases and 95 controls. Such a small number of controls in the oldest age group where the cases predominate make it difficult, especially in multivariable analysis, to be confident that age has been adequately controlled for.

Matching by age ensures that the age distribution of cases and controls is proportionately the same. However, the choice to match on age means that age cannot be examined as a risk factor, as we have forced the age groups to match. This is true for any matching criteria. Matching can be done in two different ways. In group matching, controls are selected to have proportionately the same distribution of the characteristics as the cases. If the age distribution of cases is 5% at ages 50–59, 15% at ages 60–69, 25% ages 70–79 and 55% aged 80 and over, controls are selected to be distributed in the same proportions by age. In exact matching, a control is matched individually to a case to be as close in age as possible (say within one year). These different approaches to matching require different types of statistical analysis (see Section 4.8).

Matching on several variables may make it time consuming and difficult to find controls, especially if the matching variables are not routinely available in the population registers from which the controls will be selected. There is another more important concern about matching on several variables and this is known as over-matching. Over-matching occurs when the effect of the matching makes the cases and controls too similar with respect to the exposure of interest, for example, by matching on a factor that is not a confounder but is highly correlated with the exposure of interest. For these reasons researchers, if they employ matching, prefer to match on only a few key variables such as age, which is likely to be a strong confounder of the exposure.

4.6   ASSESSMENT OF EXPOSURES

While information on exposures can come from a variety of sources, the usual method of measuring exposures in a case-control study is by interview,

using a structured questionnaire. This has the advantage that the questionnaire can be tailored to the study hypotheses. And, as we have seen, it is essential that questions on potential confounders are also included. The questionnaire may be interviewer- or self-administered. Interviewer-administered questionnaires are more demanding in terms of costs and necessity of training, but offer substantial benefits in completeness of information, with no restrictions due to illiteracy or poor vision. Information is sought on both current and past exposures using also a timeframe for past exposures. Some exposures are easier to recall than others; for example, 'ever having smoked' regularly compared to the amount smoked since starting smoking. Dietary questionnaires with up to 100 food items and nine frequency response codes make particular demands on interviewers and respondents and for reasons of recall and time usually only one period of time is assessed (for example in the last year). Questionnaires on sunlight exposure, a major putative risk factor in cataract and AMD, vary from a few questions on work- and leisure-related exposures[26] to detailed information regarding time spent outdoors or in different occupational time periods (including homecare), and in retirement up to current age, with corresponding information on use of hats and eyewear (glasses, contact lenses, sunglasses).[27] It is also important to obtain information about changes in behaviour, since these may be related to the onset of disease and hence post-date the exposure period of interest.

It is inevitable that there will be some inaccuracies in the information reported by respondents for some, if not all, of the exposures. This is not confined to case-control studies. The critical question is whether inaccuracies in the reporting of exposure are different between cases and control, known as **recall bias**. Cases, in particular, may be influenced in their answers by awareness of being a case. A question on family history of a disease may have more incorrect positive responses in cases than controls because cases are seeking an explanation of why they have the disease.

Errors can also be introduced by observers, e.g. by incorrect recording of information or variation in how interviews are conducted. Similar to recall bias, **observer bias** occurs when observer error differs proportionately between cases and controls. For example, interviewers may be more likely to stress the importance of accurate information to cases but not to controls.

How do inaccuracies in measurement affect the odds ratios? If errors by respondents or observers are proportionately similar between cases and controls (known as *non-differential measurement error*), then in general but not invariably, the odds ratio will be reduced towards null (1.0). If recall or observer bias has occurred (known as *differential measurement error*) the odds ratio will be biased upwards or downwards dependent on the direction of the bias. Unfortunately, since we do not know if recall or observer bias has occurred, we will not know if the odds ratios are biased or not. Errors in the measurement of confounders attenuate the adjustment for the effects of the confounding, resulting in 'residual confounding'. This produces a bias in either direction depending on the direction of the confounding.

Researchers try to minimize the possibility of biases and errors by tactics such as keeping interviewers, cases and controls masked with respect to the study hypotheses; by careful attention to questionnaire design and wording; and to standardization of methods if physical or biological data are being collected. Rigorous training and quality control of all concerned with collection of study data is essential.

4.7 NESTED CASE-CONTROL STUDIES

Nested case-control studies are case-control studies 'nested' within another type of study design, usually a cohort study. The main advantages are that exposures have been measured prior to becoming a case, for example through baseline data collection or stored blood samples. Controls are selected from the cohort matched on the date of the case becoming a case. An alternative approach is that controls are matched to cases from a random sample of all potential controls at baseline and are not matched on follow-up time. Because there are no advantages in nested case-control studies over

usual cohort studies in accrual of cases, the main benefit is in cost, since a smaller sample from the main study can be used.

Example 1

A nested case-control study of retinal vasculature and cardiovascular mortality was undertaken in the Beaver Dam study.[28] Cases were participants in the Beaver Dam Eye Study who died from ischaemic heart disease or stroke over a ten-year period (n = 154). Controls (n = 528) were age- and gender-matched in an approximate 1:4 ratio. Stored retinal photographs of cases and controls were analyzed. The advantage of the nested case-control study compared with a cohort study was that fewer retinal photographs needed to be read.

Example 2

A nested case-control study identified 543 men in the Physicians' Health Study (PHS) who developed cardiovascular disease over follow-up and matched them with controls.[29] The PHS was a randomized placebo-controlled trial of aspirin plus beta carotene in some 22,000 men. After excluding 252 men with a prior diagnosis of cataract or missing data, the remaining 834 men were followed for 11 years for incident cataract. Data available at baseline included stored blood samples which were analyzed for C-reactive protein. This unusual design also permitted exploration of whether the association with C-reactive protein differed according to whether the participants had a history of cardiovascular disease or not.

4.8 ANALYSIS OF CASE-CONTROL STUDIES

The calculation of an odds ratio was shown in Table 4.1; the odds ratio is sometimes called the crude or simple odds ratio because it is not adjusted for potential confounding variables. As discussed above, adjusting for the potential effect of a confounding variable on the odds ratio can be done by calculating the odds ratio separately in strata of a confounder. The Mantel–Haenszel method provides a pooled odds ratio across the strata (provided the individual odds ratios across the strata do not vary), which is the odds ratio for the exposure adjusted for the confounder. If the individual odds ratios do vary across the strata a formal test of homogeneity can be undertaken. If significant, i.e. the odds ratios are significantly different across the strata, **effect modification** is the term used, i.e. the effect of the exposure varies according to the level of some other exposure. With many variables, in a case-control analysis, a preferable approach is to use **logistic regression** and **conditional logistic regression** for an individually matched case-control study.[30] Logistic regression estimates the odds ratio (95% confidence interval and p value) for a particular exposure. If the study design used individual matching, conditional logistic regression must be used. In **multivariable logistic regression** the odds ratios are estimated for each exposure adjusted for the potential confounding effects of other exposures entered into the model. Effect modification can be tested by including an interaction term in the model. Because of the ease of computation of logistic models with present-day computers and statistical software packages, there may be a temptation for researchers to undertake multiple analyses, introducing numerous variables and interaction terms until a positive association turns up.[31] Researchers should have a clear strategy of analysis before undertaking any models, which should be based on a conceptual framework of the relations between the variables to be entered into the model.[32]

Particular issues in the statistical analysis of case-control studies in ophthalmology include the choice of one eye or both eyes for the primary outcome;[33] with the development of **generalized estimating equations** (GEE) both eyes should be used with adjustment for the correlation between eyes. This approach can increase study power, as long as the investigator is aware that the two eyes are not independent. Another area of interest is the analysis of categorical outcomes. *Multinomial logistic regression* (also called **polytomous logistic regression**) is used when there is more than one outcome and is particularly suitable for conditions with multiple discrete outcomes, such as type of cataract. If the outcomes also represent a staging of severity, for example discrete categories in a cataract grading score or different stages of age-related macular degeneration, then a proportional odds model may be appropriate. The proportional model estimates a single odds ratio across the varying categories. The main assumption of the model is that the odds ratios in different pairs of categories are the same. Caution is required in the use of the proportional odds model because assumptions that may hold for one exposure may be violated for another.

Example

Polytomous logistic regression was used in the Lens Opacity Case Control Study to examine potential risk factors across different types of cataract: pure nuclear, pure cortical, pure posterior subcapsular and mixed opacities.[34] Some factors, such as diabetes, were associated with all types of cataract except pure nuclear, while oral steroids were strongly associated only with pure posterior subcapsular opacities. Although this approach may shed light on possible differing aetiologies by cataract subtype, the fact that most cataracts were mixed raised questions of interpretation. For example, pure postcapsular opacities occurred in 72 people but a further 341 people had mixed postcapsular opacities.

4.9   REPORTING THE RESULTS OF CASE-CONTROL STUDIES

Communicating the results of case-control studies in journals requires the adequate provision of information, within the limited space available, to enable the validity of the study design, methods and results to be judged. Increasing electronic format and web-based supplementary material is a step forward in allowing the presentation of more detailed information. Variability in the quality of published studies has led to the development of guidelines for the reporting of observational studies (including case-control studies).[35] These guidelines also act as a useful checklist to researchers in designing their own research study and reviewing the results of other studies.

4.10   FUTURE DIRECTIONS

Case-control studies remain the design of choice for rare conditions, or when results are required in a short timescale, for example, because of possible harm from a policy or treatment. In the UK the Medical Research Council commissioned research into the **MMR vaccine** and autism because of public concerns about a possible link. A large case-control study (1,294 cases and 4,469 controls)[36] was mounted and published within four years — a timescale that would be impossible to achieve using other research designs. The rapid implementation of such a large study was facilitated by the availability of electronic data bases of family practitioner records. With increasing linkage of records across hospital and primary care, and enhanced inclusion of other data such as smoking and body mass index, electronic records permit the investigation of risk factors, co-morbidity and drug effects for relatively rare conditions. Large electronic records also permit the investigation of rare exposures in a case-control design (18,000 cases of AMD and 86,000 controls in a case-control study of complement associated diseases and risk of AMD).[37] Clearly, considerable care is required in the design and analysis of such studies, especially to address biases due to frequent consulters and missing information.

New methods in case-control design are being developed with the emergence of technologies which expand the opportunities to ask novel questions about disease aetiology. Geographical Information Systems (GIS) are used in spatial case-control studies to identify environmental risk factors by mapping the distribution of cases with that of controls. Case-control studies are the standard design in genetic association studies (see Chapter 6). Cost-effective platforms for genome-wide analysis make it possible to conduct the very large case-control studies that are required to detect even modest effects. Genetic epidemiology and traditional risk factor epidemiology are reintegrated in case-control studies investigating gene–environment interaction, likely to become the major area of future research using case-control or nested case-control study designs. In order to achieve the sample sizes required for gene–environment studies (from a few thousand to hundreds of thousands, dependent on allele frequency and size of effect)[38] collaborative studies with multiple investigators will be required. New study designs, such as the case-only design and population-based family

case-control studies, are also emerging to meet these challenges.[39] We are at the beginning of an exciting new era in the design and application of case-control studies.

REFERENCES

1. Paneth N, Susser E, Susser M. Origins and early development of the case-control study: Part 1, Early evolution. *Soz Praventivmed* 2002; 47:282–288.

2. Konstantopoulos A, Yadegarfar G, Elgohary M. Near-work, education, family history, and myopia in Greek conscripts. *Eye* 2008; 22:542–546.

3. Hyman LG, Lilienfeld AM, Ferris FL, 3rd, *et al*. Senile macular degeneration: a case-control study. *Am J Epidemiol* 1983; 118:213–227.

4. Pokhrel AK, Smith KR, Khalakdina A, *et al*. Case-control study of indoor cooking smoke exposure and cataract in Nepal and India. *Int J Epidemiol* 2005; 34:702–708.

5. Charliat G, Jolly D, Blanchard F. Genetic risk factor in primary open-angle glaucoma: a case-control study. *Ophthalmic Epidemiol* 1994; 1:131–138.

6. Leske MC, Warheit-Roberts L, Wu SY. Open-angle glaucoma and ocular hypertension: the Long Island Glaucoma Case-control Study. *Ophthalmic Epidemiol* 1996; 3:85–96.

7. Taylor JM. Choosing the number of controls in a matched case-control study, some sample size, power and efficiency considerations. *Stat Med* 1986; 5:29–36.

8. Bird AC, Bressler NM, Bressler SB, *et al*. An international classification and grading system for age-related maculopathy and age-related macular degeneration. The International ARM Epidemiological Study Group. *Surv Ophthalmol* 1995; 39:367–374.

9. Chylack LT, Jr., Wolfe JK, Singer DM, *et al*. The Lens Opacities Classification System III. The Longitudinal Study of Cataract Study Group. *Arch Ophthalmol* 1993; 111:831–836.

10. Topouzis F, Coleman AL, Harris A, *et al*. Factors associated with undiagnosed open-angle glaucoma: the Thessaloniki Eye Study. *Am J Ophthalmol* 2008; 145:327–335.

11. Chaine G, Hullo A, Sahel J, *et al*. Case-control study of the risk factors for age related macular

degeneration. France-DMLA Study Group. *Brit J Ophthalmol* 1998; 82:996–1002.

12. MacCarthy A, Bunch KJ, Fear NT, *et al*. Paternal occupation and retinoblastoma: a case-control study based on data for Great Britain 1962–1999. *Occup Environ Med* 2009; 66:644–649.

13. Risk factors for neovascular age-related macular degeneration. The Eye Disease Case-Control Study Group. *Arch Ophthalmol-chic* 1992; 110:1701–1708.

14. Bhatnagar R, West KP, Jr., Vitale S, *et al*. Risk of cataract and history of severe diarrheal disease in southern India. *Arch Ophthalmol* 1991; 109:696–699.

15. Krishnaiah S, Das T, Nirmalan PK, *et al*. Risk factors for age-related macular degeneration: findings from the Andhra Pradesh Eye Disease Study in South India. *Invest Ophthalmol Vis Sci* 2005; 46:4442–4449.

16. Nirmalan PK, Robin AL, Katz J, *et al*. Risk factors for age related cataract in a rural population of southern India: the Aravind Comprehensive Eye Study. *Brit J Ophthalmol* 2004; 88(8):989–994.

17. Tan GS, Wong TY, Fong CW, *et al*. Diabetes, metabolic abnormalities, and glaucoma: the Singapore Malay Eye Study. *Arch Ophthalmol* 2009; 127: 1354–1361.

18. Austin H, Flanders WD, Rothman KJ. Bias arising in case-control studies from selection of controls from overlapping groups. *Int J Epidemiol* 1989;18: 713–716.

19. Blumenkranz MS, Russell SR, Robey MG, *et al*. Risk factors in age-related maculopathy complicated by choroidal neovascularization. *Ophthalmology* 1986; 93:552–558.

20. Khan JC, Thurlby DA, Shahid H, *et al*. Smoking and age related macular degeneration: the number of pack years of cigarette smoking is a major determinant of risk for both geographic atrophy and choroidal neovascularisation. *Brit J Ophthalmol* 2006; 90:75–80.

21. AREDS. Risk factors associated with age-related macular degeneration. A case-control study in the Age-Related Eye Disease Study: Age-Related Eye Disease Study report number 3. Age-Related Eye Disease Study Research Group. *Ophthalmology* 2000; 107:2224–2232.

22. Hawkins BS. Selection of controls for clinical research studies in ophthalmology. *Arch Ophthalmol* 1988; 106:835–840.

23. Schmidt-Pokrzywniak A, Jockel KH, Bornfeld N, *et al*. Positive interaction between light iris color and ultraviolet radiation in relation to the risk of uveal melanoma: a case-control study. *Ophthalmology* 2009; 116:340–348.

24. Rothman KJ, Greenland S, Lash TL. *Modern Epidemiology*, 3rd Edition. Philadelphia: Wolters Kluwer Health/Lippincott Williams & Wilkins; 2008.

25. Mohan M, Sperduto RD, Angra SK, *et al*. India-US case-control study of age-related cataracts. India-US Case-Control Study Group. *Arch Ophthalmol* 1989; 107:670–676.

26. The Eye Disease Case-Control Study Group. Risk factors for neovascular age-related macular degeneration. *Arch Ophthalmol* 1992; 110: 1701–1708.

27. Fletcher AE, Bentham GC, Agnew M, *et al*. Sunlight exposure, antioxidants, and age-related macular degeneration. *Arch Ophthalmol* 2008; 126:1396–1403.

28. Witt N, Wong TY, Hughes AD, *et al*. Abnormalities of retinal microvascular structure and risk of mortality from ischemic heart disease and stroke. *Hypertension* 2006; 47:975–981.

29. Schaumberg DA, Ridker PM, Glynn RJ, *et al*. High levels of plasma C-reactive protein and future risk of age-related cataract. *Ann Epidemiol* 1999; 9:166–171.

30. Hosmer DW, Lemeshow S. *Applied Logistic Regression*, 2nd Edition. New York: Wiley; 2000.

31. Gotzsche PC. Believability of relative risks and odds ratios in abstracts: cross sectional study. *Brit Med J* 2006; 333:231–234.

32. Victora CG, Huttly SR, Fuchs SC, *et al*. The role of conceptual frameworks in epidemiological analysis: a hierarchical approach. *Int J Epidemiol* 1997; 26: 224–227.

33. Murdoch IE, Morris SS, Cousens SN. People and eyes: statistical approaches in ophthalmology. *Brit J Ophthalmol* 1998; 82:971–973.

34. Leske MC, Chylack LT, Jr., Wu SY. The Lens Opacities Case-Control Study. Risk factors for cataract. *Arch Ophthalmol* 1991; 109:244–251.

35. Vandenbroucke JP, Elm Ev, Altman DG, *et al*. Strengthening the Reporting of Observational Studies in Epidemiology (STROBE): Explanation and Elaboration. *Ann Intern Med* 2007; 147: 163–194.

36. Smeeth L, Cook C, Fombonne E, *et al.* MMR vaccination and pervasive developmental disorders: a case-control study. *Lancet* 2004; 364:963–969.

37. Nitsch D, Douglas I, Smeeth L, *et al.* Age-related macular degeneration and complement activation-related diseases: a population-based case-control study. *Ophthalmology* 2008; 115:1904–1910.

38. Luan JA, Wong MY, Day NE, *et al.* Sample size determination for studies of gene–environment interaction. *Int J Epidemiol* 2001; 30:1035–1040.

39. Dempfle A, Scherag A, Hein R, *et al.* Gene-environment interactions for complex traits: definitions, methodological requirements and challenges. *Eur J Hum Genet* 2008; 16:1164–1172.

Cohort studies

EMILY HERRETT AND HANNAH KUPER

5.1	What is a cohort study?	109	5.5	Alternatives to the traditional cohort design	115
5.2	Design	111			
5.3	Measuring the association between exposure and disease	113	5.6	Summary	115
			5.7	Research priorities	115
5.4	Strengths and weaknesses of a cohort design	114		References	116

5.1 WHAT IS A COHORT STUDY?

5.1.1 Introduction

This chapter provides an outline of the cohort study, a classic design that has been used since the 19th century. One of the first documented uses of the cohort design was by John Snow, who famously used it to discover the source of the 1854 cholera epidemic in London. Although the implementation of cohort studies has undergone vast improvement since the 1800s, the basic principles of the study have remained unchanged. In the past sixty years cohort studies have been used to make and check many important discoveries, particularly in non-communicable disease epidemiology. In ophthalmology, cohort studies are not yet widely used but some important examples, which have yielded valuable results, are described below.

5.1.2 Description

A cohort is a group of people, usually chosen on the basis of some common characteristic such as residence in a certain area, birth in a particular year or employment in an occupational group. The basic structure of a cohort study is shown in Fig. 5.1. It begins with a group of people who are free of the outcome of interest. Our disease-free group of people (our cohort) is then followed up over time. This means that as time passes we methodically re-assess whether the outcome of interest has occurred for each individual in the cohort. Outcomes in cohort studies are usually, but not always, specific diseases. For example, we may be interested in the progression or improvement in a condition over time (e.g. glaucoma). However, for simplicity's sake in this chapter we will refer to the outcome as a disease. We can use the findings from a cohort study to make an estimate of the incidence of disease in our group, i.e. the number of new cases that arise in our cohort during follow-up divided by either the number of people at risk (incidence) or by the person-time that has accrued (incidence rate) (these concepts are discussed in more depth in Chapter 2).

The main reason for carrying out a cohort study is to establish whether there is a link between an exposure (risk factor) and a disease. To do this we

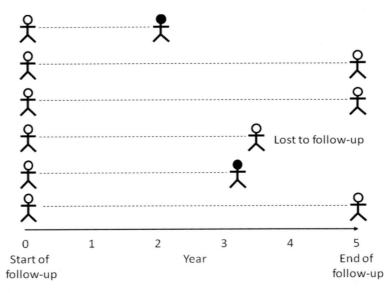

Lost to follow-up

0 1 2 3 4 5

Start of   Year   End of

follow-up   follow-up

Figure 5.1 *A simplified cohort study with five years of follow-up and six participants. At the start of the study, all participants are disease free (♀). Some participants develop the disease (♂) during follow-up, some are lost before follow-up ends and some are followed for the entire follow-up period*

would divide our cohort into a group that is 'exposed' and a group that is 'unexposed' to a risk factor of interest. Then we would compare the incidence of disease in the exposed group with that in the unexposed group. If the incidence was higher in the exposed group, then we would infer that there was a positive association between exposure and disease. This association may help us to understand the aetiology, or determinants, of the disease. The key measure of effect in a cohort study of this type is the **risk ratio**, **rate ratio**, or **relative risk** (**RR**) which measures the incidence of disease in those with the exposure compared with the incidence of disease in those without the exposure. This is discussed further below. Another reason for conducting a cohort study is to estimate the magnitude of disease incidence in our cohort. Once we know the extent of disease in the population, we can allocate appropriate resources, and plan public health interventions. For example, the incidence of cataract in a population will determine the cataract surgical rate needed.

The strength of the cohort design lies in the exclusion of people who already have the disease at baseline, that is, the prevalent cases. If we measure exposure at the start of the study, or during follow-up before the onset of disease, then we can investigate the temporal relationship between this exposure and the later onset of new 'incident' cases of disease that arise during follow-up. As we have measured exposure in a disease-free population we can be relatively certain that the measured exposure preceded, and therefore may predict, the disease. This is important because it avoids reverse causality, the situation in which the measured exposure is actually the result of disease or disease symptoms. It is this feature of cohort studies that makes the design so useful.

The Rotterdam Study is an example of a cohort study. The study participants for its ophthalmic component consisted of 6,872 people aged 55 years and over living in a suburb of Rotterdam.[1] Baseline examination occurred between March 1990 and July 1993 and included a home interview and a physical examination. The participants were then re-examined every 3–4 years to assess the occurrence of new disease. For one part of the study the outcome of interest was **primary open-angle glaucoma** (**POAG**), which meant that all participants with OAG at baseline were excluded from these analyses. The exposure of interest was diabetes. At baseline examination, all participants were defined as having diabetes (i.e. use of antidiabetic medication and/or a random or postload glucose value ≥11.1 mmol/l) or not. The participants also had their eyes examined at baseline and follow-up for the presence of OAG. The incidence of OAG during follow-up was then compared between those exposed (i.e. had diabetes) and those not exposed (i.e. not diabetic). After adjusting for age, sex and follow-up time there was no association between prevalent diabetes at baseline and the incidence of OAG during 6.5 years of follow-up (OR = 0.72, 95% CI 0.29–1.80).

Now we shall describe the cohort design in more detail.

5.2   DESIGN

5.2.1   Study population

The study population is defined as the group of people who are in the cohort. There are various ways of recruiting the study population, but typically one of three methods is used. First, studies can recruit using geographical location as a basis. For instance, members of the Salisbury Eye Evaluation and Driving Study were selected because they lived in the greater Salisbury metropolitan area, Wicomico County, USA[2] (or in Rotterdam in the study described above). Second, occupational cohorts, which recruit using as a basis employment in a particular occupation, such as the Nurses' Health Study in the United States in 1976,[3] or a French cohort of uranium processing workers.[4] Third, birth cohorts, which recruit all participants born in a certain period, for example the Millennium Cohort Study.[5]

The researchers must ensure that, once recruited to the study, the cohort participants are entirely free of the disease of interest at the start by excluding people who already have the disease or condition they are investigating (i.e. the prevalent cases). To do this, we take measurements at 'baseline' (i.e. at the start). For example, if we were conducting a study to measure the incidence of optic atrophy, our cohort members must be free of optic atrophy at baseline on examination. Only those without optic atrophy would be followed up. This ensures that during follow-up, we are only recording new incident cases.

5.2.2   Measurement of exposure

When talking about an 'exposure' in epidemiology, we mean anything that we suspect may be related to disease occurrence. This includes factors that we can control, such as smoking status or weight, and those that we cannot control, which may include our gender or ethnicity. We would normally concentrate on one main exposure of interest, but in many cases we may wish to measure and look at the effect of several exposures on disease occurrence.

If we are trying to estimate the effect of an exposure on disease occurrence, then we must measure exposure status at baseline. This can be undertaken in various ways, and investigators must choose the most efficient method to gather accurate exposure information given their available resources. For example, if we were interested in the risk factors for glaucoma, then we would consider biological measurements taken by trained study personnel to measure potential risk factors such as blood pressure or body weight. We might send questionnaires to participants to enquire about exposures such as smoking or marital status. Alternatives are genetic testing, measurement of environmental factors, or examination of medical records to look at medical history. The method depends on the type of exposure that we are interested in and on the available resources.

The cohort in the Australian Blue Mountains Eye Study consisted of 3,654 people aged 49–97 at baseline (1992–1994).[6] Eye conditions were assessed by taking a series of photographs of the eye, which were graded by specialists. Exposure information was collected by a variety of methods. Blood samples were taken and different biochemical levels were measured and genetic markers identified. Detailed questionnaires were completed about dietary intake as well as smoking and other exposures, and questions were asked about quality of life, memory and cognition and visual functioning.

Some exposures are simple to measure, and a participant can be classified only as exposed or unexposed (e.g. having diabetes or not). However, most exposures can occur at different levels, are long-lasting (chronic), or can change over time. This makes their measurement more complicated and allocation to crude 'exposed' or 'unexposed' groups is not ideal. For example, some people smoke five cigarettes per day while others smoke twenty or more per day, so it would be too simplistic to categorize them merely as 'smokers' as compared with 'non-smokers'. In order to get a better understanding of the way that smoking may be associated with the disease, we might measure smoking on a continuous scale, e.g. packs smoked per year, or else group people as 'light', 'moderate' or 'heavy' smokers. This 'continuum of exposure' is important because if we find that risk increases with increasing levels of exposure, then this is good evidence for our exposure being a determinant of disease.

Categorization of exposure according to its level at the start of follow-up is not always adequate because many exposures change over time. In studies with long follow-up duration it might be necessary to measure these changes in exposure over time. For example, in a study of OAG and caffeine consumption,[7] a first assessment of caffeine intake was made at baseline, and this was repeated up to six times during follow-up (up to 24 years).

We might also wish to investigate a 'special' exposure. By this we mean an exposure that is unique to a certain group of people. The most common example is a group of factory workers exposed to some chemical or radioactive agent, which the general population is rarely exposed to in large quantities, but that may relate to disease occurrence. The disease experience of a highly exposed cohort can show the risks of that particular exposure, which helps us to understand how the exposure might affect the general population at lower doses or smaller quantities. As an example, a cohort was constructed of US radiologic technologists (radiology technicians) to assess the risk of cataract after exposure to low doses of ionizing radiation.[8] A total of 35,705 cataract-free radiologic technologists aged 24–44 years were followed up for over 20 years (1983–2004). There was a small and non-significant increased risk of cataract in workers in the highest category (mean, 60 mGy) versus lowest category (mean, 5 mGy) of occupational dose to the lens of the eye, with an adjusted relative risk of 1.18 (0.99, 1.40). This result implies that few cases of cataract in the general population are likely to be attributable to X-ray exposure.

5.2.3   Follow-up

Follow-up, as described above, is the period of time during which we observe the cohort subjects and record disease occurrence. The duration of follow-up is important because it determines how many cases we will accumulate; follow-up for five years will inevitably lead to fewer cases than follow-up for ten years. In order to get an accurate picture of the effect of exposure on disease occurrence, it is best to accumulate as many cases as possible. Given unlimited resources we would therefore follow our cohort for many years. However, the need for maximum numbers of cases must be balanced with the feasibility of following the cohort for long periods of time and the resources available. It is costly to follow a cohort, and often investigators are keen to analyze the data and produce results quickly.

A major problem in cohort studies is keeping track of all cohort members for the duration of follow-up. Participants might change their name or migrate to new towns or even countries, making it difficult to ascertain their disease status. Attempts to trace such people are time-consuming and costly. When they can no longer be traced or are unwilling to continue participating in the study, they are termed 'lost to follow-up'. The chances of this happening increase with time, and so longer follow-up increases the number of people 'lost'. People may also be lost due to death.

Loss to follow-up can be a problem in the interpretation of the results. If those who are lost are more likely (or less likely) to have developed the disease than those who remain in the cohort, then this could introduce **bias** in our estimate of incidence. For example, if those lost were more likely to develop the disease, then we would underestimate the incidence of disease in our cohort. Of even greater concern is when loss to follow-up is higher in the exposed group compared with the unexposed group (see Section 5.4.2 below). For these reasons investigators make great efforts to maximize the follow-up of their cohort participants.

5.2.4 Outcome definition

Outcomes in cohort studies are usually diseases but could be any change in status that we believe to be associated with the exposure, such as disease progression, disease improvement or occurrence of surgical procedures.

As with the measurement of exposure, the method used for outcome ascertainment will be determined by cost and feasibility. Ideally, diseases would be measured by examination or interview of all cohort members at regular intervals throughout follow-up. However, this is costly and with a large cohort may not be possible. A cheaper and more efficient alternative might be to send each participant a postal questionnaire. This relies on self-reporting of disease, and also on participants responding to requests for information, both of which can introduce bias. An alternative to these time-consuming methods could be to use a disease register (e.g. General Practice Research Database) whereby investigators track occurrence of disease during follow-up through medical records without having to contact individual cohort participants. This depends on the outcome of interest being recorded in a disease register, which is not possible for many eye outcomes.

In the case of research into age-related macular disease (AMD) each of these methods has been used. In the Blue Mountains Eye Study AMD was assessed by repeated examination of participants.[6] In the Nurses' Health Study cases with AMD were identified by self-report in the questionnaire, and were validated from the medical records.[9] Incident cases with AMD can also be identified from the **General Practice Research Database (GPRD)** in the UK.[10]

Outcomes must be clearly defined so that we can accurately record when a member of the cohort becomes a case. For some outcomes, such as acute infections, it might be relatively easy to define this point, for instance, by the date of symptom onset. However, the definition is not always so straightforward. For example, some diseases occur on a continuous scale, such as cataracts, where at the lower end of the scale there is very little visual impairment. Therefore a decision must be made about what level of cataract we call a case in our cohort. This leads some investigators to use a more distinct outcome, such as occurrence of cataract surgery or cataract with a certain level of visual impairment, rather than assigning a cut-off in the cataract spectrum itself. In these situations, when diseases progress slowly from early, relatively symptom-free stages to more debilitating later stages, it is also difficult to assign a date of disease onset.

5.3 MEASURING THE ASSOCIATION BETWEEN EXPOSURE AND DISEASE

The analysis of a cohort study involves calculation of either the **cumulative incidence** or **incidence rate**. As mentioned above, when we are looking at the effect of an exposure on a disease, then risks or rates are calculated separately for the exposed and unexposed groups. We then use these estimates to calculate either risk ratios or rate ratios. These ratios give us an idea of how the exposure and the disease are related. Complex statistical modeling called survival analysis is often used to generate risk ratios or rate ratios for cohort study data, and also their 95% confidence intervals and p values.

When we are generating risk ratios or rate ratios, it is very important (as with any other observational study) to allow for **confounders**. Confounders are factors related to both exposure and outcome, and if we do not consider their effect in the analysis, our estimate of risk or rate could be misleading (see also Chapter 4, Section 4.4.2). In order to allow for these confounders, they must have been measured accurately at baseline. It is therefore important to consider, when initiating a cohort study, which confounders of the exposure–disease relationship might be important. Statistical models enable us to allow for confounders, provided they have been measured, and we can add them to the model along with our exposure and outcome variables. Age and sex are typical confounders and we would expect these to be accounted for in most studies.

The Beaver Dam Eye Study (BDES) investigated the association between statin use and development of nuclear cataract.[11] Among 1,299 participants in the cohort, 210 developed nuclear cataract during five years of follow-up to give a cumulative incidence (risk) of nuclear cataract of 16.2% over five years. The risk of nuclear cataract was lower among statin users (12.2%) compared with people not using statins (17.2%). This gives a risk ratio of 0.71 (95% confidence interval 0.50–1.00) for the association between statin use and risk of nuclear cataract. This association strengthened slightly after adjustment for age, sex, total cholesterol, **HDL** cholesterol, smoking and diabetes suggesting that statin use may protect from the development of nuclear cataract. Meanwhile, no association was apparent between statin use and incidence of cortical or posterior subcapsular cataract.

Unlike confounding, bias cannot be allowed for at the analysis stage in most circumstances. Bias can arise with loss to follow-up or measurement of outcome (see Section 5.4.2) and can produce an incorrect effect measure for the association between exposure and outcome (see Chapter 2). As we cannot deal with bias during the analysis, it is essential that we create measures to avoid bias when designing the study. Reducing bias means that we need to be careful to have selected our participants appropriately and tried to maximize follow-up (to avoid selection bias); we would also have collected the information from participants as accurately as possible (to avoid information bias).

Assuming that we have minimized bias and have controlled for all known confounders, we can interpret the risk or rate ratio generated by our statistical model. For example, a risk ratio of 3.5 tells us that those exposed to the risk factor are 3.5 times more likely to develop disease compared with those who are not exposed during follow-up. This tells us that the exposure is harmful. In order to assess the play of chance in our estimates, we would use 95% confidence intervals and the results of statistical tests to measure the strength of evidence for an effect of the exposure on the disease.

5.4 STRENGTHS AND WEAKNESSES OF A COHORT DESIGN

5.4.1 Strengths

A key strength of cohort studies is that exposure is assessed before the occurrence of disease, which gives us confidence that the exposure preceded the disease. Another main strength of cohort studies, compared with other observational studies, is that they can be used in connection with rare exposures. We can select a cohort of individuals with that rare exposure, thus gaining a good understanding of the incidence of disease associated with it (e.g. through an occupational cohort). In a case-control study, it would be very difficult to ascertain the effect of a rare exposure because very few of the cases would have been exposed. We can also investigate multiple outcomes in a cohort study. Again, in a case-control study, we can only investigate one outcome (our case definition), but if we were concerned that an exposure was causing several outcomes, then a cohort study would be well-placed to research this question by measuring the occurrence of several diseases during follow-up.

5.4.2 Weaknesses

While cohort studies have some important strengths, they are not appropriate for every study question. They are less useful when looking at rare diseases. For example, investigating the risk factors for childhood blindness would be extremely difficult using a cohort study, as it is such a rare condition that we would have to start with an enormous cohort of children in order to be sure of a reasonable number of outcomes. In this example, a case-control study might be more appropriate (as it is suited to the study of rare diseases).

A second weakness is the time and cost involved in follow-up. For example, the Nurses' Health Study has been running for over 30 years and now has a total of 236,000 participants. Follow-up of these nurses has involved considerable cost and effort. Time and cost can be a particular problem for birth cohorts, as we must often wait several years (or even several decades) for any outcomes to be ascertained as the participants grow older. As described above, a long duration of follow-up means that more participants are lost, and more resources are required to retain them in the cohort.

Loss to follow-up, discussed above, is often a major problem in cohort studies because we do not always know why the participants are lost. Even a well-designed study can be subject to a large loss to follow-up, thus making the results difficult to interpret. Loss to follow-up can cause bias in our estimate of the risk ratio or rate ratio if loss is related either to exposure or to outcome. Once participants are lost, we cannot determine whether their loss is related to exposure or outcome, so it is essential to develop mechanisms at the design stage that help to avoid this loss.

Many ophthalmological cohort studies are small because the most reliable information regarding eye disease is gained through physical examination of patients; on a large scale this can be costly. A small number of cases can limit the power of the analysis, which means that we may not have the ability to uncover a potential association between exposure and disease.

5.5 ALTERNATIVES TO THE TRADITIONAL COHORT DESIGN

Throughout this chapter, we have discussed the most typical kind of cohort study, which is initiated in the present; participants' baseline status is measured and then the cohort is followed up into the future. However, it may be more practical and efficient to carry out a *historical cohort study*. This means that we use exposure data *collected in the past* to define the cohort, e.g. old employment records documenting a particular occupational hazard, or birth-weight data. After the cohort participants have been chosen based on these historical exposure records, the study investigators track them, for instance through further employment records or disease registers or medical records, to ascertain their outcomes over time. This eliminates the inherent problem in cohort studies of waiting for years of follow-up to accrue. Although historical cohorts are rare in ophthalmology, there are a few notable examples. A historical cohort study was constructed including as participants people who had survived retinoblastoma (exposure) and assessing the occurrence of secondary malignancies (outcome).[12] The investigators identified from a registry cases of retinoblastoma that were diagnosed between 1945 and 2005. The register also included reports of additional cancers that occurred in these people at a later time. The median follow-up time in the registry data

was 21.9 years and this allowed the investigators to calculate the risk of second malignancies in patients with past retinoblastoma. This cohort study was historical rather than *prospective*, as all the exposure and outcome events had occurred before the investigators assembled the cohort.

Nested case-control studies are another extension of the cohort design, and are often useful to reduce the cost of the study. Here we choose all cases that occur in our cohort and a random sample of disease-free controls from the cohort, and examine these cases and controls in more detail. We are then certain that the controls are representative of the population from which the cases arose, and we have access to prospectively collected data on our cases and controls. This may be particularly relevant if detailed examination of all cohort members is costly (e.g. the need to examine medical records or perform expensive biochemical tests), making it more efficient to limit the examination to a sample of the cohort.

5.6 SUMMARY

Cohort studies are observational, and allow us to gain an understanding of the temporal relationship between an exposure and an outcome. The prospective nature of data collection is one of the main strengths of the cohort design. Cohort studies are particularly useful for investigating the effects of rare exposures or for researching multiple outcomes. However, the costs of following up a group of people for several years can be great, and care must be taken in avoiding the effects of bias and confounding in our effect estimate. While there are relatively few cohort studies specifically designed to look at ophthalmologic outcomes, a number of large cohort studies have addressed various ophthalmological outcomes.

5.7 RESEARCH PRIORITIES

There are currently few cohorts in ophthalmological research in high-income countries, but none in lower- or middle-income countries. Developing new studies would aid our understanding and could help us to address the changing burden of ophthalmological disease, particularly in these settings. Large medical databases, such as the UK's GPRD, present an excellent opportunity to study many ophthalmological outcomes. For example, the GPRD has yielded valuable research into age-related macular degeneration,[13] cataract,[14] childhood retinoblastoma[15] and glaucoma.[16] A further priority for research is the use of gene technologies; as these become cheaper and more readily available, future cohort studies should consider assessing genetic risk factors and gene–environment interactions.

REFERENCES

1. de Voogd S, Ikram MK, Wolfs RC, *et al*. Is diabetes mellitus a risk factor for open-angle glaucoma? The Rotterdam Study. *Ophthalmology*, 2006; 113: 1827–1831.

2. Valbuena M, Bandeen-Roche K, Rubin GS, *et al*. Self-reported assessment of visual function in a population-based study: the SEE project. Salisbury Eye Evaluation. *Invest Ophthalmol Vis Sci* 1999; 40:280–288.

3. Belanger, CF, Hennekens CH, Rosner B, *et al*. The nurses' health study. *Am J Nurs* 1978; 78: 1039–1040.

4. Guseva Canu I, Cardis E, Metz-Flamant C, *et al*. French cohort of the uranium processing workers: mortality pattern after 30-year follow-up. *Int Arch Occ Env Hea* 2010; 83:301–308.

5. Smith K, Joshi H. The Millennium Cohort Study. *Popul Trends* 2002; 107:30–34.

6. Tan JS, Wang JJ, Flood V, *et al*. Dietary antioxidants and the long-term incidence of age-related macular degeneration: the Blue Mountains Eye Study. *Ophthalmology* 2008; 115:334–341.

7. Kang JH, Willett WC, Rosner BA, *et al*. Caffeine consumption and the risk of primary open-angle glaucoma: a prospective cohort study. *Invest Ophthalmol Vis Sci* 2008; 49:1924–1931.

8. Chodick G, Bekiroglu N, Hauptmann M, *et al*. Risk of cataract after exposure to low doses of ionizing radiation: a 20-year prospective cohort study among US radiologic technologists. *Am J Epidemiol* 2008; 168:620–631.

9. Schaumberg DA, Hankinson SE, Guo Q, *et al*. A prospective study of 2 major age-related macular degeneration susceptibility alleles and interactions with modifiable risk factors. *Arch Ophthalmol* 2007; 125:55–62.

10. Nitsch D, Douglas I, Smeeth L, *et al*. Age-related macular degeneration and complement activation-related diseases: a population-based case-control study. *Ophthalmology* 2008; 115:1904–1910.

11. Klein BE, Klein R, Lee KE, *et al*. Statin use and incident nuclear cataract. *JAMA* 2006; 295:2752–2758.

12. Marees T, Moll AC, Imhof SM, *et al*. Risk of second malignancies in survivors of retinoblastoma: more than 40 years of follow-up. *J Natl Cancer Inst* 2008; 100:1771–1779.

13. Douglas IJ, Cook C, Chakravarthy U, *et al*. A case-control study of drug risk factors for age-related macular degeneration. *Ophthalmology* 2007; 114: 1164–1169.

14. Aina FO, Smeeth L, Hubbard R, *et al*. Hormone replacement therapy and cataract: a population-based case-control study. *Eye (Lond)* 2006; 20: 417–422.

15. Bradbury BD, Jick H. *In vitro* fertilization and childhood retinoblastoma. *Br J Clin Pharmacol* 2004; 58:209–211.

16. Zhou Z, Althin R, Sforzolini BS, *et al*. Persistency and treatment failure in newly diagnosed open angle glaucoma patients in the United Kingdom. *Br J Ophthalmol* 2004; 88:1391–1394.

Genetic epidemiology

CHRISTOPHER HAMMOND

6.1	Definition	117	6.4	Genetic epidemiology of eye diseases	126
6.2	History	117	6.5	Future developments	128
6.3	Methods	119		References	128

6.1 DEFINITION

Genetic epidemiology is a relatively new discipline, combining the elements of molecular biological techniques with the study of defined populations to ascertain the relative importance of genes and environment in the biology of disease as well as interactions between them. It has been defined as the study of the aetiology, distribution and control of disease in groups of relatives and of inherited causes of disease in populations. Perhaps a simpler definition may be that it is the study of the role of genetic factors and their interaction with environmental factors in the occurrence of disease in human populations.[1] The role of genetic epidemiology is to resolve the genetic architecture of a disease — first to define whether there is a genetic component, how large it is, and subsequently to identify specific genes involved in the aetiology, and their interaction with the environment. Many readers of this chapter may be unfamiliar with some of the genetic terminology used. The terms in bold refer to terms in the glossary at the end of this book.

The interaction between genes and environment may be complex. Mutations in genetic material (e.g. **deoxyribonucleic acid** (**DNA**), chromosome) result in an abnormal **genotype**, and this, in turn, may result in a disease **phenotype**. The environment can interact with this genetic model of disease at any stage. While many mutations are transmitted from generation to generation, the environment (in the form of ionizing radiation, for example) may cause a mutation. However, it may also interact with the genotype, and specific exposure to a certain environmental agent in the presence of a particular genotype might increase the risk of a disease phenotype (a well-known example is the combination of α-antitrypsin deficiency and smoking resulting in emphysema). There is also the traditional epidemiologic model of environmental exposure influencing the phenotype directly in a causal relationship. In addition, it is possible to have gene–gene interactions as well as gene–environment interactions.

6.2 HISTORY

The rapprochement between geneticists and epidemiologists gradually evolved as each group realized the importance of the other to the planning and design of studies as well as the relative importance of both to the overall picture of disease. The first account of 'genetics and epidemiology' was provided by Neel and Schull (1954),[2] and the first use of the term 'genetic epidemiology' seems to have been by Morton and Chung in 1978.[3] Since then there have been numerous books and articles on the subject, such as that by Khoury *et al.*, a standard text.[1]

Research into disease aetiology has been dominated in recent years by genetic research. In 1865 the Austrian monk Gregor Mendel overturned the then current theory of heredity, which was attributed to blending of parents' inherited contributions, and introduced the concept of particulate inheritance (the gene) and the rules of segregation. Molecular methods have been successfully used to identify many Mendelian diseases in ophthalmology, and while these diseases can be very damaging, most are rare and, collectively, affect only a small percentage of the population. What about the common eye diseases such as cataract and age-related macular degeneration (AMD)? It has been estimated that the lifetime risk of a genetically influenced, multifactorial disorder in Western populations is up to 60%.

The publication of the human genetic code via the Human Genome Project raised great hopes of the identification of genes involved in disease. However, the genetics of eye disease has yet to affect the majority of patients significantly. This is because most of the conditions seen are not the result of a single genetic change, which follows Mendelian inheritance, but are complex and have a multifactorial aetiology (and are therefore known as complex or multifactorial diseases). Ronald Fisher's seminal paper describing 'polygenic' inheritance was published in 1918, and recognized that the expression of many phenotypes is the result of interaction between many complex biological processes.[4] Many genes, each with **allelic** variations, contribute to the observed variability, and the phenotype results from the sum total of all the effects of contributing loci. The difficulties in the identification of susceptibility and disease-causing genes and their relative importance are legion, and there has been an explosion of statistical methods attempting to uncover the relative importance of these genetic effects. In this context, the traditional epidemiological concerns of the validity of the population under study and of selection and other biases are vital to establishing the complete picture

of disease (see also Chapters 2 and 4). It is very important, given the large geographical and temporal variation in the occurrence of many diseases, that the contexts of family and population studies are taken into account.

Once the genetics of a disease have been understood at the molecular level, the central question is to relate these changes to clinical findings or phenotypes. Theoretically, monogenic diseases (with strict Mendelian inheritance) should be the simplest to study. Numerous mutations have been identified to account for retinitis pigmentosa, but even within families with a single known mutation there is considerable phenotypic variation. Some family members are more affected than others, while yet others may be unaffected, despite the presence of a known disease-causing mutation. This **genetic heterogeneity**, both in the number of genetic mutations causing a similar phenotypic picture, and in the variation in severity of disease in individuals with the same genetic defect, currently makes it very difficult to predict outcomes in patients with a known mutation. In addition, there are many cases of retinitis pigmentosa with no apparent family history (simplex cases), suggesting that non-genetic factors may also cause the disease (known as phenocopies), although some could be caused by new mutations.

There must be other genetic and environmental determinants influencing disease status in single-gene disorders, and one of the challenges of genetic epidemiology is to clarify these determinants. The situation becomes even more complicated when considering the complex or multifactorial diseases, in which many genetic **polymorphisms** may be affecting a single phenotype.

It can therefore be seen that identification of all the genes involved in disease courtesy of the Human Genome Project will not provide all the answers to aetiology of disease. Genetic epidemiologists will be required to interpret how susceptibility genes confer risk, and how they interact with the environment. There will be both gene–environment and gene–gene interaction (**epistasis**). This relation of genotype to phenotype is the challenge for genetic epidemiology in this century, and progress is likely to be slow.

6.3   METHODS

Genetic epidemiological studies are designed to ask four questions regarding a disease or trait.

1. Is there familial aggregation?
2. Is familial clustering the consequence of shared environmental factors, biologically inherited susceptibility, or cultural inheritance of risk factors?
3. What is the genetic model of inheritance?
4. Can disease-causing or susceptibility genes be identified?

6.3.1   Is there familial aggregation?

Traditional epidemiological methods can be used to ascertain whether there is familial aggregation, either by looking at disease frequency in relatives of cases and controls, or by comparing disease frequency in relatives of cases with the frequency in the general population and computing some measure of relative risk. However, not all diseases that aggregate in a family are the result of shared genetic risk; infectious diseases, for example, are well known to cluster within families. Some single-gene disorders also give low relative risks at certain gene frequencies, particularly where there is incomplete penetrance and unaffected controls still carry the disease genotype; for example, the penetrance of the retinoblastoma gene is 90%, which means that some **heterozygotes** may not develop a tumour, but will still pass the mutant allele on to their offspring.

6.3.2   Is familial clustering the result of shared genes or shared environment?

Epidemiologic approach

The second question as to whether familial clustering is the result of shared genes or shared environment can be answered using both genetic and epidemiologic approaches, applying to both qualitative and quantitative traits. Epidemiological methods, for example, can be used to establish whether the familial aggregation has a non-genetic basis, such as clustering by calendar year versus age of onset, birth order or migration studies.

Genetic approach

Genetic methods can at the same time attempt to answer the second and third questions concerning the genetic model of inheritance and whether disease-causing or susceptibility genes can be identified, and this is discussed in the next section.

6.3.3   What is the genetic model of inheritance?

Genetic methods use either segregation analysis or multifactorial models as a common framework. These models use statistical methods of analysis of variance and path analysis to infer the degree of genetic control in both quantitative traits (such as the degree of myopia or cataract) and qualitative traits (such as presence or absence of a disease). Quantitative traits are relatively easy to analyze, as there is a continuous distribution, often transformed into as near a normal distribution as possible. Qualitative traits are more difficult to process, but can be analyzed by assuming that in a population there is an underlying continuous liability to disease, and once a certain threshold has been reached then disease is present (Fig. 6.1). The

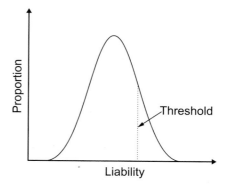

Figure 6.1 *For quantitative analysis of multifactorial diseases that can only be classified as present or absent, an underlying liability is assumed, with a normal distribution. Once a certain threshold in liability has been reached, then the disease phenotype is present.*

multifactorial model, in which the phenotype is a linear result of latent genetic and environmental factors, only allows estimation of the amount of genetic influence, but not of how many genes or which biological mechanisms are involved. These methods will be discussed further.

Segregation analysis

Segregation analysis was originally designed to test whether an observed mixture of phenotypes among offspring is compatible with Mendelian inheritance. Although largely used for sibling relationships, it can be widened to encompass more general models with pedigrees of arbitrary structure, when it is known as *complex segregation analysis*.[5] It tests explicit models of inheritance and non-genetic models on family data, selecting the model that best fits the data. In this respect it differs from the traditional epidemiological null hypothesis, where the statistical evaluation is designed to reject the null hypothesis in a 'badness-of-fit' as opposed to a 'goodness-of-fit' test. This results in a slightly different interpretation of type I and type II errors.

A criticism of model-fitting techniques such as segregation analysis is that they choose the best-fit model, even if that model fits poorly. For many complex eye diseases (with the probable exception of AMD), predictions of genes with major effects on the population for diseases such as cataract and glaucoma have not been upheld. Most genetic epidemiologists believe that there are many polymorphisms on many genes, or many significant rare mutations, each of possible major importance for the affected individual, but no single major gene responsible for the chronic, common diseases of ageing. In a disease such as retinitis pigmentosa, where a high ascertainment rate has led to efficient genetic dissection, there is a huge diversity because of both allelic and non-allelic variation. Less than one third of cases are caused by more than 600 mostly rare disease alleles at more than 55 loci. Complex diseases may be even more diverse.

Variance components analysis

The primary statistical tool used in quantitative genetics is analysis of **variance**, where the underlying assumption is a model where the phenotype is a linear function of unobserved genetic and environmental factors. That is, the variation of a trait in the population is the result of genetic and environmental factors, and the effect of each is added up for an individual to create the final measure, the phenotype. Covariances or correlations among relatives are used to partition the phenotypic variance between genetic and non-genetic factors.[6]

The observed phenotypic variance of a population (V_P) can be separated into the variance resulting from genetic and environmental components. Additive genetic variance (V_A) is the variance that results from the additive effects of alleles at each contributing locus (e.g. the **homozygous** AA might cause cataract, and aa might protect from cataract, with the heterozygote Aa in between). Dominance genetic variance (V_D) is the variance that results from the non-additive effects of two alleles at the same locus summed over all loci that contribute to the variance of the trait (in dominantly inherited conditions both AA and Aa genotypes might cause cataract, and aa might protect, so the two alleles are non-additive). Note that the analysis at no point specifies how many additive or non-additive genes are involved; as is likely in multifactorial diseases, there are probably many genes contributing to the phenotype. Shared (common) environmental variance (V_C) is the variance that results from environmental events shared by both members of a family pair (e.g. rearing, school, neighbourhood, diet). Specific (unique) environmental variance (V_E) is the variance that results from environmental effects that are not shared by family members under study and also includes measurement error. Expressing it as an equation,

$$V_P = V_A + V_D + V_C + V_E.$$

Heritability can be defined in the broad sense as the ratio of variance caused by all genetic differences among individuals relative to the total phenotypic variance. Heritability in the narrow sense is the ratio of variance contributed by the additive effects of alleles at one or more loci to the total phenotypic variance. These contributions are often reported as the standardized form, when the specific variance component is divided by the total phenotypic variance (e.g. $h^2 = V_A/V_P$, where h^2 is the narrow-sense heritability).

Maximum likelihood techniques are used to estimate the components of variance. The goal is to obtain those values of the parameters which maximize the probability of the observed data. To employ these methods, the underlying distribution for the phenotype in families must be specified, and the multivariate normal distribution is chosen to represent quantitative traits, and the normal underlying liability with threshold model used in qualitative traits (Fig. 6.1). While these are chosen with theoretical justification, nonetheless they must be recognized as arbitrary. Maximum likelihood techniques can then be used to construct a series of hierarchical models, which are then compared with a likelihood ratio test (which follows a χ^2 distribution) to select the model that fits the data most efficiently (the most parsimonious model).

Path analysis

Path analysis is an alternative approach to classic variance components modelling, but is based on the same linear model of additive genetic and environmental factors summed up to represent the final phenotype. Path analysis (or structural equation modelling) involves solving a series of simultaneous structural equations in order to estimate genetic and environmental parameters that best fit the observed family variances and covariances. It is more flexible than variance component analysis, in that covariates such as the effect of age can be introduced, and data from other family members, multiple variables and even multiple time points can be incorporated.

Family studies always involve intrinsic differences in the age and sex of relatives, and these are frequently important covariates in the common diseases of ageing. An approach to this problem is the 'family set' approach where fixed sets of relatives, all within a specified age range, are sampled and stratified by major covariates of interest. In addition, nature has provided a perfect natural experiment to control for age and sex differences, namely twins.

Twin and sib-pair studies

Monozygotic (MZ) twins share 100% of their genes, while **dizygotic (DZ)** twins share, on average, 50%

of their segregating genes. They are obviously the same age, and same-sex twins can be studied. They are usually brought up in the same environment. Therefore any greater similarity between MZ twins than DZ twins is explained as being caused by these genetic effects, assuming equal environmental influences (this major assumption of the twin model, controversial in the behavioural and social sciences, has been tested and found generally to be true[7]). In the classic method, the difference between intra-class correlations for MZ twins and those for DZ twins is doubled to estimate the heritability: this is known as the Falconer formula.[8] The remaining population variance can then be attributed to environmental effects. These estimates have low power and large standard errors and do not make use of the information available using variance component analysis and covariances. Possibly the first twin study of any disease recognising this difference related to myopia, and was published by Jablonski in 1922.[9]

In recent years, model fitting has become standard in twin research.[6] Care is required in selection of twins to avoid falsely high levels of concordance because of dual ascertainment of affected twin pairs. The MZ twins tend to be more concordant for 'environmental' risk factors, such as smoking, than DZ twins, implying a genetic component for these habits (not surprisingly, as addictive behaviour and a cellular response to nicotine and other agents may well be genetic). Therefore the 'genetic' component of diseases may include a host of factors, including behavioural and other genetic predispositions to potential environmental exposures.

Adoption studies

Another tool to examine whether there is a significant genetic effect is the adoption study: twins separated at birth and reared in different environments. This means the equal environment assumption of the classic twin study is not required. If there is greater concordance for MZ and DZ twins reared apart than for unrelated individuals, and this concordance is greater in MZ than DZ twins, a genetic aetiology is suggested. These adoption studies, however, are rare as there are few twin pairs separated at birth or shortly after.

6.3.4 How can genetic mutations be identified?

Statistical gene-mapping methods all rest on one biological phenomenon, which is **recombination** (crossing-over of chromosomes during meiosis). Loci in close proximity to each other will rarely be separated by recombination, but the farther apart two loci are, the more likely they are to be separated. The recombination fraction is therefore a measure of the genetic distance between two loci. The different methods are outlined below, and summarized in Table 6.1.

Linkage analysis

Genetic maps of the whole human chromosome have been created using DNA polymorphisms, which are known as marker loci as they lack functional significance. The most straightforward way of localizing a simple Mendelian disease gene is to investigate **haplotypes** (sequences of alleles at different loci transmitted from parent to offspring) in family pedigrees to establish which marker loci the disease gene lies near, based on the amount of recombination between the two (if the disease gene and the marker are always transmitted together, they are likely to lie close to each other on the genome map). This is known as **linkage analysis**.[10] The disease locus is usually identified using computation of maximum likelihood scores across the gene map, so-called **log of the odds (LOD)** scores. The LOD score, Z, introduced by Morton in 1955,[11] is the decimal logarithm of the likelihood ratio (or odds) that the loci are linked (with recombination fraction θ) rather than unlinked (recombination fraction 0.5). Peaks on the LOD score curve that exceed a threshold identify potential locations of disease genes (see box below). The newest marker is the **single-nucleotide polymorphism (SNP),** of which many thousands have been identified, to allow for dense-mapping of the human chromosome — in effect gene loci can be even more finely tuned. Linkage analysis is used for whole genome-wide scans.

Allele-sharing methods

Non-parametric methods are required when the mode of trait inheritance is not known, as is often

Table 6.1 *Comparison of methods in genetic epidemiology studies*

	Linkage analysis	Allele sharing methods	Candidate gene association studies	Genome-wide association studies
Study population	Families	Related cases	Unrelated cases compared with unrelated controls from a general population	Unrelated cases and controls, or quantitative trait collected in the general population
Scope of method	Identification of loci or genes causing disease by positional cloning	Applicable as linkage analysis or an association study	Contribution of mutations in candidate genes to the disease	Whole-genome common variants for common disease
A priori knowledge	Inheritance pattern	Non-parametric	Non-parametric	Non-parametric
Genetic mechanism	Monogenic to oligogenic	Monogenic to multifactorial	Multifactorial	Multifactorial
Disadvantage	No direct conclusions to general population. Families with enough meiosis required	No direct conclusions to general population. Many sib pairs and markers needed for genome screen	Not appropriate for genomic screening. Only applicable if candidate genes known	Large-scale studies required. Only common variants detected
Advantage	Very robust method for Medelian inheritance. Applicable in genetic isolates. Applicable for genomic screen	Sib pairs are easier to ascertain than families. Applicable in genetic isolates	Data collection relatively easy. Direct conclusions for general population	Agnostic approach. Direct conclusions for general population

the case with complex or multifactorial disease. Allele-sharing methods can rely on the known mode of marker inheritance, and not that of the disease, and estimate allele sharing. Results can be represented in the form of LOD scores, in a similar fashion to the parametric method.

> LOD scores are the statistical measure of the evidence for linkage. If two loci (those of the gene causing a disease [or trait] and the marker) are not linked, we would expect 50% recombinants to be formed from meioses, a recombination fraction of 0.5. It follows that all LOD scores are zero at $\theta = 0.5$ because they are then measuring the ratio of two identical probabilities, and $\log_{10}(1) = 0$. It is difficult to extract linkage information from many families because of their small size or because markers are not fully informative. However, as the overall probability of linkage in a set of families is the product of the probabilities in each individual family, the LOD scores (being logarithms) can be added up across families to achieve statistical significance.
>
> What is a significant LOD score? Obviously, there is a prior probability that two loci may be linked by chance (much debated, but probably 1 in 50). A traditional threshold LOD score used as strong evidence of linkage is 3, which corresponds to 1000:1 odds for linkage, which equates to a 5% chance of error. Linkage can be rejected if $Z < -2.0$, and figures between −2 and +3 are inconclusive. Clearly, issues surrounding multiple testing must be taken into account during analysis.
>
> As an example of calculation of LOD scores in ophthalmology, a locus for autosomal dominant familial exudative vitreoretinopathy has been mapped to chromosome 11p12–13. Statistically significant linkage was achieved, with a maximal LOD score of 6.6 at one particular marker, D11S2010.

Association studies (linkage disequilibrium)

Linkage analysis, which looks at loci of disease genes (and not any particular alleles, as there are many alleles involved at each marker locus), is restricted to family studies to examine recombinations. When populations are studied, genotype frequencies within the population are determined by allele frequencies, and this is referred to as **Hardy–Weinberg equilibrium**; for example, genotypes of marker loci are usually in this equilibrium, and this is used as a test of technical reliability in genetics laboratories. However, if a disease is associated with a particular allele more than expected by these frequencies, then there is **linkage disequilibrium (LD),** or allelic association. Consider a case-control study. If allele frequency between cases and controls is different, then there may be linkage between the allele and disease gene. It is always important to have cases and controls from the same population in relation to race and population ethnic origin, as population admixture may cause different allele frequencies, giving a false-positive association. In the past, a specific allele needed to be examined, such as a candidate gene, as the technology was unavailable to examine the whole genome.

Family controls may also be used in LD studies to test association, and the typical family structure for these types of analyses is a family 'trio' consisting of two parents and an affected offspring, to establish the transmission of an allele being studied. Special analytical methods have been developed for these studies, which offer the combination of a linkage study in the presence of association using multiple affected offspring, and in particular the transmission/disequilibrium test (TDT) developed by Spielman and Ewens.[12]

Genome-wide association studies

Genome-wide association studies (GWAS) have enabled scientists to interrogate the human genome in a comprehensive and biologically agnostic approach, in searching for unknown disease-associated variants. Unlike linkage studies, they do not require family members, and so case-control and, increasingly, population-based cohorts, have been able to be used to discover new genetic variants. The first GWAS published was in 2005, identifying the CFH gene for AMD,[13] which is discussed below, and since then there have been hundreds of GWAS, identifying novel genetic loci for many human complex diseases. Few of the identified genes or genetic loci were previously thought to be associated with the diseases. More importantly, the findings have already started providing new insights into the biological pathways of several complex diseases even when most of the disease causative variants remain to be discerned from the correlated markers in the regions.

Many methodological and technical issues that are relevant to the successful prosecution of large-scale association studies have been addressed. However, despite understandable celebration of these achievements, sober reflection reveals many challenges ahead. Compelling signals have been found, often highlighting previously unsuspected biology, but for most of the traits studied, known variants explain only a fraction of observed familial aggregation, limiting the potential for early application to determine individual disease risk. This is, in part, due to the design of association studies.

Although several hundred thousand single nucleotide polymorphism (SNP) markers are examined in a GWAS, they rely on the common disease–common variant approach. Common alleles with large effect sizes are scarce; so far, only a handful of them have been discovered by GWAS, and ironically three are ocular conditions: AMD (CFH), discussed below, exfoliation glaucoma (LOXL1),[14] and eye colour (OCA2). The majority of the risk alleles identified so far for complex diseases are common (allele frequency >5%) and confer small effect sizes (OR < 1.5). However, this observation may not really reflect the true allelic frequency spectrum of complex diseases. This is because, for any given sample size, common SNPs are easier to detect in association studies due to their higher statistical power than the rarer SNPs. In addition, the lower frequency SNPs (allele frequency <5%) are not well covered either directly or indirectly through linkage disequilibrium by the markers in the commercial genotyping arrays. As a result, they remain unexplored for disease association. The issues of unexplained or missing heritability and poor disease risk prediction have been getting considerable attention from the genetics community, leading to the scepticism of the promise of the GWAS approach to fully decipher the genetic basis of complex diseases. These issues have been discussed and debated in several perspective papers.[15,16]

Because current technology surveys only a limited subset of potentially relevant sequence variation, this should come as no surprise. Much work remains to obtain a complete inventory of the variants at each locus that contribute to disease risk and to define the molecular mechanisms through which these variants operate (Plate 6.1). The ultimate objectives — full descriptions of the susceptibility architecture of major biomedical traits and translation of the findings into clinical practice — remain distant.

Analysis of GWAS

There have been many issues relating to the design and analysis of GWAS studies. The use of small samples, which are underpowered to detect loci of realistic effect size, and over-liberal declarations of association are the main reasons why so few of the complex-trait associations that were claimed in the pre-GWAS era proved genuine. This history, together with the high dimensionality of GWA studies, their vulnerability to a range of errors and biases, and the modest effect sizes to be anticipated for most complex-trait susceptibility alleles, help to explain the pre-eminent role of replication in the evaluation of GWAS findings; all GWAS require replication cohorts. In addition, large meta-analyses (and sometimes mega-analyses) allow for pooling of several GWAS, to ascertain variants explaining smaller amounts of variation.

Some of the other issues related to analysis are detailed below.

1. Case selection. The principal issues with regard to case ascertainment revolve around the extent to which selection should be driven by manoeuvres that are designed to improve study power through enrichment for specific disease-predisposing alleles. These include efforts to minimize phenotypic heterogeneity or to focus on extreme and/or familial cases (defined, for example, by early age of onset or ascertainment from multiplex pedigrees). Because the genetic architecture of most complex traits remains poorly understood, the value of such efforts is hard to predict.

2. Control selection. Optimal selection of control samples has been controversial, although the Wellcome Trust Case Control Consortium (WTCCC) study was able to demonstrate the effectiveness of a 'common control' design in which 3,000 UK controls were compared with

2,000 cases from each of seven different diseases.[17] Although each prospective control sample must be critically evaluated, these findings suggest that a broad range of ascertainment schemes are compatible with GWA analysis, and misclassification bias is not a major concern, provided sample size is large enough.

3. Sample size. Although the first GWAS was based on 100,000 SNPs in 96 cases and 50 controls (identifying the CFH gene for AMD),[13] it is now recognized that for most common diseases, sample size of several thousand are needed, and for many quantitative traits such as refractive error this may mean 5,000+ subjects included.

4. Genotyping quality control. Before analysis of phenotypic data, genotypic data needs to be carefully examined, for hidden population stratification (using principal component analysis), for hidden relatedness of subjects (using quantile–quantile plots), for departure from Hardy–Weinberg equilibrium, and for poorly performing SNPs, which may suggest failed genotyping and which should be removed from analysis.

5. Statistical analysis: genome-wide significance. In most situations, the most powerful tool for the analysis of GWA data has been a single-point, one degree of freedom test of association, such as the Cochrane–Armitage test. Such tests allow comparison of the genotype distributions of cases and controls at each SNP in turn, and can be conducted with or without adjustment for relevant covariates. Although the Cochrane–Armitage method directly tests only one of several possible genetic models, it has the merit of being robust to modest deviations from additivity on the logistic scale (at least to those most likely to be biologically relevant). Furthermore, in situations in which the true model at the causal variant is non-additive, even modest departures from perfect LD will result in greatly reduced power to detect that non-additivity at nearby variants: in the GWA context therefore, in situations when few causal variants will be directly typed, the additive model is likely to perform well.

Historically, interpretation of genetic association findings has adopted the standard frequentist approach to the evaluation of significance.

From such a viewpoint, GWA results are compared with a single criterion of genome-wide significance. Although several benchmarks have been proposed, in European-descent GWA studies opinion is coalescing around the need to adjust for 1–2 million independent tests, which results in a target (p value) of $\sim 5 \times 10^{-8}$.

6. Functional analysis. Because of the indirect study design of GWAS, and the SNPs selection being guided by LD information and not functionality, it is more likely that the GWAS-identified SNPs are only the surrogate markers tagging for functional variants. Unlike non-synonymous SNPs, the biological effects of these SNPs are ambiguous and not directly clear, although most of them are suspected to be involved in modulating gene or transcript expression levels.

An updated list of published GWA studies can be found at the National Cancer Institute (NCI), National Human Genome Research Institute (NHGRI)'s catalogue of published genome-wide association studies (http://www.genome.gov/26525384).

6.3.5 Future technologies

The rate of gene discovery from GWAS has been exponential since 2007, but for many common diseases, large proportions of the variance attributed to genetic effects (the heritability) have not yet been explained. This partly reflects the study design of GWAS 'common disease common variant' (see Plate 6.1). There are probably many rare variants of larger effect size but affecting few people, who may be helped by new technologies such as whole genome or exome sequencing. Similarly, variants other than SNPs, such as copy number variants (CNVs), and small insertions and deletions, or inversions, may predispose individuals to disease. Similarly, little is understood at the present time about **epigenetics**, and alterations of genetic expression by environmental factors, and given these effects may be tissue-specific, will always be difficult to study in eye disease. The science of proteomics and metabolomics is new, and further advances regarding the genetic epidemiology of eye disease may be made using these technologies.

6.4   GENETIC EPIDEMIOLOGY OF EYE DISEASES

Genetic epidemiology is developing fast, and discoveries are being made on a weekly basis. AMD is the eye disease that is currently best understood, at least in part due to the large effect size of common disease variants. It will therefore serve as an example of the different methods used in understanding genetic epidemiology, ranging from family studies, segregation analysis and heritability studies, to candidate gene association studies, genome-wide linkage and association studies, and gene–environment interactions.

6.4.1   Age-related macular degeneration (AMD)

AMD has, in effect, become the 'poster boy' of genetic epidemiology of complex traits. Genes of major effect have identified new pathways involved in AMD, and are likely to result in future treatments to prevent or treat the condition. All the steps described above in understanding the genetic epidemiology of a disease have been successful in AMD. It must be noted, however, that it is likely that AMD is probably the exception rather than the rule. Current knowledge suggests that for other traits like glaucoma, cataract and refractive error, the heritability is likely to be explained by many genes of small effect.

Family history studies have demonstrated the familial aggregation of AMD. The Rotterdam Study showed that first-degree relatives of patients with late AMD had a four-fold increased risk of AMD, and that up to 23% of the population attributable risk (PAR) for AMD was explained by genetic factors.[18] The Beaver Dam Eye Study (BDES) found that a younger sibling had a two-to-ten-fold increased risk of AMD when an older sibling had AMD,[19] and a segregation analysis of 546 sibships within this cohort suggested that a single major gene could explain up to 57% of the total variability seen in cases of AMD.[20] Twin studies confirmed a heritability of AMD. The Twins UK cohort suggested a heritability of 45% for early AMD;[21] the US Veterans Twin Study estimated a heritability of 46% for any grade of AMD, and 71% for advanced AMD.[22]

Early candidate gene studies for AMD, which examined rare Mendelian disorders with phenotypes that were similar to AMD, were largely unsuccessful. Examples included looking for mutations in tissue inhibitor of metalloproteinases-3 (TIMP3), which cause autosomal dominant Sorsby fundus dystrophy, epidermal growth factor (EGF) containing fibulin-like ECM protein 1 (EFEMP1), which cause Doyne honeycomb retinal dystrophy, and endoplasmic reticulum-bound photoreceptor cell-specific factor (ELOVL4), which cause autosomal dominant Stargardt-like macular dystrophy. These studies did not find mutations that contribute to AMD. Mutations in the ATP-binding cassette, subfamily A, member 4 (ABCA4) gene, that cause autosomal recessive Stargardt disease, have been associated with AMD in some studies,[23] but not in many others, in part related to low power.

The first replicated candidate gene associated with AMD was ApoE, which is a lipophilic glycoprotein that plays an integral role in lipid and cholesterol transport. The Rotterdam Study, having identified cholesterol plaques in the carotid arteries as a risk factor for AMD, showed that the apolipoprotein gene APOE $\varepsilon 4$ allele was protective for AMD with an odds ratio 0.43 (95% CI 0.21–0.88).[24] Meta-analysis of the role of APOE in AMD concluded that there is a 20% risk attributed to $\varepsilon 2$ and a 40% protective effect for $\varepsilon 4$ in autosomal recessive and autosomal dominant roles, respectively.

Several genome-wide linkage studies of AMD, which discovered multiple loci, were published. As has been discussed, replicated loci are important, and meta-analysis identified two prominent loci: ARMD1 at chromosome 1q25–31 and age-related maculopathy susceptibility 2 (ARMS2) at 10q26.

In early 2005, three landmark papers in the journal *Science* identified complement factor H (CFH) as a gene exerting major effect in AMD. Two of these studies were a combination of fine mapping family and case-control association studies within the ARMD1 locus,[26,27] and the third study was a genome-wide association scan (GWAS), which amazingly found a highly significant signal using only 96 cases and 50 control subjects.[13] The Y402H mutation in the CFH gene resides within the heparin and CRP-binding domain and may cause complement dysregulation in AMD. In numerous studies, the TC and CC genotypes resulted in a significantly increased risk of AMD compared with the TT genotype, and a meta-analysis[28] showed that having the TC or CC genotype resulted in a 2.5- to 6-fold increased risk of AMD, implying a possible multiplicative effect. The estimated PAR for the CFH gene has been reported to range from 22% to 54%; as expected from the common disease, common variant approach, around 40% of Caucasian populations have a high-risk allele for AMD. As a result of the CFH gene discovery, further research into complement has identified other polymorphisms in complement cascade genes such as C2, C3 and C5, which have been proved, and replicated, to be associated with AMD.

The second locus (ARMS2) on chromosome 10q26 contains LOC387715. The LOC387715 (A69S) polymorphism has a strong association with AMD; a single serine confers a two-to-three-fold increase in the odds of AMD, and two serines, a six-to-twelve-fold increase, and risk of AMD seems additive to CFH allele-risk, and smoking.[29,30] The estimated PAR for LOC387715 has been reported between 34.3% and 57%. Adjacent to LOC387715, within ARMS2, is HtrA serine peptidase 1 (HTRA1), which is a heat shock serine protease found in drusen. Mutations and variants in the promoter region of HTRA1 have been found to significantly increase the risk of late AMD, and particularly exudative AMD within Chinese populations, with a PAR of 22% in American and 53% in Chinese cohorts.

Further genetic pathways continue to be unravelled in AMD. Larger GWAS studies, adjusting for the effects of the two main loci described above, have identified polymorphisms in lipid-regulating genes which are involved in regulation of high-density lipoprotein cholesterol levels, such as the hepatic lipase gene (LIPC).[31]

Gene–gene interaction and Gene–environment interaction

With risk alleles now specified, it is possible to examine gene–gene interaction and gene–environment interaction. Risks for the CFH, LOC387715 and other genes associated with AMD aetiology seem to be additive, and do not interact. Gene–environment interaction with smoking has been demonstrated; the CC genotype and smoking result in a 144-fold increased risk of AMD over the CT or TT genotype. Future studies will examine other environmental risk factors in relation to the risk genotypes for AMD.

It is now possible, with relatively few SNP markers, to predict an individual's lifetime risk of AMD, and thus deliver the promise of genomic 'personalized medicine'[32] (Plate 6.2). It remains to be tested whether knowledge of risk can be transferred into prevention of disease, or alter individual behaviour, but certainly new treatments will emerge, and the prospects for intervention in the most common cause of blindness in the developed world have altered with the new genetic knowledge.

6.4.2   Glaucoma

Numerous whole genome linkage scans using familial glaucoma and the affected sib-pair design have identified susceptibility loci, but few genes have been identified. In 1997, Stone and 14 colleagues from seven laboratories reported the identification of a gene (TIGR, now named MYOC after myocilin, the protein product of the gene found in the trabecular meshwork) associated with familial juvenile open-angle glaucoma. Screening of adults with primary open-angle glaucoma revealed that 2–4% also carried a mutation of the coding region of this gene.[33]

The LOXL1 gene was identified as a major susceptibility gene for pseudoexfoliation and its associated glaucoma using a genome-wide association scan in the Icelandic population.[14] The risk variant explains a large proportion of pseudoexfoliation.

Other genes associated with primary open-angle glaucoma have been difficult to find, but examination of the endophenotypes, or intermediate traits, associated with glaucoma such as optic disc size, intraocular pressure, and central corneal thickness have identified genetic variants, and large-scale collection of cases and controls for GWAS continues.

6.4.3 Cataract

The first gene associated with age-related cataract was reported by two groups in 2008 and 2009, namely the EPHA2 gene, and particularly associated with cortical lens opacities.[34,35] Further research into the genetic epidemiology of cataract, which twin studies suggest has a heritability of 50–60%,[36] continues.

6.4.4 Refractive error

Numerous twin studies have identified a high heritability, of the order of 80%, for refractive error. The largest, involving over 2,000 pairs of twins, suggested a heritability of 77%; shared, common family environment explained 7% of variance, and individual (unique) environment 17%.[37] Despite 20 myopia linkage loci being identified, specific genetic variants associated with myopia and refractive errors have been difficult to identify. The implication is that, like human height (another highly heritable trait), there are likely to be numerous genes each associated with small effect size. The first GWA Studies have identified genetic variants, and large-scale meta-analyses are likely to identify more.

6.5 FUTURE DEVELOPMENTS

The future of genetic epidemiology will concern the identification and characterization of population-level processes and structures that contribute to the emergence and maintenance of disease. Greater integration of molecular, physiological, genetic, pharmacological and epidemiological studies will be required to dissect out the relative roles of genes and environment for both single-gene and multi-factorial diseases. The explosion of technology and statistical procedures has resulted in vast amounts of data, but the fundamental concepts of good epidemiological study design remain to ensure that susceptibility genes identified are valid and representative. Studies need to be large enough to have sufficient power to detect relatively small genetic influences, and further research into the 'missing heritability' is required.

REFERENCES

1. Khoury MJ, Beaty TH, Cohen BH. *Fundamentals of Genetic Epidemiology.* New York: Oxford University Press; 1993.

2. Neel JV, Schull WJ. *Human Heredity.* Chicago: The University of Chicago Press; 1954, pp. 283–306.

3. Morton NE, Chung CS (eds.). *Genetic Epidemiology.* New York: Academic Press; 1978, pp. 3–11.

4. Fisher RA. The correlation between relatives on supposition of Mendelian inheritance. *Trans Roy Soc Edinburgh* 1918; 52:399–433.

5. Pairitz Jarvik G. Complex segregation analysis: uses and limitations. *Am J Hum Genet* 1998; 63: 942–946.

6. Neale MC, Cardon LR. *Methodology for Genetic Studies of Twins and Families.* Dordrecht: Kluwer Academic Publishers; 1992.

7. Kyvik KO. Generalisability and assumptions of twin studies. In: *Advances in Twin and Sib-Pair Analysis,* Spector TD, Snieder H, MacGregor AJ (eds.). London: Greenwich Medical Media Ltd; 2000.

8. Falconer DS. *Introduction to Quantitative Genetics.* 3rd Edition. Harlow: Longman; 1989.

9. Jablonski W. Ein Beitrag zur Vererbung der Refraktion menschlicher Augen. *Arch Augenheilk* 1922; 91:308.

10. Elston RC. Methods of linkage analysis — and the assumptions underlying them. *Am J Hum Genet* 1998; 63:931–934.

11. Morton NE. Sequential tests for the detection of linkage. *Am J Hum Genet* 1955; 7:277–318.

12. Spielman RS, Ewens WJ. The TDT and other family-based tests for quantitative traits. *Am J Hum Genet* 1996; 59:983–989.

13. Klein RJ, Zeiss C, Chew EY, *et al.* Complement factor H polymorphism in age-related macular degeneration. *Science* 2005; 308:385–389.

14. Thorleifsson G, Magnusson KP, Sulem, *et al.* Common sequence variants in the LOXL1 gene confer susceptibility to exfoliation glaucoma. *Science* 2007; 317:1397–1400.

15. Goldstein DB. Common genetic variation and human traits. *N Engl J Med* 2009; 360:1696–1698.

16. McCarthy MI, Abecasis GR, Cardon LR, *et al.* Genome-wide association studies for complex traits: consensus, uncertainty and challenges. *Nat Rev Genet* 2008; 9:356–369.

17. Wellcome Trust Case Control Consortium. Genome-wide association study of 14,000 cases of seven common diseases and 3,000 shared controls. *Nature* 2007; 447:661–678.

18. Klaver CC, Wolfs RC, Assink JJ, *et al.* Genetic risk of age-related maculopathy. Population-based familial aggregation study. *Arch Ophthalmol* 1998; 116:1646–1651.

19. Klein BE, Klein R, Lee KE, *et al.* Risk of incident age-related eye diseases in people with an affected sibling: the Beaver Dam Eye Study. *Am J Epidemiol* 2001; 154:207–211.

20. Heiba IM, Elston RC, Klein BE, *et al.* Sibling correlations and segregation analysis of age-related maculopathy: the Beaver Dam Eye Study. *Genet Epidemiol* 1994; 11:51–67.

21. Hammond CJ, Webster AR, Snieder H, *et al.* Genetic influence on early age-related maculopathy: twin study. *Ophthalmology* 2002; 109:730–736.

22. Seddon JM, Cote J, Page WF, *et al.* The US twin study of age-related macular degeneration: relative roles of genetic and environmental influences. *Arch Ophthalmol* 2005; 123:321–327.

23. Stone EM, Webster AR, Vandenburgh K, *et al.* Allelic variation in ABCR associated with Stargardt disease but not age-related macular degeneration. *Nat Genet* 1998; 20:328–329.

24. Klaver CC, Kliffen M, van Duijn CM, *et al.* Genetic association of apolipoprotein E with age-related macular degeneration. *Am J Hum Genet* 1998; 63: 200–206.

25. Fisher SA, Abecasis GR, Yashar BM, *et al.* Meta-analysis of genome scans of age-related macular degeneration. *Hum Mol Genet* 2005; 14:2257–2264.

26. Edwards AO, Ritter R, 3rd, Abel KJ, *et al.* Complement factor H polymorphism and age-related macular degeneration. *Science* 2005; 308:421–424.

27. Haines JL, Hauser MA, Schmidt S, *et al.* Complement factor H variant increases the risk of age-related macular degeneration. *Science* 2005; 308:419–421.

28. Thakkinstian A, Han P, McEvoy M, *et al.* Systematic review and meta-analysis of the association between complement factor H Y402H polymorphisms and age-related macular degeneration. *Hum Mol Genet* 2006; 15:2784–2790.

29. Jakobsdottir J, Conley YP, Weeks DE, *et al.* Susceptibility genes for age-related maculopathy on chromosome 10q26. *Am J Hum Genet* 2005; 77:389–407.

30. Tuo J, Ross RJ, Reed GF, *et al.* The HtrA1 promoter polymorphism, smoking, and age-related macular degeneration in multiple case–control samples. *Ophthalmology* 2008; 115:1891–1898.

31. Neale BM, Fagerness J, Reynolds R, *et al.* Genome-wide association study of advanced age-related macular degeneration identifies a role of the hepatic lipase gene (LIPC). *Proc Natl Acad Sci USA* 2010; 107:7395–7400.

32. Maller J, George S, Purcell S, *et al.* Common variation in three genes, including a noncoding variant in CFH, strongly influences risk of age-related macular degeneration. *Nat Genet* 2006; 38: 1055–1059.

33. Stone EM, Fingert JH, Alward WL, *et al.* Identification of a gene that causes primary open angle glaucoma. *Science* 1997; 275:668–670.

34. Shiels A, Bennett TM, Knopf HL, *et al.* The EPHA2 gene is associated with cataracts linked to chromosome 1p. *Mol Vis* 2008; 14:2042–2055.

35. Jun G, Guo H, Klein BE, *et al.* EPHA2 is associated with age-related cataract in mice and humans. *PLoS Genet* 2009; 5:Epub 2009 Jul 31.

36. Hammond CJ, Snieder H, Spector TD, *et al.* Genetic and environmental factors in age-related nuclear cataracts in monozygotic and dizygotic twins. *N Engl J Med* 2000; 342:1786–1790.

37. Lopes MC, Andrew T, Carbonaro F, *et al.* Estimating heritability and shared environmental effects for refractive error in twin and family studies. *Invest Ophthalmol Vis Sci* 2009; 50:126–131.

7

Clinical trials

MAUREEN MAGUIRE

7.1	Introduction	131
7.2	Key design elements	132
7.3	Data analysis and monitoring data and safety	141

7.4	Reporting results	142
7.5	Future directions	142
	References	144

7.1 INTRODUCTION

7.1.1 Historical perspective

Clinical trials — experiments testing treatments on human subjects — have had a major impact on nearly every area in the field of ophthalmology. Meinert has traced the history of clinical trials beginning with a passage from the Bible.[1] Experiments using humans were conducted over the centuries; however, the era of modern clinical trials in medicine did not begin until the early 1930s with the first reports of randomized treatment assignment and the creation of the Therapeutic Trials Committee, appointed by the Medical Research Council of Great Britain. In 1976, the **Diabetic Retinopathy Study (DRS)** Research Group reported on the results of the first large-scale, multicentred, randomized clinical trial in ophthalmology.[2,3] Panretinal photocoagulation of eyes of diabetic patients with defined levels of proliferative disease was shown to decrease dramatically the risk of severe loss of vision. Despite the years that have passed, the DRS results continue to guide the management of patients.

The success of the DRS inspired the application of clinical trials methodology to several other questions about the management of patients with specific ocular diseases. Most of the largest trials have been sponsored by the United States National Eye Institutes of the **National Institutes of Health (NIH)** and the medical research councils of other countries. Many clinical trials have been sponsored by the pharmaceutical industry because the process to approve a new drug generally requires a series of clinical trials.

7.1.2 Types of clinical trial in the development of drugs

Although regulatory agencies in different countries have different specific requirements, the sequence of testing a new drug in humans typically follows the general approach used by the Center for Drug Evaluation and Research, **Food and Drug Administration (FDA)** of the United States (http://www.fda.gov/cder/handbook).

➤ Phase 1 clinical trials involve the first application of a new drug to humans. These studies typically are conducted in 20 to 80 healthy volunteer subjects who are closely monitored. Usually, neither randomized nor concurrent controls are included. The main goal of Phase 1 trials is to determine the metabolic and pharmacologic actions of the drug, the side effects associated with increasing doses, and, if possible, to gain early evidence on effectiveness.

➤ Phase 2 clinical trials are conducted to obtain preliminary data on the effectiveness of a drug in patients with the targeted disease or condition. Phase 2 trials may incorporate a comparison group of randomized controls, a historical control group, or no control patients. The patients participating in the trials are closely monitored for short-term side effects.

➤ Phase 3 clinical trials usually involve patients with the targeted disease or condition who are randomly assigned to the new drug or an appropriate control treatment (placebo or active treatment that is considered standard therapy). Based on preliminary evidence of efficacy in Phase 2 trials, Phase 3 trials are designed to gather the additional information about effectiveness and safety that is needed to evaluate the overall risk — benefit relationship of the drug.

Although Phase 1 and Phase 2 trials have an important role in the development of new treatments, the remainder of this chapter will be directed towards Phase 3 drug trials and **randomized clinical trials** (**RCTs**) of surgery and medical devices.

7.2   KEY DESIGN ELEMENTS

Designing a clinical trial requires that several key elements be addressed in an integrated way (Table 7.1). Modification of one element may have major implications on the best choice for other

Table 7.1 *Major study design elements for clinical trials*

7.2.1	Objective of the trial
7.2.2	Treatments/interventions
7.2.3	Study population
7.2.4	Treatment assignment
7.2.5	Outcome measures
7.2.6	Follow-up
7.2.7	Sample size
7.2.8	Masking and other practices to strengthen trail design

elements. Several excellent textbooks provide guiding principles for all clinical trials.[1,4,5] The following sections will address the application of those guiding principles to clinical trials in ophthalmology.

7.2.1   Objective of the trial

All of the design elements of a clinical trial are directed at achieving a specific objective of the particular trial. However, the objective is usually refined or modified in the process of making choices for the other elements: for example, a new drug may be promising for slowing lens opacification. The initial objective of the clinical trial may be to evaluate whether administration of the drug is beneficial. Designers of the clinical trial may decide that at least three years of daily administration is necessary to have an impact on the lifelong process of cataract formation. Also, they may decide that preventing the formation of clinically significant lens opacity among patients with no or minimal signs of lens opacity would provide definitive evidence that the drug actually affected lens opacification. These choices would modify the original objective of the trial to the evaluation of whether long-term administration of the drug decreases the incidence of clinically significant lens opacity.

7.2.2   Treatments/interventions

7.2.2.1   *Choice of comparison groups*

Once the decision has been made to evaluate a particular treatment (the test treatment), the most appropriate comparison group needs to be chosen. For conditions with no currently accepted treatment, the only choice is a no-treatment group.

Use of placebos and sham procedures in no-treatment groups

Clinical trials involving drugs in liquid, tablet or capsule form, topical eye drops and ointments should have placebos given to the no-treatment group. Care needs to be taken to ensure that the placebo and test medication appear identical. If they are distinguishable, the theoretical advantages of their use are lost. Use of sham procedures should be considered for clinical trials involving interventions such as surgical procedures, radiotherapy, devices and behavioural programmes. The degree of subjectivity of the outcome measures may increase or decrease the need for a sham treatment. Risks of the sham procedure itself, cost of the procedure, time and effort of patients and investigators, expenditure of scarce resources, and the degree of **masking** actually achieved need to be evaluated when considering a sham procedure. For example, a sham intravitreal injection (no penetration of the globe) and sham photodynamic therapy (intravenous infusion of saline rather than photoreactive dye) were used in a trial of intravitreal ranibizumab versus photodynamic therapy with verteporfin for treatment of predominantly classic choroidal neovascularization associated with age-related macular degeneration.[6] All patients received either an intravitreal injection of ranibizumab or a sham injection. In addition, the maculae of all patients were exposed to laser light. Because of the subjective component of visual acuity testing, investigators believed that the relatively low risks associated with an intravenous infusion of saline and the exposure to a low level of light were justified to achieve the masking of the patients.

Comparison group when there is a proven treatment

Clinical trials that involve comparison of a new treatment with a proven treatment ('active control') are becoming more common as the number of conditions with effective treatments increases. However, there may be some instances when comparing a new treatment to a no-treatment group may be reasonable. If the proven treatment involves high cost that impedes widespread administration, or great pain or inconvenience to patients, then a no-treatment comparison group may be ethical, especially if the proven treatment has only a small beneficial effect. After the publication of the results of the efficacy of photodynamic therapy,[7] health agencies in several countries decided that the costs of repeated sessions of photodynamic therapy were not warranted in view of its relatively small impact on preserving visual

acuity. Thus, clinical trials of new treatments for predominantly classic choroidal neovascularization with a no-treatment group could have been considered because the proven treatment was not available for most patients in the country, and cheaper, effective treatments were needed.

7.2.2.2 *Standardization of treatment*

Patient management in each treatment group, including groups assigned to 'observation', needs to be explicitly defined. For medications, the formulation, the dose taken upon each administration, the schedule of administration, and the duration of use need to be specified. For trials of surgical interventions, including laser treatment, all aspects of the procedure that might affect clinical outcome need to be specified. Balancing this need with the preferences of each surgeon may be difficult. However, if the surgery is ever to be recommended, other surgeons must be able to replicate the procedure in all aspects that affect the clinical outcome. In a clinical trial of a laser treatment it might be important to specify the number, location, intensity, power and duration of laser burn applications while allowing surgeon preferences on the exact type of anaesthesia, contact lens, and brand of laser.

Treatment if there are signs of toxicity or adverse events

Patient management after signs of possible toxicity and adverse events needs to be specified. In placebo-controlled trials, an attempt should be made to respond to signs of toxicity without unmasking the treatment assignment. Typically, patients are managed assuming that they are receiving the active drug unless appropriate medical treatment of the adverse event depends on revealing the treatment assignment. Depending on the drug and the side effects, the amount or frequency of study drug (active drug or placebo) administration can be decreased. In some cases of signs of toxicity, the patient may simply discontinue the study drug (active drug or placebo), be treated for the condition as needed, and continue to be followed. The management of adverse events should be similar in that efforts should be made to treat the patient for the adverse event without revealing the treatment assignment if the trial involves masking and providing guidelines for care; for example, in a trial of a steroidal intravitreal implant, there should be guidelines with respect to medical treatment and early removal of the implant for patients who have an elevation in intraocular pressure.

Treatment if disease progresses

Standard procedures may be needed for handling patients whose disease has progressed to the point where additional measures must be taken to protect the patient. If a drug is being tested to see whether it controls intraocular pressure and prevents progression of glaucomatous visual field defect, then provisions need to be in place for handling patients who suffer visual field deterioration, regardless of the treatment group to which they are assigned. If possible, such patients should be treated in a way that does not require unmasking the treatment assignment, perhaps by supplementing or replacing the study drugs (active drug or placebo) with a surgical treatment. In a prevention trial, once eyes develop the targeted condition, patients should have the same options for treatment of their condition as patients outside of the clinical trial.

7.2.3   Study population

The participants in a clinical trial should be representative of the patients to whom the results are intended to apply. The desirable property of including a broad group of patients with a particular eye condition, so that the results can be applied widely, competes with the desirable property of including only those patients who are likely to benefit from the treatment. Often the larger sample size required to show a treatment effect in a broadly defined population, in comparison to the sample size required in a more homogeneous group, forces the choice of the more limited study population because of logistical and resource utilization issues. Alternatively, reducing the utilization

of resources by simplifying trial procedures may allow inclusion of, and generalization to, a broad group of patients.[8]

7.2.3.1   *Eligibility criteria*

Inclusion criteria

Participants in a clinical trial must possess certain qualities for the objectives to be met. Enrolled patients should meet the following criteria:

➤ They should have the eye condition of interest. A case definition must be constructed to specify the constellation of signs and symptoms that must be present to confirm the presence of the eye condition. Limits for the acceptable stages of the disease process need to be demarcated. A case definition for a clinical trial of a drug for slowing progression of diabetic retinopathy might require the patient to have **type 1** or **type 2 diabetes mellitus** as defined by the World Health Organization, and diabetic retinopathy in at least one eye within a given range of the **Early Treatment for Diabetic Retinopathy Study** (**ETDRS**) fundus grading scale (see Chapter 21).

➤ They must be able to complete the testing needed for eligibility determination and assessment of outcomes. Patients need to be able to complete diagnostic tests and evaluations needed to confirm eligibility. Patients who cannot sustain the appropriate pose for the duration of automated visual field examination cannot be entered into trials that require demonstration of a specific visual field defect or use visual field deterioration as the primary outcome measure.

➤ They should have a high likelihood of being available for the duration of follow-up. Patients with a terminal disease and lifestyles that preclude complying with the scheduled follow-up visits should not be enrolled.

➤ They should be capable of providing informed consent to enroll in the clinical trial. To provide informed consent, patients need to be able to understand the implications of joining a clinical trial and to evaluate the risks and benefits of participation. Children and patients with diminished mental capacity may have guardians who can take on the responsibility of making the decision to enroll for them; investigators need to consult with their local institutional review boards or ethics committees about guidelines for consent by the guardian and assent by the patient before enrolling such patients.

Exclusion criteria

Participants in a clinical trial should not have certain conditions:

➢ Conditions that strongly influence the outcome measures. Patients who have other ocular conditions that can strongly influence the outcome measures, independent of the treatment applied, should not be enrolled. In some clinical trials, this statement must be balanced with the desirable property of including the full range of patients to whom the treatment will be applied if it is shown to be beneficial.

➢ Conditions that contra-indicate or preclude one of the treatments. Patients who have medical conditions that contra-indicate one of the treatments should not be entered into the study. Similarly, patients who have a condition that makes administration of a treatment impossible should not be enrolled. The **Multicenter Uveitis Steroid Treatment** (**MUST**) Trial compares local therapy, with a fluocinolone acetonide intraocular implant, with systemic corticosteroid therapy.[9] Patients with uncontrolled glaucoma are excluded because of the risk of visual field loss resulting from steroid-related intraocular pressure elevation. Patients should be questioned before randomization about conditions that would interfere with application of any of the treatments in the study.

7.2.3.2   Determination and confirmation of eligibility

Determining the eligibility for enrolment in a clinical trial can be solely the responsibility of the examining clinician or a shared responsibility with a central review group. In the **Age-Related Eye Disease Study** (**AREDS**) (see Chapter 22), clinical centre staff were responsible for ensuring that the majority of the eligibility criteria were met; however, the staff of a central fundus photograph reading centre determined whether certain of the criteria involving the appearance of the fundus were met, based on colour stereo photographs.[10] This procedure had the benefit of providing uniform interpretation across the clinical centres and avoided enrolling patients who did not have photographic evidence to fulfil the eligibility criteria. The disadvantages were that the central evaluation delayed enrolment into the trial and now clinicians have sole responsibility for identifying patients with the requisite drusen characteristics. An alternative to central determination of eligibility is central confirmation of eligibility. Patients are determined as eligible by the examining clinician, but the agreement of the clinician's opinion with central review can be assessed as a quality control measure. The disadvantage of this process is that incorrect judgments by examining clinicians may result in enrolment and analysis of patients who do not truly meet the eligibility criteria, as well as erroneous exclusion of eligible patients.

7.2.4   Treatment assignment

7.2.4.1   Treatment assignment by person or by eye?

Clinical trials of eye disease can raise interesting questions about the unit of treatment assignment. When the eye condition typically affects only one eye of a patient at a time, such as vein occlusion or amblyopia, assigning a patient to a treatment group is equivalent to assigning an eye to a treatment group. When both eyes are typically affected simultaneously by an eye condition, assigning one eye to one treatment group and the contralateral eye to the other treatment group is appealing from both design and ethical perspectives. Because disease incidence and progression are often strongly correlated between eyes of the same person, comparing treatments within patients is statistically efficient and usually requires lower numbers of patients than comparing treatment across a group of people. Treatment assignment by eye also allows one eye to receive the better treatment, if indeed there are differences in the clinical effects of the two treatments. In the DRS, one eye was assigned panretinal photocoagulation and the other eye was observed.[2,3]

However, a paired-eye design as described above may not be possible or desirable. Some treatments are administered systemically so that it is impossible to treat only one eye, as in dietary supplements for prevention of advanced age-related macular degeneration.[10] Treatments that are administered locally to only one eye may have systemic activity that causes a contralateral effect. In the **Glaucoma Laser Trial** (**GLT**), one eye received topical medication first while the other eye received argon laser trabeculoplasty first in a clinical trial to assess the relative efficacy of the two treatments in preventing additional deterioration of the visual field.[11] However, timolol maleate, a topical beta-blocker which is absorbed systemically and slightly lowers intraocular pressure in the contralateral eye, was one of the topical medications. Interpretation of the trial results was complicated by the crossover effect of timolol. Finally, some outcome measures are not eye-specific. Even if two treatments could be applied locally without crossover effects, their effects on health-related quality of life could not be ascertained.

7.2.4.2   Randomized treatment assignment

Treatment assignments in a clinical trial should always be randomized. Simple randomization without stratification or **blocking** should provide, over the long run, treatment groups that are balanced on all factors affecting outcome measures. However, clinical trials involve finite numbers of patients and imbalance on influential factors can happen by chance. Often randomization schedules are stratified by clinical centre and over recruitment time to ensure balance on these two important factors. Despite efforts to standardize procedures, clinical centre effects and temporal trends in the outcome measures are often substantial. Methods for generating random treatment assignments may be found in the textbook by Meinert.[1] One commonly used method of random treatment allocation is to generate

a separate randomization schedule for each clinical centre and use a permuted block system, with randomly selected block sizes, within each clinical centre. In some trials, randomization schedules are further stratified based on risk of progression as assessed at baseline or based on the expected magnitude of treatment benefit. However, stratification on too many factors may actually increase the probability of imbalance.

Randomizing treatment assignment between the two eyes of the same patient

There are many ways of accommodating a paired design in a randomized treatment schedule. One simple method is to designate, according to a fixed rule, one of the eyes as the eye to be randomized. The rule may be as simple as 'Designate the right eye'. Then assign the designated eye to one of the treatments using the methods described above. The contralateral eye is then automatically assigned the alternative treatment.

Securing the treatment assignment until the time of randomization

Patients and clinical centre staff should not know the next treatment assignment before the patient is enrolled into the study. Whether a website, central telephone service, envelope system, or secured randomization notebook is used for allocating treatment assignments, there should be no way to discover the next treatment assignment.[12] Well-intentioned people have tried to manipulate the allocation system because they believed that a particular patient was especially well suited for one of the treatment groups or preferred one treatment over the other. Use of quasi-random practices, such as assigning treatment groups based on the terminal digit of an identification number, or on the order of presentation at the clinical centre, or on the day of the week or month allows clinical staff and/or patients to calculate the next treatment assignment and to manipulate the system to yield a desired treatment assignment. Because of their great potential to create damaging imbalances between treatment groups, these quasi-random practices should not be used.

7.2.4.3 *Timing of treatment assignment*

Good analysis of data from clinical trials requires that all patients who are enrolled and assigned a treatment in a clinical trial be followed and analyzed in the treatment group to which they were assigned. Analysis by 'intention to treat' means that a patient assigned to surgery has their outcome measures included with all other patients assigned to surgery, even if surgery was never performed. All eligibility criteria must be verified before requesting a randomized treatment assignment so that there is no reason not to administer the assigned treatment. Treatment should be as soon as possible after the assignment is revealed to minimize the chance of the patient failing to receive the assigned treatment. In some clinical trials of laser treatment, the treatment assignments were not released unless the patient was present and a laser room was available in case the patient was assigned to this treatment.

7.2.5 Outcome measures

Outcome measures are qualitative or quantitative measures of the characteristics of the patient that the study treatments may affect. In most clinical trials, one outcome measure is designated as the *primary outcome measure* because it best captures the intended effect of the treatment. Other outcome measures are designated as *secondary outcome measures* because they supplement the primary outcome measure in evaluating the treatments fully.

7.2.5.1 *Primary outcome measure*

The choice of a primary outcome measure is very important, as it strongly influences the interpretation of the clinical trial as well as eligibility criteria, follow-up procedures and sample size.

Desirable properties of primary outcome measures

➤ *Definitive with respect to the condition under study.* An outcome measure is definitive if differences in the measure in groups of patients are clinically meaningful, and provide convincing evidence that one group is 'better off' than the other.

➤ *Objective.* The measure should be as independent as possible of influence by the expectations, motivation, hopes, fears and so on, of the patient and evaluator.

➤ *Reliable or reproducible.* If a patient's condition remains constant the outcome measure should be constant under repeated testing at different times or by different examiners.

➤ *Well defined.* The required conditions for measurement, the method of measurement and the summarization of the measurement need to be explicit.

➤ *Not subject to floor and ceiling effects.* For continuous outcome measures, patients in the trial with different levels of the characteristic being measured should have different scores and both improvement and deterioration should be possible.

Visual acuity is the most commonly used outcome measure in clinical trials for eye conditions. For many retinal diseases, visual acuity is a definitive measure because a patient group with better visual acuity is considered 'better off' than an otherwise comparable group of patients. However, visual acuity measurement can be influenced by the expectations and emotions of patients and evaluators and, therefore, may not be constant under repeated testing. Highly structured protocols for lighting, testing distances, refractive correction, chart design and interpretation of patient responses have been developed so that the measurement is well defined. The impact of subjectivity of visual acuity measurement can be decreased by masking patients and examiners to treatment assignment, and by strict adherence to the protocol for instructing the patient and for interpreting responses from the patient. Similarly, a detailed protocol on administering the test of visual acuity can increase the reproducibility of the measurement by decreasing intra-observer and inter-observer variation.[13] Floor and ceiling effects may be avoided, by testing materials that cover the full range of visual acuity expected at both baseline and follow-up.

The importance of selecting a definitive primary outcome measure cannot be overemphasized. Berson and colleagues presented results of a randomized, double-masked clinical trial of vitamin supplementation for patients with retinitis pigmentosa.[14] The primary outcome measure was **electroretinogram** (**ERG**) amplitude. Although patients receiving vitamin A supplementation had a statistically significant slower rate of decline in ERG amplitude, vitamin A supplementation for patients with retinitis pigmentosa remains controversial to this day. Many researchers believed that the definitive measure should have been based on visual field area and that the results on ERG decline were not clinically meaningful. Differences between treatment groups on visual field area were not statistically significant.

Further specification of the primary outcome measure

Additional aspects may need to be specified to characterize fully the primary outcome measure for the main comparison of treatment groups. If the primary outcome measure is the development of a particular condition, such as incident disease in a prevention clinical trial or graft rejection in a trial for recipients of a corneal transplant, then the remaining important issue is taking into account the time over which the condition developed. One straightforward approach is to use the cumulative proportion that develops the condition by a given time after enrolment. As an example, the great majority of corneal grafts that fail do so within two years of surgery. Therefore, the two-year failure rate would be expected to capture any effect of a new treatment. Alternatively, especially when a high proportion of patients in each treatment group is expected to develop the condition, summarizing the time to the event in each group through survival curves may better capture an effect of a treatment. The early trials of treatment for cyto-megalovirus retinitis in patients with autoimmune deficiency syndrome used the time to progression of retinal damage as the primary outcome variable.

Primary outcome measures that depend on a continuous scale require additional decisions. As an example, if visual acuity is measured on charts that are scaled logarithmically with an equal number of optotypes per line, the number of letters read correctly is used as the score. For a particular trial, two of the questions that need to be addressed are:

1. What better captures the desired effect of the treatment — the level of visual acuity at follow-up or the change in visual acuity relative to the baseline value?
2. Which summary measure of the continuous distribution should be used — mean, median or percentage of patients exceeding a particular level? In general, statistical comparisons of treatment groups will be more powerful if the means or medians of the distributions are compared rather than proportions formed after dividing the distribution into observations above or below a particular level.[15] However, many believe that the proportion of individual patients who have a clinically meaningful change in vision needs to be different between treatment groups for there to be evidence of treatment benefit or harm. Also, differences in means and medians of data that do not follow a 'normal' distribution may be especially insensitive to differences in the 'tail areas' (the best and worst visual acuity outcomes). For these reasons, three-line loss in visual acuity (doubling of the visual angle) and six-line loss (quadrupling of the visual angle) are commonly used primary outcome measures.

7.2.5.2 Secondary outcome measures

Secondary outcome measures complement the primary outcome measure and enrich the interpretation of the clinical trial. Areas typically addressed with secondary outcome measures are:

➢ Visual function;
➢ Incidence and severity of complications of treatment and/or side-effects;
➢ Changes related to the eye condition under study in the physical status of the eye;
➢ Pharmacologic activity of drugs;
➢ Health- and vision-related quality of life;

> Activities required to administer the treatment according to the trial protocol;
> Costs associated with the treatment.

The desirable properties and detailed specification of primary outcome measures also apply to secondary outcome measures. Results on the secondary outcome measures provide information on mechanisms responsible for the effects of treatments and the resources required to apply the treatment. In the Anti-**VEGF** Antibody for the Treatment of Predominantly Classic Choroidal Neovascularization in Age-Related Macular Degeneration (ANCHOR) trial, secondary outcome measures allowed the advantages and disadvantages of the treatment to be considered comprehensively.[6] The secondary outcome measures of the proportions with 20/40 (6/12, 0.5) or better visual acuity and with 20/200 (6/60, 0.1) or worse visual acuity provided descriptive information on vision that complement the primary outcome measure of the proportion of patients with less than a 15-letter loss in visual acuity. The increase in the area of neovascularization in the group treated with photodynamic therapy and decrease in area in the groups treated with intravitreal ranibizumab supported the dramatic differences in visual acuity. The percentage of patients in each group with arterial thromboembolic events, which were side effects of another intravenously administered anti-VEGF agent, provided information on the magnitude of increased risk, if any, in the ranibizumab groups.

7.2.6 Follow-up

The frequency and duration of follow-up are governed by the eye condition and treatment under study. Follow-up examinations should be proportional to the rate of change expected in the eye condition as characterized by the outcome measures. For conditions such as bacterial keratitis that usually either progress or heal completely within a few weeks, examinations need to be every few days initially and then tapered over four or six weeks to obtain a final status. Alternatively, in a prevention

trial of a slowly progressive disease such as glaucoma, the duration of follow-up needs to be years, and the frequency of examination may be as low as every six or twelve months.

Extreme efforts should be made to obtain complete follow-up on all patients, including those who do not have their eligibility confirmed, refuse treatment, or are non-compliant with study procedures. Failure to return for a scheduled follow-up visit may be related to the trial outcome measures. Some patients are inclined to discontinue follow-up because their vision is good and they are experiencing no side effects, whereas other patients may be inclined to discontinue follow-up because they have suffered loss of vision or side-effects. Clinical trials with high loss to follow-up can yield biased results leading to incorrect conclusions about treatment effects.

7.2.7 Sample size

For clinical trials designed to detect differences between treatment groups, the number of patients needed for analysis depends on four key quantities:

1. The minimum size of the difference on the primary outcome measure believed to be clinically meaningful.
2. The standard deviation of the primary outcome measure in the patient population to be studied.
3. The type I error level to be used for statistical testing in the final analysis.
4. The desired statistical power to detect the designated difference.

Clinicians and statisticians need to work together because making realistic choices for these quantities often requires judgement and, sometimes, educated guesses. Note that a **type I error**, also known as **alpha (α) error**, is a conclusion that a difference exists between treatment groups when none truly exists. Type I error is controlled by setting the level of statistical significance (p-value) required to conclude that a difference exists. Statistical **power** is the probability of detecting a difference between treatment groups when a difference of the selected magnitude truly exists. Failure to conclude that a difference exists when one truly does exist is a **type II error**, also known as **beta (β) error**. The level of statistical power can be expressed as $1-\beta$.

$$N \approx \left[\frac{2\left[(Z_{\alpha/2} + Z_{\beta}) * (\text{Standard Deviation})\right]}{(\text{Difference})^2} \right]^2$$

where:

N is the number of subjects per treatment group
$Z_{\alpha/2}$ is the value of the point on the abscissa (x-axis) of a standard Normal curve with $100(\alpha/2)\%$ of the area under the curve to the right (e.g. for an alpha level of 0.05, $Z_{0.025} = 1.96$)
Z_{β} is the value of the point on the abscissa (x-axis) of a standard Normal curve with $100(\beta)\%$ of the area under the curve to the right (e.g. for a power level of 0.80, $Z_{0.20} = 0.84$).

Inspection of a simplified form of the basic formula for sample size required when comparing the two means or proportions reveals important facts about the size of the required sample. The required sample size increases if:

➤ The level of α is decreased [e.g. using p = 0.01 ($Z_{\alpha/2} = 2.576$) as the criterion for statistical significance rather than p = 0.05 ($Z_{\alpha/2} = 1.96$)].
➤ The level of power is increased [e.g. using 90% power ($\beta = 0.10$; $Z_{\beta} = 1.28$) rather than 80% power ($\beta = 0.20$; $Z_{\beta} = 0.84$)].
➤ The standard deviation of the outcome measure is increased (using a less precise method of measurement).
➤ The difference between groups is decreased (considering a smaller difference as meaningful).

Full discussion of the issues involved in sample size determination and the formulas for calculations are provided in the textbooks mentioned earlier,[1,4,5] as well as in articles specifically addressing applications in ophthalmology.[16,17] Clinical trials involving two eyes of the same person, either both in one treatment group or one eye in each of two treatment groups, must use methods that accommodate the correlation between eyes in the outcome measure.

Some points about sample size determination warrant special emphasis. The size of the sample is extremely sensitive to the magnitude of the difference between treatment groups. Choosing an unrealistically large difference between groups that yields a small sample size will provide low power for detecting smaller, but clinically meaningful differences. Few treatments are dramatically effective. A reasonable starting point for discussion of the size of the difference to be detected is a 33% relative reduction, such as 30% risk reduced to 20%. Whether the difference should be larger or smaller depends on the severity of the vision loss as well as the risks and costs of treatment. Although 80% power is standard in many areas of investigation, higher levels of power are often used in clinical trials because failing to identify a truly effective treatment is a serious error. Also, the calculated sample size must allow for deaths and losses to follow-up.

Some clinical trials are designed to show that two treatments are 'equivalent'. A treatment with proven efficacy may be associated with high costs, pain, side effects or some other undesirable property. In these instances, identifying a replacement treatment of similar efficacy is important. The approach to sample size calculation for equivalency trials is different from the traditional approach described above.[18]

7.2.8 Masking and other practices to strengthen trial design

Clinical trials incorporate many procedures to minimize bias and increase precision in the comparison of treatment groups. **Masking** patients, evaluators, and those managing patient care to the assigned treatment group is a powerful tool in reducing the possibility of bias. As mentioned above, placebo medications and sham treatments can be used. If these procedures cannot be used, clinical evaluators of patients may be masked by having different people responsible for assigning the treatment and evaluating the patient. Information identifying the treatment group is removed from all material available to evaluators, and patients are requested not to reveal their treatment assignment to the evaluators. Those evaluating laboratory results, fundus photographs, or other images are easily masked by labelling materials with only identification numbers and codes unrelated to treatment group. Well-defined protocols for all outcome assessments not only reduce the opportunity for biased ascertainment, but also decrease the magnitude of random measurement error. Quality control procedures, such as certification of clinical centre staff in protocol procedures, assessment of intra-observer and inter-observer variation in evaluations, and ongoing review of incoming data to identify evidence of non-protocol practices, contribute to the standardization that reduces bias and increases precision.

7.3 DATA ANALYSIS AND MONITORING DATA AND SAFETY

7.3.1 Statistical methods for data analysis

Most data from well-designed and executed clinical trials require only simple statistical methods for the analysis of independent or paired (correlated) data. Methods for comparison of independent groups (χ^2 test of independence, t-test, Wilcoxon Rank Sum test, logrank test) may be used for clinical trials involving only one eye per person and those involving a person-specific outcome measure (e.g. quality of life score). Methods for comparison of correlated groups (McNemar's test for paired proportions, paired t-test, Wilcoxon Signed Rank test,) may be used for trials involving treatment of one eye with one treatment and the contralateral eye with the alternative treatment. When both eyes of the patient are assigned the same treatment and the outcome measure may be assessed on each eye, either one person-specific score may be used (the average of two eyes, or worst eye, or composite score) or the score from each eye may be analyzed using methods that account for the correlation between eyes. The choice of approach should be tied to the exact objective of the trial and the formulation of the primary outcome measure. Fortunately, there have been many advances incor-

porated into the major statistical software packages to deal with the analysis of correlated data.[19,20]

Recruitment of patients may take place over months or years so that patients have varying length of follow-up. Survival analysis methods, such as the **Kaplan–Meier** method and **Cox proportional hazards regression**, accommodate varying lengths of follow-up. The outcome measure must be specified as a binary event and the methods are valid only on the assumption that the reason for the varying length of follow-up is not related to the outcome, so that missed visits and loss to follow-up are not to be related to whether the patient's status is good or bad. Recent advances in the analysis of repeated measures data, continuous or categorical, also accommodate varying lengths of follow-up.[21]

7.3.2 Data analysis by 'intention to treat'

Data analysis by 'intention to treat' means that data from patients (eyes) should be analyzed in the group to which the patient (eye) was assigned. This applies to patients who never received an assigned active treatment, were administered the alternative treatment, were non-compliant, had extraordinary events that affected their outcome measures, were unmasked, or deviated in any other way from the protocol. These departures from the trial protocol compromise the interpretation of the results, no matter how the data are analyzed. However, alternatives to intention-to-treat data analysis are subject to inducing greater bias in the comparison of treatment groups. Patients who fall into these categories often have outcomes that are very different from other patients and excluding them or reassigning them can have substantial impact on results. Note that in order to complete an intention-to-treat analysis, all patients must continue to be followed for outcomes after their departure from the study protocol.

7.3.3 Rationale for data and safety monitoring

Data from clinical trials that have long periods of recruitment and/or follow-up are reviewed periodically by a group of methodologists, clinicians and others concerned with the patients as research subjects. Guidelines for committees have been promulgated by the **USA Food and Drug Administration (FDA)**[a] as well as the **National Institutes of Health (NIH)**.[b] The primary purpose of the review is to evaluate the evidence of harm or benefit in any of the treatment groups and, as needed, recommend changes to the protocol or stopping the trial. Patients and investigators participate in randomization of treatment groups on the assumption that none of the treatments is superior. Once there is clear evidence that a treatment is either beneficial or harmful, no patients should be assigned to the inferior treatment group.

7.3.4   Statistical implications of multiple analyses over time

Examining the data several times as they accumulate with the potential for stopping enrolment has an impact on the probability of declaring a difference between groups when one does not exist. Conventional experimental design assumes that there will be one analysis of the data. However, with interim monitoring, the more frequently the data are examined with the possibility of stopping the trial, the greater the chance of observing a large difference by chance, thereby increasing the chance of type I (α) error. Sequential analysis plans, interim analysis plans, α spending functions, and stochastic curtailment are some of the many statistical approaches to this problem. Most involve requiring very strong evidence of a treatment effect (very low p-values) early in the trial to designate the difference as statistically significant.

7.3.5   Other considerations for stopping early

Strong evidence of a treatment effect, as measured by the primary outcome variable, is just one of the factors influencing whether a clinical trial should be stopped early. Trends in secondary outcome measures that are not consistent with the primary outcome measure may indicate that additional patients and follow-up are needed to fully judge the treatment. Similarly, treatment effects that are not consistent over important subgroups of patients or that appear only in patients enrolled during a specific time period or a subset of clinical centres, large amounts of missing data, the possibility of reversal in effect with longer observation, the possibility of late complications, and conflicting results from other similar clinical trials may each warrant continuation of the clinical trial.

7.4   REPORTING RESULTS

In order for the results of clinical trials to have the appropriate impact on clinical practice, the design, conduct, analysis, and interpretation must be presented clearly and in sufficient detail to allow readers to judge the validity of the results and conclusions. An international group of leaders in clinical trial methodology and editors of medical journals have developed the **Consolidated Standards of Reporting Trials (CONSORT)** statement to help authors prepare manuscripts reporting on randomized clinical trials[22] (Table 7.2). The statement provides a checklist of key points in the design and conduct of the trial and a flow diagram providing the numbers of patients assessed for eligibility, randomized to each treatment group, followed in each treatment group, and analyzed in each treatment group. Reasons for patients not having been followed or analyzed must be supplied by the authors of the manuscript. The items on the checklist address areas that may produce biased estimates of treatment effect and/or affect the reliability or relevance of the findings. Editors of most of the major journals in ophthalmology now require that a completed CONSORT statement be submitted with the manuscripts.

7.5   FUTURE DIRECTIONS

Clinical trials in the future are likely to retain the key design elements of past trials. However, the

---

[a] http://www.fda.gov/downloads/RegulatoryInformation/ Guidances/UCM126578.pdf

[b] http://grants.nih.gov/grants/guide/notice-files/not98-084.html

Table 7.2 *CONSORT table*

CONSORT Statement 2001 Checklist
Items to include when reporting a randomized trial

PAPER SECTION and topic	Item	Descriptor
TITLE & ABSTRACT	1	How participants were allocated to interventions (e.g. 'random allocation', 'randomized', or 'randomly assigned').
INTRODUCTION		
Background	2	Scientific background and explanation of rationale.
METHODS		
Participants	3	Eligibility criteria for participants and the settings and locations where the data were collected.
Interventions	4	Precise details of the interventions intended for each group and how and when they were actually administered.
Objectives	5	Specific objectives and hypotheses.
Outcomes	6	Clearly defined primary and secondary outcome measures and, when applicable, any methods used to enhance the quality of measurements (e.g. multiple observations, training of assessors).
Sample size	7	How sample size was determined and, when applicable, explanation of any interim analyses and stopping rules.
Randomization — Sequence generation	8	Method used to generate the random allocation sequence, including details of any restrictions (e.g. blocking, stratification).
Randomization — Allocation concealment	9	Method used to implement the random allocation sequence (e.g. numbered containers or central telephone), clarifying whether the sequence was concealed until interventions were assigned.
Randomization — Implementation	10	Who generated the allocation sequence, who enrolled participants, and who assigned participants to their groups.
Blinding (masking)	11	Whether or not participants, those administering the interventions, and those assessing the outcomes were blinded to group assignment. If done, how the success of blinding was evaluated.
Statistical methods	12	Statistical methods used to compare groups for primary outcome(s); Methods for additional analyses, such as subgroup analyses and adjusted analyses.
RESULTS		
Participant flow	13	Flow of participants through each stage (a diagram is strongly recommended). Specifically, for each group report the numbers of participants randomly assigned, receiving intended treatment, completing the study protocol, and analyzed for the primary outcome. Describe protocol deviations from study as planned, together with reasons.
Recruitment	14	Dates defining the periods of recruitment and follow-up.
Baseline data	15	Baseline demographic and clinical characteristics of each group.
Numbers analyzed	16	Number of participants (denominator) in each group included in each analysis and whether the analysis was by 'intention-to-treat'. State the results in absolute numbers when feasible (*e.g.* 10/20, not 50%).
Outcomes and estimation	17	For each primary and secondary outcome, a summary of results for each group, and the estimated effect size and its precision (e.g. 95% confidence interval).
Ancillary analyses	18	Address multiplicity by reporting any other analyses performed, including subgroup analyses and adjusted analyses, indicating those pre-specified and those exploratory.
Adverse events	19	All important adverse events or side effects in each intervention group.
DISCUSSION		
Interpretation	20	Interpretation of the results, taking into account study hypotheses, sources of potential bias or imprecision and the dangers associated with multiplicity of analyses and outcomes.
Generalizability	21	Generalizability (external validity) of the trial findings.
Overall evidence	22	General interpretation of the results in the context of current evidence.

From Moher D, Schulz KF, Altman DG. The CONSORT statement: revised recommendations for improving the quality of reports of parallel-group randomised trials. *Lancet* 2001; 357(9263):1191-1194.

The CONSORT Statement 2001 checklist is intended to be accompanied with the explanatory document that facilitates its use. For more information, visit www.consort-statement.org.

orientation of the objectives, outcome measures, and interpretation are likely to move more towards consideration of the impact of adopting a treatment in the general practice of ophthalmology. Expenditure of funds and other resources, the magnitude of the treatment benefit, and the ability of the healthcare system to deliver the treatment will receive greater attention in the design of clinical trials. As more treatments for the major conditions are established as at least minimally efficacious, there will be more trials of new, candidate treatments versus the currently available treatment with the aim of showing that the new treatment is equivalent to or better than the currently available treatment. The trials in the United States, United Kingdom and several European countries comparing ranibizumab and bevacizumab for treatment of neovascular age-related macular degeneration are examples of such clinical trials. Advances in technology will provide the ability to capture data and images from nearly every clinical care facility so that more investigators may participate easily in clinical trials. The challenge with widespread participation will be in assuring that evaluation of eligibility criteria, treatment of patients, and assessment of outcome measures are performed with sufficient adherence to the protocol.

REFERENCES

1. Meinert CL. *Clinical Trials: Design, Conduct, and Analysis*. New York: Oxford University Press; 1986.

2. Diabetic Retinopathy Study Research Group. Preliminary report on effects of photocoagulation therapy. *Am J Ophthalmol* 1976; 81:383–397.

3. Diabetic Retinopathy Study Research Group. Photocoagulation treatment of proliferative diabetic retinopathy: the second report of Diabetic Retinopathy Study findings. *Ophthalmology* 1978; 85:82–106.

4. Friedman LM, Furberg CD, Demets DL. *Fundamentals of Clinical Trials*, 3rd Edition. New York: Springer Science + Business Media; 1998.

5. Piantadosi S. *Clinical Trials: A Methodologic Perspective*, 2nd Edition. New York: John Wiley & Sons; 2005.

6. Brown DM, Kaiser PK, Michels M, *et al*. Ranibizumab versus verteporfin for neovascular age-related macular degeneration. *N Engl J Med* 2006; 355:1432–1444.

7. Treatment of Age-related Macular Degeneration With Photodynamic Therapy (TAP) Study Group. Photodynamic therapy of subfoveal choroidal neovascularization in age-related macular degeneration with verteporfin: one-year results of 2 randomized clinical trials — TAP report 1. *Arch Ophthalmol* 1999; 117:1329–1345.

8. Peto R, Baigent C. Trials: the next 50 years. Large scale randomised evidence of moderate benefits. *Br Med J* 1998; 317:1170–1171.

9. Multicenter Uveitis Steroid Treatment (MUST) Trial — ClinicalTrials.gov. Web 18 Oct 2009. (http://clinicaltrials.gov/ct2/show/NCT00132691.)

10. Age-Related Eye Disease Study Research Group. A randomized, placebo-controlled, clinical trial of high-dose supplementation with vitamins C and E, beta carotene, and zinc for age-related macular degeneration and vision loss: AREDS report no. 8. *Arch Ophthalmol* 2001; 119: 1417–1436.

11. Glaucoma Laser Trial Research Group. The Glaucoma Laser Trial (GLT): 4. Contralateral effects of timolol on the intraocular pressure of eyes treated with ALT. *Ophthalmic Surgery* 1991; 22:324–329.

12. Schulz KF. Subverting randomization in controlled trials. *JAMA* 1995; 274:1456–1458.

13. Beck RW, Moke PS, Turpin AH, *et al*. A computerized method of visual acuity testing: adaption of the Early Treatment of Diabetic Retinopathy Study testing protocol. *Am J Ophthalmol* 2003; 135:194–205.

14. Berson EL, Rosner B, Sandberg MA, *et al*. A randomized trial of vitamin A and vitamin E supplementation for retinitis pigmentosa. *Arch Ophthalmol* 1993; 111:761–772.

15. Bailey IL, Bullimore MA, Raasch TW, *et al*. Clinical grading and the effects of scaling. *Invest Ophthalmol Vis Sci* 1991; 32:422–432.

16. Javitt JC. When does the failure to find a difference mean that there is none? *Arch Ophthalmol* 1989; 107:1034–1040.

17. Gauderman WJ, Barlow WE. Sample size calculations for ophthalmologic studies. *Arch Ophthalmol* 1992; 110:690–692.

18. Roebruck P, Kuhn A. Comparison of tests and sample size formulae for proving therapeutic equivalence based on the difference of binomial probabilities. *Stat Med* 1995; 14:1583–1594.

19. Glynn RJ, Rosner B. Accounting for the correlation between fellow eyes in regression analysis. *Arch Ophthalmol* 1992; 110:381–387.

20. Therneau TM, Grambsch PM, Fleming TR. Martingale-based residuals for survival models. *Biometrika* 1990; 77:147–160.

21. Zeger SL, Liang K-Y. Longitudinal data analysis for discrete and continuous outcomes. *Biometrics* 1986; 42:121–130.

22. Moher D, Schutz KF, Altman DG, for the CONSORT Group. The CONSORT statement: revised recommendations for improving the quality of reports of parallel-group randomised clinical trials. *Lancet* 2001; 357:1191–1194.

Screening in ophthalmology

RICHARD WORMALD AND ROBERT LINDFIELD

8.1   Introduction   147
8.2   Definition of screening   147
8.3   Principles of screening   148
8.4   Planning a programme   150
8.5   Quality assurance of screening   150
      programmes
8.6   Evaluation of screening programmes   151
8.7   Specific issues in ophthalmology   156
8.8   Future research priorities   164
8.9   Conclusion   165
      References   165

8.1   INTRODUCTION

Preventing disease is vital to secure health. Prevention can be broken down into three separate approaches: *primary* (preventing occurrence of disease), *secondary* (preventing the effects of disease) and *tertiary* (restoring function lost as a results of disease). Screening is an important weapon in the armoury of secondary prevention.

Screening exposes many healthy individuals to an examination to identify a few who may have disease. Clear thinking and a careful evaluation are essential when any screening programme is undertaken. An understanding of the principles of screening and how they apply to the specific condition targeted is mandatory. These principles and their application to some of the main areas of blindness prevention are considered in this chapter.

8.2   DEFINITION OF SCREENING

'Screening is a process of identifying apparently healthy people who may be at increased risk of a disease or condition. They can then be offered information, further tests and appropriate treatment to reduce their risk and/or any complications arising from the disease or condition.'[1]

If the presence of the condition is confirmed, then effective treatment should lead to a better outcome than that associated with presentation later in the clinical course of the disease (when it has become symptomatic). Such an improved outcome may impinge not just on the individual but also on his/her immediate associates or on the population as a whole (e.g. identifying and treating people for diabetic retinopathy reduces the cost of blindness to society).

Screening is a public health intervention intended to reduce the population burden of a condition or its consequences.[2] It is often confused with opportunistic testing, sometimes termed case finding, when a screening test may be used. An example of case finding is the routine testing of intraocular pressure amongst people presenting with an eye problem other than glaucoma. Opportunistic case finding occurs when a test is offered to an individual without symptoms of the disease when he/she presents to a health care practitioner for reasons unrelated to that disease.

A population-based screening programme is an organized integrated process where all activities along the screening pathway are planned, coordinated, monitored and evaluated through a quality assurance framework. All of these activities must be resourced adequately to ensure benefits are maximised.

It is now well recognized that effects of screening may not always be beneficial and that harmful outcomes can occur. These arise as a result of errors of the screening test: mistaken designation as being disease-free or affected (i.e. both false-negative and false-positive test results) that can have serious consequences. The test itself may also potentially be harmful (see below).

An important consideration of screening is that it is a health intervention imposed on the population, and so has important ethical implications. Traditionally, medical care is provided for those who seek help. Screening aims to provide healthcare before help is sought in order to identify and treat illness at an earlier stage in its natural history and thereby achieve a better outcome. Individuals must not be coerced, yet their participation is essential if the programme is to be effective. This can only be achieved by convincing the public that being screened offers real benefits to the individual or the community. The benefits must be tangible and well understood by the public without causing undue alarm or anxiety.

Public anxiety can be allayed in part through a robust quality assurance process. This ensures that specific standards are maintained throughout the screening programme, which must have a continuous programme quality assurance.

Different countries approach screening in different ways. Screening for a variety of different diseases has been established throughout the United Kingdom (UK). Currently there are eleven screening programmes in the UK covering cancer, antenatal and newborn, child health, sexually transmitted diseases and vascular disease and it includes a national screening programme for diabetic retinopathy (see Box 8.2). A **National Screening Committee (NSC)** oversees the activities of these screening programmes.

8.3   PRINCIPLES OF SCREENING

A World Health Organization (WHO) working paper published in 1968 considered various aspects of screening and determined a number of principles that will always be relevant to any screening programme in any health environment.[3] However, as with many such principles, they cannot all be universally applied to all situations, and exceptions occur, as will be seen below. After taking into account international work on the appraisal of screening programmes, particularly from Canada and the United States of America (USA), the NSC has added to the original principles. The principles concern the condition itself, the screening test, the treatment and the screening programme, and are detailed in Box 8.1.

Box 8.1   *United Kingdom National Screening Committee principles for screening*

The Condition:

- The condition should be an important health problem.
- The epidemiology and natural history of the condition, including development from latent to declared disease, should be adequately understood and there should be a detectable risk factor, disease marker, latent period or early symptomatic stage.
- All the cost-effective primary prevention interventions should have been implemented as far as practicable.
- If the carriers of a mutation are identified as a result of screening the natural history of people with this status should be understood, including any psychological implications.

The Test:

- There should be a simple, safe, precise, reliable, robust, and validated screening test.
- The distribution of test values in the target population should be known and a suitable cut-off level defined and agreed.

(Continued)

(*Continued*)

- The test should be acceptable to the population.
- There should be an agreed policy on the further diagnostic investigation of individuals with a positive test result and on the choices available to them.
- If the test is for mutations, if all possible known mutations are not being tested, the criteria used to select the subset of mutations to be covered by screening, should be clearly set out.

The Treatment:

- There should be an effective treatment or intervention for patients identified through early detection, with evidence of early treatment leading to better outcomes than late treatment.
- There should be agreed evidence-based policies covering which individuals should be offered treatment and the appropriate treatment to be offered.
- Clinical management of the condition and patient outcomes should be optimised in all health care providers prior to participation in a screening programme.

The Screening Programme:

- There should be evidence from high quality Randomised Controlled Trials that the screening programme is effective in reducing mortality or morbidity. Where screening is aimed solely at providing information to allow the person being screened to make an 'informed choice' (e.g. Down's syndrome, cystic fibrosis carrier screening), there must be evidence from high quality trials that the test accurately measures risk. The information that is provided about the test and its outcome must be of value and readily understood by the individual being screened.
- There should be evidence that the complete screening programme (test, diagnostic procedures, treatment/intervention) is clinically, socially and ethically acceptable to health professionals and the public.

(*Continued*)

- The benefit from the screening programme should outweigh the physical and psychological harm (caused by the test, diagnostic procedures and treatment).
- The opportunity cost of the screening programme (including testing, diagnosis and treatment, administration, training and quality assurance) should be economically balanced in relation to expenditure on medical care as a whole (i.e. value for money). Assessment against these criteria should have regard to evidence from cost–benefit and/or cost-effectiveness analyses and have regard to the effective use of available resources.
- All other options for managing the condition should have been considered (e.g. improving treatment, providing other services), to ensure that no more cost-effective intervention could be introduced or current interventions increased within the resources available.
- There should be a plan for managing and monitoring the screening programme and an agreed set of quality assurance standards.
- Adequate staffing and facilities for testing, diagnosis, treatment and programme management should be available prior to the commencement of the screening programme.
- Evidence-based information, explaining the consequences of testing, investigation and treatment, should be made available to potential participants to assist them in making an informed choice.
- Public pressure for widening the eligibility criteria for reducing the screening interval, and for increasing the sensitivity of the testing process, should be anticipated. Decisions about these parameters should be scientifically justifiable to the public.

[The principles are specific to the UK but are relevant to most screening programmes in other countries. However, differing historical backgrounds to the ethical debate in other countries may result in different decisions about the implementation and application of screening.]

This information is available on the NSC website at http://www.nsc.nhs.uk/

8.4   PLANNING A PROGRAMME

There are specific stages in the development of a screening programme. This needs careful planning before implementation.

8.4.1   Justifying the screening programme

A justification in terms of opportunity cost and the public health significance of the disease should be clearly laid out. The target population and its enumeration should be defined precisely. This should normally be based on high quality evidence of the effectiveness of screening as a public health intervention in the relevant setting, including cost-effectiveness analysis. More than one and preferably several independent randomized trials of screening included in a systematic review with meta-analysis when appropriate (see Chapter 9 on meta-analysis) provide the ideal evidence base for justifying a screening programme.

8.4.2   Identifying people to be screened

The target population is defined by specific characteristics including age (e.g. newborn), gender (e.g. cervical cancer) or condition (e.g. diabetic, pregnant). People with these characteristics are referred to the screening programme according to specific criteria.

Referral criteria should be agreed upon, and be acceptable to all clinicians who will receive the referrals. Channels of communication for referral and feedback should be established with clearly defined mechanisms for follow-up of non-attendees (so called call/recall mechanisms). Facilities for the diagnosis and treatment of detected cases should be in place before the programme commences, and the policy regarding who to treat and how should be agreed by all clinical participants.

A coherent plan for the systematic coverage of the population by invitation, testing and follow-up must be constructed with adequate administrative support. Appropriate measures to deal with non-responders, such as the number of further invitations and reminders, need planning.

8.4.3   Setting up the screening service

Screening sites should be chosen to maximize uptake. Once identified, the necessary equipment and trained personnel must be supplied to each site. A single team can move round a number of sites to save on costs. When all is in place, invitations for screening can be delivered and examinations commenced.

8.4.4   Ensuring quality

Mechanisms for the prospective evaluation of the programme, which should include both process and outcome measures, should be in place. Monitoring of false-positive referrals is straightforward but it is more difficult to define false-negative or missed cases. Two methods are available. A random or systematic sample of test-negative cases may be referred for verification of their case-negative status at the diagnostic centre. The sample size for this will depend on the estimated false-negative rate and the precision of the estimate of sensitivity, as in sample survey methodology. Monitoring of true-positive referrals from subsequent screening of the target population should attempt to determine whether such cases are newly incident since the previous test, or whether they were missed cases at the previous examination. This may be determined by the stage at which the disease is detected and by a re-examination of the results of the previous test.

8.5   QUALITY ASSURANCE OF SCREENING PROGRAMMES

Quality assurance (QA) is a system of monitoring and maintaining the standards of every aspect of a screening programme. Every screening programme needs a robust QA process to ensure that standards set at the beginning are being met throughout the programme.

There are two types of QA, internal and external:

1. Internal QA is a continuous check of the process and outcomes of each screening programme to ensure that it is meeting and maintaining standards. It is conducted by staff employed by the screening programme. The resulting statistics are reported to an overarching body responsible for quality assurance, but the programme staff should use the information to monitor the programme and make appropriate changes where necessary.
2. External QA is a regular but infrequent review of a screening programme using staff external to the screening programme to assess whether the programme is meeting standards. The overarching body responsible for quality assurance receives the report and necessary changes are implemented.

8.6 EVALUATION OF SCREENING PROGRAMMES

A screening programme can be evaluated by reviewing:

1. The process of screening.
2. The outcome of screening.

Process measures of screening evaluate the activity of the screening programme, whereas outcome measures are concerned with the impact of the programme on the health of the target population.

8.6.1 Process measures

Process measures include:

- Validity of the screening test — sensitivity and specificity.
- Reliability of the screening test — measurement of within and between observer variation.
- Yield of screening.
- Cost per case detected and successfully treated.
- Coverage of screening.

The **validity** of a test is its ability to differentiate correctly between those who have the disease and

Table 8.1 *2 × 2 table for the sensitivity, specificity and predictive value of a screening test*

	Disease-Positive	Disease-Negative	Total
Test-positive	A	B	A + B
Test-negative	C	D	C + D
Total	A + C	B + D	A + B + C + D

those who do not. Two kinds of error, *false-positive* and *false-negative*, may occur, both of which are important in a screening programme. They are best examined with a traditional 2 × 2 table analysis. In practice, the most important parameters are the **sensitivity** (sometimes termed detection rate) and the **positive predictive value (PPV)**, which depends on the prevalence of the disease in the target population.

When drawing the table (Table 8.1) it is essential to adhere to the convention and to place the gold standard findings (disease-positive and disease-negative) in the columns and the test findings in the rows, otherwise confusion and error are inevitable.

Sensitivity (detection rate) is the proportion of persons with the disease that the test correctly identifies [$= A/(A + C)$ in Table 8.1] usually expressed as a percentage. Thus the sensitivity of a test is a measure of its ability to detect disease in those who are affected.

Specificity (true-negative rate) is the proportion of persons who are disease-free whom the test identifies as normal [$= D/(B + D)$ in Table 8.1]. Thus the specificity of a test is a measure of its ability to identify correctly those who are disease-free.

The computation of these test parameters depends upon the existence of a gold standard that can determine the truth with regard to the disease status of the participants. This can be problematic in some situations, for example when it is hard to categorize individuals clearly as diseased and non-diseased, or when the case definition is imprecise. This is particularly true for glaucoma. In nature, few diseases demonstrate a clear step from being disease-free to being affected. Usually there is a continuum between health and disease, particularly for chronic or degenerative disease. Thus, an arbitrary judgment based on practical considerations must be made in order to decide when the transition from health to disease has occurred.

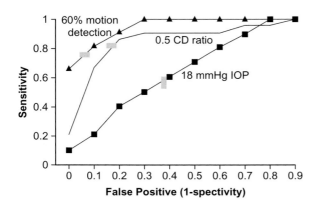

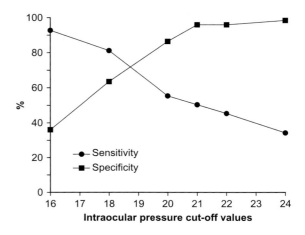

Figure 8.1 *Receiver operating characteristic (ROC) curve for sensitivity and specificity of three screening tests used in the Roscommon glaucoma survey[4] for differing cut-off points of intraocular pressure (IOP), cup–disc ratio (CD) and motion-sensitivity testing. Optimum cut-off points for each test are shown as shaded boxes*

Figure 8.2 *Sensitivity and specificity plotted for different values of a test (intraocular pressure for Caucasian participants in the Baltimore Eye Survey)[6]*

The relation between sensitivity and specificity is important. Increasing the sensitivity of a test will usually be at the expense of specificity, and vice versa. This is best described by plotting the sensitivity of a test parameter (y axis) against 1 — specificity (x axis) for different cut-off values of the test (Fig. 8.1). The closer the curve is to the top left-hand corner of the graph, the better or more discriminating the test. The area under each curve quantifies differences between tests. The method was first described by researchers examining the sensitivity of radar to detect signals, and was termed the '**receiver operating characteristic' curve** (**ROC**), a term still used to describe such plots.[5]

An alternative is simply to plot sensitivity and specificity against different values of the test-parameter outcome. The lines of each cross at the point where sensitivity and specificity values are optimal (Fig. 8.2), although this is not necessarily the best point at which to set the test value. Implications of false-positive and false-negative findings have to be considered carefully in order to achieve the right balance.

Positive predictive value (**PPV**) is the probability of being disease-positive if the test is positive. This is an important parameter [= A/(A + B)] because it reveals the amount of work the screening test will generate at the referral centres

and the number of persons who will be unnecessarily referred for further examination. It is determined by the false-positive rate (B) but also influenced by the prevalence of the disease. PPV can also be described in Bayesian terms[7] as the conditional probability of being disease-positive if the test is positive. This can be expressed as:

$$PPV = \frac{sensitivity \times prevalence}{probability\ of\ a\ positive\ test}$$

It is the combined probability of the test detecting a case when among known cases (i.e. the sensitivity) and the probability of the individual being a case in the target population (the prevalence) divided by the overall probability of a test being positive in the population. Thus even when the test sensitivity is high, if the prevalence is low, so also will be the PPV (see worked example in box below). The Bayesian concepts behind this are explored in some good statistical texts.[7]

Negative predictive value (**NPV**) is the probability of being disease-negative if the test is negative [=D/(C + D)]. This is relevant to the concerns of screened individuals, and influences the degree of assurance that the screened negative person can assume when the test is negative. Like PPV, it is prevalence-dependent. When the prevalence is low, the NPV will tend to be high, even though the test may be quite insensitive. In the worked example below, the NPV is 8950/8955, which is negligibly different from 1.

Yield is the number of persons screened to detect one case and is also dependent on prevalence of disease in the population [= (A + B + C + D)/A]. Yield can be extended to include cost per yield and further, cost per yield who are then successfully treated.

The stage at which the disease is detected is a useful way of examining the progress of the screening programme over time. In the example of diabetic eye disease, severe retinopathy should become increasingly rare with each screen of the population as the condition is detected earlier in its natural history (see Chapter 21).

Prevalence is the proportion of true cases in the population [= (A + C)/(A + B + C + D)] and is an important consideration in any screening programme because of its effect on PPV; but it is also a measure of the public health importance of the disease. A reasonably precise estimate of the prevalence of a disease is required before screening can be implemented. Screening is not an appropriate method for estimating prevalence, although screening tests may be used in a sample survey to estimate prevalence.

Worked example

In a hypothetical population of 10,000 with a disease prevalence of 0.5%, the 2 × 2 table can be drawn up as in Table 8.2.

Because the PPV is the sensitivity of the test multiplied by the prevalence divided by the probability of a positive test (0.9 × 0.005/0.1045 = 0.043) and is 4.3%, one can calculate the number of false-positives in cell B as 1,000 and the specificity of the test [(8950/9950) × 100], which is 90%. One might assume that a test with a 90% sensitivity and specificity would perform well, but with a low prevalence, large numbers of false-positives have to be assessed in order to find one true case. In this example, it is 22 false-positives for every true-positive (i.e. the yield is low).

The **reliability** of a test measures variability of the test results, whereas validity deals with the ability of the test to distinguish normal from abnormal. A reliable test gives consistent results when repeated on the same individual. It depends on the variation inherent in the test itself, which may be random or biological (sometimes termed reproducibility), and that introduced by the observer who conducts the test, which may be both random and systematic (intra-(within) and inter-(between) observer variation).

There are two sources of this variation, namely the subject and the instrument.

The subject. Some biological parameters are notoriously variable. An example is the intraocular pressure (IOP), which varies with diurnal rhythm, with each cardiac cycle, with posture, and possibly also seasonally. Similarly, responses to luminous stimuli at threshold in visual field testing are subject to short- and long-term fluctuation. A wide variance in responses as a result of this has a deleterious influence on a screening test, reducing its sensitivity and PPV. This type of variation is hard to control. Biological measurements, which are subject to wide variations, manifest a phenomenon known as the regression to the mean. Single measurements have a certain probability of being an outlying or atypical finding, which increases with the variability of the measurement. Repeated measurements of the same parameter will tend to regress to the mean value (either above or below), and so give a more representative result. Thus one way of dealing with this type of variation is to repeat the measurement on several occasions. This can be problematic in screening, when there may be only one opportunity to apply the test.

The instrument. The precision of a measurement made by any instrument depends upon its powers of discrimination in the detection of relevant biological changes. Recent interest in optical scanning of the **nerve fibre layer** (**NFL**) as a way of

Table 8.2 Worked example of a 2 × 2 table

	Disease-Positive	Disease-Negative	Total
Test-positive	45	1000	1045
Test-negative	5	8950	8955
Total	50	9950	10000

detecting glaucoma, by measuring its thickness, is limited by the machine's ability to detect small changes in a way that is reproducible, that is, by its signal-to-noise ratio. Repeated measures on the same area of the neuroretina must vary significantly less than the degree of change that would constitute clinical relevance. When these changes are a matter of a few microns, extreme demands are made of the precision of such instruments. Instruments vary in their consistency and, depending on the field conditions of the screening programme, may require more or less frequent calibration. The more robust the test, the less frequent will be the need for a calibration but, whatever the circumstances, regular calibration of instruments used in screening is essential.

Inter- and intra-observer variations. One component of the reproducibility of repeated observations in the above example will be that introduced by the operator of the instrument. For example, small random variations in the determination of the end-point in applanation tonometry or the angle of incidence of the air jet on the cornea in pneumo-tonometry may be the cause. Because the dials of the Goldmann and Perkins tonometers are graded in 2 mmHg steps, digit preference, with even numbers being recorded more frequently than odd, is often observed in IOP measurements. In the course of a screening programme, an observer's methods may also drift systematically with time. Using standard controls repeatedly throughout the programme can help to maintain consistency, limiting the tendency to drift and controlling intra-observer (i.e. within observer) variation.

Inter-observer variation (i.e. between-observer variation) can also be controlled. This source of variation tends to be more important because it can be systematic rather than random. It is reduced by clear instructions and training, with frequent calibration. The best way to measure agreement (or concordance) between observers is a matter of some statistical controversy, and a number of different approaches have been described. The simplest is to record the percentage agreement for all observations made by two or more observers. Statisticians have pointed out that this approach is inadequate because it makes no allowance for chance agreement. When the number of possible outcomes is small, the possibility of chance agreement is high. The most frequently quoted statistic for the measurement of agreement is the **kappa statistic** (κ). This compensates for chance agreement by observing the proportion of observed agreements that occur in excess of (or less than) those expected by chance alone. The kappa statistic is therefore a value that ranges from 1 to –1. Zero denotes no agreement beyond that expected by chance; 1 is perfect agreement; and –1 is perfect disagreement. The standard error of κ can be calculated, which enables its precision to be quantified by confidence limits. Kappa can be further refined by weighting for discordance, when the observations are ranked categorical measures, so that more weight is given to disagreements beyond one ranked category and less to disagreement within one category. This is called the *weighted κ statistic.*

The acceptable level of kappa depends on the nature of the observations and the implications of misclassification, but generally a level of 0.75 or more represents very good agreement. The method of calculating κ can be found in several good statistical texts.[8]

For a screening programme to have its desired effect on the population at risk, the great majority of that population should be tested. **Coverage** is the proportion of the population at risk, including those with the disease who are undiagnosed, who are screened during any one trawl. The case-detection rate will always be limited by the number of cases who fail to attend the screening procedure. The actual detection rate will depend on the biases influencing the response to screening. In general, a healthy volunteer effect is observed, with those at a relatively low risk of the disease responding to the invitation for screening, while those at a higher risk decline. Thus the prevalence of disease in those tested is lower than the true prevalence and the PPV adversely affected. Occasionally, bias works in the opposite direction when an increased genetic risk may lead to greater uptake. Persons with a family history of glaucoma, for example, may be more likely to respond to an invitation for screening.

For screening to be successful a special effort must therefore be made to encourage response.

Here the acceptability of the screening test is of importance. An unpleasant, painful or invasive test will deter response. The target population must be properly informed about the nature and purpose of the screening test so that all can clearly understand that there is a real benefit to be derived from attending. Access to the screening site must be optimal. Long and costly travel to the site will deter attendance. Ideally, screening should be available within the community of the target population, outside the hospital setting (which is associated with fear and disease), and preferably in the primary care setting where individuals are used to having contact with healthcare services. Feedback, explanation and reassurance about the outcome of the examination are essential for all individuals so that the word spreads in the community that attending the screen is a positive experience.

8.6.2   Outcome measures

As the main aim of screening is to reduce the morbidity of a given condition, the principal outcome should be a measure of the impact of the screening process. The success of a programme of screening for diabetic retinopathy should therefore be a measure of the reduction of visual impairment from that cause which can be attributable to the earlier detection and successful treatment. For example, the expressed goal of the WHO working party on diabetes in the St Vincent declaration of 1990 was to reduce diabetic blindness by one third by the year 2000.[9] For this to be possible, some mechanism for monitoring visual impairment in the target population has to be in place. It must also be realized that any decrease in visual impairment due to DR might be due to better management of the disease and attribution to the screening programme should be made with due caution.

Randomized trials of screening

When a large-scale and expensive screening programme is being considered, the best way of establishing whether or not it is justified and worthwhile is by conducting a randomized trial of screening.

Individuals or small communities are randomized to screening or no screening. Clearly defined and carefully measured outcomes can then be ascertained in groups with confidence that any differences are not explained by confounding factors, which will have been controlled for in the randomization process. The same cannot be said for non-randomized observational or natural history studies.

A number of randomized trials have been undertaken in the USA and Scandinavia for mammography screening for breast cancer, which clearly and consistently demonstrate a reduction in mortality in the screened group.[10] However, a subsequent systematic review of these trials suggests that all but one trial (which showed no effect) were at substantial risk of bias. There is now a controversy, with those in favour of screening attacking the reviewers for undermining the screening programme, and others casting doubt on the safety and effectiveness of the programme. This situation highlights the importance of good quality evidence on which to base screening initiatives.

Observational studies

Evidence of the effectiveness of screening can sometimes be gleaned from observational studies. It may be possible to examine temporal changes in statistics, or to compare geographical areas where screening has or has not been practised. Case-control studies can be used to examine the protective effect of screening on individuals with and without the adverse outcome that screening is intended to prevent.[11] In all these studies, and especially in case-control studies, great care must be taken to anticipate possible confounding factors. The weakness of all these methods is that the unknown confounder can never be controlled for.

Bias in screening studies

Two particular forms of bias may arise in the evaluation of screening, namely lead-time bias and length bias.

Lead-time bias may occur when there is an apparent increase in survival or onset of morbidity (like blindness) in a screened population compared with an unscreened one. Screening tends to lead to earlier detection of the disease, which in turn leads to an apparent increase in survival or increase in time free from morbidity because the earlier detected cases carry the diagnosis for longer. Their real times from onset of the disease to death or blindness may, in fact, be no different, but the screened cases are detected closer to onset than the unscreened cases.

Length bias is a similar but separate concern. Diseases may progress at different rates in different individuals. Some may have an aggressive disease progressing rapidly from onset to termination, whereas others may have an indolent or slowly progressive condition. Screening at specific time intervals (e.g. every three years) will tend to detect more indolent than aggressive cases because the indolent cases contribute more person-time at risk of being detected. A rapidly progressing disease may start and finish within the interval between the two screenings. This might equally explain why persons presenting late with glaucoma are at a great risk of blindness, late presentation being a marker for a rapidly progressive and severe disease. Screening will detect a greater proportion of milder or less aggressive disease, and thus give an erroneous or biased impression of benefit, and potentially lead to unnecessary treatment.

8.7 SPECIFIC ISSUES IN OPHTHALMOLOGY

8.7.1 Diabetic retinopathy

Different nations have different strategies to prevent blindness in persons with diabetes. In the USA, where eye care professionals are abundant, the **American Academy of Ophthalmology (AAO)** recommends regular comprehensive examination by a specialist, the frequency depending on the estimated level of risk.[12]

In the UK, the NSC has recommended implementation of national standards of screening for retinopathy using digital cameras. Although this entails an expensive initial capital cost, the use of cameras provides the basis of ongoing evaluation and quality control (see Box 8.2).

There is has been no randomized trial of diabetic screening, and the decision to implement national standards in the UK was made by a multidisciplinary consensus group. Screening was already taking place across the UK but in a variable and inconsistent way. It is, of course, only justified where adequate resources exist for the treatment of diabetic retinopathy; if, therefore, no laser equipment is available for retinal photocoagulation, no ground exists for screening for retinopathy. It becomes less important than the need for facilities for the optimum control of diabetes, which itself reduces the risk of developing retinopathy.

The population at risk

The key to a successful programme for the prevention of sight loss in patients with diabetes is the identification of persons at risk of having retinopathy, that is, all patients with diabetes in a defined population. This is best achieved by the establishment of a local diabetes register, which should be maintained carefully by a responsible team. Each newly diagnosed person with diabetes is added and each deceased or migrated patient removed. The register is then used to prompt the annual eye examination of each patient with diabetes, and a record is made of the outcome. Dedicated computer software is now available for the establishment of such registers.

A key issue in the screening of diabetes is the coverage of the programme. Those at greatest risk of sight loss are those with poor long-term control, for example teenagers and young adults, and these are also likely to be poorly compliant with other aspects of their treatment. Additionally, other complications of long-standing diabetes, such as peripheral vascular disease and amputation, may make it physically more difficult for these high-risk cases to attend an eye screening facility.

The screening test

The screening test may consist of a complete examination of the fundus through dilated pupils by an individual who is fully trained to recognize sight-threatening changes.

However the use of retinal photography, based on seven stereo fields, has been shown to be more effective than a clinical examination at detecting disease. For screening at least two 45° fields, one centred on the disk and the other on the macula, are required. More views may provide additional sensitivity, although at a trade-off of an increased cost. The advent of digital retinal cameras may facilitate screening, storage, transmission and retrieval of images. There is ongoing debate about the use of non-mydriatic digital cameras, which have the convenience of portability and have been used successfully in rural settings. Using non-mydriatic photos with three fields has been shown, in some studies, to be as sensitive and specific as standard seven field photographs, but result in more referrals because of ungradable pictures.

Structure

Depending on the structure of the screening programme, criteria for referral can be at two different levels. Simple single-level screening requires a larger measure of skill in order for the screener to judge whether or not sight-threatening retinopathy is present. A two-level process is an alternative, often employed in the UK, where the primary screener is required simply to determine whether any retinopathy is present. If so, the person is referred to the secondary level where the severity of the retinopathy is assessed, and subsequent referral on to an ophthalmologist is made when treatment is deemed necessary. The secondary level is provided by a diabetes physician who justifies the extra level, (and consequent cost), with the argument that those with any retinopathy require a full examination by a physician for any associated diabetic complications. This assumes that the physician is proficient in the detection of a retinopathy requiring the attention of an ophthalmologist. Such alternatives are relevant in countries where there are relatively few ophthalmologists, whose time has to be used with maximum efficiency; however, there is limited evidence for their effectiveness.

In most western European countries, there are sufficient ophthalmologists to provide primary screening. In low-income countries, visual impairment from diabetic retinopathy does not yet feature as a major priority in the prevention of blindness because there are few persons with diabetes, and those few rarely survive long enough to acquire retinopathy. In middle-income countries where economic development has been rapid, as in parts of India or the Gulf states, diabetes can be extremely common and visual impairment a common complication. Identification and treatment of sight-threatening diabetic retinopathy is increasingly important in these countries; however, the feasibility of large-scale screening programmes has yet to be established.

Frequency of screening

All maturity-onset patients should be screened at diagnosis and at regular intervals. Type 1 juvenile-onset cases need not be screened until five years after the onset of the condition, then regularly (between one and three years), because its onset is acute, and no significant damage is inflicted on the retinal vasculature in the first few years. Conversely, maturity-onset cases may have an occult onset, and approximately 5% of them will present with retinopathy, more if the cases are Latino (16%).

> **Box 8.2 *Description of the UK screening programme for diabetic retinopathy***
>
> The national screening programme for diabetic retinopathy was set up in the UK in 2004. Each country — England, Scotland, Northern Ireland and Wales — has its own programmes. Each has the same aim (to eliminate blindness due to diabetic retinopathy) and overall objectives, but some details of the specific country programmes differ. This section describes the English programme.
>
> The English DR screening programme was established in 2005. It has been gradually developed and expanded over time. The programme developed a set of specific objectives. These included an aim to screen 100% of registered diabetics in England by the end of 2007.
>
> *(Continued)*

(Continued)

Every diabetic over the age of 12 in England is eligible for inclusion. Each general practice has a register of persons with diabetes that generates a list for invitation to attend screening. Screening is organised by a local screening programme. There should be one screening programme per 12,000 persons with diabetes.

Every person with diabetes should receive a two-view digital image of their retina each year. This image is graded by qualified graders, and the patient is referred for further investigation and treatment if necessary. Each screening programme has a system in place to ensure that patients are called and re-called at the correct times.

There are four models of delivering the photography service:

- Static photography: The patient visits a centre where a digital camera is based.
- Mobile photography: A mobile van with a digital camera moves around the area and the patient visits the van on specific dates at a certain location.
- Optometry service: Digital imaging takes place at optometry practices.
- Mixed: A combination of any of the first three methods.

The digital photos are sent electronically to a screening centre where they are graded.

Grading

A consistent, repeatable, valid method of screening for diabetic retinopathy was developed in 1984, and called the Airlie House Classification. Its purpose was to ensure that scientific studies had a consistent way of measuring DR. The Airlie House Classification was modified into the Early Treatment of Diabetic Retinopathy Scale (ETDRS). The ETDRS used six grades of DR per eye (eleven grades in total for both eyes) and has been widely used in epidemiological studies including in the UK.

It was felt that, whilst the ETDRS method was useful for academic studies, it was too

(Continued)

(Continued)

complicated for population-based screening programmes. Consequently the UK DR Screening Committee adopted a simpler approach (See Table 8.3).

Quality Assurance

The quality of the screening programme is monitored by a quality assurance process. The QA process can be internal (regular, repeated testing of the service which informs the screening programme of any issues) or external, where an organization with overall responsibility for screening programmes in England reviews the programme with an external audit team.

Internal quality assurance includes regular assessment of photographic quality, competence of grading staff (with repeated tests of ability to grade different levels of diabetic retinopathy), and the monitoring of any screening failures, such as where a patient with DR requiring further investigation has been missed.

Criteria for Internal QA include:

- Continual training and accreditation of screeners.
- Audit by ophthalmologist to determine false-positive rate.
- Collection of adverse event data.
- Regrading by camera or ophthalmoscopy to detect false-negatives.

The QA process is an integral part of any screening programme as it determines whether the screening process is being conducted effectively thereby ensuring that standards are high, and false-positives and false-negatives are kept to a minimum.

Cost

Economic analyses of DR Screening have suggested that the process is economically viable. However, there has, as yet, been no health economic assessment of whether the overall programme is cost-effective.

Table 8.3   *Description of the UK grading system for diabetic retinopathy*

Retinopathy	Description	Outcome
R0 (no visible retinopathy)	No diabetic retinopathy anywhere.	Rescreen 12 months.
R1 (mild)	Background diabetic retinopathy — mild. The presence of at least one of any of the following features anywhere: • dot haemorrhages • microaneurysms • hard exudates • cotton wool spots • blot haemorrhages • superficial/ flame shaped haemorrhages	Rescreen 12 months.
R2 (observable background)	Background diabetic retinopathy — observable. Four or more blot haemorrhages in one hemi-field only (inferior and superior hemi-fields delineated by a line passing through the centre of the fovea and optic disc).	Rescreen 6 months (or refer to ophthalmology if this is not feasible).
R3 (referable background)	Background diabetic retinopathy — referable. Any of the following features: • four or more blot haemorrhages in both inferior and superior hemi-fields • venous beading • IRMA (intraretinal microvascular abnormalities)	Refer ophthalmology. These patients may be kept under surveillance and will not necessarily receive immediate referral.
R4 (proliferative)	Proliferative diabetic retinopathy. Any of the following features: • active new vessels • vitreous haemorrhage	Refer ophthalmology. These patients are likely to receive laser treatment or another intervention.
R6 (inadequate)	Not adequately visualized. Retina not sufficiently visible for assessment.	Technical failure. Arrange alternative screening examination. This will be automatic within the screening programme.

8.7.2   Primary open-angle glaucoma (POAG)

Although many people instinctively feel that glaucoma is a disease that should be screened for because of its insidious nature, the argument is far more complex than for diabetic retinopathy. This is because of two problems:

1. The lack of a clear understanding of the natural history of the disease.
2. The need for a suitable screening test.

There exists an enormous body of literature on the subject of screening for glaucoma, and much of it is flawed. At least one textbook on general epidemiology cites chronic glaucoma as an example of a condition for screening using **Intra Ocular Pressure** (**IOP**) testing. The flaw is an erroneous assumption about the discriminating ability of the test, based on hypothetical distributions of the IOP in diseased and non-diseased states.[13] The assumption that 'no glaucoma is associated with a pressure below 22 mmHg' is erroneous, as at least half of patients with glaucoma are now known to have 'normal' eye pressure. A substantial **Health Technology Assessment** (**HTA**) review highlights the large volume of literature on the subject and the paucity of good quality research, particularly on diagnostic test accuracy. The review concludes that, on the current level of evidence, screening cannot be justified and that high quality randomized screening trials are needed.[14] This is not to say that opportunistic testing for glaucoma should not continue as currently practised by community-based ophthalmologists and optometrists. In this case, practitioners may consider that they are performing screening tests on patients although the process does not constitute a formal screening programme. The population at risk is not formally identified nor called for screening at regular intervals. The tests applied are not screening but diagnostic tests, requiring not only a relatively complex technology but, what is even more important, also a considerable level of technical skill and clinical judgment.

8.7.2.1   *The population at risk*

Increasing age, raised intraocular pressure, black African ethnic origin and a family history of glaucoma are the main and undisputed risk factors for chronic open-angle glaucoma. Mongoloid races carry a greater risk of angle-closure. Age interacts with race; black African people acquire glaucoma at a younger age than Caucasians, and are at a considerably greater risk of glaucoma blindness.[15] However, it is likely that the risk varies between different populations in black Africa. Family history is unreliable. None of these factors facilitates the identification of a population subgroup to be selected for screening, although they may be used to encourage those at increased risk to seek testing.

8.7.2.2   *The screening tests*

The three tests necessary for the diagnosis of glaucoma, namely an IOP measurement, an optic disk examination and a visual field assessment, all perform poorly as single screening tests, with low sensitivity. The combination of IOP and disk assessment only marginally improves the validity,[5] and the current view of the AAO is that all three tests should be performed routinely in the comprehensive eye examination.[16]

Intraocular pressure (IOP)

Despite it being clearly shown in 1966 by Hollows and Graham that the IOP is inadequate as

a screening index,[17] opportunistic testing for glaucoma in many circumstances relies on pressure measurement. Its performance as a test is illustrated above, using data from the Baltimore Eye Study (Fig. 8.2). Given these findings, it is not surprising that most surveys show that, for every diagnosed case, there is another undiagnosed one in the community. It comes also as no surprise that cases continue to present late in the course of the disease with a poor prognosis for vision.

Surveys also find that a significant proportion of previously diagnosed and treated cases show no evidence of having the disease.[18] Presumably these persons, having been found to have a raised IOP, have been diagnosed as having glaucoma without any corroborating evidence of an optic disk change or a visual field loss. Nevertheless, it remains true that, after age, a raised IOP is the single most significant risk factor for glaucoma. When found, a high IOP needs treating and the risk of developing glaucoma (if not already present) should be carefully assessed.

Corneal thickness

In recent years, mainly as a result of evidence from the **Ocular Hypertension Treatment Study** (**OHTS**),[19] corroborated in some subsequent studies, such as the **European Glaucoma Prevention Study** (**EGPS**),[20] central corneal thickness appears in multivariate analysis to be a risk factor modifying the influence of IOP. Elevated IOP in the presence of a thick cornea is less of a concern than in people with thinner corneas. The actual mechanism of this relationship is likely to be complex. The central corneal thickness and corneal rigidity affect the accuracy of the pressure measurement whether it is by contact or non-contact tonometric methods so that a thicker more rigid cornea will lead to the IOP being overestimated, and a thinner one underestimated. But corneal thickness is itself influenced by other glaucoma risk factors such as age (it gets thinner with increasing age) and race (African-Americans and African-Caribbeans have thinner corneas). Independent causal relationships are postulated such as a correlation between a thinner cornea and a greater vulnerability of the optic nerve head perhaps due to weaker protection of the nerve fibres to the effects of pressure.

Optic discs

Ophthalmologists have long relied on the appearance of the disc as a method of detecting glaucoma, based on the aphorism that, if the disk is normal, there can be no glaucoma, whatever the IOP. A better understanding of optic-disc anatomy means that we cannot be so certain. The presence and extent of cupping of the optic disc is, to a large extent, a function of disc size. A large disc will have a large cup, and a small disc a small cup.[21] Therefore, a reliance on disk appearance alone can give rise to both kinds of error, false-positive and false-negative: a large disc in the former case and a small disc in the latter. The findings of the Baltimore survey are evidence of how poorly disc appearances alone function as criteria for screening. Because disc size is in no way influenced by IOP, combining the two parameters provides little improvement in validity, as was also shown in the Baltimore study.

Disc changes in glaucoma, other than cup–disc ratio, can be extremely subtle, and are the domain of experienced glaucoma specialists who can detect potentially pathognomonic change. However, these changes are too subtle for use in screening, and agreement between specialists in recognizing these changes has been shown to be variable.[22]

Nerve fibre layer (NFL) changes

Some commentators believe that imaging of the nerve fibre layer in glaucoma may be a useful screening tool.[23] The presence of a definite groove or defect in the nerve fibre layer, which can be sometimes seen with direct or indirect ophthalmoscopy (and better with a red-free filter), is best demonstrated using specialized photographic techniques. Such a defect is a strong predictor of glaucoma and is very unlikely to be a false-positive finding, even though it may precede the appearance of a definite abnormality of visual function. But the absence of a visible defect does not exclude glaucoma. Detection of an NFL defect requires good clarity of the optical media and usually a dilated pupil, although the successful use of the non-mydriatic camera has been reported.[24] To visualize an NFL groove easily may also require that the nerve fibre damage is focal and that the rest of the NFL is thick, young and healthy. None of these conditions make this technique likely to be suitable for screening in the community, although technological developments in this area may change this. New technology using scanning laser technology (Heidelberg Retinal Tomograph and **Ocular Computerized Tomography (OCT)**) and analysis of reflected polarized light from the nerve fibre layer (GDX) are thought to offer new avenues for glaucoma screening, but have yet to be shown to be useful. None of them offers the simple inexpensive and robust technology usually required for screening in the primary care sector.

New imaging technologies

In recent years there has been much interest in imaging technologies such as the Heidelberg Retinal Tomograph, the GDX and the OCT, which may provide the basis for diagnostic structural analysis of the optic nerve head and nerve fibre layer thickness. Literature on these has been extensively reviewed in the HTA report,[14] and so far no conclusive evidence either of superiority of one device over another or over expert human evaluation has emerged.

Visual field testing

The reliable demonstration of an abnormal visual function in screening for glaucoma is probably the best hope for the development of a screening tool, although to some this may seem like accepting defeat. Because accumulating evidence indicates that a substantial proportion of nerve fibres are lost before defects in the visual field can be reliably detected, the ideal objective is to detect the disease before any loss of function has occurred, that is, primary rather than secondary prevention. Given that no treatment for the disease is without side effects or potential harm, intervention has to be justifiable by the high probability that the situation will deteriorate if nothing is done. The identification of persons who may require intervention should therefore be based on the presumptive identification of a functional impairment at a stage when it causes no disability. The diagnostic process should then confirm the presence of that functional impairment, and that it is (or is very likely to be) progressive before treatment is started. On the basis of this argument, it is logical to develop a screening tool, which is capable of detecting definite abnormalities of visual function reliably without too much concern for suspects who may or may not later develop glaucoma.

Visual function is traditionally assessed in glaucoma by plotting the visual field, and numerous methods now exist for the execution of this test, from simple and subjective confrontation testing to fully automated and computerized full-threshold measurements with a wide range of stimuli (see Chapter 13 on Glaucoma).

The rigorous requirements of a screening test impose restrictions on what it is possible to achieve in visual field screening, but much work has been done to overcome some of these difficulties. A major problem arises from the fluctuation in retinal sensitivity, which is a normal feature of visual function. This variation is accentuated in glaucoma patients. The process of identifying the threshold of perception is an arduous task, which requires many repetitions. These and other reasons are enough to exclude threshold testing as a possible screening tool, but supra-threshold techniques have been widely tested and show promise.

The principle of this strategy is to reduce the false-positive rate by looking only for marked focal reductions in retinal sensitivity. The price is some loss of sensitivity to the detection of early defects. Henson has developed a testing strategy using automated tangent screen technology for which these parameters have been calculated on samples of known cases and controls.[25] Sponsel and others have implemented this strategy with some success in the Save Sight America campaign.[26] The cost of this dedicated technology is relatively high, and alternatives are being developed using low-cost technology, for example the Damato campimeter, which uses an oculokinetic technique.[27] With computers becoming widespread in clinical practice, much research is being carried out on the development of simple software-based tests which can be run on any compatible personal computer. Examples include the Ophthimus 'high pass resolution perimetry'[28] and motion sensitivity testing.[29] A more recent addition to the technology is the frequency doubling perimeter, which uses phase contrast stimuli of larger areas of the visual field. While this shows promise, it is yet to be formally tested in a population-based setting. This is promising in that it is relatively easy to use and not too expensive, but the HTA review[14] found insufficient evidence to draw firm conclusions about the best available visual function testing screening device.

8.7.2.3 *Structure*

No formal screening for open-angle glaucoma appears to be taking place in any developed or developing country. Case finding is facilitated in the UK by the provision of free sight testing by optometrists for persons with a positive family history of glaucoma and persons over 65 years of age.

Persons of African origin are at substantially increased risk of both the disease and blindness as a result of it, and there is some justification for implementing targeted health awareness programmes to encourage use of services (perhaps specifically provided) for the detection of glaucoma. However, great care must be taken not to stigmatize a racial ethnic minority, and any such programme must be clearly owned by the targeted population.

8.7.3   Screening children

Screening children for defective vision is widely practised throughout the world. In the UK, every local organization responsible for healthcare has a different approach to the problem, and there is no consistent national policy on the subject.[30] It is a good example of an area where screening has been planned and executed without a structure of clear aims, outcomes or evaluation. The arguments for and against screening children are complex and to some extent vary according to local conditions.

Although the detection and treatment of amblyopia and refractive error overlap, they are best dealt with separately.

8.7.3.1 *Amblyopia*

When it is difficult to be precise about the case definition of a disease, screening for it will inevitably be problematic. Case definitions of **amblyopia** vary widely but nearly all depend on the presence of defective vision, which does not improve through correction of refractive errors. The exact mechanism for amblyopic visual loss is not fully understood, and different mechanisms may act in different types of amblyopia, for instance in strabismus and in refractive errors. Although treatment for amblyopia is widely practised, there is limited evidence of its efficacy. Occlusion therapy of the unaffected eye is its mainstay, although stimulation of the affected eye is sometimes used. There is also some debate about the public health significance of amblyopia. Amblyopia is common in Western populations, and up to 5% of children can be affected.[31] However, it is rarely the cause of severe visual impairment because it nearly always affects one eye only, certainly in its commonest form caused by strabismus or anisometropia (unequal refraction in the two eyes). It can only be a contributory cause when sight is lost in the other eye from another cause. A surveillance-based study in the UK suggested that lifetime risk of vision loss in the second eye of an individual with amblyopia was approximately 1.2%.[32]

Most severe forms of strabismus and sight loss from other causes in children will be evident early in life. It is common practice to check the red reflex of infants at birth to eliminate the possibility of congenital cataract, although this probably does not constitute formal screening. Attentive parents rarely miss a deviating eye, and it is important that all children with new squints are seen by an ophthalmologist to exclude more sinister underlying pathology, such as uniocular congenital cataract or retinoblastoma. Children with squint can be helped greatly by treatment, and amblyopia is frequently reduced or eliminated and the eye aligned. A compliant family and many hospital visits are required. Profound amblyopia with very poor vision may not respond to treatment, especially when established for some time. Strabismic and anisometropic amblyopia behave differently, because with strabismus there appears to be a

sensitive period until the age of seven or eight years, after which the loss of cerebral plasticity prevents effective treatment of the condition. Apparently, this does not apply to anisometropic amblyopia.

It is generally thought to be the case that the younger the age at which amblyopia is detected, the better the outcome of the treatment (good quality clinical trial evidence for this assumption is lacking, although a number of trials are now in place). This has led to the principal concern of those wishing to screen for amblyopia, namely that of achieving the right balance of test validity and reliability and age at screening. A test of visual acuity remains essential for screening for amblyopia, but the younger the age, the less valid this test becomes. In the UK, it is thought difficult to achieve a reliable routine test before three and a half years of age, and children enter infant school usually before the age of five years.

A Cochrane systematic review has not found high quality evidence to support the screening of children for amblyopia.[33]

8.7.3.2 *Pre-school vision screening*

A series of studies in the USA (Vision in Preschoolers studies) have shown that identifying a valid, reliable and readily applicable screening test is problematic in this age group.

Several other issues in pre-school screening have also been identified:

1. There is no evidence that it is safe and effective to treat refractive error in pre-school age children.[34]
2. Screening for amblyopia and strabismus does not appear to be cost effective.[35]
3. It has been shown that there is poor uptake of pre-school screening by those most at risk.[36]

8.7.3.3 *Refractive error and school vision screening*

It is the normal practice in many countries to test children's vision regularly while they are at school. This constitutes a screening procedure, and should be subject to the same constraints as all screening efforts with regard to the evaluation of both process and outcome measures. It is probably more important where access to optometric expertise is limited, prevalence of uncorrected refractive error is high (e.g. certain Asian countries) and a child may become (sometimes severely) disabled at school as a result of an uncorrected refractive error. Training teachers to test vision has been quite successful in certain parts of India, but only because it is linked to a follow-up facility of ophthalmic medical assistants who can refract and prescribe the necessary spectacles.[37]

It should be noted that this sort of screening does not fulfil all the formal requirements from the public health point of view. Early detection may not influence materially the prognosis of the condition, in this case myopia. Evidence from studies on primates has given rise to the concern that avid and certainly overcorrection of refractive error may worsen the condition by inhibiting natural 'emmetropization'.[38] In the light of what is apparently an epidemic of myopia in the school and university populations of South-East Asia,[39] we should remain keenly aware that correcting the refractive error, whilst limiting impairment, is not curing the problem or dealing with the cause. Behavioural factors, particularly in relation to prolonged near-vision tasks, may be important in progression of myopia (see Chapter 11) and evidence suggests that outdoor activity with its emphasis on distance vision tasks may be protective.

The UK NSC recommends that all children have visual acuity tested between the ages of four and five by a trained individual (orthoptist or supervised by an orthoptist). This is in addition to testing the red reflex in all neonates. No screening for visual loss in secondary school age children is recommended.

A Cochrane systematic review has not found high quality evidence to support the screening of school children for refractive error[40] indicating that more operational research is required.

8.7.4   Defective vision in the elderly

Poor vision in elderly persons is a common problem, which is often remediable and most frequently caused by cataract (see Chapter 10). Loss of sight leads to deterioration in quality of life, loss of economic potential and increased morbidity from falls. Despite this, many elderly persons do not complain of sight loss nor seek help when it is available. This is a well described problem in India, being addressed by 'eye-screening camps' and motivational strategies in which successfully operated persons encourage those who are blind as a result of cataract to take up the offer of help. Socio-cultural barriers have to be overcome and people's expectations changed.

Similar problems exist among the elderly in the UK.[41] Many elderly persons may develop sight loss from a variety of causes, including cataract, but do not seek help, perhaps believing that it is the inevitable accompaniment of old age. They are not aware that quality of life can be greatly improved by surgery or simple refraction. General practitioners are required to offer assessment of sensory function on an annual basis for all patients over 75 years, although many are poorly trained and equipped to do this.[42] Access to an ophthalmologist is usually via a GP but is often initiated following a sight test by an optometrist. If an elderly person does not feel the need for new spectacles and, in particular, wishes to avoid the expense, then the sight loss will often remain undetected.[43] Routine screening of older people for visual impairment has been advocated but there is no evidence to support the effectiveness of this approach. A cluster randomized trial to assess whether formal sight testing of those over 75 years of age by GPs did not find any improvement in vision amongst the target group after screening.

8.8   FUTURE RESEARCH PRIORITIES

8.8.1   Diabetic retinopathy

Research is urgently needed to deal with the rapidly emerging problem of diabetic sight loss in countries where economic development has been rapid and both the prevalence of maturity onset diabetes and survival with the condition are increasing. The assumption that models developed for Western nations are appropriate elsewhere may not be correct. Digital photography may fail in the face of much more frequent media opacity, and the technology may not be sustainable. Studies in the Middle East, on the Indian subcontinent and on some Pacific islands are indicated.

8.8.2 Primary open-angle glaucoma (POAG)

With the rapid growth of genetic research, specific genetic abnormalities for POAG may soon be known. This will lend a new dimension to the screening for glaucoma. Carriers of specific genetic abnormalities will become the target population at risk who will require regular testing. The possibility of automated self-testing devices should be explored but there will still be the need to demonstrate that such a strategy can save sight. The problem with POAG is that its natural history under treatment is as much as 30 years. Surrogate outcomes in terms of prevention of development of early field loss or progression will be necessary. Variability of measurements of function needs to be reduced so that trials become more feasible.

8.8.3 Prevention of amblyopia

The results of current research, which will soon be published, will deal with questions about the public health significance of the condition as well as effectiveness of treatment. It will then be possible to make evidence-based policy decisions on the opportunity cost and, if indicated, organize coherent national strategies. Photorefractive technology may offer an efficient detection system if the costs can be justified.

8.9 CONCLUSION

Screening is a potentially powerful public health intervention, which has its place in the natural development of the epidemiological foundations of any discipline. A forerunner of screening is the population-based survey, in which visual impairment by cause is quantified, and potential screening tests can

be evaluated. In this way, population subgroups that might be targeted by screening can be identified. For rarer diseases, case-control studies can estimate levels of risk as well as the groups at risk. Randomized controlled trials demonstrate the benefit and sometimes the cost-benefit of treatment. The same method can demonstrate the efficacy or otherwise of screening.

It follows therefore that much groundwork is required before screening for a disease is considered; this groundwork may not have the immediate appeal of screening, but it is essential to provide the assurance that such an enormous effort will be worthwhile.

REFERENCES

1. NHS. What is screening? Available from http://www.screening.nhs.uk/screening [last accessed 1st Feb 2010].
2. Wilson JM, Jungner YG. *Screening for Disease.* Geneva: WHO; 1968.
3. Courtright P, Johnson GJ (eds). *Prevention of Blindness in Leprosy.* Proceedings of a symposium sponsored by WHO through its Programmes for Leprosy and Prevention of Blindness, revised edition. London: The International Centre for Eye Health; 1991.
4. Coffey M, Reidy A, Wormald R, *et al.* Prevalence of glaucoma in the west of Ireland. *Br J Opthalmol* 1993; 77:17–21.
5. Murphy JM, Berwick DM, Weinstein MC, *et al.* Performance of screening and diagnostic tests. Application of receiver operating characteristic analysis. *Arch Gen Psych* 1987; 44:550–555.
6. Tielsch JM, Katz J, Singh K, *et al.* A population-based evaluation of glaucoma screening: the Baltimore Eye Survey. *Am J Epidemiol* 1991; 134:1102–1110.
7. Dunn G, Everitt B. *Clinical Biostatistics.* London: Arnold; 1995.
8. Altman DG. *Practical Statistics for Medical Research.* London: Chapman & Hall; 1995.
9. St Vincent Working Party Report. The Acropolis Affirmation Diabetes Care — St Vincent in progress. Statement from St Vincent Declaration meeting, Athens, Greece, March 1995. *Diabet Med* 1995; 12:636.

10. Tabar L, Fagerberg G, Day NE, *et al.* The Swedish two-county trial of mammographic screening for breast cancer: recent results on mortality and tumor characteristics. *Pathol Biol* (Paris) 1992; 39:846.

11. Friedman DR, Dubin N. Case-control evaluation of breast cancer screening efficacy. *Am J Epidemiol* 1991; 133:974–984.

12. American Academy of Ophthalmology. Screening for Diabetic Retinopathy. Available from: http://one.aao.org/CE/PracticeGuidelines/Clinical Statements_Content.aspx?cid=ed55ed3c-b34b-4f10-ae1309e063d8d773 [last accessed 1st Feb 2010].

13. Mausner JS, Kramer S (eds). *Epidemiology: An Introductory Text*, 2nd Edition. Philadelphia: WB Saunders; 1985.

14. Burr JM, Mowatt G, Hernández R, *et al.* The clinical effectiveness and cost-effectiveness of screening for open angle glaucoma: a systematic review and economic evaluation. *Health Technol Assess* 2007; 11:iii–iv, ix–x, 1–90.

15. Sommer A, Tielsch JM, Katz J, *et al.* Racial differences in the cause-specific prevalence of blindness in east Baltimore. *N Eng J Med* 1991; 325:1412–1417.

16. American Academy of Ophthalmology. Primary Open Angle Glaucoma. Preferred Practice Pattern. San Francisco: American Academy of Ophthalmology; 2000.

17. Hollows FC, Graham PA. Intra-ocular pressure, glaucoma, and glaucoma suspects in a defined population. *Br J Ophthalmol* 1966; 50:570–586.

18. Klein BE, Klein R, Sponsel WE, *et al.* Prevalence of glaucoma. The Beaver Dam Eye Study. *Ophthalmology* 1992; 99:1499–1504.

19. Brandt JD, Beiser JA, Kass MA, *et al.* Central corneal thickness in the Ocular Hypertension Treatment Study (OHTS). *Ophthalmology* 2001; 108:1779–1788.

20. European Glaucoma Prevention Study Group. Central corneal thickness in the European Glaucoma Prevention Study. *Ophthalmology* 2007; 114:454–459.

21. Jonas JB, Fernandez MC, Naumann GO. Correlation of the optic disc size to glaucoma susceptibility. *Ophthalmology* 1991; 98:675–680.

22. Schwartz JT. Methodologic differences and measurement of cup–disk ratio: an epidemiologic assessment. *Arch Ophthalmol* 1976; 94:1101–1105.

23. Hitchings RA, Poinoosawmy D, Poplar N, *et al.* Retinal nerve fibre layer photography in glaucomatous patients. *Eye* 1987; 1:621–625.

24. Airaksinen PJ, Nieminen H, Mustonen E. Retinal nerve fibre layer photography with a wide angle fundus camera. *Acta Ophthalmol* 1982; 60:362–368.

25. Henson DB. Visual field screening and the development of a new screening program. *J Am Optom Assoc* 1989; 60:893–898.

26. Sponsel WE, Ritch R, Stamper R, *et al.* Prevent Blindness America visual field screening study. The Prevent Blindness America Glaucoma Advisory Committee. *Am J Ophthalmol* 1995; 120:699–708.

27. Mutlukan E, Damato BE, Jay JL. Clinical evaluation of a multi-fixation campimeter for the detection of glaucomatous visual field loss. *Br J Ophthalmol* 1993; 77:332–338.

28. Frisén L. High-pass resolution perimetry. A clinical review. *Doc Ophthalmol* 1993; 83:1–25.

29. Wu X, Wormald RP, Fitzke F, *et al.* Laptop computer perimetry for glaucoma screening. *Invest Ophthalmol Vis Sci* 1991; 32:810.

30. Stewart-Brown SL, Haslum MN, Howlett B. Preschool vision screening: a service in need of rationalisation. *Arch Dis Child* 1988; 63:56–359.

31. Thompson JR, Woodruff G, Hiscox FA, *et al.* The incidence and prevalence of amblyopia detected in childhood. *Public Health* 1991; 105:455–462.

32. Rahi JS, Logan S, Timms C, *et al.* Risk, causes, and outcomes of visual impairment after loss of vision in the non-amblyopic eye: a population-based study. *Lancet* 2002; 360: 597–602.

33. Powell C, Hatt SR. Vision screening for amblyopia in childhood. *Cochrane Database of Systematic Reviews* 2009, Issue 3. Art. No. CD005020. DOI: 10.1002/14651858.CD005020.pub3.

34. Kulp MT. Vision in Preschoolers (VIP) Study Group. Findings from the Vision in Preschoolers (VIP) Study. *Optom Vis Sci* 2009; 86:619–623.

35. Carlton J, Karnon J, Czoski-Murray C, *et al.* The clinical effectiveness and cost-effectiveness of screening programmes for amblyopia and strabismus in children up to the age of 4–5 years: a systematic review and economic evaluation. *Health Technol Assess* 2008; 12:iii, xi–194.

36. Castanes MS. Major review: The under-utilization of vision screening (for amblyopia, optical anomalies and strabismus) among preschool age children. *Binocul Vis Strabismus Q* 2003; 18:217–232.

37. Kumar R. Ophthalmic manpower in India — need for a serious review. *Int Ophthalmol* 1993; 17:269–275.

38. Hung LF, Crawford ML, Smith EL. Spectacle lenses alter eye growth and the refractive status of young monkeys. *Nature Med* 1995; 1:761–765.

39. Chew SJ, Chia SC, Lee LK. The pattern of myopia in young Singaporean men. *Singapore Med J* 1988; 29:201–211.

40. Powell C, Wedner S, Hatt SR. Vision screening for correctable visual acuity deficits in school-age children and adolescents. *Cochrane Database of Systematic Reviews* 2004, Issue 4. Art. No.: CD005023. DOI: 10.1002/14651858.CD005023.pub2.

41. Wormald RP, Wright LA, Courtney P, *et al.* Visual problems in the elderly population and implications for services. *Br Med J* 1992; 304:1226–1229.

42. Fink A, Wright L, Wormald R. Detection and prevention of treatable visual failure in general practice: room for improvement? *Br J Gen Pract* 1994; 44:587–589.

43. Reinstein DZ, Dorward NL, Wormald RP *et al.* Correctable undetected visual acuity deficit in patients aged 65 and over attending an accident and emergency department. *Br J Ophthalmol* 1993; 77:293–296.

9

Research synthesis

JENNIFER EVANS AND RICHARD WORMALD

9.1   Introduction   169
9.2   The process of a systematic review   170
9.3   Types of research synthesis   172
9.4   Conclusions   173
9.5   Future research needs   173
      References   173

9.1   INTRODUCTION

Reviewing the state of the literature on a given question before going on to make new observations or to conduct new prospective research is the accepted standard in academic undertakings. In a thesis, for example, the first chapter is usually a literature review that summarizes the state of knowledge from which the new hypothesis is to be constructed. To be excellent, such reviews have to be thorough and inclusive, but until recently, little attention has been given to the scientific validity of this process, and usually no formal effort is made to summarize and, where possible, synthesize the findings of previous work.

Traditional expert reviews allow an author to collect and select evidence to support the prior beliefs held by that expert. In contrast, a systematic review should be conducted without prejudice. The type and quality of evidence for a clearly defined question is investigated in order to answer a specific clinical question. Over the last decade, an ideal standard for the summary and synthesis of knowledge has been established, using methodology that aims to control bias and assess the reliability of the evidence.[1]

This methodology is necessary for a number of reasons. First, no single study, however perfect in its design, conduct and analysis, can be free of the possibility of being wrong just by chance. The larger and more representative the research, the less this is likely, but it will always be possible. The study provides an estimate of the truth and, if it stands alone, cannot be compared with any other estimate. When several studies ask the same question, we can see a pattern emerging whereby the results cluster around what we can begin to be more confident is a true estimate. Thus synthesizing research allows us to obtain a better estimate of the truth by reducing the random error of effect estimates.

The second reason is subtly different. Small studies may lack **power** individually to detect moderate effects. By combining these studies, sufficient power is generated to enable us to observe a statistically significant effect. This is because the pooled estimates are now providing a better estimate of the truth than the individual studies, none of which on its own is conclusive.

Third, the volume of published medical literature is now too large for any individual practitioner realistically to keep up to date with current research by reading individual studies and assess the balance of evidence.

By formally organizing and summarizing studies that attempt to answer the same or a similar question, risk of **bias** in individual studies can be assessed systematically. Consequently, the overall strength of an estimated effect or parameter can be graded in terms of quality of evidence. Properly judged decisions can then be made on whether to implement findings or commission new research.

9.2　THE PROCESS OF A SYSTEMATIC REVIEW

The systematic review process begins with forming the question for which an answer is sought. Key features of this question include the population and outcome measure (for reviews of prevalence); intervention and comparison (for reviews of intervention studies); and case definition, test type and location (for diagnostic test accuracy studies). We will discuss the process of doing a systematic review by using intervention trials as an example.

The second step is to create a protocol for answering the question. In essence, a systematic review is an observational study of the trials addressing a particular clinical or scientific question. As for primary studies, reporting the methods in detail before commencing the research is important. A detailed protocol should give information on the procedures for identifying relevant trials, inclusion and exclusion criteria, and the methods for assessing the quality of included trials.

The protocol should set out *a priori* which outcomes are to be analyzed and how they are to be analyzed. The choice of outcome measures and length of follow-up should be selected on the basis of relevance to patients, rather than simply summarizing all the outcomes reported in the individual trials. Consumer or patient groups can be involved in the choice of outcomes at the protocol stage.[2] The implicit purpose behind having a detailed protocol is that the conduct of the review should be as objective as possible, particularly since the review authors will likely be aware of the results of some of the published trials.

The protocol should address in detail the way in which the review authors plan to identify relevant studies. A good search strategy will use several different databases and include all studies, irrespective of language. Ideally an information specialist should be involved in designing the search strategies, as this is a specialized field. Searches need to be reasonably sensitive, that is, likely to pick up all relevant studies, without generating too many unnecessary references. The importance of methods to identify studies is not often appreciated or addressed properly in traditional reviews. Similarly, methods of collecting and extracting data, paying attention to minimizing the number of data extraction errors by duplicate extraction and entry, are important. In summary, a systematic review is a research project, similar to primary data collection, and needs to have the same rigour and attention to detail.

Systematic reviews usually are based on published aggregate data but can also use individual participant data.[3] This method can have considerable benefits, particularly because it involves more collaboration with investigators of the individual studies, provides more flexibility in the analysis, and enables better quality control of the data. It is considered the gold standard approach but does require considerable extra time and effort. As for published data, the original randomization must be preserved when pooling the data, and heterogeneity between studies should be assessed.

9.2.1　Assessing the risk of bias

The results of systematic reviews depend on the quality of the trials included in the review. Pooling the results of a sample of poor quality trials, for example, may lead to incorrect conclusions being drawn. Therefore, assessing the risk of bias of individual studies is a critical part of the systematic review process. Many systems have been designed to grade study quality. In general, domain-based grading scales are clearer and more transparent than summary scores. The **Cochrane Collaboration**'s tool for assessing the risk of bias considers allocation of treatment, masking, incomplete outcome data and selective outcome reporting separately (Box 9.1).[4]

Box 9.1   *Cochrane Collaboration's tool for assessing the risk of bias in individual studies*

- ➤ **Sequence generation:** Was the allocation sequence adequately generated?
- ➤ **Allocation concealment:** Was allocation adequately concealed?
- ➤ **Blinding (masking) of participants, personnel and outcome assessors:** *Assessments should be made for each main outcome (or class of outcomes).* Was knowledge of the allocated intervention adequately prevented during the study?
- ➤ **Incomplete outcome data:** *Assessments should be made for each main outcome (or class of outcomes).* Were incomplete outcome data adequately addressed?
- ➤ **Selective outcome reporting:** Are reports of the study free of suggestion of selective outcome reporting?
- ➤ **Other sources of bias:** Was the study apparently free of other problems that could put it at a high risk of bias?

www.cochrane-handbook.org

Several well-recognized potential biases may affect systematic reviews. Trials that have statistically significant results are more likely to be published and, within published trials, statistically significant outcomes are more likely to be reported.[5] If studies showing no effect for a particular outcome are selectively excluded from the meta-analysis, the overall effect of treatment will be exaggerated. Currently this *publication bias* and *outcome reporting bias* is difficult to avoid as it is not always possible to identify and obtain access to unpublished data. Current efforts to ensure that all trials are registered at inception,[6] and better access to trial protocols[7] will improve future reviews. However, reviewers should try to identify unpublished studies, for example by searching conference abstracts, and contact investigators directly for data on outcomes that are not reported adequately.

Structured assessment of individual study quality can feed into an overall assessment of the quality of the evidence for each outcome. Again many published schemes for grading quality of evidence are available but one particularly useful approach is that offered by GRADE (http://www.gradeworkinggroup.org/). The scheme takes into account study quality and publication bias as well as the consistency, precision and directness of the evidence. This assessment provides a transparent and systematic approach to assessing the overall quality of the evidence and, thus, facilitates evidence-based conclusions as to the effects of treatment.

9.2.2   Pooling data (meta-analysis)

Meta-analysis refers to the combined analysis of the results of the studies included in the review to produce a pooled estimate of treatment effect. The key point is that the original randomization must be preserved when pooling the data; it is not correct simply to treat all the different trials as one large study. A weighted average of the results of the individual trials is calculated with larger trials being given more weight. The quality and validity of the meta-analysis results depends on the methods used to do the systematic review. Meta-analysis of a biased sample of poor quality trials, for example, may be precise but will be wrong.

Two conceptual models underlie the statistical methods in a meta-analysis: fixed and random effects models. The fixed effects model assumes all studies are estimating a fixed true effect, while the random model assumes the effect being estimated is not fixed for all studies but varies randomly for each study conducted. This assumption leads to wider confidence limits around pooled estimates but still assumes that the studies are essentially repetitions of the same experiment.

Usually results of meta-analysis are plotted in the form of a *forest plot*. Fig. 9.1 shows a forest

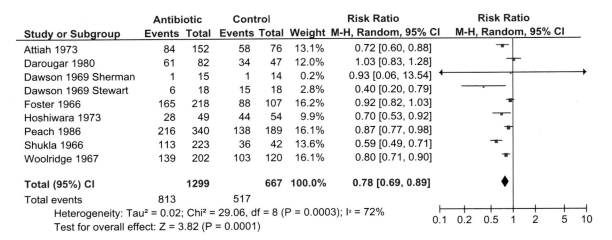

Figure 9.1 *Meta-analysis of trials of antibiotics versus control for treatment of active trachoma*

plot of the results of individual trials of antibiotic treatment for trachoma on the outcome 'active trachoma at three months'. The pooled estimate of effect is shown at the bottom of the graph in the diamond shape, the size of which represents the confidence intervals of the pooled estimate.

9.2.3   Assessing heterogeneity

Combining the results of multiple studies increases the power of the analysis and gives a more precise measure of effect. However, if there is considerable variation in the results of individual studies (heterogeneity), reporting one pooled estimate of treatment effect may not be appropriate. Heterogeneity arises due to differences in patient populations, interventions or study design, and should be investigated if possible. For example, the studies can be divided up into groups that are more similar and the analyses repeated.

Heterogeneity is a critical issue in meta-analysis and it is wrong to attempt to combine the results of research that are not homogeneous, i.e. that are not asking the same question about the same parameter in the same population. A well-known adage is that it is not appropriate to compare the effects of apples and oranges unless one is interested in the generic effects of fruit.

9.3   TYPES OF RESEARCH SYNTHESIS

It is only worth synthesizing the highest quality evidence, hence the emphasis in systematic reviews on the type and quality of study and the way they are conducted. Reviews of the effect of interventions will usually only include well-designed randomized controlled trials, since only they provide an effect estimate based on a fair comparison with a control group and can, if they are properly designed and executed, reliably control bias and confounding. Synthesizing studies of disease prevalence or incidence should only include representative randomly sampled survey populations using appropriate adjustments for clustering if necessary.

In recent years, summaries of the burden of eye disease on both global and national scales, using systematic review methods and meta-analytic techniques, have been published. Pooling data from different prevalence studies can provide a very useful summary of prevalence. There are a number of different examples for visual impairment and eye disease.[8–12]

Synthesizing observational studies for risk factors for disease is much more difficult and more prone to serious bias than synthesizing clinical trial results. This is in part because observational studies are more difficult to interpret anyway, in particular the effects of uncontrolled confounding are very difficult to address. But also publication and selective outcome reporting bias are likely to be even more of a problem with these studies, as the conduct of clinical trials is much more regulated than for observational studies. Similarly, synthesizing case series and reports is also very likely to be biased. An emerging field deals with systematic reviews of studies of diagnostic test accuracy. These reviews, however, need to be conducted carefully with clear criteria for study selection and identification of potential sources of bias. The number of genetic studies published is increasing; hence, the importance of their systematic reviews is increasing.[13]

9.4 CONCLUSIONS

Drawing together the results of different studies is a scientific endeavour and needs to be performed within a framework that aims to minimize the risk of bias and improve precision. The overarching aim of these reviews is to identify the 'true' answer to the question posed.

9.5 FUTURE RESEARCH NEEDS

Active research into the science of systematic reviews is ongoing. This research focuses on the impact of bias on the outcome of reviews, for example, the impact of outcome reporting bias.[14] Such research usually covers a broader medical field than just ophthalmology. It is important that eye health care researchers aiming to conduct systematic reviews keep up to date with methodological developments for this type of study.

REFERENCES

1. Egger M, Smith DG, Altman DG. *Systematic Reviews in Health Care: Meta-analysis in Context*, 2nd Edition. London: BMJ Publishing Group; 2001.
2. Evans J, Virgili G, Gordon I, *et al. Interventions for neovascular age-related macular degeneration. Cochrane Database of Systematic Reviews.* New York: John Wiley & Sons; 2009.
3. Stewart LA, Tierney JF. To IPD or not to IPD? Advantages and disadvantages of systematic reviews using individual patient data. *Eval Health Prof* 2002; 25:76–97.
4. Higgins JPT, Altman DG. Assessing the risk of bias in included studies. In: Higgins JPT, Green S, (eds). *Cochrane Handbook for Systematic Reviews of Interventions.* The Cochrane Collaboration, 2008. Available from www.cochrane-handbook.org.
5. Dwan K, Altman DG, Arnaiz JA, *et al.* Systematic review of the empirical evidence of study publication bias and outcome reporting bias. *PLoS ONE* 2008; 3:e3081.
6. Laine C, Horton R, DeAngelis CD, *et al.* Clinical trial registration: looking back and moving ahead. *JAMA* 2007; 298:93–94.
7. Chan AW. Bias, spin, and misreporting: time for full access to trial protocols and results. *PLoS Med* 2008; 5:e230.
8. Congdon N, O'Colmain B, Klaver CC, *et al.* Eye Diseases Prevalence Research Group. Causes and prevalence of visual impairment among adults in the United States. *Arch Ophthalmol* 2004; 122: 477–485.
9. Congdon N, Vingerling JR, Klein BE, *et al.* Eye Diseases Prevalence Research Group. Prevalence of cataract and aphakia/pseudophakia among adults in the United States. *Arch Ophthalmol* 2004; 122: 487–494.
10. Friedman DS, O'Colmain BJ, Munoz B, *et al.* Prevalence of age-related macular degeneration in the United States. *Arch Ophthalmol* 2004; 122: 564–572.
11. Owen CG, Fletcher AE, Donoghue M, *et al.* How big is the burden of visual loss caused by age related macular degeneration in the United Kingdom? *Br J Ophthalmol* 2003; 87:312–317.
12. Friedman DS, Wolfs RC, O'Colmain BJ, *et al.* Eye Diseases Prevalence Research Group. Prevalence of open-angle glaucoma among adults in the United States. *Arch Ophthalmol* 2004; 122:532–538.
13. Thakkinstian A, Han P, McEvoy M, *et al.* Systematic review and meta-analysis of the association between complement factor H Y402H polymorphisms and age-related macular degeneration. *Hum Mol Genet* 2006; 15:2784–2790.
14. Kirkham JJ, Dwan KM, Altman DG, *et al.* The impact of outcome reporting bias in randomised controlled trials on a cohort of systematic reviews. *Br Med J* 2010; 340:c365.

SECTION 3

SPECIFIC ENTITIES

10

Age-related cataract

EMILY GOWER AND SHEILA WEST

10.1	Introduction	177	10.5	Risk factors for cataract	184
10.2	Cataract subtypes and mechanisms for cataract development	177	10.6	Medications	188
			10.7	Genetics	189
10.3	Cataract grading systems: characterization of phenotypes	178	10.8	Cataract and mortality	189
			10.9	Summary and future directions	190
10.4	Burden of disease	178		References	190

10.1 INTRODUCTION

Age-related cataract is the leading cause of blindness and low vision worldwide, accounting for nearly 50% of all world blindness (with best correction), with an estimated 18 million people blind from the disease.[1] During the past decade, availability of cataract surgical services has increased dramatically both in the developed world and in many developing countries; however, many countries still have limited access to surgical services. Cataract surgery is the most commonly performed surgical procedure in the United States with more than two million procedures performed annually. Despite the high rate of surgery, even in the developed world, where cataract surgical services are widely available, lens opacity is still an important cause of low vision, and even blindness in some populations. With most populations ageing, estimates suggest that the prevalence of cataract will increase substantially in the coming decades.

10.2 CATARACT SUBTYPES AND MECHANISMS FOR CATARACT DEVELOPMENT

The subtypes of cataract are divided clinically into three categories, based on anatomical location: cortical, nuclear and **posterior subcapsular** (**PSC**) cataract (Plates 10.1–10.5). The lens is surrounded by a capsule. The nucleus is the centre of the lens and contains the embryonic nucleus. Lens fibres in the nucleus contain proteins present since infancy, and are subjected to life-long insults. Because of their location, nuclear lens fibres are unable to readily repair damaged lens proteins. The nucleus is surrounded by the lens cortex, which contains anteriorly a thin layer of epithelial cells (the only cells with a nucleus, since lens fibres lose their organelles as they mature and elongate). The cortical and subcapsular regions are closest to the anterior chamber and vitreous, where nutrients are exchanged and photo-oxidative damage is most likely. Nuclear cataract is typically the most common form of cataract. It begins as a clouding of the lens, resulting from protein aggregation that reflects the ageing process. Cortical cataract is typically the second most common type. It appears in the form of wedge or spoke-shaped opacities within the cortex that become visually disabling when they reach the visual axis. PSC cataract is typically the least common cataract, and is likely to result from and consist of damaged cells that migrate to the posterior subcapsular area. Mixed opacities, where two or more subtypes co-exist, are common. Each of these subtypes is an important cause of blindness and visual impairment. The relative prevalence and risk factors for each of these types are described below.

10.3 CATARACT GRADING SYSTEMS: CHARACTERIZATION OF PHENOTYPES

Rigorous investigations into the aetiology of cataract have been considerably enhanced by the development of valid and reliable classification systems to identify the presence and severity of the different lens opacity types. Differentiation of nuclear, cortical, and PSC lens opacities is important for two reasons. First, a careful phenotypic description of the type of cataract permits better characterization of the distribution of cataract types in populations and, subsequently, clues into possible aetiological factors. Second, as the different types have been associated with different aetiologies, precision in characterization of cataract is critical in epidemiological studies.

Several grading systems are in use for categorizing cataract type and severity. They are based on photographic images of the lens taken in standardized fashion, and largely rely on graders who compare features of the images to standard photographs in order to grade severity. The systems differ largely in the standard photographs used to differentiate severity of the lens opacity.[2–6] Occasionally, these systems are used in research to grade cataracts clinically instead of basing them on photographs; but rigorous testing for **validity** and inter- and intra-observer **reliability** is necessary

prior to starting the project in order to ensure the grading is comparable with photographs and from one clinical grader to another. Unfortunately, many of the major cataract epidemiological studies have used different grading schemes, and, more importantly, different cut-offs to define opacification, which makes cross-study comparisons difficult. The World Health Organization has developed a clinical tool for the simple assessment of cataract type with the slit lamp, which may be useful for population surveys, although to date most have assessed blindness due to cataract without reference to type.[7]

Automating image analyses has been attempted several times, with varying results. Quantifying the density of nuclear opacification has been the most successful, despite the need to rely on grader specification of the nuclear region. A recent report using **anterior segment ocular coherence tomography** (**AS-OCT**) to determine the degree of nuclear opalescence showed some promise since OCT removes some of the variability in slit lamp and flash settings in subjective assessment of nuclear density.[8] Further work is needed to test the value of cortical and PSC assessment by AS-OCT, especially since multiple scans in several meridians are needed, and the report noted the production of artifacts in the anterior surface.

Analysis of the loss of retinal image clarity is associated with cataract severity, but this approach cannot determine the type of cataract, and does not detect early change. Further investigations of automated grading systems, and better, low-cost digital image capture systems for cortical and PSC cataracts are warranted, as this would substantially reduce the cost of cataract research.

10.4 BURDEN OF DISEASE

10.4.1 Incidence and prevalence worldwide

Reports on the prevalence and incidence of cataract amongst populations differ across studies based on the definitions and cut-offs used to define visually significant cataract, the grading systems used to identify the subtypes and severity, and the differences in race, gender and age distribution within the population being studied. Typically, cataract prevalence tends to increase with increasing age, and in most studies, the prevalence of each subtype also increases with increasing age.

Distribution of lens opacity types in populations

Differences in the distribution of the cataract subtypes within racial or ethnic populations point to potential differences in genetic or genetic/environment or environmental exposures that could be exploited for aetiological research. For example, population-based studies in Barbados and Salisbury, Maryland, have shown that African Americans/Caribbeans have a higher prevalence of cortical cataract as compared with Caucasians, and lower prevalence of nuclear and PSC opacities (Tables 10.1–10.3).[9,10] Incidence rates of cortical opacities are also high in African Americans/Caribbeans, confirming that the difference with Caucasians is real.[11] In the **Salisbury Evaluation Eye Study** (**SEE**), this difference was not explained by differences in sunlight exposure,

diabetes, or gender, suggesting other exposures and/or a strong genetic component may be important.[12]

Some studies in Asian populations have reported PSC rates that are substantially higher than the rates seen in African-derived populations and Caucasians. Two Asian studies that used clinical grading rather than image assessment reported rates of PSC that are higher in Chinese ethnic groups.[13,14] Two more recent large-scale lens opacity studies among Asian ethnic groups provide very different rates of PSC. The Beijing Eye Study (in Chinese) reports PSC rates similar to Caucasians; however, the **Singapore Malay Eye Study** (**SiMES**) reports PSC rates that are more than double the rates in the Beijing Eye Study (Table 10.4).[15] The SiMES study also suggests higher rates of cortical cataract in Asian populations as compared with Caucasians. In each of these studies, image assessment was used to classify cataract subtypes; however, different grading systems were used. The Beijing Eye Study used a cut-off of AREDS grade 3 for defining nuclear cataract. If grade 3 was considered normal, the overall prevalence of nuclear cataract would drop

Table 10.1 *Prevalence of nuclear cataract by age and gender (%)*

	Barbados	Beaver Dam Wisconsin	Blue Mountains Australia	Salisbury, Maryland Black	Salisbury, Maryland White	Melbourne VIP Australia	SiMES Singapore	Beijing Eye Study
Dates of study	1988–1992	1988–1990	1992–1994	1990–1993	1993–1995	1991–1998	2004–2006	
Participants	4,191	4,631	2,489	567	1,543	4,602	2,896	4,439
Grading system used	LOCS II	Wisconsin	Wisconsin	Wilmer	Wilmer	Wilmer	Wisconsin	AREDS
Age (years)								
40–49	0	0.4	—	—	—	0.2	0.2	2.9
50–54	0.2	0.5	1.6	—	—	0.4	1.5	7
55–59	0.6	3.2	2.3	—	—	2.8	7.4	35.8
60–64	2.6	9.2	5.3	—	—	6.6	21.6	63.6
65–69	6.2	21.9	17.2	8.3	16.8	17.6	39.8	85.4
70–74	13.3	33.2	27.6	11.5	28.1	26.5	67.8	94.4
75–79	23.9	50.1	44.9	16.7	48.8	46.2	83.3	98.2*
80–84	35.9	63.3	54.5	43.8	59.9	70.1	—	—
85+	—	90.3	66.2	—	—	80.4	—	—
Gender								
Female	5.7	20.8	19.6	18	35.8	13.9	14.4**	80.1
Male	5.9	12.5	17.7	11.8	27.6	8.9	10.9**	82.9

* persons aged 75+.
** adjusted.

Table 10.2 *Prevalence of cortical cataract by age and gender (%)*

	Barbados	Beaver Dam Wisconsin	Blue Mountains Australia	Salisbury, Maryland Black	Salisbury, Maryland White	Melbourne VIP Australia	SiMES Singapore	Beijing Eye Study
Dates of study	1988–1992	1988–1990	1992–1994	1990–1993	1993–1995	1991–1998	2004–2006	2001
Participants	4,191	4,631	2,489	567	1,543	4,602	2,896	4,439
Grading system used	LOCS II	Wisconsin	Wisconsin	Wilmer	Wilmer	Wilmer	Wisconsin	
Age (years)								
40–49	1	0.1	—	—	—	0.9	4.2	1.1
50–54	3.3	0.3	0.7	—	—	2.8	14	3.2
55–59	12.6	0.3	1.7	—	—	4.8	30.6	7.2
60–64	20.4	2	2.9	—	—	11.8	46.5	13.4
65–69	28.5	5.6	7.5	7.9	1.4	18.4	54.2	21.9
70–74	38.8	8.6	8.9	23.8	1.7	27.9	60.5	31.5
75–79	47.5	12.5	11.4	17.6	3.9	33.9	63.9	35.7*
80–84	56.4	20.6	18.1	26.8	6.1	43.2	—	
85+	—	13.3	16.7	—	—	41.4	—	
Gender								
Female	20.4	5.9	8	20.7	2.8	12.7	22.8	11.0
Male	14.1	2.9	4.3	12.2	2.4	9.9	18.3**	8.1

* 75 years and older
** age adjusted

Table 10.3 *Prevalence of posterior subcapsular cataract (PSC) by age and gender (%)*

	Barbados	Beaver Dam Wisconsin	Blue Mountains Australia	Melbourne VIP Australia	Salisbury, Maryland Black	Salisbury, Maryland White	SiMES Singapore	Beijing Eye Study
Dates of study	1988–1992	1988–1990	1992–1994	1990–1993	1993–1995	1991–1998	2004–2006	2001
Participants	4,191	4,631	2,489	567	1,543	4,602	2,896	4,439
Grading system used	LOCS II	Wisconsin	Wisconsin	Wilmer	Wilmer	Wilmer	Wisconsin	
Age (years)								
40–49	0.6	1.2	—	—	—	1.9	1.4	1.2
50–54	1.6	1.7	2.9	—	—	1.9	3.1	1.8
55–59	1.1	2.4	2.9	—	—	3.1	6.1	2.7
60–64	3	5.3	4.5	—	—	3.6	9.7	4.6
65–69	5.4	5.9	6.3	2.5	4.8	4.9	18.3	6.8
70–74	7.3	8.3	6.8	4.4	5	5	24.1	9
75–79	8.4	8.5	11.4	0	6.7	11.7	39.7	27.3*
80–84	24.6	16.2	12.3	2.9	6.7	16.3	44.1	—
85+	—	6.9	19.6	—	—	17.2	—	—
Gender								
Female	4.1	5	6.2	2.6	4.9	4	9.8**	4.0
Male	3.6	4.9	6.5	2.6	6.2	4.3	10.3**	4.4

* 75 years and older
** age adjusted, ANY psc

Table 10.4 Prevalence and proportion of blindness and low vision associated with age-related cataract in recent population-based studies

	Baltimore		Beaver Dam	Blue Mountains	Salisbury		Barbados	Proyecto VER	SiMES	Beijing Eye Study
	White	Black	White	White	White	Black	Black	Hispanic		Northern China
At risk (n)	2,913	2,395	4,866	3,625	1,853	666	4,303	4,766	3,089	4,439
Low vision WHO (n)	30	22	114	106	50	35	—	92	86	43
Blind US (n)	19	24	23	24	10	11	130	14	22	nr
Blind WHO (n)	9	16	17	17	3	4	71	11	16	17
All vision impaired	49	46	137	130	60	46	—	106	132	not reported
Low vision WHO due to cataract (%)	70.0	77.3	—	64.2	42.0	45.7	—	46.7	81.4	36.7
Blind US due to cataract (%)	15.8	33.3	4.3	8.1	0.0	9.1	40.8	14.3	63.6	—
Blind WHO due to cataract (%)	11.1	25.0	5.9	7.1	0.0	0.0	31.0	18.2	68.8	38.5
Vision impairment due to cataract (%)	49.0	54.3	—	53.8	35.0	37.0	—	42.5	71.2	nr

from 50.3% to 13.6%,[15,16] demonstrating the importance in defining cut-offs and the necessity of ensuring comparability of grading systems when one tries to compare rates across populations. While the SiMES study used a system with a minimal opacity definition for early cortical cataract, the rates of cortical cataract were higher in this study than in studies of other populations using the same grading system, suggesting that this ethnic group is likely also to have higher rates of PSC cataract. Whether these rates differ due to differences in use of cataract services, or other factors, warrants further exploration.

Meaningful comparisons of differences in specific cataract subtypes between Latinos living in the United States and Caucasians are somewhat hampered, since the Latino studies relied strictly on clinical grading without use of image-based cataract assessment systems. With this caveat in mind, Latinos in Los Angeles appear to have higher rates of posterior subcapsular cataract compared with Caucasians, but this difference may also be due to differential access to cataract surgical services.[17,18]

The prevalence and incidence of lens opacities differ between the sexes, with women having consistently higher rates of cortical opacities compared with men.[12,19] This gender difference is not explained by any difference in diabetes, sunlight exposure, or age.[20] Ten-year, age-adjusted incidence rates of nuclear and cortical opacities were higher in females compared with males in the Caucasian populations of Blue Mountain, Australia,[21] and ten- and fifteen-year, age-adjusted incident nuclear opacities were higher in females in Beaver Dam, Wisconsin (**BDES**).[22,23] However, a strong gender difference in PSC cataract does not appear to exist. The reason(s) for a gender difference in nuclear and cortical cataract are not clear. However, differences in expression of the lens proteomes between male and female rats suggested potential differences in oxidative stress regulation that deserves further research.[24]

These population and sex differences in cataract prevalence may provide clues regarding aetiology, and reasons why such differences exist should be explored further.

Cataract blindness

Data on the prevalence and incidence of cataract blindness within a population may vary, depending on the survey methodology and specifically how the primary cause of blindness is defined. The World Health Organization defines blindness as vision worse than 20/400 (3/360) in the better-seeing eye (see Chapter 1), while the definition in the USA is based on vision worse than 20/200 (6/60). Furthermore, some individuals are blind from multiple ocular conditions, and correction of one condition would not alter the visual status. For example, if an individual with severe optic nerve damage from glaucoma or retinal damage from diabetic retinopathy had cataract surgery, he/she would likely still have poor vision following cataract surgery. Thus, the prevalence of blindness due to cataract would differ depending on how the cause of blindness was defined. Data from population studies suffer from small numbers, but suggest cataract as a cause of blindness is not common in developed countries (Table 10.4), but as a cause of visual impairment.

The WHO has developed relatively simple, inexpensive rapid assessment methodologies for evaluating blindness in developing countries (see Chapters 1 and 3). These **Rapid Assessments of Cataract Surgical Services (RACSS)** and **Rapid Assessment of Avoidable Blindness (RAAB)** are useful in evaluating programmatic issues, and for providing general data on cataract blindness. They do not, however, include sufficient depth of information to identify the type of cataract or to rule out other causes of blindness. Another limitation of these studies is the methodology for classifying primary cause of blindness. When an individual presents with dense lens opacity, evaluation of the retina and optic nerve is not feasible. Thus, the primary cause of blindness is attributed to cataract, regardless of whether other co-morbid ocular conditions may be present.

Numerous RACSS/RAAB studies have been conducted in Africa,[25–29] Asia,[30–43] and South America.[44–47] The data reported differ slightly across studies; in some studies age- and gender-adjusted rates of blindness are provided, while in others the prevalence of blindness among survey participants is

Table 10.5 RACSS

Continent	Country	State	Year	# Examined (% of enumerated)	Adjusted*** % bilateral blindness	% Adjusted bilateral blindness due to cataract (95% confidence interval)	% of bilateral blind due to cataract
Africa	Nigeria	Kebbi state	2006	2,424 (93.6%)	4.4 (4.1–4.7)	2.1 (1.5–2.7) U	46
	Kenya	Embu District	2007	3,376 (99.2%)	2 (1.5–2.5)U	not reported	40
	Cameroon	Muyuka	early 2000s	1,787 (89.3%)	1.4 (0.9–2.0)	0.9 (0.4–1.4)	60
South America	Argentina		early 2000s	4,302 (93.5%)	1 (0.7–1.3)	0.5 (0.4–0.8)%	54
	Guatamala	4 districts	early 2000s	4,806 (98.1%)	3.5 (3.0–4.2)	2.3 (1.8–3.0)	66
	Paraguay	Not reported	Not reported	2,136 (89%)	3.14 (2.2–4.4)	2.01 (1.3–3.0)%	64
Asia	Myanmar	Meiktila Division	2005	2,076 (83.7%)	5.3 (4.0–6.6)	not reported	53
	Timor–Leste		2005	1,414 (96.2%)	4.1 (3.1–5.1)	not reported	79
	Philippines	Negros Island and Antique District	2005–2006	5,951 (79%)	2.5 (1.9 to 3.1)	not reported	54–63
	New Guinea	Papua	2004–2005	1,174 (98.6%)	3.9 (3.4–6.1)	2.9 (1.7–3.4)%	73
	Bangladesh	Satkhira	2005	4,868 (91.9%)	2.9 (2.4–3.4)	not reported	79
	Pakistan	Chakwal District	not reported	1,505 (94.1%)	3.1 (2.3–4.1)	1.8 (1.0–3.0)	47
	Pakistan	Orakzai Agency	not reported	1,549 (97%)	5.9 (4.7–7.0)U	4.8 (3.8–5.9)U	82U
	India	Gujarat	1995	1,962 (95.8%)	2.9	1.2	<50
	India	Karnataka State	1995	2,195 (84%)	7.4 U	4.93 (4.52– 5.34)	–
	Turkmenistan	entire country	1996	6,011 (98.2%)	1.3 (1.0–1.7)	0.6 (0.4–0.9)	45

Blindness: < 3/60 in better eye

U: unadjusted

*** adjusted for age and gender unless otherwise noted

reported. Table 10.5 reports data on studies that defined blindness according to the WHO definition (vision worse than 3/60 in the better seeing eye), and data were available for both bilateral blindness overall and blindness due to cataract. Across these RACSS/RAAB studies, the reported prevalence of bilateral blindness due to cataract ranged from 0.5% to roughly 5% of the population aged 50 years and older, while the overall rate of bilateral blindness was as high as 7%. The percent of bilateral blindness due to cataract ranged from 40% to approximately 80% of all blindness. The difference in the rates of blindness attributable to cataract likely varies largely based on the availability of cataract surgical services in these areas.

10.4.2 Impact of the disease on quality of life

While the incidence and prevalence of cataract are important indicators to quantify what proportion of a population is affected, the impact of the disease on cataract patients' lives is the primary indicator of the burden of cataract in society. Several studies have evaluated different aspects of how cataract adversely impacts daily life. The development of self-reported quality of life tools for use in studying the impact of visual impairment in general began with research on cataract surgery patients, indicating the significant potential of cataract in causing visual impairment, and the resulting benefit of cataract surgery on visual function.[48] The original tool, **Activities of Daily Vision Scale (ADVS)**, was followed by the development of shorter sets of questions specifically for cataract surgery, such as the **VF-14**.[49] These questionnaires have been used to document patient complaints due to cataract, and specifically complaints that are not necessarily captured by tests of visual acuity or contrast sensitivity. Recognition of the broad impact of cataract on patient function led to a change in surgery best practices. The USA Preferred Practice Guidelines for cataract surgery now state that cataract surgery is also indicated when a patient reports that his/her function is compromised, regardless of acuity deficits.[50]

Studies have reported the substantial independent impact of cataract on reduced quality of life, after adjusting for other factors.[51] A recent study, conducted in three developing countries, reported that individuals with vision-impairing cataract are significantly less likely to participate in both 'work-related' and 'leisure-related' activities than their normal-sighted counterparts.[52] Several studies have used the VF-14 or ADVS to compare quality of life before and after cataract surgery, and most have shown an improvement in multiple aspects of quality of life following surgery among patients with good post-surgical visual outcomes.[48,53,54]

Several studies have demonstrated an association between cataract and vehicle crash risk, and some studies have shown that cataract progression can be the primary motivator in driving cessation among the elderly. Owsley *et al.* were among the first researchers to report the relationship between cataract and increased crash risk. In their prospective observational study, patients who underwent cataract surgery were nearly 50% less likely to have a motor vehicle accident in the next four to six years than individuals who had cataract but declined surgery.[55] This study and other longitudinal observational studies in the elderly also highlight the problems in evaluating single outcomes, since patients who undergo cataract surgery are likely to be healthier and to have less co-morbidity than individuals who decline surgery, despite similarity in the level of visual impairment.

10.5 RISK FACTORS FOR CATARACT

An exhaustive review is beyond the scope of this chapter; this section will cover highlights and recent literature. Readers are also directed to previous reviews.[12,19]

10.5.1 Smoking

Cigarette smoking is one of the most consistently reported risk factors for age-related cataract development. Numerous studies have demonstrated an association between cigarette smoking and both nuclear and posterior subcapsular (PSC) cataract,[12,19,56–60] and several studies have shown a dose-dependent relationship between pack-years of use and degree of opacification.[58–63] Smoking cessation appears to reduce the risk of cataract;[59] however, much of the reduction in risk may be attributed to the lower cumulative pack-years smoked by individuals who stopped smoking. Some of the reduction, however, may result from reversing of damage.[61] The consistency of the association dose-response relationship and findings of change after cessation provide strong evidence for causality, with smoking now a well-accepted risk for nuclear opacity. In 2004, cataract was added to the USA Surgeon General's report on health effects of smoking, the first ocular condition to have this dubious distinction.[64] An estimated 20% of cataract cases in the USA may be attributable to smoking, and in countries such as China, where smoking is more common, cataract is, and will continue to be, an epidemic.

10.5.2   Diabetes

More than fifty years ago, researchers suspected that diabetes was a risk factor for cataract development, based on data from diabetic rat models. The first known mechanisms by which diabetes can affect cataract formation relate to how elevated levels of glucose affect the sorbitol pathway and how increased free radical production leads to oxidative damage.[65] More recently, studies have suggested a link between calpains (a family of cysteine proteases) and cataractogenesis.[66,67] Research suggests that the increased production of calcium resulting from diabetes stimulates over-production of various calpains, and this increase results in lenticular and epithelial cell damage.[68]

Population-based studies have identified an excess risk of cortical and PSC lens opacities in persons with diabetes,[15,20,69–71] and the risk appears to increase with increasing duration of diabetes.[72] In two prospective studies, diabetes mellitus was associated with an increased five-year incidence of both cortical and PSC cataract. Early diagnosis of diabetes and maintaining tight control are likely to help reduce the risk of age-related cataract, since

the level of diabetic control, measured by the level of glycated haemoglobin, is related to prevalence, onset and progression of lens opacity.[69,70,73] An interaction has also been noted in some studies where an association between glycated haemoglobin and cataract was seen only in diabetics.[70,73] Such a result may indicate that tight glucose control can minimize the risk of cataract in those with diabetes, as has been demonstrated with other diabetes-associated ocular conditions.[74]

Research has suggested that the effect estimates for diabetes on cataract formation decrease with age. This finding has been repeated in a number of studies.[75–77] A diminishing effect of diabetes on cataractogenesis in older age groups may indicate either an increasing influence of other factors, which may overwhelm the effect of diabetes or, more likely, a survivor bias wherein severe diabetes leads to early mortality, leaving only healthier survivors in the older age groups.

No study to date has reported on differential effects of the influence of diabetes on cataract formation across different ethnicities. The **attributable risk** of cataract due to diabetes in Africans/Caribbeans is estimated at 14%, but the attributable risk among other populations may be different, depending upon the prevalence of diabetes and the level of control.[76]

10.5.3   Radiation exposures: sunlight and other sources of radiation

Early work on animal models identified exposure to optical radiation as a cataractogenic agent, with an action spectrum that clearly implicated **ultraviolet light B** (**UVB, 290–320 nm**).[78,79] Recent work in rabbit lenses suggests that the cumulative effect of repeated UVB radiation is more harmful to the lens metabolic profile than the same dose in a single irradiation.[80] Oxidative damage resulting from UVB exposure is hypothesized to be the mechanism through which UVB exposure may induce cataract. The anterior cortical surface probably receives the most radiant energy, explaining the predominant findings of higher cortical cataract risk with increased sun exposure, with less or no effect on rates of nuclear cataract and PSC.[76] Furthermore, three studies characterized the distribution of the position of opacities, and each found increased risk of cortical cataract in the lower nasal quadrant compared with other areas of the lens.[78–80] Researchers hypothesize that the lower nasal quadrant of the lens would be the most affected by solar UV exposure, given the angle of the sun during peak UV hours.

Geographical differences in cataract risk have long been associated with differences in ambient sunlight. Population-based surveys over large geographical areas, using latitude as the marker of exposure, found elevated risk of cataract where ambient UVB exposure was highest.[81,82] However, such studies are subject to bias known as 'ecological fallacy', wherein many other risk factors could vary along with ambient sunlight producing a spurious association.

The imprecision of the measure of ocular exposure to UV light has been a hindrance to more precise research in human populations, with many studies using ambient UV or number of skin sunburns as surrogate markers. However, ocular exposure is more dependent on behavioural characteristics, such as time spent outside in sunlight and use of sunglasses and brimmed hats, which makes ambient exposure a poor marker. Sunburn is also highly subject to skin type, while the crystalline lens does not have a similar known variation amongst individuals with different skin types.

Methods of estimating ocular exposure in a more precise way were developed[83–85] using a Maryland Sun Year (MSY) as a unit of measure. This metric was tied to the average amount of UVB light that falls on a flat plane in Maryland in a year, using averages based on measurements made over several years. Ocular exposure to UVB was estimated, factoring in hat use, glasses use, time outside during particular seasons, time of day and geographical location. This detailed assessment of cumulative ocular exposure to ultraviolet light in a highly exposed group, Maryland fishermen, showed a dose–response relationship between exposure and risk of cortical opacities.[86] While this research demonstrated proof of principle, extrapolation of risk to the kind of exposures experienced by a general population, which includes other ethnic groups and females, was not possible. A subsequent evaluation in a population-based study in the same geographical area demonstrated an increased risk of cortical opacity with increasing ocular exposure to UVB varying with sex and race.[20]

The public health ramifications of the association between ultraviolet light exposure and lens opacity extend to global warming, and increases in lens opacity have been modelled under various scenarios attributable to the ozone hole.[87] However, exposure to UVB can be limited through very simple measures of wearing plastic glasses or sunglasses when outside, and wearing a brimmed hat. These measures have become part of the sun awareness campaigns carried out in Australia, Canada and in the USA by the Environmental Protection Agency's SunWise program.[88–90]

Other radiation exposure

Ionizing radiation is a cataractogenic stimulus.[91] Fortunately, the earth's atmosphere filters ionizing radiation, and human populations are not exposed to solar sources. Exposure to ionizing radiation in human populations has been man-made, and research into cataracts resulting from such exposure has been conducted on atomic bomb survivors, nuclear reactor disaster survivors, and populations exposed through low doses received during radiological exposure.

Early reports on atomic bomb survivors in Japan suggested that the minimum dose required to produce a detectable cataract from a single exposure was 1.5 Gy.[92,93] Such data supported the recommendations of the National Council on Radiation Protection (NCRP), which state that 2 Gy (single dose) or 5 Gy as a fractionated dose is the minimum dose required to produce a detectable cataract.[94,95] However, a recent re-analysis of cataract prevalence among the atomic bomb survivors in Japan suggests no evidence for a threshold effect.[96]

Moreover, recent data from exposed populations challenge the threshold recommendations. Cataract among the 8,607 clean-up workers at the nuclear site in Chernobyl was assessed at 12 and 14 years after exposure. PSC and cortical cataract rates were present in a dose-dependent fashion, and suggest a threshold under 1 Gy.[97] Using cataract extraction as a surrogate for cataract, a study in 35,705 radiologic technologists, followed for 20 years, found that those reporting three or more X-ray exposures to the head and neck were 25% more likely to have had cataract extraction.[98] In addition, the technologists who worked in the highest category of exposure (mean 60 mGy) were 18% more likely to have cataract extraction compared to those in the lowest category of exposure (mean 5 mGY), though the latter difference was not statistically significant. Nevertheless, these differences suggest that there may be no threshold, or at least that the threshold is considerably lower than NCRP recommendations.[94]

10.5.4 Oxidative stress and antioxidants

Unlike most ocular tissues, which are vascularized and supplied with ample levels of oxygen, the lens cells are normally hypoxic. Animal models suggest that the lens may have difficulty controlling the consumption of oxygen, and increasing oxygen to the posterior lens surface is associated with increasingly higher consumption of oxygen by the lens.[99] Such a scenario may lead to increased production of reactive oxygen species, known to contribute to opacification.

One mechanism by which increasing levels of oxygen may reach the posterior lens is through breakdown in vitreous, or removal of vitreous altogether. Vitrectomies are associated with rapid development of nuclear opacities, and posterior lens exposure to higher than normal levels of oxygen is felt to be the mechanism that leads to cataract development.[100] It may also explain age-related nuclear opacification, if an association of age-related vitreous liquefaction and nuclear opalescence can be shown.[101] The observational studies that have shown a relationship between early onset myopia (not myopic shift due to nuclear cataract) and nuclear cataract development, may also be explained by the association of myopia with vitreous syneresis.[102,103] However, not all studies have found an association of myopia with nuclear cataract, and some report another cataract type, PSC, to be related to myopia.[104,105]

If oxidative stress is cataractogenic, then theoretically, prevention or amelioration of the stress should be protective. This theory has been used to explain why the anterior chamber fluid has such high levels of vitamin C, an anti-oxidant, and why the lens has a number of anti-oxidant enzymes, like glutathione reductase. Oxidative stress is also the underlying biologic mechanism to postulate that increased intake of anti-oxidant nutrients, vitamins or supplements may be protective against cataractogenesis. Epidemiological studies of such a hypothesis are notoriously difficult to carry out for several reasons. First, intake levels of dietary or supplemental anti-oxidants may not be reflected in serum or ocular levels. For example, while increased dietary intake of vitamin C seems to correlate with increased ocular levels of vitamin C, vitamin E intake appears to be regulated so that increased intake is not associated with higher ocular vitamin E levels. Second, recall of dietary intake has measurement error, and serum measurements reflect a single point in time, which may not represent long-term patterns.

Numerous interventional studies have attempted to demonstrate a protective effect of anti-oxidant nutrients, vitamins and supplements against cataract, with no clear, consistent findings.[12,19,106] Several clinical trials of anti-oxidant vitamins in diverse populations have notably failed to demonstrate any consistent, protective effect for cataract.[107–109] The **Age Related Eye Disease (AREDS)** clinical trial followed 4,629 patients randomized to four combinations of anti-oxidants plus zinc and placebo.[107] No protective effect was seen on incidence or progression of lens opacities. A more recent study of 1,020 participants randomized to multivitamin versus placebo, using the same AREDS grading scheme, found a protective effect of supplementation for nuclear opacity, and a two-fold increased risk for PSC.[110] A clinical trial in an Indian population was carried out to address the concern that populations in Europe or North America are already anti-oxidant replete and supplementation would have no added benefit whereas a less well-nourished population may experience protection. However, thrice weekly observed supplementation with beta-carotene, vitamin C and E compared with placebo appeared to provide no protection against progression of nuclear, cortical or PSC opacities over a five-year period.[108] Many of these trials have been criticized for not including the correct supplement dosing, and for too short a period of time, or being conducted in study populations that are already taking supplements outside the trial. Considering the huge investment in research in this area, and the conflicting findings across many different populations and study designs, this field deserves a thorough and careful review with recommendations of promising approaches before further research can be justified.

10.6   MEDICATIONS

10.6.1   Steroids

Among a number of medications that have been suggested as causing or promoting lens opacity, corticosteroids have likely the strongest association with cataract formation. This class of drug includes topical drops, systemic oral medication and inhalers. Oral steroids, particularly high doses or with prolonged use, have long been implicated in posterior subcapsular cataract.[12] Early studies suggested an absence of risk with inhaled corticosteroids, but were criticized for being conducted primarily in young populations or confounded by oral steroid use as well.[19] Several studies have now reported a risk of cataract among users of inhaled steroids,[111–113] which may well be a risk factor both for PSC and nuclear opacity. One study reported a dose–response relationship, with the heaviest users of inhaled steroids having nearly a ten-fold increased risk of PSC compared with non-users.[111] However, a recent study examining the relationship between oral and inhaled corticosteroid and cataract development showed that inhaled corticosteroids increased cataract risk only among those participants who reported prior use of oral corticosteroids.[114]

It should be noted that several factors may complicate the detection of small effects due to inhaled steroids. The particular lesions associated with steroid use may have a reversible component and

can be difficult to detect since they rarely affect vision.[58,115] In addition individual susceptibility may vary substantially, and synergism with other cataractogenic factors may ultimately determine any individual's PSC outcome.[58,59,116]

10.6.2   Topical intra-ocular pressure lowering medications

A population-based study of African Caribbean persons in Barbados reported an association between use of topical medications for lowering intraocular pressure (IOP) and increased incident nuclear opacity.[76] Within this group, the primary IOP lowering medications were topical beta-blockers, and after careful adjustment to exclude high intraocular pressure itself as the risk factor, a consistent elevated risk with treatment was observed. This finding led to the addition of cataract components to two glaucoma clinical trials, the **Ocular Hypertensive Treatment Study (OHTS)** and **Early Manifest Glaucoma (EMG)** clinical trials, in an effort to verify a potentially damaging consequence of glaucoma medication, which has considerable clinical relevance when treating older, at risk persons. The EMG trial confirmed this association but the OHT Study did not.[77,117] Although the OHT Study reported no treatment effect on increasing the risk of lens opacity, this lack of an association could be attributed to the cross-sectional assessment of cataract, after a higher proportion of persons in the medication treatment arm had already had cataract surgery.[117] Recently the finding of an association has been confirmed in another longitudinal study.[118]

10.6.3   Medications evaluated for their potential to prevent cataract formation

A large body of evidence suggests that across racial groups, women have higher rates of cataract, even after adjusting for women's greater longevity.[20,69,119–124] Postmenopausal oestrogen decline was hypothesized to play a role. Despite early evidence of a protective role of hormone replacement therapy based on prevalence data in the Salisbury (SEE) and Beaver Dam (BDES) populations,[125,126] prospective, longitudinal data from these populations failed to show a beneficial effect.[127,128] It is likely that other endogenous hormonal effects are implicated in cataractogenesis in women.[127]

The promise of medication to prevent or retard cataract growth among the general population has proved elusive. Initial hopes for aspirin or non-steroidal anti-inflammatory agents as anti-cataract agents have not been supported. Two reports of protective effect of long-term statin use against nuclear cataract or any cataract are intriguing, owing to its anti-inflammatory and anti-oxidant effects.[129,130] However, the findings are in a small sample of the remainder of the Beaver Dam population, and the remainder of the Blue Mountains population (in the latter there was insufficient power to evaluate cataract subtypes), and thus deserve confirmation in other studies evaluating the effect of statins specifically.[131]

As cataract surgery continues to become cheaper and more accessible to populations worldwide, the role of medications targeted at preventing cataract formation has become less important. In order to be practical, such a drug would need to be very inexpensive, safe for long-term use, and easy to administer.

10.7 GENETICS

The likelihood of a genetic pre-disposition to nuclear and cortical cataract has been evaluated in several population studies (see also Chapter 6). In studies of monozygotic and dizygotic Caucasian twins in the UK, the heritability of nuclear cataract was estimated at 48%, with unique environmental factors estimated to account for another 14% of the variability.[132] The heritability in sibling pairs has been estimated at 36% after adjusting for smoking in an older cohort in Salisbury.[133] In extensive analyses in the Beaver Dam cohort pedigrees that included smoking control, the data suggest contributions to nuclear cataractogenesis from multiple genes, characteristic of a complex disorder.[64] Promising work has been carried out investigating

mutations in the crystalline genes, using congenital or **autosomal dominant** (**AD**) nuclear cataract cases, but further work linking these to age related cataract is needed.

Similarly, cortical cataract appears to have a strong genetic component. In the UK Twin Study, additive and dominant genes accounted for 53%–58% of the variability in cortical cataract, with unique environmental factors accounting for 26%–37%.[134] The heritability for cortical cataract in the SEE sibling pairs was 24%.[135] Gamma S crystalline gene mutation has been reported causing a dominant cortical cataract in a Chinese family,[136] and a unique locus on a chromosome not formerly linked to cataract has been identified using data from Beaver Dam.[137] To date, much research has identified polymorphisms and mutations that are associated with **autosomal** dominant or **recessive** (**AR**) congenital cataracts, with some work in age-related cataract, and this field is growing and will continue to evolve. Fascinating work on the crystalline genes has provided not only leads into cataractogenesis, but also associations with other neurological, cardiac, and muscular disorders that will likely provide insights into the ageing process.

10.8 CATARACT AND MORTALITY

Data are accumulating that suggest cataract, especially nuclear opacities and mixed opacities that include nuclear, are independent predictors of mortality.[138–145] Cataract shares risk factors such as age and smoking with systemic diseases known to cause early mortality, and is also associated with co-morbid conditions like diabetes that lead to early mortality. Thus, a question can be raised whether cataract is just a surrogate marker for these other factors. However, the increased risk of mortality generally persists, even after adjustment for age, smoking, diabetes and other co-morbid conditions, suggesting cataract is an independent indicator of mortality. The association has been observed in a variety of populations,[138,139,142,144] lending further credence to the finding.

However, not all population-based studies have found this association, although the characterization of lens status in these studies was often less than ideal.[146–148] For example, two studies that did not find the association defined cataract as lens opacity graded clinically in individuals with vision loss of worse than 6/12 or 6/18.[146,147] Thus a sizeable fraction of those with lens opacities but without vision loss are left in the comparison group, with the potential to attenuate any association.

The specific cellular processes that portend accelerated mortality may be mirrored in the opacification of the lens. It is tempting to speculate that factors leading to altered proteins or aggregation in the lens are also factors involved in early death, but further research is needed to identify such an ageing process. However, if there is a similar process that occurs in the ocular lens, as well as systemically, then the risk of death may be most pronounced in the years closest to the lens assessment. Longer follow-up (while including a greater number of deaths) may weaken the association unless the development of new opacities is also considered.

Attempts to refine the association by determining whether cataract is associated with a specific cause of death have not been conclusive. One study found nuclear cataract associated with death from stroke, but not cancer,[145] while another found cataract in women associated with cardiovascular, respiratory and other non-cancer deaths, but again not related to cancer.[141] However, two other studies found an increase in deaths related to cancer.[138,142] If the ageing changes that are evident in the lens as well as systemically are markers of processes that simply pre-dispose an individual to early death, then it may be that no one cause will be associated with cataract.

Nevertheless, this association suggests exciting avenues of research into the ageing process that can use known pathways in lens opacification to investigate cellular pathways for premature senescence.

10.9 SUMMARY AND FUTURE DIRECTIONS

Prevalence data have been accumulated for a substantial proportion of the world's population, and numerous risk factors have been identified for cataract development. Questions such as why women have higher rates of cataract formation than men, and why blacks have higher rates of nuclear cataract but lower rates of cortical and PSC cataract remain unanswered. Perhaps the future answers to cataract prevention lie within the clues provided by these classic epidemiologic data.

10.9.1 Research priorities

1. Testing of automatic grading systems, including AS-OCT, for assessment of cataract subtypes — particularly in the case of cortical and PSC cataracts.
2. Exploration for the reasons for gender differences in prevalence of nuclear and cortical subtypes, and also differences in prevalences of all three cataract subtypes in different ethnic populations.
3. Before further intervention studies of antioxidant nutrients, vitamins and supplements in the prevention or delay of cataract development can be justified, a thorough and careful review of past studies must be undertaken, with recommendations for any further promising approaches if they exist.
4. Reports of a protective effect against cataract of long-term statin use deserve confirmation.
5. The association of cataract with mortality suggests avenues of research into the ageing process, using known pathways in lens opacification.

REFERENCES

1. Resnikoff S, Pascolini D, Etya'ale D, *et al*. Global data on visual impairment in the year 2002. *Bull World Health Organ* 2004; 82:844–851.
2. Chylack LT Jr., Leske MC, Sperduto R, *et al*. Lens Opacities Classification System. *Arch Ophthalmol* 1988; 106:330–334.
3. Foster A, Resnikoff S. The impact of Vision 2020 on global blindness. *Eye* 2005; 19:1133–1135.
4. Sparrow JM, Bron AJ, Brown NA, *et al*. The Oxford Clinical Cataract Classification and

Grading System. *Int Ophthalmol* 1986; 9:207–225.

5. Taylor HR, West SK. The clinical grading of lens opacities. *Aust N Z J Ophthalmol* 1989; 17:81–86.

6. West SK, Rosenthal F, Newland HS, *et al.* Use of photographic techniques to grade nuclear cataracts. *Invest Ophthalmol Vis Sci* 1988; 29:73–77.

7. Thylefors B, Chylack LT Jr., Konyama K, *et al.* A simplified cataract grading system. *Ophthalmic Epidemiol* 2002; 9:83–95.

8. Wong AL, Leung CK, Weinreb RN, *et al.* Quantitative assessment of lens opacities with anterior segment optical coherence tomography. *Br J Ophthalmol* 2009; 93:61–65.

9. Leske MC, Connell AM, Wu SY, *et al.* Prevalence of lens opacities in the Barbados Eye Study. *Arch Ophthalmol* 1997; 115:105–111.

10. West SK, Munoz B, Schein OD, *et al.* Racial differences in lens opacities: the Salisbury Eye Evaluation (SEE) project. *Am J Epidemiol* 1998; 148:1033–1039.

11. Leske MC, Wu SY, Nemesure B, *et al.* Nine-year incidence of lens opacities in the Barbados Eye Studies. *Ophthalmology* 2004; 111:483–490.

12. West SK, Valmadrid CT. Epidemiology of risk factors for age-related cataract. *Surv Ophthalmol* 1995; 39:323–334.

13. Seah SK, Wong TY, Foster PJ, *et al.* Prevalence of lens opacity in Chinese residents of Singapore: the Tanjong Pagar Survey. *Ophthalmology* 2002; 109:2058–2064.

14. Tsai SY, Hsu WM, Cheng CY, *et al.* Epidemiologic study of age-related cataracts among an elderly Chinese population in Shih-Pai, Taiwan. *Ophthalmology* 2003; 110:1089–1095.

15. Xu L, Cui T, Zhang S, *et al.* Prevalence and risk factors of lens opacities in urban and rural Chinese in Beijing. *Ophthalmology* 2006; 113: 747–755.

16. Jonas JB, Xu L, Wang YX. The Beijing Eye Study. *Acta Ophthalmol* 2009; 87:247–261.

17. Varma R, Torres M. Prevalence of lens opacities in Latinos: the Los Angeles Latino Eye Study. *Ophthalmology* 2004; 111:1449–1456.

18. Broman AT, Hafiz G, Munoz B, *et al.* Cataract and barriers to cataract surgery in a US Hispanic

population: Proyecto VER. *Arch Ophthalmol* 2005; 123:1231–1236.

19. Abraham AG, Condon NG, West GE. The new epidemiology of cataract. *Ophthalmol Clin North Am* 2006; 19:415–425.

20. West SK, Duncan DD, Munoz B, *et al.* Sunlight exposure and risk of lens opacities in a population-based study: the Salisbury Eye Evaluation project. *JAMA* 1998; 280:714–718.

21. Kanthan GL, Wang JJ, Rochtchina E, *et al.* Ten-year incidence of age-related cataract and cataract surgery in an older Australian population. The Blue Mountains Eye Study. *Ophthalmology* 2008; 115:808–814.

22. Klein BE, Klein R, Lee KE. Incidence of age-related cataract over a 10-year interval: the Beaver Dam Eye Study. *Ophthalmology* 2002; 109: 2052–2057.

23. Klein BE, Klein R, Lee KE, *et al.* Incidence of age-related cataract over a 15-year interval. The Beaver Dam Eye Study. *Ophthalmology* 2008; 115: 477–482.

24. Guest PC, Skynner HA, Salim K, *et al.* Detection of gender differences in rat lens proteins using 2-D-DIGE. *Proteomics* 2006; 6:667–676.

25. Rabiu MM. Cataract blindness and barriers to uptake of cataract surgery in a rural community of northern Nigeria. *Br J Ophthalmol* 2001; 85:776–780.

26. Oye JE, Kuper H, Dineen B, *et al.* Prevalence and causes of blindness and visual impairment in Muyuka: a rural health district in South West Province, Cameroon. *Br J Ophthalmol* 2006; 90:538–542.

27. Rabiu MM, Muhammed N. Rapid assessment of cataract surgical services in Birnin-Kebbi local government area of Kebbi State, Nigeria. *Ophthalmic Epidemiol* 2008; 15:359–365.

28. Mathenge W, Kuper H, Limburg H, *et al.* Rapid assessment of avoidable blindness in Nakuru district, Kenya. *Ophthalmology* 2007; 114:599–605.

29. Mathenge W, Nkurikiye J, Limburg H, *et al.* Rapid assessment of avoidable blindness in Western Rwanda: blindness in a post-conflict setting. *PLoS Med* 2007; 4:e217.

30. Wadud Z, Kuper H, Polack S, *et al.* Rapid assessment of avoidable blindness and needs assessment of cataract surgical services in Satkhira

District, Bangladesh. *Br J Ophthalmol* 2006; 90:1225–1229.

31. Anjum KM, Qureshi MB, Khan MA, *et al.* Cataract blindness and visual outcome of cataract surgery in a tribal area in Pakistan. *Br J Ophthalmol* 2006; 90:135–138.

32. Nirmalan PK, Thulasiraj RD, Maneksha V, *et al.* A population based eye survey of older adults in Tirunelveli district of south India: blindness, cataract surgery, and visual outcomes. *Br J Ophthalmol* 2002; 86:505–512.

33. Amansakhatov S, Volokhovskaya ZP, Afanasyeva AN, *et al.* Cataract blindness in Turkmenistan: results of a national survey. *Br J Ophthalmol* 2002; 86:1207–1210.

34. Garap JN, Sheeladevi S, Shamanna BR, *et al.* Blindness and vision impairment in the elderly of Papua New Guinea. *Clin Exp Ophthalmol* 2006; 34:335–341.

35. Ramke J, Palagyi A, Naduvilath T, *et al.* Prevalence and causes of blindness and low vision in Timor-Leste. *Br J Ophthalmol* 2007; 91:1117–1121.

36. Limburg H, Kumar R. Follow-up study of blindness attributed to cataract in Karnataka State, India. *Ophthalmic Epidemiol* 1998; 5: 211–223.

37. Zainal M, Ismail SM, Ropilah AR, *et al.* Prevalence of blindness and low vision in Malaysian population: results from the National Eye Survey 1996. *Br J Ophthalmol* 2002; 86:951–956.

38. Haider S, Hussain A, Limburg H. Cataract blindness in Chakwal District, Pakistan: results of a survey. *Ophthalmic Epidemiol* 2003; 10:249–258.

39. Shaikh SP, Aziz TM. Rapid assessment of cataract surgical services in age group 50 years and above in Lower Dir District, Malakand, Pakistan. *J Coll Physicians Surg Pak* 2005; 15:145–148.

40. Edussuriya K, Sennanayake S, Senaratne T, *et al.* The prevalence and causes of visual impairment in central Sri Lanka. The Kandy Eye study. *Ophthalmology* 2009; 116:52–56.

41. Eusebio C, Kuper H, Polack S, *et al.* Rapid assessment of avoidable blindness in Negros Island and Antique District, Philippines. *Br J Ophthalmol* 2007; 91:1588–1592.

42. Limburg H, Vasavada AR, Muzumdar G, *et al.* Rapid assessment of cataract blindness in an urban district of Gujarat. *Indian J Ophthalmol* 1999; 47:135–141.

43. Casson RJ, Newland HS, Muecke J, *et al.* Prevalence and causes of visual impairment in rural Myanmar: the Meiktila Eye Study. *Ophthalmology* 2007; 114:2302–2308.

44. Duerksen R, Limburg H, Carron JE, *et al.* Cataract blindness in Paraguay — results of a national survey. *Ophthalmic Epidemiol* 2003; 10:349–357.

45. Beltranena F, Casasola K, Silva JC, *et al.* Cataract blindness in four regions of Guatemala: results of a population-based survey. *Ophthalmology* 2007; 114:1558–1563.

46. Oliveira DF, Lira RP, Lupinacci AP, *et al.* Cataract surgery complications as a cause of visual impairment in a population aged 50 and over. *Cad Saude Publica* 2008; 24:2440–2444.

47. Nano ME, Nano HD, Mugica JM, *et al.* Rapid assessment of visual impairment due to cataract and cataract surgical services in urban Argentina. *Ophthalmic Epidemiol* 2006; 13:191–197.

48. Mangione CM, Phillips RS, Lawrence MG, *et al.* Improved visual function and attenuation of declines in health-related quality of life after cataract extraction. *Arch Ophthalmol* 1994; 112: 1419–1425.

49. Cassard SD, Patrick DL, Damiano AM, *et al.* Reproducibility and responsiveness of the VF-14. An index of functional impairment in patients with cataracts. *Arch Ophthalmol* 1995; 113:1508–1513.

50. O'Day DM. Management of cataract in adults. Quick reference guide for clinicians. The Cataract Management Guideline Panel of the Agency for Health Care Policy and Research. *Arch Ophthalmol* 1993; 111:453–459.

51. Nirmalan PK, Tielsch JM, Katz J, *et al.* Relationship between vision impairment and eye disease to vision-specific quality of life and function in rural India: the Aravind Comprehensive Eye Survey. *Invest Ophthalmol Vis Sci* 2005; 46:2308–2312.

52. Polack S, Kuper H, Eusebio C, *et al.* The impact of cataract on time-use: results from a population based case-control study in Kenya, the Philippines and Bangladesh. *Ophthalmic Epidemiol* 2008; 15:372–382.

53. Desai P, Reidy A, Minassian DC, *et al.* Gains from cataract surgery: visual function and quality of life. *Br J Ophthalmol* 1996; 80:868–873.

54. Mangione CM, Phillips RS, Seddon JM, *et al*. Development of the 'Activities of Daily Vision Scale'. A measure of visual functional status. *Med Care* 1992; 30:1111–1126.

55. Owsley C, McGwin G, Jr., Sloane M, *et al*. Impact of cataract surgery on motor vehicle crash involvement by older adults. *JAMA* 2002; 288:841–849.

56. Christen WG, Manson JE, Seddon JM, *et al*. A prospective study of cigarette smoking and risk of cataract in men. *JAMA* 1992; 268:989–993.

57. DeBlack SS. Cigarette smoking as a risk factor for cataract and age-related macular degeneration: a review of the literature. *Optometry* 2003; 74:99–110.

58. Flaye DE, Sullivan KN, Cullinan TR, *et al*. Cataracts and cigarette smoking. The City Eye Study. *Eye* 1989; 3(Pt 4):379–384.

59. West S, Munoz B, Emmett EA, *et al*. Cigarette smoking and risk of nuclear cataracts. *Arch Ophthalmol* 1989; 107:1166–1169.

60. West S, Munoz B, Schein OD, *et al*. Cigarette smoking and risk for progression of nuclear opacities. *Arch Ophthalmol* 1995; 113:1377–1380.

61. Christen WG, Glynn RJ, Ajani UA, *et al*. Smoking cessation and risk of age-related cataract in men. *JAMA* 2000; 284:713–716.

62. Hankinson SE, Willett WC, Colditz GA, *et al*. A prospective study of cigarette smoking and risk of cataract surgery in women. *JAMA* 1992; 268:994–998.

63. Hiller R, Sperduto RD, Podgor MJ, *et al*. Cigarette smoking and the risk of development of lens opacities. The Framingham studies. *Arch Ophthalmol* 1997; 115:1113–1118.

64. Klein AP, Duggal P, Lee KE, *et al*. Polygenic effects and cigarette smoking account for a portion of the familial aggregation of nuclear sclerosis. *Am J Epidemiol* 2005; 161:707–713.

65. Varma SD. Aldose reductase and the aetiology of diabetic cataracts. *Curr Top Eye Res* 1980; 3:91–155.

66. Biswas S, Harris F, Dennison S, *et al*. Calpains: enzymes of vision? *Med Sci Monit* 2005; 11:RA301–RA310.

67. Harris F, Biswas S, Singh J, *et al*. Calpains and their multiple roles in diabetes mellitus. *Ann N Y Acad Sci* 2006; 1084:452–480.

68. Biswas S, Harris F, Singh J, *et al*. Role of calpains in diabetes mellitus-induced cataractogenesis: a mini review. *Mol Cell Biochem* 2004; 261: 151–159.

69. Hennis A, Wu SY, Nemesure B, *et al*. Risk factors for incident cortical and posterior subcapsular lens opacities in the Barbados Eye Studies. *Arch Ophthalmol* 2004; 122:525–530.

70. Klein BE, Klein R, Lee KE. Diabetes, cardiovascular disease, selected cardiovascular disease risk factors, and the 5-year incidence of age-related cataract and progression of lens opacities: the Beaver Dam Eye Study. *Am J Ophthalmol* 1998; 126:782–790.

71. Saxena S, Mitchell P, Rochtchina E. Five-year incidence of cataract in older persons with diabetes and pre-diabetes. *Ophthalmic Epidemiol* 2004; 11:271–277.

72. Klein BE, Klein R, Moss SE. Prevalence of cataracts in a population-based study of persons with diabetes mellitus. *Ophthalmology* 1985; 92:1191–1196.

73. Miglior S, Bergamini F, Migliavacca L, *et al*. Metabolic and social risk factors in a cataractous population. A case-control study. *Dev Ophthalmol* 1989; 17:158–164.

74. Cundiff DK, Nigg CR. Diet and diabetic retinopathy: insights from the Diabetes Control and Complications Trial (DCCT). *Med Gen Med* 2005; 7:3.

75. Ederer F, Hiller R, Taylor HR. Senile lens changes and diabetes in two population studies. *Am J Ophthalmol* 1981; 91:381–395.

76. Leske MC, Wu SY, Hennis A, *et al*. Diabetes, hypertension, and central obesity as cataract risk factors in a black population. The Barbados Eye Study. *Ophthalmology* 1999; 106:35–41.

77. Tavani A, Negri E, La VC. Selected diseases and risk of cataract in women. A case-control study from northern Italy. *Ann Epidemiol* 1995; 5:234–238.

78. Pitts DG, Cullen AP, Hacker PD. Ocular effects of ultraviolet radiation from 295 to 365 nm. *Invest Ophthalmol Vis Sci* 1977; 16:932–939.

79. Pitts DG, Cameron LL, Jose JG, *et al*. Optical radiation and cataracts, In: Waxler M, Hitchens V, eds. *Optical Radiation and Visual Health*, CRC Press; 1986:13–41.

80. Fris M, Cejkova J, Midelfart A. The effect of single and repeated UVB radiation on rabbit lens. *Graefes Arch Clin Exp Ophthalmol* 2008; 246:551–558.

81. Brilliant LB, Grasset NC, Pokhrel RP, *et al.* Associations among cataract prevalence, sunlight hours, and altitude in the Himalayas. *Am J Epidemiol* 1983; 118:250–264.

82. Hollows F, Moran D. Cataract – the ultraviolet risk factor. *Lancet* 1981; 2:1249–1250.

83. Duncan DD, Schneider W, West KJ, *et al.* The development of personal dosimeters for use in the visible and ultraviolet wavelengths regions. The Salisbury Eye Evaluation Team. *Photochem Photobiol* 1995; 62:94–100.

84. Duncan DD, Munoz B, Bandeen-Roche K, *et al.* Visible and ultraviolet-B ocular-ambient exposure ratios for a general population. Salisbury Eye Evaluation Project Team. *Invest Ophthalmol Vis Sci* 1997; 38:1003–1011.

85. Duncan DD, Munoz B, Bandeen-Roche K, *et al.* Assessment of ocular exposure to ultraviolet-B for population studies. The Salisbury Eye Evaluation Project Team. *Photochem Photobiol* 1997; 66: 701–709.

86. Taylor HR, West SK, Rosenthal FS, *et al.* Effect of ultraviolet radiation on cataract formation. *N Engl J Med* 1988; 319:1429–1433.

87. West SK, Longstreth JD, Munoz BE, *et al.* Model of risk of cortical cataract in the US population with exposure to increased ultraviolet radiation due to stratospheric ozone depletion. *Am J Epidemiol* 2005; 162:1080–1088.

88. SunWise Program: Region 1: EPA New England. U.S. Environmental Protection Agency. 12–30–2008. 9–1–2009.

89. SunSmart Victoria. 4–24–2009. 9–1–2009.

90. Sun Safety. 7–3–2008. Health Canada.

91. Rohrschneider W. Studies on the formation and morphology of Rontgen-radiation cataract in humans. *Arch F Augen* 1932; 106:221–254.

92. Otake M, Schull WJ. The relationship of gamma and neutron radiation to posterior lenticular opacities among atomic bomb survivors in Hiroshima and Nagasaki. *Radiat Res* 1982; 92:574–595.

93. Nefzger MD, Miller RJ, Fujino T. Eye findings in atomic bomb survivors of Hiroshima and Nagasaki: 1963–1964. *Am J Epidemiol* 1969; 89:129–138.

94. Limitations of exposure to ionizing radiation. National Council on Radiation Protection and Measurements. 116. 1–1–1993. Bethesda, MD.

95. 1990 Recommendations of the International Commission on Radiological Protection. *Ann ICRP* 1991; 21:1–201.

96. Nakashima E, Neriishi K, Minamoto A. A reanalysis of atomic-bomb cataract data, 2000–2002: a threshold analysis. *Health Phys* 2006; 90:154–160.

97. Worgul BV, Kundiyev YI, Sergiyenko NM, *et al.* Cataracts among Chernobyl clean-up workers: implications regarding permissible eye exposures. *Radiat Res* 2007; 167:233–243.

98. Chodick G, Bekiroglu N, Hauptmann M, *et al.* Risk of cataract after exposure to low doses of ionizing radiation: a 20-year prospective cohort study among US radiologic technologists. *Am J Epidemiol* 2008; 168:620–631.

99. Shui YB, Fu JJ, Garcia C, *et al.* Oxygen distribution in the rabbit eye and oxygen consumption by the lens. *Invest Ophthalmol Vis Sci* 2006; 47:1571–1580.

100. Holekamp NM, Shui YB, Beebe DC. Vitrectomy surgery increases oxygen exposure to the lens: a possible mechanism for nuclear cataract formation. *Am J Ophthalmol* 2005; 139:302–310.

101. Harocopos GJ, Shui YB, McKinnon M, *et al.* Importance of vitreous liquefaction in age-related cataract. *Invest Ophthalmol Vis Sci* 2004; 45:77–85.

102. Kubo E, Kumamoto Y, Tsuzuki S, *et al.* Axial length, myopia, and the severity of lens opacity at the time of cataract surgery. *Arch Ophthalmol* 2006; 124:1586–1590.

103. Younan C, Mitchell P, Cumming RG, *et al.* Myopia and incident cataract and cataract surgery: the Blue Mountains Eye Study. *Invest Ophthalmol Vis Sci* 2002; 43:3625–3632.

104. Chang MA, Congdon NG, Bykhovskaya I, *et al.* The association between myopia and various subtypes of lens opacity: SEE (Salisbury Eye Evaluation) project. *Ophthalmology* 2005; 112: 1395–1401.

105. Lim R, Mitchell P, Cumming RG. Refractive associations with cataract: the Blue Mountains Eye Study. *Invest Ophthalmol Vis Sci* 1999; 40:3021–3026.

106. Wu SY, Leske MC. Antioxidants and cataract formation: a summary review. *Int Ophthalmol Clin* 2000; 40:71–81.

107. A randomized, placebo-controlled, clinical trial of high-dose supplementation with vitamins C and E and beta carotene for age-related cataract and vision loss: AREDS Report No. 9. *Arch Ophthalmol* 2001; 119:1439–1452.

108. Gritz DC, Srinivasan M, Smith SD, *et al.* The Antioxidants in Prevention of Cataracts Study: effects of antioxidant supplements on cataract progression in South India. *Br J Ophthalmol* 2006; 90:847–851.

109. McNeil JJ, Robman L, Tikellis G, *et al.* Vitamin E supplementation and cataract: randomized controlled trial. *Ophthalmology* 2004; 111:75–84.

110. Maraini G, Sperduto RD, Ferris F, *et al.* A randomized, double-masked, placebo-controlled clinical trial of multivitamin supplementation for age-related lens opacities. Clinical trial of nutritional supplements and age-related cataract report no. 3. *Ophthalmology* 2008; 115:599–607.

111. Cumming RG, Mitchell P. Inhaled corticosteroids and cataract: prevalence, prevention and management. *Drug Saf* 1999; 20:77–84.

112. Jick SS, Vasilakis-Scaramozza C, Maier WC. The risk of cataract among users of inhaled steroids. *Epidemiology* 2001; 12:229–234.

113. Smeeth L, Boulis M, Hubbard R, *et al.* A population based case-control study of cataract and inhaled corticosteroids. *Br J Ophthalmol* 2003; 87:1247–1251.

114. Wang JJ, Rochtchina E, Tan AG, *et al.* Use of inhaled and oral corticosteroids and the long-term risk of cataract. *Ophthalmology* 2009; 116: 652–657.

115. Gracy RW, Yuksel KU, Jacobson TM, *et al.* Cellular models and tissue equivalent systems for evaluating the structures and significance of age-modified proteins. *Gerontology* 1991; 37:113–127.

116. Limburg H, Foster A, Vaidyanathan K, *et al.* Monitoring visual outcome of cataract surgery in India. *Bull World Health Organ* 1999; 77: 455–460.

117. Herman DC, Gordon MO, Beiser JA, *et al.* Topical ocular hypotensive medication and lens opacification: evidence from the ocular hypertension treatment study. *Am J Ophthalmol* 2006; 142: 800–810.

118. Kanthan GL, Wang JJ, Rochtchina E, *et al.* Use of antihypertensive medications and topical beta-blockers and the long-term incidence of cataract and cataract surgery. *Br J Ophthalmol* 2009; 93:1210–1214.

119. Cheng CY, Liu JH, Chen SJ, *et al.* Population-based study on prevalence and risk factors of age-related cataracts in Peitou, Taiwan. *Zhonghua Yi Xue Za Zhi* (Taipei) 2000; 63:641–648.

120. Klein BE, Klein R, Linton KL. Prevalence of age-related lens opacities in a population. The Beaver Dam Eye Study. *Ophthalmology* 1992; 99:546–552.

121. Leske MC, Wu SY, Nemesure B, *et al.* Incidence and progression of lens opacities in the Barbados Eye Studies. *Ophthalmology* 2000; 107:1267–1273.

122. McCarty CA, Mukesh BN, Fu CL, *et al.* The epidemiology of cataract in Australia. *Am J Ophthalmol* 1999; 128:446–465.

123. Mitchell P, Cumming RG, Attebo K, *et al.* Prevalence of cataract in Australia: the Blue Mountains eye study. *Ophthalmology* 1997; 104:581–588.

124. Sperduto RD, Hiller R. The prevalence of nuclear, cortical, and posterior subcapsular lens opacities in a general population sample. *Ophthalmology* 1984; 91:815–818.

125. Freeman EE, Munoz B, Schein OD, *et al.* Hormone replacement therapy and lens opacities: the Salisbury Eye Evaluation project. *Arch Ophthalmol* 2001; 119:1687–1692.

126. Klein BE, Klein R, Ritter LL. Is there evidence of an estrogen effect on age-related lens opacities? The Beaver Dam Eye Study. *Arch Ophthalmol* 1994; 112:85–91.

127. Freeman EE, Munoz B, Schein OD, *et al.* Incidence and progression of lens opacities: effect of hormone replacement therapy and reproductive factors. *Epidemiology* 2004; 15:451–457.

128. Klein BE, Klein R, Lee KE. Reproductive exposures, incident age-related cataracts, and age-related maculopathy in women: the Beaver Dam Eye Study. *Am J Ophthalmol* 2000; 130:322–326.

129. Klein BE, Klein R, Lee KE, *et al.* Statin use and incident nuclear cataract. *JAMA* 2006; 295: 2752–2758.

130. Tan JS, Mitchell P, Rochtchina E, *et al.* Statin use and the long-term risk of incident cataract: the Blue Mountains Eye Study. *Am J Ophthalmol* 2007; 143:687–689.

131. Leske MC. Nuclear cataract: do statins reduce risk? *Arch Ophthalmol* 2007; 125:401–402.

132. Hammond CJ, Snieder H, Spector TD, *et al.* Genetic and environmental factors in age-related nuclear cataracts in monozygotic and dizygotic twins. *N Engl J Med* 2000; 342:1786–1790.

133. Congdon N, Broman KW, Lai H, *et al.* Nuclear cataract shows significant familial aggregation in an older population after adjustment for possible shared environmental factors. *Invest Ophthalmol Vis Sci* 2004; 45:2182–2186.

134. Hammond CJ, Duncan DD, Snieder H, *et al.* The heritability of age-related cortical cataract: the twin eye study. *Invest Ophthalmol Vis Sci* 2001; 42:601–605.

135. Congdon N, Broman KW, Lai H, *et al.* Cortical, but not posterior subcapsular, cataract shows significant familial aggregation in an older population after adjustment for possible shared environmental factors. *Ophthalmology* 2005; 112:73–77.

136. Sun H, Ma Z, Li Y, *et al.* Gamma-S crystallin gene (CRYGS) mutation causes dominant progressive cortical cataract in humans. *J Med Genet* 2005; 42:706–710.

137. Iyengar SK, Klein BE, Klein R, *et al.* Identification of a major locus for age-related cortical cataract on chromosome 6p12-q12 in the Beaver Dam Eye Study. *Proc Natl Acad Sci USA* 2004; 101:14485–14490.

138. West SK, Munoz B, Istre J, *et al.* Mixed lens opacities and subsequent mortality. *Arch Ophthalmol* 2000; 118:393–397.

139. Hennis A, Wu SY, Li X, *et al.* Lens opacities and mortality: the Barbados Eye Studies. *Ophthalmology* 2001; 108:498–504.

140. Cugati S, Cumming RG, Smith W, *et al.* Visual impairment, age-related macular degeneration, cataract, and long-term mortality: the Blue Mountains Eye Study. *Arch Ophthalmol* 2007; 125:917–924.

141. Reidy A, Minassian DC, Desai P, *et al.* Increased mortality in women with cataract: a population based follow up of the North London Eye Study. *Br J Ophthalmol* 2002; 86:424–428.

142. Clemons TE, Kurinij N, Sperduto RD. Associations of mortality with ocular disorders and an intervention of high-dose antioxidants and zinc in the Age-Related Eye Disease Study: AREDS Report No. 13. *Arch Ophthalmol* 2004; 122:716–726.

143. Nucci C, Cedrone C, Culasso F, *et al.* Association between lens opacities and mortality in the Priverno Eye Study. *Graefes Arch Clin Exp Ophthalmol* 2004; 242:289–294.

144. Williams SL, Ferrigno L, Mora P, *et al.* Baseline cataract type and 10-year mortality in the Italian-American Case-Control Study of age-related cataract. *Am J Epidemiol* 2002; 156:127–131.

145. Knudtson MD, Klein BE, Klein R. Age-related eye disease, visual impairment, and survival: the Beaver Dam Eye Study. *Arch Ophthalmol* 2006; 124:243–249.

146. Borger PH, van LR, Hulsman CA, *et al.* Is there a direct association between age-related eye diseases and mortality? The Rotterdam Study. *Ophthalmology* 2003; 110:1292–1296.

147. Thiagarajan M, Evans JR, Smeeth L, *et al.* Cause-specific visual impairment and mortality: results from a population-based study of older people in the United Kingdom. *Arch Ophthalmol* 2005; 123:1397–1403.

148. Xu L, Wang YX, Wang J, *et al.* Mortality and ocular diseases: the Beijing Eye Study. *Ophthalmology* 2009; 116:732–738.

11

Epidemiology of refractive errors and presbyopia

LESLIE HYMAN AND ILESH PATEL[a]

11.1	Introduction	197		11.9	Associated factors	209
11.2	Public health significance	198		11.10	Preventive and/or control strategies; controlled trials	214
11.3	Classification/Grading systems	198				
11.4	Prevalence	199		11.11	Summary	214
11.5	Incidence/Progression	205		11.12	Suggestions/Priorities for future epidemiological research	214
11.6	Distribution by age, gender and ethnicity	206				
11.7	Geographical distribution (urban versus rural)	207		11.13	Presbyopia	215
					References	219
11.8	Changes in prevalence or distribution with time	208				

11.1 INTRODUCTION

Refractive errors (**ametropias**) are ocular conditions that result from an imbalance between refractive power and axial length of the eye and can be rectified by corrective lenses or refractive surgery. The most common types of refractive error, myopia, hyperopia and astigmatism, occur in an unaccommodated eye when parallel light rays are not brought into sharp focus precisely on the retina, thus producing a blurred retinal image. Presbyopia, an additional type of refractive condition in which the ability to accommodate (change the lens to focus on nearby objects) is reduced or lost, is generally associated with ageing and is considered to be physiological rather than pathological, occurring almost universally. As commonly occurring conditions, refractive errors are a cause of public health and economic concerns, with high costs associated with their correction.[1,2] Refractive errors, even at moderate levels, are associated with other ocular complications and visual impairment.[3]

Within the past 15 years, over 30 epidemiologic studies, conducted with children and adults in different populations worldwide, have provided valuable information on the prevalence of refractive errors and possible associated factors. This chapter summarizes major findings regarding: (a) public health significance; (b) prevalence and its changes over

[a] Acknowledgements: The authors gratefully acknowledge the administrative and editorial assistance of Ms Jayme Mendelsohn, BA, in preparing this chapter, and the editorial comments of Suh-Yuh Wu, MS, M Cristina Leske, MD MPH and Thomas Norton, PhD.

time; (c) associated factors and (d) control strategies. Fewer studies have addressed the epidemiology of presbyopia, which is reviewed in Section 11.13.

11.1.1   Clinical descriptions

Myopia or nearsightedness is the condition that occurs when parallel rays of light from distant objects are brought to focus in front of the retina; this error inhibits clear distance vision and is corrected by a minus lens. **Hyperopia**, farsightedness or **hypermetropia** occurs when parallel light rays from a distant object are brought to sharp focus behind the retina, leading to blurred vision which is corrected by a plus lens. **Astigmatism** is an optical defect in which corneal or lenticular refractive power is not uniform in all meridians, i.e. parallel light rays are bent unequally by different meridians, preventing a sharp point of focus on the retina. Astigmatism is classified as 'with the rule' when the refractive power of the vertical meridian is the greatest, as 'against the rule' when the refractive power of the horizontal meridian is greatest, and 'oblique' when the two principal meridians are neither horizontal nor vertical.

11.2   PUBLIC HEALTH SIGNIFICANCE

Uncorrected refractive error is a leading cause of global blindness and visual impairment. Worldwide, uncorrected refractive error has been estimated to account for 18.2% of blindness (presenting visual acuity worse than 3/60 in the better eye) and more than half of visual impairment (presenting visual acuity less than 6/18 in the better eye). It causes blindness in an estimated 5 to 8.2 million persons and visual impairment in 145 million.[4] In studies of children ranging in age from 3 to 15 years, the proportion of visual impairment due to uncorrected refractive error varies from 72.6% in Sydney, Australia[5] to 75% in Beijing, China,[6] 76.8% in Sao Paulo, Brazil,[7] and as high as 94.9% in Guangzhou, China.[8]

Uncorrected refractive errors in children may hinder school performance and lead to the development of **amblyopia**. In adults, they may reduce occupational productivity and quality of life. Although refractive errors cannot be prevented, they can be easily diagnosed and treated. Corrective lenses, in particular, are cost effective interventions to administer.

In recent studies with adults, uncorrected refractive error accounted for at least one third of presenting impairment.[9–12] A recent report estimated a 5.3% prevalence of visual impairment due to uncorrected refractive errors in the United States,[13] projecting that more than 11 million Americans could have vision improved to 20/40 or better with refractive correction.[13] This study also found that persons with correctable visual impairment were more likely to be of non-white ancestry, poor, less educated or to lack private health insurance, pointing towards healthcare access as a barrier to obtaining proper optical correction.[13] A higher prevalence of uncorrected refractive error, 15.1%, was observed in a population-based study of Mexican-Americans.[14] The extent of uncorrected refractive error across the globe is a major observation to emerge from a public health perspective, particularly because decreased visual acuity due to refractive errors can be improved for a relatively small cost. Some investigators in rural China and Tanzania have begun to explore potential barriers to spectacle use in children.[15–16] Further attention should be given to overcome these barriers and develop strategies to provide refractive correction to those affected.

11.3   CLASSIFICATION/GRADING SYSTEMS

Refractive error is measured on a continuous scale in **dioptres (D)**, a unit that measures the degree to which light converges or diverges; positive values represent the correction for the condition that occurs when rays of light converge behind the retina (**hyperopia**), zero indicates convergence on the retina (**emmetropia**) and negative values represent the correction for convergence in front of the retina (**myopia**). **Astigmatism** requires the use of a toric lens, which consists of a spherical and cylindrical lens, to customize corrections for the major meridians. These measurements are frequently summarized by **dioptric spherical** equivalent (SE) values, the average power of a corrective lens, defined as the sum of the spherical power plus half the cylindrical power.

Definitions for each refractive condition are based on specified dioptric cut-off values. Although positive refractive error measurements are considered hyperopic and negative measurements as myopic, standard criteria for classification as mild, moderate and severe levels of myopia or hyperopia have not been established. Cut-off points for mild myopia can vary from −0.50 D down to −1.00 D and for high myopia from −5.0 D to −6.0 D, limiting comparisons across studies. Another complicating factor is whether or not refractive measures are made after accommodation is blocked with a cycloplegic agent, particularly for hyperopic eyes that may appear emmetropic unless accommodation is paralyzed. A study conducted on 1,334 Chinese schoolchildren in Singapore, seven to nine years of age, attempted to define myopia by determining a refractive error value that corresponds to a level of uncorrected logMAR VA of >0.3, a common criterion for a driver's license in the USA.[17] This sensitivity analysis suggested cut-off points of −0.50 D or −0.75 D for myopia; such approaches provide practical guidelines for classification and should be explored further. Astigmatism is most commonly measured in dioptric units by manifest refraction as total or refractive astigmatism, but can also be evaluated by keratometry to measure corneal or internal (i.e. lenticular) astigmatism.

Refractive error has been measured in different studies by objective and subjective methods, with and without cycloplegia. Cycloplegia is important in studies of refractive error in children, as noncycloplegic autorefraction measurements may overestimate myopia and underestimate hyperopia,[18] but may not be necessary in adults,[19] perhaps because accommodative ability lessens with age.

11.4   PREVALENCE

11.4.1   Overview

The refractive state of the eye changes throughout life, beginning at birth. Infants tend to have hyperopic eyes that may shift towards emmetropia during the first years of life. During school age years, in some children, refractive status may shift towards myopia. This shift is followed by a period of rapid myopization (school age or juvenile onset myopia) that tends to plateau in mid to late teenage years;[20] additional and more modest progression may occur during early adulthood before fully stabilizing. The refractive state in mid-life tends to shift if an underlying hyperopia becomes manifest as the range of accommodation decreases; and in older adults it can change again towards myopia, possibly due to change in lenticular refraction. Because of these variations at different stages of life, information in this chapter is presented by age category and type of refractive error. Except for pre-school age children, comparisons across studies for school age children and adults in different populations are limited by differences in definitions, data collection methods and age ranges studied.

11.4.2   Pre-school age children

Three population-based studies conducted on different ethnic groups have provided cross-sectional data on refractive error in pre-school age children from six to 72 months, using similar methods.[21–23] The availability of these data permits the first comparisons to be made across populations at these young ages when refractive development is occurring. The prevalence of myopia and hyperopia varies by study and ethnicity (Table 11.1). Myopia was most prevalent in African-Americans in Baltimore and Los Angeles and in the Chinese children in Singapore; prevalence was lowest in Hispanics in Los Angeles and in Baltimore whites. In contrast, hyperopia was most frequent in Baltimore whites and Hispanic children in Los Angeles and lowest in Singapore. These cross-sectional data suggest that children with myopia have a general shift towards emmetropia from infancy to six years of age. Hyperopia prevalence decreased after 6 to 11 months of age in Baltimore whites, Los Angeles Hispanics and Chinese Singaporeans but remained fairly constant in each subsequent age group. In African-Americans, the pattern was less consistent. Similar rates of myopia and hyperopia in males and females were reported in Singapore.

Table 11.1 Prevalence of myopia* and hyperopia** in pre-school age children in Baltimore, Maryland,[21] Los Angeles, California[22] and Singapore by ethnicity[23]

Age (Months)	Baltimore					Los Angeles					Singapore		
		Myopia		Hyperopia			Myopia		Hyperopia			Myopia	Hyperopia
	n = (AA, W)	AA %	White %	AA %	White %	n = (AA, Hisp)	AA %	Hisp %	AA %	Hisp %	n = Chinese	Chinese %	Chinese %
6–11	(83,84)	9.6	0.0	4.8	23.8	(277,296)	13.7	6.4	7.6	15.9	165	4.8	3.0
12–23	(181,175)	7.5	2.3	7.4	12.1	(549,543)	9.1	7.2	6.9	10.1	450	6.4	1.6
24–35	(248,189)	10.5	1.1	6.3	13.0	(545,572)	6.4	4.0	7.7	9.8	441	10.2	0.91
36–47	(240,210)	5.9	0.0	6.3	9.6	(532,532)	5.5	1.5	10.5	14.1	513	4.7	0.39
48–59	(261,201)	6.2	1.5	8.5	14.0	(548,543)	4.2	1.8	11.1	12.2	540	3.9	2.6
60–72	(245,171)	6.6	1.2	7.8	12.9	(543,544)	4.1	2.4	8.1	11.8	530	2.5	0.94
TOTAL	(1268,1030)	7.4	1.1	6.9	13.2	(2994,3030)	6.6	3.7	8.8	12.0	2,639	5.3	1.4

* myopia defined as ≤ –1 D.
** hyperopia defined as ≥ +3 D.
AA = African American.
Hisp = Hispanic.

The studies found lower rates of myopia among pre-school age children than in older children and adults, with variability across ethnic groups. These findings are consistent with previously observed patterns of early emmetropization in young pre-school age children prior to reaching the age when myopia onset is likely to occur. The continued presence of hyperopia in the Baltimore and Los Angeles populations may suggest a different pattern for young children with this refractive error type.

11.4.3   School age children/adolescents

11.4.3.1   *Myopia*

Myopia is the most common type of refractive error, affecting up to an estimated 33% of adults in the USA who are 20 years and older,[24] and its prevalence appears to be increasing in younger birth cohorts.[25–26] Over the past 30 years, myopia prevalence is estimated to have increased by 66% in the USA.[27–28] In Asian populations, prevalence is even higher, with rates as high as 40% by age nine years in Chinese children in Singapore.[29] Concerns about the increasing rates have led to recent studies in children that include various school based samples[29–33] and a series of cluster-based samples in different countries as part of the Refractive Error Study in Children (RESC), which used a standard protocol.[8,27,34–39] Some, but not all, studies have also investigated hyperopia and astigmatism. Table 11.2 provides prevalence data based on cycloplegic autorefraction for studies that defined myopia as SE ≤ −0.5 D, hyperopia as SE ≥2.0 D and astigmatism as cylinder ≥0.75 D in either eye. Although comparisons are limited by differences in definitions, data collection methods and age ranges, myopia prevalence is consistently highest in East Asian children from Singapore,[29] Hong Kong,[30] Malaysia[35] and China[8,40] and lowest in children in India,[34] Australia[32,41] and rural Mongolia.[42] In Singapore, myopia prevalence in 7–9-year-old children was 36.3%, which is over three-fold the prevalence in Australian children 11–15 years old.[29]

11.4.3.2   *Hyperopia*

For comparative purposes, Table 11.2 includes studies defining hyperopia as spherical equivalent ≥2.0 D, a more clinically meaningful cut-off. Based on this definition, hyperopia prevalence was generally found in all studies to be low in children, with some variability across populations.[8,29–32,34–35,37–40,43]

11.4.3.3   *Astigmatism*

Astigmatism appears to be more prevalent in infants and young children than in adults, but this observation is based on samples that are not population-based. The presence of against the rule astigmatism in infants has been associated with the development and progression of school age myopia in a non-population-based cohort.[44] However, epidemiologic data on astigmatism in children are limited. Using a definition of astigmatism as cylinder ≥0.75 D in either eye, prevalence varied widely, ranging from over 40% in Singapore[29] and Guangzhou, China[8] to a low of 9.5% and 9.8% in Shunyi District, China[39] and Andhra Pradesh, India.[34]

11.4.4   Young adults (myopia)

Although the majority of myopia develops in school age children usually between eight to 14 years old[45] and stabilizes in teenage years, studies conducted in selected populations of university students or occupational groups[46] indicate that myopia may also begin at later ages, contributing to the overall prevalence in adults. The National Research Council Committee on Vision and Working Group on Myopia Prevalence and Progression reviewed over 500 articles, mostly published between 1950 and 1986; it concluded that myopia can start and increase after age 16, although it is less severe than myopia that develops in school age children, and seems limited to a smaller proportion of myopes. The report also estimated that up to 40% of low hyperopes and emmetropes entering colleges, military academies or performing occupations requiring extensive near-work are likely to become myopic before age 25.[20] Since the available studies have used different criteria, it is unclear whether the

Table 11.2 *Refractive error in school age children in different populations*

Author, year of publication	Country/ Subgroup	Age range (Years)	Year of study	Sample size	Prevalence (%) Myopia SE ≤ −0.5 D	Hyperopia SE ≥ 2.0 D	Astigmatism (Cyl ≥ 0.75 D in either eye)
Fan, 2004[30]	Hong Kong	5–16	1998–2000	7,560	36.7	4.0	
Saw, 2006[29]	Singapore	7–9	1999–2001	1,962	36.3	1.7	42.6
	Malay			1,245	22.1	3.4	44.3
	Chinese			285	40.1	1.2	42.5
	Indian			152	34.1	2.4	41.3
	Malaysia	7–9	2003	1,752	13.4	2.9	22.2
	Malay			348	9.2	2.9	18.7
	Chinese			1,467	30.9	1.8	34
	Indian			126	12.5	3.9	22.4
Goh, 2005[35]	Malaysia	7–15	2003	4,634	20.7	1.6	
	Malay			3,257	15.4	1.5	
	Chinese			764	46.4	1.1	
	Indian			412	16.2	2.0	
Zhao, 2000[39]	China (Shunyi District)	5–15	1988–1998	5,884	21.6	2.7	9.5
He, 2004[8]	Urban China (Guangzhou)	5–15	2002–2003	4,364	38.1	4.6	42.8
He, 2007[40]	China (Yangxi)	12–18	2005	2,454	42.4	1.2	25.3
	Urban				50	1.51	26.6
	Rural				33	0.82	23.6
Congdon, 2008[31]	Rural China (Xichang)	11–17	2007	1,892	62.3*	0.2	1.7+
Naidoo, 2003[38]	Durban, South Africa	5–15	2002	4,890	4.0	2.6	14.6
Murthy, 2002[37]	Urban India (New Delhi)	5–15	2000–2001	6,447	7.4	7.4	14.6
Dandona, 2002[34]	Rural India (Andhra Pradesh)	7–15	2000–2001	4,074	5.6	0.68	9.8
Ojaimi, 2005[32] Ip, 2008[78] Ip, 2008[41] Huynh, 2007[43]	Australia		2003–2005				
	Younger	5–8		1,724	1.43	13.2	
	Older	11–15		2,340	11.9	5.0	13.6
Kleinstein, 2003[33]	US	5–17	1997–1998	2,523	10.5		
	African-American			534	8.6		
	Asian			491	19.8		
	Hispanic			463	14.5		
	White			1,035	5.2		

➢ myopia defined as <−0.5 D in both eyes.
➢ +astigmatism defined as >+0.75 D in both eyes.

factors influencing onset in young adults differ from those for school age myopia.

11.4.5 Older adults (myopia/ hyperopia/astigmatism)

This section focuses on population-based studies among adults ages 40 years and older[10,12,47–65] which provided information on prevalence, changes and risk factors for refractive errors. Estimates from the Eye Diseases Prevalence Research Group,[66] which applied standard definitions and pooled data from six studies, indicate a USA prevalence among adults of 25% for myopia, defined as ≤−1.0 D SE and 10% for hyperopia, defined as ≥3.0 D SE,[66] a clinically meaningful level. Table 11.3 presents prevalence from studies

Table 11.3 *Refractive error in adults in different populations*

Author, year of publication	Ethnicity/Location/Study name	Age range (years)	Year of study	Sample size	Myopia		High myopia ≤-5.0D	Hyperopia		Astigmatism	
					<-0.5 D	≤-1.0D	≤-5.0D	>+0.5 D	≥+3.0 D	<-0.5 D	≤-1.0 D
ASIAN											
Wong, 2000[52]	Singapore/Tanjong Pagar Eye Study	40–79	1997–1998	1232	35.0	28.0[a]		35.9		43.9	
Saw, 2008[69]	Singapore/Singapore Malay Eye Study	40–80	2004–2006	2974	24.6	18.0[a]	3.5[c]	35.3		39.4	
Xu, 2005[80]	China/Beijing Eye Study	40–90	2001	4319	22.9	16.9[a]					
He, 2009[71]	China/Liwan Eye Study	≥50	2003–2004	1269	32.3		5.0[c]	40.0			
Liang, 2009[183]	China/Handan Eye Study	≥30	2006–2007	6491	26.7	13.5[a]	1.8	15.9		24.5	
		≥40	2006–2007	5300	18.8	9.5[a]	1.5	23.1			
		≥50	2006–2007	4005	18.2	11.9[a]	2.6	35.6			
Cheng, 2003[57]	Taiwan/Shihpai Eye Study	≥65	1999–2000	1361	18.3	13.6[a]		60.1		73.4	43.1[b]
Sawada, 2008[68]	Japan/Tajimi Eye Study	≥40	2000–2001	3021	41.8	32.4[a]	8.2[c]	27.9		54.0	26.4[b]
Gupta, 2008[67]	Myanmar/Meiktila Eye Study	≥40	2005	1863	51.0	42.7[a]					30.6[b]
Bourne, 2004[58]	Bangladesh/National Blindness and Low Vision Survey of Bangladesh	≥30	1999–2000	11,189	22.1[d]	12.5	1.8	20.6		32.4[e]	
Shah, 2008[70]	Pakistan/National Blindness and Visual Impairment Survey	≥30	2002–2003	14,490	36.5		4.6	27.1	1.7[f]	27.1[g]	
Dandona, 1999[59]	India/Andhra Pradesh Eye Study	≥15	1996–1997	2321	19.4	15.20		9.83		12.9	9.8
Raju, 2004[47]	India/Tamil Nadu Eye Study	≥40	2001–2003	2508	27.0		3.7[c]			54.8	

(Continued)

Table 11.3 (Continued)

Author, year of publication	Ethnicity/Location/Study name	Age range (years)	Year of study	Sample size	Myopia <-0.5 D	Myopia ≤-1.0D	High myopia ≤-5.0D	Hyperopia >+0.5 D	Hyperopia ≥+3.0 D	Astigmatism <-0.5 D ≤ -1.0 D
AFRICAN										
Wu, 1999[53]	West Indies/Barbados Eye Study	40–84	1987–1992	4709	21.9	15.8[a]		46.9		
EUROPEAN										
Attebo, 1999[12]	Australia/Blue Mountains Eye Study	49–97	1992–1994	3654	14.4	12.6	1.8	57.0	7.7	
Wensor, 1999[51]	Australia/M-VIP[h]	≥40	1992–1994	4744	17	15.8	2.5	37.0	6.4	
Hofman, 1991[62]	The Netherlands/Rotterdam Eye Study	≥55	1991–1995			17.59	3.96		17.6	
Wang, 1994[50]	USA/Beaver Dam Eye Study	43–84	1988–1990	4533		26.5	3.8		11.5	
LATINO										
Munoz, 2002[10]	Arizona, USA/P-VER	≥40	1997–1999			18.0	2.5		7.2	
Tarczy-Hornoch, 2006[49]	California, USA/LALES	≥40	1999–2003	5927		16.8	2.4			
US NATIONAL SAMPLE										
Vitale, 2008[24]	USA/NHANES[i]	≥40	1999–2004	7357	41.0[g]	31.0	6.0		5.3	31.0
	Non-hispanic black				36.5[g]	26.4	4.3		3.5	32.3
	Non-hispanic white				42.6[g]	33.0	6.4		5.4	31.1
	Mexican-American				36.4[g]	23.8	3.3		4.2	30.5

[a]Myopia defined as <-1.0 D; [b]Astigmatism defined as <-1.0 D; [c]High myopia defined as <-5.0 D; [d]Myopia defined as ≤-0.5 D; [e]Astigmatism >0.5 D; [f]Hyperopia >+5.0 D; [g]Astigmatism <-0.75 D; [h]Melbourne Visual Impairment Project; [i]National Health And Nutrition Examination Study.

with common definitions for myopia and high myopia, hyperopia and astigmatism. For purposes of discussion, and to include Asian populations, the comparisons that follow will be limited to studies of adults 40 years and older that used a definition of −1.0 D SE for myopia and 0.5 D for hyperopia.

Myopia frequency varies and, as observed with children, appears to be most frequent in Asian populations. The highest prevalence rates of 42.7%, 32.4% and 28% were observed in Myanmar, a population of multiple Asian ancestries,[67] in Japan[68] and in a population of Chinese ancestry in Singapore.[52] However, a high prevalence of 26.5% was also observed in Beaver Dam, Wisconsin,[65] a population of predominantly European descent. Prevalence observed in the other studies was more consistent, ranging from 12.5% to 18%.[10,12,49,51,53,55,62,69–70] Severe myopia worse than −5 D was also most frequent in the Asian populations in Japan (8%),[68] and in Guangzhou, China(5%).[71]

Hyperopia prevalence also varies, with the highest rate of 57% observed in the Blue Mountains Eye Study[12] and the lowest rate in Japan of 27.9%, a reverse pattern to that seen for myopia. Astigmatism >−0.5 D appears to be frequent in Asian population;[52,68–69] however, few comparable studies exist, limiting conclusions.

11.5 INCIDENCE/PROGRESSION

This section summarizes available information on myopia incidence and progression in children and incidence of myopia and hyperopia in adults.

11.5.1   Children

11.5.1.1   *Myopia incidence*

Limited epidemiological data are available on myopia incidence in children. Despite methodological differences, studies have documented the high risk of myopia development in Asian populations.[30,72–73] In children in Beijing, China, aged 5–13 years at baseline, myopia incidence was 18.5% after 28.5 months,[73] and a one-year incidence of 14.4% was observed in Hong Kong among 4,973 children

aged 6–15 years.[30] In both studies incidence was higher for females than for males and increased with age up to early adolescence. A three-year cumulative myopia incidence of 42.7% was found in 569 children from seven to nine years at baseline in the **Cohort Study of Risk Factors of Myopia (SCORM)** conducted in Singapore. Unlike the other studies, incidence decreased with increasing age from seven to eight/nine years, ranging from 47.7% to 38.45 and 32.4%, respectively, suggesting that in this population, susceptibility to myopia development appears to be highest in the younger children. No statistically significant difference by sex was found, but the three-year incidence of myopia was higher in children of Chinese (49.5%) than non-Chinese (27.2%) ancestry.[72]

11.5.1.2   *Myopia progression*

Comparable data on myopia progression are available from SCORM and a cohort of 469 children with myopia who participated in the **Correction of Myopia Evaluation Trial (COMET)**, a multicentre clinical trial conducted in the USA.[74] Both studies observed faster progression in females compared with males and a consistent decrease in progression with increasing age. For each age group (six to seven years, eight years and nine years) progression was higher in children in SCORM than COMET, further documenting the relative severity of myopia in Asian populations, even at younger ages.[72,74]

11.5.2   Adults

Longitudinal refractive changes in adults have been observed in several population-base studies.[54,60–61,64–65] A shift towards hyperopia has been observed in middle-aged adults younger than 70 years old and a myopic shift in adults 70 years and older, most likely due to increasing nuclear opacity. Myopia incidence increases with increasing age; in the Barbados and the **Beaver Dam Eye Studies (BDES)**, nine and ten-year cumulative incidence was low in adults between 40–60 years (3–4%) and increased to 28.4% and 14.5% respectively in adults 70 years and older. As would be expected, hyperopia incidence decreased with increasing age in both studies; the nine- and ten-year incidence was higher in those who were 40–60 years old at baseline than those who were 70 years and older (26.3% versus 9.6% in Barbados and 25% versus 13% in Beaver Dam).[54]

11.6 DISTRIBUTION BY AGE, GENDER AND ETHNICITY

11.6.1 School age children/ adolescents

11.6.1.1 *Myopia*

Myopia prevalence in children increases substantially from seven to 17 years in East Asian populations[30,29,75,40] and to a small extent in Malaysia,[35] India[34,37] and South Africa[38] (Fig. 11.1). Patterns by sex are less consistent. Some studies found a higher myopia prevalence in girls[31,33–34,39–40] while others observed a higher prevalence in boys[35] or similar rates for both sexes.[30,35,37]

As mentioned previously, myopia prevalence is consistently higher in children from Asian populations than from South Africa, or urban and rural areas of India, a pattern observed at all ages (Fig. 11.1). The lowest myopia rates were observed in Australian children. Interestingly, although six to seven-year-old children of Chinese ancestry in the Sydney Myopia Study had over a four-fold higher prevalence of myopia than children of European Caucasian ethnicity (3% versus 0.7%),[76] their prevalence was substantially lower than children of Chinese ancestry in Singapore, who had a prevalence of 29%.[77] This observation suggests that differences in environmental or lifestyle factors between Sydney (Australia) and Singapore may have a stronger influence on myopia development than being of Chinese descent.

11.6.1.2 *Hyperopia*

From the available data on hyperopia in children it appears that its prevalence may decrease during younger school age years and then stabilize during adolescence. For example, hyperopia prevalence decreased between ages six to seven years and 9–12 years in populations in Australia,[78] Singapore and Malaysia,[29] but remained constant throughout teenage years in a rural Chinese population.[40]

The relationship between hyperopia and gender in children is unclear. In China and in Australia, hyperopia is more frequent in younger females than males, but the difference is not seen after age nine in China and at 12 years of age in Australia, while in New Delhi, hyperopia was more prevalent in females ages 11–13 years.[37] Higher prevalence is observed in children of European Caucasian ancestry[78] than of Asian descent.[29,40]

11.6.1.3 *Astigmatism*

No consistent age patterns have been observed for astigmatism. In urban China and in rural India, where astigmatism prevalence ≥0.75 D was approximately 10%, it was associated with older ages.[34,39] Prevalence increased from 21.6% to 33% at ages 13–17 years[40] in rural China, while a small decrease in prevalence was observed between ages seven to nine years in Singapore and Malaysia.[29] In contrast, prevalence was similar for six- and 12-year-old children in Sydney, Australia.[43]

Patterns of astigmatism by gender are also unclear. Studies in China[31,39–40] and India[34,37,59] observed higher astigmatism prevalence in middle school age girls than boys, using different definitions, while other studies found no differences.[8,30,43,79]

Prevalence varies among ethnic groups, with highest rates in the young Asian populations in Singapore[29] and in Guangzhou, China,[8] and lowest in Australia. In Malaysia, prevalence was higher among children of Chinese than Malay or Indian ancestry. In a study conducted among different ethnic groups for different regions in the USA, astigmatism was most frequent in the Hispanic and Asian children and lowest in African Americans.[33] Prevalence patterns also vary according to type of astigmatism, e.g. refractive or corneal.

11.6.2 Adults

A general pattern has been observed for changes in refractive error by age in men and women,

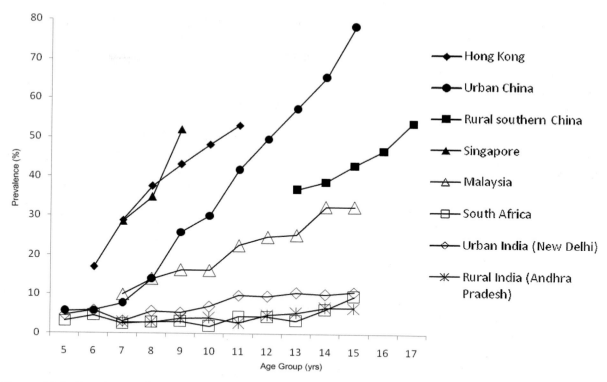

Figure 11.1 *Myopia prevalence in children aged 5–17 years*

Note: Hong Kong,[31] urban China,[9] Rural southern China,[41] Singapore,[30] Malaysia,[36] South Africa,[39] urban India (New Delhi),[38] Rural India (Andhra Pradesh).[35]

i.e. myopia prevalence decreases[12,49–53,63,66] and hyperopia increases with increasing age up to approximately 65–75+ years of age.[12,52–53,63,66] An increase in myopia prevalence at older ages also has been noted,[47,49,51–53,57–58] and is thought to be related, at least in part, to the development of lens opacities, an association that is discussed further in Section 11.9. Figure 11.2 illustrates the changes in prevalence of myopia and hyperopia by age in females for studies with similar definitions and age ranges.[52,53,63,71] This figure shows a shift towards hyperopia beginning around age 40–50 years that levels off and is eventually followed by an increase in myopia at older ages. The general consistency of this pattern across studies, and for men and women, suggests that there may be changes in the eye with time, due to ageing.

In general, myopia prevalence appears to be similar in males and females in some,[12,49–51,53,66] but not all, studies[69,80] but this pattern varies by age group. In contrast, high myopia is higher in females than males regardless of the sex distribution of moderate myopia in the same population.[52,80] Hyperopia has been consistently observed to be more prevalent in females,[12,47,53,59] with some exceptions.[24,68] Astigmatism prevalence did not differ by gender in studies in Singapore, Japan and India reporting this information,[47,68,69] while prevalence in a USA national sample, was higher for men 60 years of age and older.

11.7 GEOGRAPHICAL DISTRIBUTION (URBAN VERSUS RURAL)

As mentioned above, myopia prevalence in adults varies by country and ethnic origin, with the highest prevalence occurring in East Asian populations. Rates of myopia were frequently observed

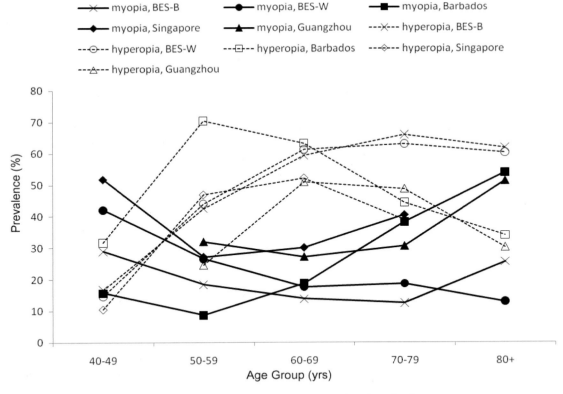

Figure 11.2 *Prevalence of myopia (<−0.5 D) and hyperopia (>0.5 D) in females by age*

Note: BES-B = Baltimore Eye Survey-Black;[63] BES-W = Baltimore Eye Survey-White;[63] Barbados = Barbados Eye Study;[54] Singapore = Tanjong Pagar district in Singapore;[52] Guangzhou = Liwan District, Guangzhou, China.[71]

to be higher in urban than in rural areas (Tables 11.2 and 11.3, Fig. 11.1) among children and adults,[8,29,30,34,38,40,52,53,59,68,71,81] lending support to the hypothesis that factors associated with urbanization may contribute to myopia development.

11.8 CHANGES IN PREVALENCE OR DISTRIBUTION WITH TIME

In Asian populations, where reported myopia prevalence in Chinese children aged 15 years and younger is over 35%,[30,31,40,82] factors such as increasing urbanization and more intensive near-work demands are believed to contribute to the high rates. The higher rates in children than in adults also suggest a true increase in prevalence over time. A study based on annual survey examinations

of school age children attending kindergarten through high school in Nara, Japan documented an increase in myopia prevalence between 1984 and 1996 for students aged seven through 17 years.[83] Similar results were observed in a series of 13 nationally-based prevalence surveys in Israeli young adults (16–22 years of age) where myopia prevalence increased by almost 40% from 20.3% in 1990 to 28.3% in 2002.[25] A comparison of **National Health and Nutrition Examination Study (HANES)** data collected in 1971–1972 and 1999–2004 documented an overall increase in myopia prevalence of 60% over the past 30 years in US adults 20 years and older;[28] this increase was observed in males and females, blacks and whites for each age group. In contrast, myopia prevalence has decreased in Danish conscripts from 1964 to 2004.[84] While an increase in myopia prevalence over time is documented in some populations, similar data on changes in hyperopia or astigmatism prevalence were not identified.

In adults, the question raised by cross-sectional data is whether the observed lower prevalence of myopia in the older ages (60 years) compared with younger ages (40 years) is due to longitudinal changes or a cohort effect. It is possible that the changes in prevalence occur as part of the ageing process. Investigators from several studies have reported their data longitudinally[54,56,60,61,64,65] and by birth cohort to attempt to address this question.[54,65] The analyses from the Beaver Dam Eye Study cohort provide the strongest evidence to date that the observed changes by age are likely to be due to both longitudinal changes and cohort effects, at least in this white population from Beaver Dam, Wisconsin.[65]

11.9 ASSOCIATED FACTORS

11.9.1 Overview

Refractive error is a continuum and changes in refraction may occur throughout life. Refractive changes result from a complex interplay of developmental, genetic, internal and external factors that influence eye growth, size and shape which also change throughout life and remain largely unknown. Furthermore, factors that influence the development of refractive error in pre-school age children may differ from those that play a role in school age children or later in life. For example, in young children who experience rapid eye growth, the level of refractive error may be more susceptible to influences by genetic or environmental factors, particularly those that may occur in the visual environment, that influence eye growth, corneal shape or lens thickness. Normal ageing, accompanied by loss of accommodation, may play a larger role in the hyperopic shift that occurs in middle ages, while mechanical factors such as the development of lens opacities may be responsible for the increase in myopia prevalence at older ages. Studies investigating genetic and environmental factors for possible associations with refractive errors in children and adults have focused on myopia as the type

of refractive error that is most frequent and more likely to be associated with other sight threatening ocular complications. In addition, although various studies have investigated factors associated with refractive error, many suffer from methodological limitations such as insufficient sample sizes, selected populations and inconsistent methods of data collection. Therefore, this section emphasizes recent studies with adequate sample size and standard protocols for data collection. While potential associated factors for each refractive error type are addressed, the emphasis is on myopia. Where relevant, school age children and adults are discussed separately.

11.9.2 Biometry

The final refractive state of the eye, e.g. dioptric power, is a function of ocular biometric components including axial length, lens thickness, lens position and corneal shape. In addition, it is determined by the refractive state of the lens. Therefore, an individual's refractive state is affected by factors that influence changes in these ocular components. Refractive state is determined primarily by axial length; an increase in axial elongation is a major source of myopia in children and adults; conversely a shorter eye is related to hyperopia. Because of the relationship between refractive state and biometric components, recent studies in children and adults have examined biometry measurements along with refraction data to better understand these interrelationships. In Singaporean Chinese children, seven to nine years old and in COMET, which included children six to 12 years old at baseline, myopia progression was highly correlated with change in axial length, driven primarily by an increase in vitreous chamber depth.[82,74] One dioptre of myopia progression was associated with 0.5 mm of axial elongation in the COMET cohort[74] over a three-year period. Three recent prevalence studies in adults, the Tanjong Pagar Survey in Singapore,[85] **Los Angeles Latino Eye Study (LALES)**,[86] and the Liwan Eye Study in China,[71] also collected biometric measurements to evaluate the hypothesis that differences in axial length may explain the variation in refractive error among adults.[86,87] Results from Tanjong Pagar and LALES suggest that axial length and vitreous chamber depth are each correlated with refractive error in all age groups and corneal power is correlated with refractive error, at least until 80 years of age. A significant, but weaker association was observed between nuclear opalescence and a myopic shift after ages 50 to 60 years. This relationship was stronger in persons 60 years and older, which may explain the levelling off of the hyperopic shift at these older ages.[86,87] The Liwan Eye Study also found that axial length was the major determinant of spherical equivalent refractive error, followed by corneal power. In this study, the relationship between refractive error and axial length differed for those with axial length ≤ 23 mm and axial length >23 mm; axial length explained 12% of the variation in SE in shorter eyes and 70% in the longer eyes, suggesting that refractive error may be more dependent on axial length in myopic than in non-myopic eyes.[71] In addition, males had longer eyes, flatter corneas, deeper anterior chambers and thinner lenses.[71]

In summary, these studies have documented that axial length is a major determinant of refractive error in large samples of children and adults, and suggest that the strength of the relationship varies in persons older and younger than 60 years old, with a stronger association in those younger than 60 years. The weaker association in older persons may result from the influence of lens changes on refractive error and the rigidity of the sclera.

11.9.3   Genetics

11.9.3.1   *Molecular genetics*

Myopia and hyperopia are complex traits that result from a combination of genetic and environmental factors, including gene–gene and gene–environment interactions (see Chapter 6). Although a genetic component to refractive error is believed to exist, and numerous investigations have attempted to identify a specific genetic link, efforts have had limited success. Understanding the genetics of refraction also requires understanding of the genetic determinants of the biometric components (e.g. axial length, corneal curvature, anterior chamber depth, lens thickness) each of which can be assessed as a quantitative trait, related to the clinical phenotype of refractive error type. Most of the positive molecular genetics findings for myopia have been derived from studies of relatively small numbers of families with high myopia.[88] Fourteen high myopia loci have been identified, but no candidate gene has been found for moderate amounts of myopia and most data are inconsistent. However, heritability estimates for myopia range from 50% to 96% and for axial length from 40% to 94% across studies, providing support for a genetic component for myopia and eye size.[88,89] Several review articles have summarized the current literature on the genetics of overall refractive error or myopia.[88–91] These articles indicate that myopia susceptibility genes currently are unknown and no candidate gene investigated for moderate myopia has been confirmed. The fact that no gene has yet been implicated for moderate levels of myopia supports the belief that the role of genetics in moderate myopia is more complicated and perhaps not as big as the role of external factors. Large genome-wide association studies are needed to increase the likelihood of identifying specific genes or genetic loci, clarify specific genetic factors and evaluate gene–environment interactions.

11.9.3.2   *Familial factors*

The role of genetics in myopia also has been explored in multiple familial aggregation studies, twin and sibling studies, school-based samples (SCORM), and population-based samples,[92–105] which provide the most consistent evidence for a genetic role in refractive error. Studies investigating parental refraction and refractive error in their children have repeatedly found a positive association between parental myopia and the incidence, prevalence and progression of myopia, longer eyes and changes in axial length in their children,[72,106–115] supporting a role for heredity in myopia susceptibility, progression and eye growth. Among 12-year-old children with myopia in the Sydney Myopia Study, parental myopia was associated with larger amounts of myopia and longer axial length, with a stronger association observed in East Asian compared with European Caucasian children.[115] No association between axial length and parental myopia was observed in the non-myopic children in this study,[115] suggesting that parental refraction is more influential in determining the eye size of children with than without myopia. In COMET, a clinical trial investigating the effect of *progressive addition lenses* (*PALs*) compared with *single vision lenses* (*SVLs*) on myopia progression, it was found that among children with two myopic parents, less myopia progression and axial length changes occurred in the group assigned to PALs than SVLs. These analyses, which were based on a subset of participants, suggest that the success of spectacle interventions to slow myopia progression in children may be influenced by the number of myopic parents. This factor might be considered when targeting groups most amenable to such interventions.[111] In summary, parental refraction has been well documented as a risk factor for myopia and supports a role for genetics. The nature of this role requires further clarification and shared environmental factors within families need to be identified.

11.9.4　Environmental factors

11.9.4.1　*Near-work*

Compelling evidence to indicate that refractive error can be influenced by factors in the visual environment comes from studies in chicks, tree shrews, macaque monkeys and other species, where myopia was experimentally induced by placing a translucent diffuser over an eye to create form deprivation (form deprivation myopia) or by using negative lenses to shift the focal plane of the eye.[116] These observations have led to interest in exploring the role of the visual environment in human myopia, particularly in children. Although the relevance of the animal findings to humans has not been proven, a consistent line of reasoning was suggested by Gwiazda.[107] She observed that myopic children with insufficient accommodation may experience defocus when doing near-work that could lead axial elongation and an increase in myopia as seen in many animal species. This 'blur

hypothesis' suggests that axial elongation occurs in children in response to the hyperopic defocus that occurs when they under-accommodate to near targets. In combination with the increased ocular demands caused by near-work, especially in urban populations, this hypothesis provides a rationale for a relationship between near-work and myopia. Intensive near-work activity has been the environmental factor most commonly investigated for a possible association with myopia, but a direct assessment of this relationship has been difficult to ascertain.

Most of these initial investigations were conducted in selected populations, and interpretation is limited by methodological issues, including selection bias and small sample sizes.[117] One study, conducted by Zylberman *et al.*, compared myopia prevalence between Israeli 14- and 18-year-old male and female teenagers attending a general school and an Orthodox school, to evaluate the association between myopia and the sustained near vision and frequent accommodation changes, resulting from a swaying habit while studying, and the variety of text print sizes used in the Orthodox training. The males attending Orthodox schools had a three-fold increase in myopia prevalence and an average of 2.4 D more myopia than males in the general schools, lending some credibility to the hypothesis that increased ocular demand may result in more myopia.[118] The possible relationship between near-work and myopia has been studied using different approaches to quantify time spent in near-work activities. This included number of books read/week, hours of reading/day and 'dioptre-hours', a unit that takes into account the hours spent in near-work tasks (e.g. reading, computer use, video games) with different weights assigned to each activity; but results have been inconsistent. No association between myopia and time spent on near-activities was found in the Xichang Pediatric Refractive Error Study,[119] yet a small but significant association between myopia and dioptre-hours/week was found in the Orinda Longitudinal Study of Myopia.[109] In a comparison of Singapore schoolchildren seven to nine years old with children from Xiamen, China, Saw *et al.* observed that the number of books read/day was associated with higher myopia of at least 3 D.[120] Reading more than two books/week was also related to higher myopia in a cross-sectional analysis of the SCORM data,[75] but not to myopia incidence in this same cohort.[114] In the Sydney Myopia Study, close reading distance and continuous reading, but not the amount of time spent in near-work activities, were associated with higher myopia prevalence.[121] These varied findings may reflect the lack of an accurate and meaningful assessment of near-work in relationship to myopia, or that near-work may not play as significant a role as suggested by the animal studies.

Intelligence, school performance, parental education, urban schooling and urbanization have also been investigated as independent factors or possible surrogates for near-work. Higher IQ scores were associated with higher myopia incidence and prevalence in Singapore and the USA.[122] Increased scores on school-based standardized assessment tests for reading and mathematics were associated with higher myopia incidence[106] in a large cohort of children in Avon, south-west UK. In studies in South Africa,[38] India[34,37] Malaysia[35] and urban China[8] higher parental education was associated with greater myopia prevalence in their children. Urban schooling was associated with myopia in a rural Chinese population[40] as was urbanization in Sydney, Australia.[123] In contrast, years of schooling were inversely associated with hyperopia in children in New Delhi[37] and with higher parental education in urban China.[8] Although these studies may implicate a role for these near-work-related factors and native intelligence, their interrelationship with genetic factors and the home environment is difficult to disentangle and remains unclear.

Using surrogate measures of education and occupation, studies in adults have observed relationships between myopia and higher education levels and professional occupations, lending some additional support to the proposed role for increased near-work activity or other related factors resulting from these exposures.[49,51,52,58,61,63,64,124] Conversely, hyperopia was associated with lower educational levels and non-professional occupation.[63,64] Despite these suggestive observations and their consistency with results from the studies of children, the role of near-work in refractive error requires further investigation.

11.9.4.2   *Outdoor exposure*

Increased time spent outdoors or in sports activities have been explored as possible protective factors for myopia development, a possibility supported by the low rates in Australia, where the culture emphasizes outdoor sport activities, compared with other countries. While one study reported a protective association between outdoor activities and myopia in males only,[125] and another found no association,[119] other studies have reported positive findings for both sexes. Thus the Sydney Myopia Study found that more time spent outdoors, but not sports activity, was associated with less myopia and a more hyperopic mean refraction;[76] a protective effect of more time spent outdoors was also observed in SCORM teenagers.[126] In cross-sectional and longitudinal analyses of the Orinda Longitudinal Study of Myopia,[109,110] less time spent in sports activity and less time spent outdoors were associated with myopia, and in the longitudinal analysis, this association was stronger in children with two compared with one or no myopic parents. The risk of becoming myopic was lowest in children with no myopic parent and the highest amount of sports/outdoor activity, suggesting an interaction between parental myopia and the role of outdoor activity in myopia.[110] Despite the lower myopia rates in Sydney, the Chinese children in Sydney reported performing significantly more near-work activities than those in Singapore, but the largest difference between groups was in the number of hours spent weekly in outdoor/sports activity (13.75 hours in Sydney versus three hours in Singapore).[77] A two-year longitudinal study of 158 first-year medical students in Copenhagen reported that increased physical activity decreased the risk of myopia development and progression in these young adults, lending further support for a protective role of these factors in myopia.[127] Proposed mechanisms to explain a protective effect of increased outdoor activity include low accommodative demand at distance, higher outdoor light intensity causing pupil restriction, greater depth of field and less image blur, but remain unclear. Further study is required to confirm or better understand the relative importance of increased outdoors activities compared with near-work activities in myopia.

11.9.4.3   *Lighting levels*

A possible role for the influence of lighting levels on myopia has been investigated by evaluating season of birth, number of daylight hours and nightlight use for young children, with no evidence to confirm such an association.[128–133]

11.9.5   Anthropometric parameters and dietary changes

Since axial length, which is a major determinant of refractive error, has been hypothesized to be positively correlated with body size, this variable has been explored in children and adults for possible relationships with refractive error and axial length. An additional rationale to investigate body stature stems from the speculation that changing dietary patterns involving intake of higher glycemic indices and protein consumption, and lower intake of fat and carbohydrates, may contribute to the recent increases in myopia prevalence. The premise is that the dietary changes may be associated with increases in height and may deregulate the control of eye growth, suggesting that myopes would be taller, heavier and have higher **body mass index** (**BMI**).[134] Increased height was associated with longer eyes and refraction in Singaporean schoolchildren[113] and with longer axial length, but not refraction in adults in Singapore[135] and in Australian or rural Chinese children.[32,136] A positive association between myopia and heavier weight, but not height or BMI was observed in a cohort of 1,224 twins aged 18 to 86 years.[137] In the Singaporean children, increased weight and higher BMI, but not height, were associated with a more hyperopic refraction,[113] and in the Sydney Myopia Study cohort hyperopia was associated with shorter height, but not weight or BMI.[78] A cross-sectional evaluation showed that higher saturated fat and cholesterol intake were associated with longer axial length, but not refractive error in Singaporean children.[138] The inconsistency among these results may reflect different populations or methodology, but also may indicate that a relationship between body stature and refraction, if one exists, is modest.

11.9.6   Ocular factors

11.9.6.1   *Children*

Faster progression, amount of myopia and eye growth have been observed in children who have myopia at younger ages.[74,82] Increased axial myopia was associated with decreased macular volume and thickness in SCORM, a finding that should be corroborated.[139] Hyperopia may occur more frequently in children with other ocular conditions such as amblyopia or abnormal convergence.[37]

11.9.6.2   *Adults*

Nuclear lens opacities and posterior subcapsular cataracts have been associated with myopia consistently in cross-sectional studies,[47,51,53,58,85,87,140–143] and are believed to be related to the myopic shift that occurs in older ages. However, the association between nuclear opacities and myopia in longitudinal studies has been less consistent[54,61,64–65,87,141] and may vary with lens opacity type.[54,140,144] This association may reflect increasing nuclear sclerosis of the lens with age, leading to a myopic shift in refraction.[85] It may be that the myopic shift in older adult eyes is due to the increased refractive index of the lens along with changes in the shape and size of the lens. However, it is unclear whether the lens opacities cause the myopia or the myopia induces lens thickening, and further study is needed to better understand the underlying mechanism(s) of this relationship. Hyperopia has been associated with a decrease in lens opacities[47,58] and with moderate nuclear opacities.[65]

Glaucoma and elevated intraocular pressure also have been associated with myopia,[53,54,145,146] but the direction and the mechanism for this relationship need clarification. Hyperopia also has been associated with age-related maculopathy,[147] but this finding has not been consistent across studies.[148,149]

11.10 PREVENTIVE AND/OR CONTROL STRATEGIES; CONTROLLED TRIALS

Refractive errors are corrected by refocusing light on the retina using optical corrections such as eyeglasses and contact lenses, or by refractive surgery which changes the shape of the cornea and is performed in adult eyes once the level of refractive error has stabilized. Refractive surgery, of which the most popular type is **Laser Assisted In Situ Keratomileusis (LASIK)** is one of the most commonly performed surgical procedures in the USA. Despite its popularity, limited information is available about long-term risks or complications. Neither lens- nor surgical-corrections change eye size; therefore, persons with myopia remain at risk for other ocular conditions caused by excessive axial elongation. There is no strategy known to prevent myopia or hyperopia and most therapeutic approaches have aimed to slow down myopia progression, which is the focus of this discussion. Treatments for myopia progression in children that have been evaluated recently in randomized clinical trials fall into two main categories: (1) corrective lenses including single vision lenses, bifocals or progressive addition lenses (PALs), or contact lenses, e.g. rigid permeable lenses, and (2) pharmacologic agents, e.g. atropine and pirenzipine. Such treatments do not slow eye growth or limit the physiological changes associated with axial elongation, thus the risks for sight-threatening complications remain. Although methods for the studies have varied, e.g. power and type of lens used, eligibility criteria including age range and level of myopia, and length of follow-up, the results have been generally consistent. Most studies have shown a modest treatment benefit ranging from 0.20 D to 0.98 D that occurs in the first year and is sustained for up to three years in some studies.[150–154] These findings indicate that although the interventions tried to date have shown some benefit, the magnitude of the effect noted is not sufficient to change clinical practice. In addition, the pharmacologic agents have significant side effects. Larger treatment effects have been observed in some subgroups of children with larger accommodative deficits suggesting that treatment benefits may vary for different groups of children.[155–157]

11.11 SUMMARY

Refractive errors are common, multi-factorial conditions, caused by a complex interaction of genetic and environmental factors. Genetic and environmental factors related to eye size and shape are similar, but not identical, to those related to refractive status, reflecting the complex relationship between these ocular characteristics. Refractive error frequencies vary across populations of different ancestral origins. Rates of myopia are increasing and are especially high in East Asian populations that have experienced rapid, recent urban development, suggesting that urbanization factors play a role in these populations. Some studies suggest a role for near-work in myopia due to increased ocular demand. Yet, inconsistent results between myopia and various direct and surrogate measures of near-work also highlight the difficulties in its accurate assessment and raise the possibility that near-work may not be as significant a factor in myopia as indicated by animal studies. The recent observation of a protective effect of increased outdoor activity warrants further investigation. There is consistent evidence from different studies that longitudinal changes in refractive error do occur; these may be part of an ageing process and the increase in myopia at older ages appears primarily due to lens changes. While no therapeutic intervention has shown a large enough benefit to warrant new clinical recommendations to treat myopia in children, the modest but consistent effect across studies, and the larger treatment benefits observed in some subgroups, i.e. with lower accommodation, raises a possibility that with better understanding of the underlying mechanism for the positive effect, more effective interventions can be developed.

11.12 SUGGESTIONS/PRIORITIES FOR FUTURE EPIDEMIOLOGICAL RESEARCH

To advance understanding of the epidemiology of refractive errors, the following suggestions for future directions and opportunities are offered.

1. Use standard methods and definitions to facilitate comparisons across available and future studies.

2. Develop strategies to identify and overcome barriers to providing best-corrected refractions.

3. Explain the ethnic differences in the prevalence of refractive errors, specifically the factors that account for the high myopia rates in Asian populations.

4. Clarify the temporal relationship between refractive errors and other age-related ocular conditions such as lens opacities and glaucoma.

5. Clarify the relationship between refractive changes and changes in ocular components (e.g. lens, anterior chamber, vitreous, corneal curvature) as well as overall axial length. Specific topics include understanding:

   (a) the role of defocus or accommodation in myopia onset, progression and eventual stabilization,

   (b) whether the genetic and environmental factors influencing refractive changes differ from those for ocular components, and

   (c) whether the interactions of the gene–environment mechanisms influencing refractive changes differ from those that influence changes in each ocular component and how these relationships change throughout life.

6. Develop novel, cost-effective interventions to prevent myopia onset or to slow progression and identify subgroups most likely to benefit from spectacle interventions.

7. Monitor the future impact on long-term eye health of the large number of refractive surgeries, one of the most frequently performed operations in the USA.[158] It is important to develop strategies for systematically monitoring these procedures, including the identification of those groups most likely to benefit and those most likely to be at risk of complications.

11.13   PRESBYOPIA

11.13.1   Introduction

Presbyopia is the age-related loss of lens accommodation that results in an inability to focus at near distances. It is the most common physiological change occurring in the adult eye and is thought to cause universal near-vision impairment with advancing age.

The predominant theory for the development of presbyopia suggests that as the lens ages, it becomes increasingly hard and less malleable in response to the shape-changing forces exerted by the ciliary body and zonules. As a result, the ability of the lens to change shape and therefore power is diminished with age. Additionally, age-related changes in capsular and ciliary body elasticity and structural changes in the shape of the ciliary body have been observed. Thus, the aetiology of presbyopia is likely to be multifactorial with changes in numerous anterior segment structures implicated.

11.13.1.1   Definitions

There is no universally accepted definition of presbyopia and no standard technique for its measurement. Presbyopia is measured in dioptres and requires a plus lens for its correction. In the developed world, the N5 optotype has been used as the endpoint for near-vision testing.[159] Recent studies in developing countries have used the N8 optotype, which was selected to match the type size for newsprint in many developing countries.[160–161] These studies have also standardized near-vision measurement by placing the near chart 16 inches (40 cm) away from the subject.

A person's distance refractive state also affects their near-vision status. Those with near-vision impairment may include hyperopes even though they may have some accommodation. Conversely, those without near-vision impairment may include myopes despite having lost their accommodative ability. Hence, West and colleagues have suggested classification of presbyopia as (1) 'functional' presbyopia to represent those persons who have near-vision impairment in their usual distance visual state and (2) 'objective' presbyopia to represent persons in whom near vision is impaired with distance-vision corrected, if needed.[160]

Recent studies have defined participants as objective presbyopes if all of the following are true:

➢ They are unable to read the N8 optotype at 16 inches with distance correction, if needed, in place.

➢ They have at least one line improvement with the addition of a plus lens.
➢ At least 1 dioptre of additional power ('add') was needed to improve near vision.

11.13.2   Prevalence

Most studies of refractive error have been limited to distance vision and the prevalence of presbyopia has not been well studied. There are few studies that have used a population-based approach and most have been conducted in developing countries. Prevalence data are available from four large population-based studies that were conducted in Brazil, India, Tanzania and Timor-Leste using standard protocols. Incidence data are not available.

In a rural Tanzanian population aged ≥ 40 years old the prevalence of objective and functional presbyopia was 62% and 59% respectively.[160] In southern India, Nirmalan *et al.* found an objective presbyopia prevalence of 55% in subjects ≥ 30 years old.[161] Duarte in Brazil estimated the prevalence of functional presbyopia in 3,000 adults ≥ 30 years old at 55%.[162] In Timor-Leste, the prevalence of functional presbyopia in adults aged ≥ 40 years was 44%.[163] Data from these studies are summarized in Table 11.4.

A survey of ocular morbidity in rural Ugandan adults found presbyopia to be the most common cause of vision impairment for which treatment was sought.[164]

11.13.3   Distribution by age and gender

In rural Tanzania, India and Brazil, the prevalence of presbyopia increased with age to a plateau.

In Tanzania, age-adjusted data showed a higher prevalence among females than males. In a multivariate analysis after adjusting for age, education and residence in town/village, females had 46% higher odds of being presbyopic. Nirmalan[161] and Duarte[162] also reported higher prevalence among females. In Tanzania, females also had more severe presbyopia than males across all age groups.[160] Pointer observed presbyopia to affect women earlier than men in his clinic-based study.[165]

11.13.4   Geographical distribution

Several studies have correlated variations in the age at onset of presbyopia with latitude and ambient temperature. Rambo drew attention to the geographical variation in the ages at which various populations sought help from opticians, with persons in the tropics presenting earlier than those in northern regions.[166] However, observational studies show the age of onset of presbyopia in the

Table 11.4 *Population-based studies of presbyopia*

	STUDY			
	Brazil[162]	Tanzania[160]	India[161]	Timor-Leste[163]
Ancestry	White 81% Indigenous 19%	African	Indian	Melanesian-Papuan
Sample size	3007	1562	5587	1414
Lower age limit (years)	30	40	30	40
Participation rate (%)	93	84	NA	96
End-point for near-vision testing	N4	N8	N8	N8
Prevalence (%) by presbyopia type				
Functional	55	59		44
Objective		62	55	

NA — not available.

high Andes was similar to that in the United Kingdom,[167] whereas presbyopia occurred much earlier in a native population in the Bolivian plains, which is at much the same latitude as the Andes.[168] Hence, Miranda and Weale have speculated that higher ambient temperatures, rather than latitude, were more likely to be associated with earlier onset of presbyopia.[169,170] Data from Jain's case series of 800 presbyopes in India concur with this view.[171]

11.13.5 Risk factors

Studies have implicated a variety of risk factors for presbyopia. Among them, ancestry has received the most attention.

11.13.5.1 *Ancestry*

Studies of patients presenting to hospital eye clinics and optometry practices suggest that African-derived populations develop presbyopia earlier[172–175] and may have more severe presbyopia across age groups than European-derived populations.[173,176] However, these data are from patients presenting to hospital or optometrists and the findings could be affected by selection bias.

Kragha and Hofstetter derived data from optometry practices. They compared Canadian and Puerto Rican subjects between 45 and 60 years old and found Puerto Ricans had more severe presbyopia at a specific age.[177]

In Hong Kong, Edwards's study of Hong Kong Chinese subjects between the ages of 11 and 65 years old found that Chinese lost their accommodative power earlier[178] than in Duane's study of Caucasians.[179]

11.13.5.2 *Other factors*

In Tanzania, West found secondary education and residence in town (as opposed to a village) were significantly associated with a higher prevalence of presbyopia.[160] In southern India, Nirmalan found rural residence (as opposed to a city), nuclear opacity of the lens, myopia and hyperopia were independently associated with presbyopia.[161]

11.13.6 Public health significance/quality of life

Presbyopia poses an important public health issue for maintaining quality of life and economic viability in middle-aged and older persons. Recent data have highlighted the importance of near vision for quality of life in adults. McDonnell used the National Eye Institute Refractive Error Quality of Life Instrument to evaluate the association of presbyopia with vision-targeted health-related quality of life in patients across the USA. The instrument scores indicated that in this population presbyopia was associated with substantial negative effects on vision-targeted health-related quality of life.[159] In contrast, a small study in a spectacle-corrected sample of 110 presbyopes in the USA showed only a nominal decrease in quality of life with presbyopia using time trade-off utility analyses.[180] Here, a comparison was made between perfect near vision and presbyopia using time as the trade-off variable.

For a long time, it was thought that presbyopia affected quality of life in developed countries only, where reading and writing are the main near-vision tasks undertaken. However, Patel showed that in rural communities in Tanzania, where near-vision tasks other than reading and writing are predominant, uncorrected presbyopia also had a substantial impact on quality of life.[181] For example, near vision was used for winnowing grain, sorting rice, weeding, sewing, cooking food, dressing children and lighting and adjusting lamps. Men and women had different needs for near vision but equally demonstrated loss of quality of life with presbyopia. In Brazil, Duarte showed that 58% of presbyopes reported requiring near vision for their routine daily tasks, further documenting the need for near vision in a developing country setting.[162]

Presbyopia may also affect the productivity of individuals, particularly during prime working years and hence can hamper economic development of nations. The World Health Organization has placed increasing emphasis on adult literacy to improve attainment of development goals, but people require good near vision to be able to benefit from programmes to improve literacy. Also, as more transactions are done in writing, adults without good reading vision will be at an economic disadvantage.

11.13.6.1   *Spectacle use*

There are limited data on the prevalence of spectacle use for presbyopia. In developed countries, it is likely that obtaining adequate near correction is within the economic means of the average citizen. However, this may not be the case in developing countries. Only 6% of the subjects with presbyopia in rural Tanzania had corrective spectacles.[160] In Timor-Leste, among those who were presbyopic, only 31% of men and 21% of women had spectacle correction.[163] In southern India, Nirmalan found only a third of presbyopes had correction.[161]

Patel and colleagues gave spectacles to subjects with functional presbyopia in the study in rural Tanzania. After two months, 92% of presbyopes reported using the near-vision spectacles with half using them a few times a week and another 18% using them daily. This gives an indication of the utility of adequate near vision in this population in rural Tanzania where many subjects did not routinely undertake reading and writing tasks. Better near vision after the use of these spectacles resulted in reported improvements in quality of life.[182]

11.13.6.2   *Barriers to correction*

Research on the determinants of and barriers to near spectacle use, though limited, has focused on affordability and availability.

(1) *Affordability*

In Tanzania, 70% of subjects were able to afford spectacles at a price that covered the cost and shipping of the spectacles (US$2). Males were more likely to be able to afford spectacles, whereas a higher proportion of women needed to rely on another person to help them pay for spectacles. An appreciation of the usefulness of having adequate near vision made subjects willing to pay for spectacles and obtain replacements if the need arose.[182] By contrast, in Timor-Leste, 25% of men and 15% of women were willing to pay US$3 for spectacles.[163]

In India, Nirmalan's study found 18% of presbyopes cited financial reasons as the principal factor for not obtaining correction.

(2) *Accessibility*

The lack of knowledge of refractive services and cost and time to access them pose additional burdens on the individual.

The majority of subjects in West's study in Tanzania did not know where to get spectacles. Women were less likely to know than men. A third of subjects could not afford the means to travel to a location where spectacles could be obtained. Once again, women were less likely to be able to afford the travel.[182]

(3) *Awareness of presbyopia*

Nirmalan's study showed that amongst presbyopes without correction 24% reported they had no significant problem while a further 24% reported they were able to see at near adequately.[161] In Tanzania, West reports that many subjects were not aware that correction could return adequate near vision to them. Because presbyopia is a gradual process, many had forgotten the value of having good near vision.[182]

Good data on the availability and affordability of near-vision refractive services, including a system for efficient dispensation of good-quality, affordable spectacles, are still awaited.

11.13.7   Summary

Women have a higher prevalence of, and more severe, presbyopia. Despite this, women in developing countries are less likely to have spectacle correction. Men and women have different needs for near vision but are equally likely to report problems with daily activities due to near-vision impairment. However, women are less likely to be able to afford correction and less likely to know where to get spectacles.

As developing countries undergo the demographic transition to an ageing population, the number of people with presbyopia will increase. The impact on quality of life for older persons is now established. Clearly, presbyopia poses an important public health issue and effective solutions are needed to combat this burgeoning problem.

11.13.8 Preventive or control strategies/trial

Assessment and correction of presbyopia require modest expertise and can be undertaken independently of fixed optical services. Such an approach can be an independent but integrated part of a comprehensive eye health solution, as it may be the first point of contact for persons with other eye problems and could identify those in need of further eye care services.

11.13.9 Suggestions/priorities for future epidemiological research

➢ Further work to determine why women appear to have a higher prevalence of presbyopia and more severe presbyopia at a specific age is warranted.
➢ Racial and geographical variations in presbyopia need to be better understood as well.
➢ Incidence data need to be collected, as do prevalence data from other regions.
➢ The social and economic impact of correction needs to be assessed to justify intervention programmes.
➢ A sustainable model to distribute good quality, low-cost near-vision spectacles that accommodates barriers to correction in urban and rural settings needs to be developed.
➢ Programmes to raise community awareness of presbyopia also need to be developed.

REFERENCES

1. Lim MC, Gazzard G, Sim EL, *et al.* Direct costs of myopia in Singapore. *Eye* May 2009; 23:1086–1089.
2. Rein DB, Zhang P, Wirth KE, *et al.* The economic burden of major adult visual disorders in the United States. *Arch Ophthalmol* 2006; 124:1754–1760.
3. Saw SM, Gazzard G, Shih-Yen EC, *et al.* Myopia and associated pathological complications. *Ophthalmic Physiol Opt* 2005; 25:381–391.
4. Resnikoff S, Pascolini D, Mariotti SP, *et al.* Global magnitude of visual impairment caused by uncorrected refractive errors in 2004. *Bull World Health Organ* 2008; 86:63–70.
5. Robaei D, Huynh SC, Kifley A, *et al.* Correctable and non-correctable visual impairment in a population-based sample of 12-year-old Australian children. *Am J Ophthalmol* 2006;142:112–118.
6. Lu Q, Zheng Y, Sun B, *et al.* A population-based study of visual impairment among pre-schoolchildren in Beijing: the Beijing study of visual impairment in children. *Am J Ophthalmol* 2009; 147:1075–1081.
7. Salomao SR, Cinoto RW, Berezovsky A, *et al.* Prevalence and causes of visual impairment in low-middle income schoolchildren in Sao Paulo, Brazil. *Invest Ophthalmol Vis Sci* 2008; 49:4308–4313.
8. He M, Zeng J, Liu Y, *et al.* Refractive error and visual impairment in urban children in Southern China. *Invest Ophthalmol Vis Sci* 2004;45:793–799.
9. Tielsch JM, Sommer A, Witt K, *et al.* Blindness and visual impairment in an American urban population. The Baltimore Eye Survey. *Arch Ophthalmol* 1990; 108:286–290.
10. Munoz B, West SK, Rodriguez J, *et al.* Blindness, visual impairment and the problem of uncorrected refractive error in a Mexican-American population: Proyecto VER. *Invest Ophthalmol Vis Sci* 2002; 43:608–614.
11. Munoz B, West SK, Rubin GS, *et al.* Causes of blindness and visual impairment in a population of older Americans: The Salisbury Eye Evaluation Study. *Arch Ophthalmol* 2000; 118:819–825.
12. Attebo K, Ivers RQ, Mitchell P. Refractive errors in an older population: the Blue Mountains Eye Study. *Ophthalmology* 1999; 106:1066–1072.
13. Vitale S, Cotch MF, Sperduto RD. Prevalence of visual impairment in the United States. *JAMA* 2006; 295:2158–2163.
14. Varma R, Mohanty SA, Deneen J, *et al.* Burden and predictors of undetected eye disease in Mexican-Americans: the Los Angeles Latino Eye Study. *Med Care* 2008; 46:497–506.
15. Congdon N, Zheng M, Sharma A, *et al.* Prevalence and determinants of spectacle nonwear among rural Chinese secondary schoolchildren: the Xichang Pediatric Refractive Error Study Report 3. *Arch Ophthalmol* 2008; 126:1717–1723.

16. Odedra N, Wedner SH, Shigongo ZS, *et al.* Barriers to spectacle use in Tanzanian secondary school students. *Ophthalmic Epidemiol* 2008; 15: 410–417.

17. Luo HD, Gazzard G, Liang Y, *et al.* Defining myopia using refractive error and uncorrected logMAR visual acuity >0.3 from 1334 Singapore schoolchildren ages 7–9 years. *Br J Ophthalmol* 2006; 90:362–366.

18. Fotedar R, Rochtchina E, Morgan I, *et al.* Necessity of cycloplegia for assessing refractive error in 12-year-old children: a population-based study. *Am J Ophthalmol* 2007; 144:307–309.

19. Krantz EM, Cruickshanks KJ, Klein BE, *et al.* Measuring refraction in adults in epidemiological studies. *Arch Ophthalmol* 2010; 128:88–92.

20. National Research Council (U.S.). Working Group on Myopia Prevalence and Progression. *Myopia: Prevalence and Progression.* Washington, DC: National Academy Press; 1989.

21. Giordano L, Friedman DS, Repka MX, *et al.* Prevalence of Refractive Error among Preschoolchildren in an Urban Population: The Baltimore Pediatric Eye Disease Study. *Ophthalmology* 2009; 116:739–746.

22. Prevalence of myopia and hyperopia in 6- to 72-month-old African American and Hispanic children: the multi-ethnic pediatric eye disease study. *Ophthalmology* 2010; 117:140–147; e143.

23. Dirani M, Chan YH, Gazzard G, *et al.* Prevalence of refractive error in Singaporean Chinese children — the strabismus, amblyopia and refractive error in young Singaporean children (STARS) study. *Invest Ophthalmol Vis Sci* 2009; epub.

24. Vitale S, Ellwein L, Cotch MF, *et al.* Prevalence of refractive error in the United States, 1999–2004. *Arch Ophthalmol* 2008; 126:1111–1119.

25. Bar Dayan Y, Levin A, Morad Y, *et al.* The changing prevalence of myopia in young adults: a 13-year series of population-based prevalence surveys. *Invest Ophthalmol Vis Sci* 2005; 46:2760–2765.

26. Rose K, Smith W, Morgan I, *et al.* The increasing prevalence of myopia: implications for Australia. *Clin Exp Ophthalmol* 2001; 29:116–120.

27. Pokharel GP, Negrel AD, Munoz SR, *et al.* Refractive Error Study in Children: results from Mechi Zone, Nepal. *Am J Ophthalmol* 2000; 129:436–444.

28. Vitale S, Sperduto RD, Ferris FL, 3rd. Increased prevalence of myopia in the United States between 1971–1972 and 1999–2004. *Arch Ophthalmol* 2009; 127:1632–1639.

29. Saw SM, Goh PP, Cheng A, *et al.* Ethnicity-specific prevalences of refractive errors vary in Asian children in neighbouring Malaysia and Singapore. *Br J Ophthalmol* 2006; 90:1230–1235.

30. Fan DS, Lam DS, Lam RF, *et al.* Prevalence, incidence, and progression of myopia of schoolchildren in Hong Kong. *Invest Ophthalmol Vis Sci* 2004; 45:1071–1075.

31. Congdon N, Wang Y, Song Y, *et al.* Visual disability, visual function, and myopia among rural chinese secondary schoolchildren: the Xichang Pediatric Refractive Error Study (X-PRES) report 1. *Invest Ophthalmol Vis Sci* 2008; 49:2888–2894.

32. Ojaimi E, Rose KA, Morgan IG, *et al.* Distribution of ocular biometric parameters and refraction in a population-based study of Australian children. *Invest Ophthalmol Vis Sci* 2005; 46:2748–2754.

33. Kleinstein RN, Jones LA, Hullett S, *et al.* Refractive error and ethnicity in children. *Arch Ophthalmol* 2003; 121:1141–1147.

34. Dandona R, Dandona L, Srinivas M, *et al.* Refractive error in children in a rural population in India. *Invest Ophthalmol Vis Sci* 2002; 43:615–622.

35. Goh PP, Abqariyah Y, Pokharel GP, *et al.* Refractive error and visual impairment in school-age children in Gombak District, Malaysia. *Ophthalmology* 2005; 112:678–685.

36. Maul E, Barroso S, Munoz SR, *et al.* Refractive Error Study in Children: results from La Florida, Chile. *Am J Ophthalmol* 2000; 129:445–454.

37. Murthy GV, Gupta SK, Ellwein LB, *et al.* Refractive error in children in an urban population in New Delhi. *Invest Ophthalmol Vis Sci* 2002; 43:623–631.

38. Naidoo KS, Raghunandan A, Mashige KP, *et al.* Refractive error and visual impairment in African children in South Africa. *Invest Ophthalmol Vis Sci* 2003; 44:3764–3770.

39. Zhao J, Pan X, Sui R, *et al.* Refractive Error Study in Children: results from Shunyi District, China. *Am J Ophthalmol* 2000; 129:427–435.

40. He M, Huang W, Zheng Y, *et al.* Refractive error and visual impairment in schoolchildren in rural southern China. *Ophthalmology* 2007; 114:374–382.

41. Ip JM, Huynh SC, Robaei D, *et al.* Ethnic differences in refraction and ocular biometry in a

population-based sample of 11–15 year-old Australian children. *Eye* 2008; 22:649–656.

42. Morgan A, Young R, Narankhand B, *et al.* Prevalence rate of myopia in schoolchildren in rural Mongolia. *Optom Vis Sci* 2006; 83:53–56.

43. Huynh SC, Kifley A, Rose KA, *et al.* Astigmatism in 12-year-old Australian children: comparisons with a 6-year-old population. *Invest Ophthalmol Vis Sci* 2007; 48:73–82.

44. Gwiazda J, Grice K, Held R, *et al.* Astigmatism and the development of myopia in children. *Vision Res* 2000; 40:1019–1026.

45. Morgan I, Rose K. How genetic is school myopia? *Prog Retin Eye Res* 2005; 24:1–38.

46. McBrien NA, Adams DW. A longitudinal investigation of adult-onset and adult-progression of myopia in an occupational group. Refractive and biometric findings. *Invest Ophthalmol Vis Sci* 1997; 38:321–333.

47. Raju P, Ramesh SV, Arvind H, *et al.* Prevalence of refractive errors in a rural South Indian population. *Invest Ophthalmol Vis Sci* 2004; 45:4268–4272.

48. Saw SM, Gazzard G, Koh D, *et al.* Prevalence rates of refractive errors in Sumatra, Indonesia. *Invest Ophthalmol Vis Sci* 2002; 43:3174–3180.

49. Tarczy-Hornoch K, Ying-Lai M, Varma R. Myopic refractive error in adult Latinos: the Los Angeles Latino Eye Study. *Invest Ophthalmol Vis Sci* 2006; 47:1845–1852.

50. Wang Q, Klein BE, Klein R, *et al.* Refractive status in the Beaver Dam Eye Study. *Invest Ophthalmol Vis Sci* 1994; 35:4344–4347.

51. Wensor M, McCarty CA, Taylor HR. Prevalence and risk factors of myopia in Victoria, Australia. *Arch Ophthalmol* 1999; 117:658–663.

52. Wong TY, Foster PJ, Hee J, *et al.* Prevalence and risk factors for refractive errors in adult Chinese in Singapore. *Invest Ophthalmol Vis Sci* 2000; 41:2486–2494.

53. Wu SY, Nemesure B, Leske MC. Refractive errors in a black adult population: the Barbados Eye Study. *Invest Ophthalmol Vis Sci* 1999; 40:2179–2184.

54. Wu SY, Yoo YJ, Nemesure B, *et al.* Nine-year refractive changes in the Barbados Eye Studies. *Invest Ophthalmol Vis Sci* 2005; 46:4032–4039.

55. Xu L, Li J, Cui T, *et al.* Visual acuity in northern China in an urban and rural population: the Beijing Eye Study. *Br J Ophthalmol* 2005; 89:1089–1093.

56. Bengtsson B, Grodum K. Refractive changes in the elderly. *Acta Ophthalmol Scand* 1999; 77:37–39.

57. Bourne RR, Dineen BP, Ali SM, *et al.* Prevalence of refractive error in Bangladeshi adults: results of the National Blindness and Low Vision Survey of Bangladesh. *Ophthalmology* 2004; 111:1150–1160.

58. Cheng CY, Hsu WM, Liu JH, *et al.* Refractive errors in an elderly Chinese population in Taiwan: the Shihpai Eye Study. *Invest Ophthalmol Vis Sci* 2003; 44:4630–4638.

59. Dandona R, Dandona L, Naduvilath TJ, *et al.* Refractive errors in an urban population in Southern India: the Andhra Pradesh Eye Disease Study. *Invest Ophthalmol Vis Sci* 1999; 40:2810–2818.

60. Gudmundsdottir E, Arnarsson A, Jonasson F. Five-year refractive changes in an adult population: Reykjavik Eye Study. *Ophthalmology* 2005; 112:672–677.

61. Guzowski M, Wang JJ, Rochtchina E, *et al.* Five-year refractive changes in an older population: the Blue Mountains Eye Study. *Ophthalmology* 2003; 110:1364–1370.

62. Hofman A, Grobbee DE, de Jong PT, *et al.* Determinants of disease and disability in the elderly: the Rotterdam Elderly Study. *Eur J Epidemiol* 1991; 7:403–422.

63. Katz J, Tielsch JM, Sommer A. Prevalence and risk factors for refractive errors in an adult inner city population. *Invest Ophthalmol Vis Sci* 1997; 38:334–340.

64. Lee KE, Klein BE, Klein R. Changes in refractive error over a 5-year interval in the Beaver Dam Eye Study. *Invest Ophthalmol Vis Sci* 1999; 40: 1645–1649.

65. Lee KE, Klein BE, Klein R, *et al.* Changes in refraction over 10 years in an adult population: the Beaver Dam Eye study. *Invest Ophthalmol Vis Sci* 2002; 43:2566–2571.

66. Eye Disease Prevalence Research Group. The prevalence of refractive errors among adults in the United States, Western Europe, and Australia. *Arch Ophthalmol* 2004; 122:495–505.

67. Gupta A, Casson RJ, Newland HS, *et al.* Prevalence of refractive error in rural Myanmar: the Meiktila Eye Study. *Ophthalmology* 2008; 115:26–32.

68. Sawada A, Tomidokoro A, Araie M, *et al.* Refractive errors in an elderly Japanese population: the Tajimi study. *Ophthalmology* 2008; 115:363–370; e363.

69. Saw SM, Chan YH, Wong WL, *et al*. Prevalence and risk factors for refractive errors in the Singapore Malay Eye Survey. *Ophthalmology* 2008; 115:1713–1719.

70. Shah SP, Jadoon MZ, Dineen B, *et al*. Refractive errors in the adult Pakistani population: the national blindness and visual impairment survey. *Ophthalmic Epidemiol* 2008; 15:183–190.

71. He M, Huang W, Li Y, *et al*. Refractive error and biometry in older Chinese adults: the Liwan eye study. *Invest Ophthalmol Vis Sci* 2009; 50:5130–5136.

72. Saw SM, Tong L, Chua WH, *et al*. Incidence and progression of myopia in Singaporean schoolchildren. *Invest Ophthalmol Vis Sci* 2005; 46:51–57.

73. Zhao J, Mao J, Luo R, *et al*. The progression of refractive error in school-age children: Shunyi district, China. *Am J Ophthalmol* 2002; 134:735–743.

74. Hyman L, Gwiazda J, Hussein M, *et al*. Relationship of age, sex, and ethnicity with myopia progression and axial elongation in the correction of myopia evaluation trial. *Arch Ophthalmol* 2005; 123:977–987.

75. Saw SM, Chua WH, Hong CY, *et al*. Nearwork in early-onset myopia. *Invest Ophthalmol Vis Sci* 2002; 43:332–339.

76. Rose KA, Morgan IG, Ip J, *et al*. Outdoor activity reduces the prevalence of myopia in children. *Ophthalmology* 2008; 115:1279–1285.

77. Rose KA, Morgan IG, Smith W, *et al*. Myopia, lifestyle, and schooling in students of Chinese ethnicity in Singapore and Sydney. *Arch Ophthalmol* 2008; 126:527–530.

78. Ip JM, Robaei D, Kifley A, *et al*. Prevalence of hyperopia and associations with eye findings in 6- and 12-year-olds. *Ophthalmology* 2008; 115:678–685; e671.

79. Tong L, Saw SM, Carkeet A, *et al*. Prevalence rates and epidemiological risk factors for astigmatism in Singapore schoolchildren. *Optom Vis Sci* 2002; 79:606–613.

80. Xu L, Li J, Cui T, *et al*. Refractive error in urban and rural adult Chinese in Beijing. *Ophthalmology* 2005; 112:1676–1683.

81. He M, Zheng Y, Xiang F. Prevalence of myopia in urban and rural children in mainland China. *Optom Vis Sci* 2009; 86:40–44.

82. Saw SM, Chua WH, Gazzard G, *et al*. Eye growth changes in myopic children in Singapore. *Br J Ophthalmol* 2005; 89:1489–1494.

83. Matsumura H, Hirai H. Prevalence of myopia and refractive changes in students from 3 to 17 years of age. *Surv Ophthalmol* 1999; 44 (Suppl 1):S109–115.

84. Jacobsen N, Jensen H, Goldschmidt E. Prevalence of myopia in Danish conscripts. *Acta Ophthalmol Scand* 2007; 85:165–170.

85. Wong TY, Foster PJ, Johnson GJ, *et al*. Refractive errors, axial ocular dimensions, and age-related cataracts: the Tanjong Pagar survey. *Invest Ophthalmol Vis Sci* 2003; 44:1479–1485.

86. Shufelt C, Fraser-Bell S, Ying-Lai M, *et al*. Refractive error, ocular biometry, and lens opalescence in an adult population: the Los Angeles Latino Eye Study. *Invest Ophthalmol Vis Sci* 2005; 46:4450–4460.

87. Wong TY, Foster PJ, Ng TP, *et al*. Variations in ocular biometry in an adult Chinese population in Singapore: the Tanjong Pagar Survey. *Invest Ophthalmol Vis Sci* 2001; 42:73–80.

88. Young TL. Molecular genetics of human myopia: an update. *Optom Vis Sci* 2009; 86:E8–E22.

89. Young TL, Metlapally R, Shay AE. Complex trait genetics of refractive error. *Arch Ophthalmol* 2007; 125:38–48.

90. Hornbeak DM, Young TL. Myopia genetics: a review of current research and emerging trends. *Curr Opin Ophthalmol* 2009; 20:356–362.

91. Tang WC, Yap MK, Yip SP. A review of current approaches to identifying human genes involved in myopia. *Clin Exp Optom* 2008; 91:4–22.

92. Han W, Yap MK, Wang J, *et al*. Family-based association analysis of hepatocyte growth factor (HGF) gene polymorphisms in high myopia. *Invest Ophthalmol Vis Sci* 2006; 47:2291–2299.

93. Hammond CJ, Snieder H, Gilbert CE, *et al*. Genes and environment in refractive error: the twin eye study. *Invest Ophthalmol Vis Sci* 2001; 42:1232–1236.

94. Dirani M, Shekar SN, Baird PN. The role of educational attainment in refraction: the Genes in Myopia (GEM) twin study. *Invest Ophthalmol Vis Sci* 2008; 49:534–538.

95. Guggenheim JA, Pong-Wong R, Haley CS, *et al*. Correlations in refractive errors between siblings in the Singapore Cohort Study of Risk factors for Myopia. *Br J Ophthalmol* 2007; 91:781–784.

96. Klein AP, Suktitipat B, Duggal P, *et al*. Heritability analysis of spherical equivalent, axial length,

corneal curvature, and anterior chamber depth in the Beaver Dam Eye Study. *Arch Ophthalmol* 2009; 127:649–655.

97. Zhu G, Hewitt AW, Ruddle JB, *et al.* Genetic dissection of myopia: evidence for linkage of ocular axial length to chromosome 5q. *Ophthalmology* 2008; 115:1053–1057; e1052.

98. Simpson CL, Hysi P, Bhattacharya SS, *et al.* The Roles of PAX6 and SOX2 in Myopia: lessons from the 1958 British Birth Cohort. *Invest Ophthalmol Vis Sci* 2007; 48:4421–4425.

99. Fotouhi A, Etemadi A, Hashemi H, *et al.* Familial aggregation of myopia in the Tehran eye study: estimation of the sibling and parent offspring recurrence risk ratios. *Br J Ophthalmol* 2007; 91:1440–1444.

100. Hur YM, Zheng Y, Huang W, *et al.* Comparisons of refractive errors between twins and singletons in Chinese school-age samples. *Twin Res Hum Genet* 2009; 12:86–92.

101. Ciner E, Ibay G, Wojciechowski R, *et al.* Genome-wide scan of African-American and white families for linkage to myopia. *Am J Ophthalmol* 2009; 147:512–517; e512.

102. Hall NF, Gale CR, Ye S, *et al.* Myopia and polymorphisms in genes for matrix metalloproteinases. *Invest Ophthalmol Vis Sci* 2009; 50:2632–2636.

103. Khor CC, Grignani R, Ng DP, *et al.* cMET and refractive error progression in children. *Ophthalmology* 2009; 116:1469–1474, 1474; e1461.

104. Wojciechowski R, Congdon N, Bowie H, *et al.* Heritability of refractive error and familial aggregation of myopia in an elderly American population. *Invest Ophthalmol Vis Sci* 2005; 46:1588–1592.

105. Klein AP, Duggal P, Lee KE, *et al.* Support for polygenic influences on ocular refractive error. *Invest Ophthalmol Vis Sci* 2005; 46:442–446.

106. Williams C, Miller LL, Gazzard G, *et al.* A comparison of measures of reading and intelligence as risk factors for the development of myopia in a UK cohort of children. *Br J Ophthalmol* 2008; 92:1117–1121.

107. Gwiazda J, Thorn F, Bauer J, *et al.* Myopic children show insufficient accommodative response to blur. *Invest Ophthalmol Vis Sci* 1993; 34:690–694.

108. Pacella R, McLellan J, Grice K, *et al.* Role of genetic factors in the aetiology of juvenile-onset myopia based on a longitudinal study of refractive error. *Optom Vis Sci* 1999; 76:381–386.

109. Mutti DO, Mitchell GL, Moeschberger ML, *et al.* Parental myopia, near work, school achievement, and children's refractive error. *Invest Ophthalmol Vis Sci* 2002; 43:3633–3640.

110. Jones LA, Sinnott LT, Mutti DO, *et al.* Parental history of myopia, sports and outdoor activities, and future myopia. *Invest Ophthalmol Vis Sci* 2007; 48:3524–3532.

111. Kurtz D, Hyman L, Gwiazda JE, *et al.* Role of parental myopia in the progression of myopia and its interaction with treatment in COMET children. *Invest Ophthalmol Vis Sci.* 2007; 48:562–570.

112. Zadnik K, Satariano WA, Mutti DO, *et al.* The effect of parental history of myopia on children's eye size. *JAMA* 1994; 271:1323–1327.

113. Saw SM, Chua WH, Hong CY, *et al.* Height and its relationship to refraction and biometry parameters in Singapore Chinese children. *Invest Ophthalmol Vis Sci* 2002; 43:1408–1413.

114. Saw SM, Shankar A, Tan SB, *et al.* A cohort study of incident myopia in Singaporean children. *Invest Ophthalmol Vis Sci* 2006; 47:1839–1844.

115. Ip JM, Huynh SC, Robaei D, *et al.* Ethnic differences in the impact of parental myopia: findings from a population-based study of 12-year-old Australian children. *Invest Ophthalmol Vis Sci* 2007; 48:2520–2528.

116. Norton TT, Metlapally R, L. YT. *Chapter 27: Myopia in Pathobiology of Ocular Disease: A Dynamic Approach*, 2nd Edition. New York: Marcel Dekker; 1994.

117. Rosenfield M, Gilmartin B. *Myopia & Nearwork.* Woburn, MA: Butterworth–Heinemann; 1998.

118. Zylbermann R, Landau D, Berson D. The influence of study habits on myopia in Jewish teenagers. *J Pediatr Ophthalmol Strabismus* 1993; 30:319–322.

119. Lu B, Congdon N, Liu X, *et al.* associations between near work, outdoor activity, and myopia among adolescent students in rural China. *Arch Ophthalmol* 2009; 127:769–775.

120. Saw SM, Zhang MZ, Hong RZ, *et al.* Near-work activity, night-lights, and myopia in the Singapore-China study. *Arch Ophthalmol* 2002; 120(5): 620–627.

121. Ip JM, Saw SM, Rose KA, *et al.* Role of near work in myopia: findings in a sample of Australian schoolchildren. *Invest Ophthalmol Vis Sci* 2008; 49: 2903–2910.

122. Saw SM, Tan SB, Fung D, *et al.* IQ and the association with myopia in children. *Invest Ophthalmol Vis Sci* 2004; 45:2943–2948.

123. Ip JM, Rose KA, Morgan IG, *et al.* Myopia and the urban environment: findings in a sample of 12-year-old Australian schoolchildren. *Invest Ophthalmol Vis Sci* 2008; 49:3858–3863.

124. Shimizu N, Nomura H, Ando F, *et al.* Refractive errors and factors associated with myopia in an adult Japanese population. *Jpn J Ophthalmol* 2003; 47:6–12.

125. Parssinen O, Lyyra AL. Myopia and myopic progression among schoolchildren: a three-year follow-up study. *Invest Ophthalmol Vis Sci* 1993; 34:2794–2802.

126. Dirani M, Tong L, Gazzard G, *et al.* Outdoor activity and myopia in Singapore teenage children. *Br J Ophthalmol* 2009; 93:997–1000.

127. Jacobsen N, Jensen H, Goldschmidt E. Does the level of physical activity in university students influence development and progression of myopia? A 2-year prospective cohort study. *Invest Ophthalmol Vis Sci* 2008; 49:1322–1327.

128. Saw SM, Wu HM, Hong CY, *et al.* Myopia and night lighting in children in Singapore. *Br J Ophthalmol* 2001; 85:527–528.

129. Quinn GE, Shin CH, Maguire MG, *et al.* Myopia and ambient lighting at night. *Nature* 1999; 399: 113–114.

130. Zadnik K, Jones LA, Irvin BC, *et al.* Myopia and ambient night-time lighting. CLEERE Study Group. Collaborative Longitudinal Evaluation of Ethnicity and Refractive Error. *Nature* 2000; 404:143–144.

131. Gwiazda J, Ong E, Held R, *et al.* Myopia and ambient night-time lighting. *Nature* 2000; 404:144.

132. McMahon G, Zayats T, Chen YP, *et al.* Season of birth, daylight hours at birth, and high myopia. *Ophthalmology* 2009; 116:468–473.

133. Mandel Y, Grotto I, El-Yaniv R, *et al.* Season of birth, natural light, and myopia. *Ophthalmology* 2008; 115:686–692.

134. Cordain L, Eaton SB, Brand Miller J, *et al.* An evolutionary analysis of the aaetiology and pathogenesis of juvenile-onset myopia. *Acta Ophthalmol Scand* 2002; 80:125–135.

135. Wong TY, Foster PJ, Johnson GJ, *et al.* The relationship between ocular dimensions and refraction with adult stature: the Tanjong Pagar Survey. *Invest Ophthalmol Vis Sci* 2001; 42:1237–1242.

136. Sharma A, Congdon N, Gao Y, *et al.* Height, stunting, and refractive error among rural Chinese schoolchildren: the See Well to Learn Well project. *Am J Ophthalmol* 2010; 149:347–353; e341.

137. Dirani M, Islam A, Baird PN. Body stature and myopia — The Genes in Myopia (GEM) twin study. *Ophthalmic Epidemiol* 2008; 15(3):135–139.

138. Lim LS, Gazzard G, Low YL, *et al.* Dietary factors, myopia, and axial dimensions in children. *Ophthalmology* 2010; 117:993–997.

139. Luo HD, Gazzard G, Fong A, *et al.* Myopia, axial length, and OCT characteristics of the macula in Singaporean children. *Invest Ophthalmol Vis Sci* 2006; 47:2773–2781.

140. Chang MA, Congdon NG, Bykhovskaya I, *et al.* The association between myopia and various subtypes of lens opacity: SEE (Salisbury Eye Evaluation) project. *Ophthalmology* 2005; 112:1395–1401.

141. Panchapakesan J, Rochtchina E, Mitchell P. Myopic refractive shift caused by incident cataract: the Blue Mountains Eye Study. *Ophthalmic Epidemiol* 2003; 10:241–247.

142. Pesudovs K, Elliott DB. Refractive error changes in cortical, nuclear, and posterior subcapsular cataracts. *Br J Ophthalmol* 2003; 87:964–967.

143. Wong TY, Klein BE, Klein R, *et al.* Refractive errors and incident cataracts: the Beaver Dam Eye Study. *Invest Ophthalmol Vis Sci* 2001; 42:1449–1454.

144. Younan C, Mitchell P, Cumming RG, *et al.* Myopia and incident cataract and cataract surgery: the Blue Mountains Eye Study. *Invest Ophthalmol Vis Sci* 2002; 43:3625–3632.

145. Mitchell P, Hourihan F, Sandbach J, *et al.* The relationship between glaucoma and myopia: the Blue Mountains Eye Study. *Ophthalmology* 1999; 106:2010–2015.

146. Wong TY, Klein BE, Klein R, *et al.* Refractive errors, intraocular pressure, and glaucoma in a white population. *Ophthalmology* 2003; 110:211–217.

147. Xu L, Cui T, Yang H, *et al.* Prevalence of visual impairment among adults in China: the Beijing Eye Study. *Am J Ophthalmol* 2006; 141:591–593.

148. Wang JJ, Jakobsen KB, Smith W, *et al.* Refractive status and the 5-year incidence of age-related maculopathy: the Blue Mountains Eye Study. *Clin Exp Ophthalmol* 2004; 32:255–258.

149. Wong TY, Klein R, Klein BE, *et al*. Refractive errors and 10-year incidence of age-related maculopathy. *Invest Ophthalmol Vis Sci* 2002; 43:2869–2873.

150. Walline JJ, Jones LA, Mutti DO, *et al*. A randomized trial of the effects of rigid contact lenses on myopia progression. *Arch Ophthalmol* 2004; 122:1760–1766.

151. Fulk GW, Cyert LA, Parker DE. A randomized trial of the effect of single-vision vs. bifocal lenses on myopia progression in children with esophoria. *Opt Vis Sci* 2000; 77:395–401.

152. Gwiazda J, Hyman L, Hussein M, *et al*. A randomized clinical trial of progressive addition lenses versus single vision lenses on the progression of myopia in children. *Invest Ophthalmol Vis Sci* 2003; 44:1492–1500.

153. Leung JT, Brown B. Progression of myopia in Hong Kong Chinese schoolchildren is slowed by wearing progressive lenses. *Opt Vis Sci* 1999; 76: 346–354.

154. Shih YF, Hsiao CK, Chen CJ, *et al*. An intervention trial on efficacy of atropine and multi-focal glasses in controlling myopic progression. *Acta Ophthalmol Scand* 2001;79:233–236.

155. Hasebe S, Ohtsuki H, Nonaka T, *et al*. Effect of progressive addition lenses on myopia progression in Japanese children: a prospective, randomized, double-masked, crossover trial. *Invest Ophthalmol Vis Sci* 2008; 49:2781–2789.

156. Cheng D, Schmid KL, Woo GC, *et al*. Randomized trial of effect of bifocal and prismatic bifocal spectacles on myopic progression: two-year results. *Arch Ophthalmol* 2010; 128:12–19.

157. Gwiazda JE, Hyman L, Norton TT, *et al*. Accommodation and related risk factors associated with myopia progression and their interaction with treatment in COMET children. *Invest Ophthalmol Vis Sci* 2004; 45:2143–2151.

158. Aaron MM, Aaberg TM. Ophthalmology resident training in refractive surgery. *Am J Ophthalmol* 2001; 131:241–243.

159. McDonnell PJ, Lee P, Spritzer K, *et al*. Associations of presbyopia with vision-targeted health-related quality of life. *Arch Ophthalmol* 2003; 121:1577–1581.

160. Burke AG, Patel I, Munoz B, *et al*. Population-based study of presbyopia in rural Tanzania. *Ophthalmology* 2006; 113:723–727.

161. Nirmalan PK, Krishnaiah S, Shamanna BR, *et al*. A population-based assessment of presbyopia in the state of Andhra Pradesh, south India: the Andhra Pradesh Eye Disease Study. *Invest Ophthalmol Vis Sci* 2006; 47:2324–2328.

162. Duarte WR, Barros AJ, Dias-da-Costa JS, *et al*. [Prevalence of near vision deficiency and related factors: a population-based study] [Article in Portuguese]. *Cad Saude Publica* 2003; 19: 551–559.

163. Ramke J, du Toit R, Palagyi A, *et al*. Correction of refractive error and presbyopia in Timor-Leste. *Br J Ophthalmol* 2007; 91:860–866.

164. Kamali A, Whitworth JA, Ruberantwari A, *et al*. Causes and prevalence of non-vision impairing ocular conditions among a rural adult population in sw Uganda. *Ophthalmic Epidemiol* 1999; 6: 41–48.

165. Pointer JS. The presbyopic add. II. Age-related trend and a gender difference. *Ophthalmic Physiol Opt* 1995; 15:241–248.

166. Rambo VC. Further notes on the varying ages at which different peoples develop presbyopia. *Am J Ophthalmol* 1953; 36:709–710.

167. Sargent JP. High-altitude ophthalmology. *A Inst Barraquer* 1968; 8:158–174.

168. Weale R. *A Biography of the Eye, Development, Growth, Age*. London: H. K. Lewis; 1982.

169. Weale RA. Epidemiology of refractive errors and presbyopia. *Surv Ophthalmol* 2003; 48:515–543.

170. Miranda MN. The geographic factor in the onset of presbyopia. *Trans Am Ophthalmol Soc* 1979; 77: 603–621.

171. Jain IS, Ram J, Gupta A. Early onset of presbyopia. *Am J Optom Physiol Opt* 1982; 59:1002–1004.

172. Adefule AO, Valli NA. Presbyopia in Nigerians. *East Afr Med J* 1983; 60:766–772.

173. Covell LL. Presbyopia; comparative observations of white and Negro populations. *Am J Ophthalmol* 1950; 33:1275–1276.

174. Hofstetter HW. Further data on presbyopia in different ethnic groups. *Am J Optom Arch Am Acad* 1968; 45:522–527.

175. Nwosu SN. Ocular problems of young adults in rural Nigeria. *Int Ophthalmol* 1998; 22:259–263.

176. Kaimbo K, Maertens K, Missotten L. [Study of presbyopia in Zaire] [Article in French]. *Bull Soc Belge Ophtalmol* 1987; 225 Pt 2:149–156.

177. Kragha IK, Hofstetter HW. Bifocal adds and environmental temperature. *Am J Optom Physiol Opt* 1986; 63:372–376.

178. Edwards MH, Law LF, Lee CM, *et al.* Clinical norms for amplitude of accommodation in Chinese. *Ophthalmic Physiol Opt* 1993; 13:199–204.

179. Duane A. Normal values of the accommodation at all ages. *JAMA* 1912; 59:1010–1013.

180. Luo BP, Brown GC, Luo SC, *et al.* The quality of life associated with presbyopia. *Am J Ophthalmol* 2008; 145:618–622.

181. Patel I, Munoz B, Burke AG, *et al.* Impact of presbyopia on quality of life in a rural African setting. *Ophthalmology* 2006; 113(5):728–734.

182. Patel I, Munoz B, Mkocha H, *et al.* Change in function and spectacle-use 2 months after providing presbyopic spectacles in rural Tanzania. *Br J Ophthalmol* 2010; 94:685–689.

183. Liang YB, Wong TY, Sun LP, *et al.* Refractive errors in a rural Chinese adult population: the Handan Eye Study. *Ophthalmology* 2009; 116: 2119–2127.

The epidemiology of low vision

GARY RUBIN

12.1 Introduction 227
12.2 Prevalence of low vision 227
12.3 The relationship between visual 230
    impairment and low vision
12.4 Causes of low vision 232

12.5 Low-vision rehabilitation 233
12.6 Global issues 236
12.7 Future research needs 237
    References 237

12.1 INTRODUCTION

The terms 'low vision' and 'visual impairment' are often used interchangeably. However, here we are using 'visual impairment' to refer to loss of organ function as defined by subjective criteria such as reduced visual acuity or restricted visual field. 'Low vision', on the other hand, refers to an inability to perform everyday visual tasks, such as reading or recognizing faces, resulting from a visual impairment. Within the framework of the WHO terminology low vision is a disability[1] or activity limitation[2] as opposed to an impairment.[a] One consequence of the distinction between impairment and disability is that while it makes sense to consider unilateral versus bilateral visual impairment, no such distinction applies to low vision. Eyes may be visually impaired but people have low vision.

The concept of low vision was popularized by Eleanor Faye in the 1970s to identify persons who might benefit from vision rehabilitation services but would not be considered blind. The WHO subsequently adopted low vision as a classification of people with vision worse than normal but better than legal blindness. In Britain this is referred to as 'partial sight'. A common definition of low vision is a 'visual disability that cannot be corrected by conventional spectacles or with medical or surgical treatment', which precludes reduced vision from refractive error or treatable conditions such as cataract.

12.2 PREVALENCE OF LOW VISION

There is an extensive epidemiology of visual impairment worldwide, much of which is reviewed earlier in this book (refer to Chapter 1), but the epidemiology of low vision is not so well established. Although low vision is a consequence of visual impairment, we cannot simply use visual impairment data to establish the prevalence of low vision. One complication is that low vision excludes those with treatable disorders. It is estimated that as much as one half of visual impairment among the elderly in the USA could be eliminated by refractive correction or surgical treatment.[3] The proportion is even greater for segments of the population who have less access to health

---

[a] It is surprising, therefore, that in the WHO International Classification of Disease 'low vision' refers to a level of visual acuity worse than 6/18 (20/60), which is an impairment rather than a disability.

care,[4] and for populations with a higher prevalence of refractive error (e.g. Malaysians and other Asian groups).[5] A second problem is that current definitions of visual impairment (largely based on acuity) fail to capture a significant proportion of the population who are visually disabled. We examine this problem in greater detail below.

Low vision may be defined objectively by task performance or subjectively by self-reported task difficulty. Estimates of the prevalence of low vision vary widely according to the definition of the disability and methods of assessment. Available data from population-based studies are summarized in Table 12.1. Most of the epidemiological studies of visual disability have relied entirely on self-report. The Rand Health Insurance Study[6] reported that 20% of their sample were unable to read newsprint, but this high proportion is misleading as it included all those who required glasses to read. The National Center for Health Statistics' Health Interview Survey[7] estimated that 2% of the US population had difficulty reading ordinary newsprint and 5% of the population had difficulty seeing even when wearing glasses. The Lighthouse National Survey on Vision Loss[8] reported that 9% of the adult population could not recognize a nearby face or read newsprint, or described themselves as having poor or very poor vision even with glasses. An additional 8% could not recognize a face across a room or had other trouble seeing even with glasses. The **EPESE** study (**Established Populations for Epidemiologic Studies of the Elderly**)[9] reported that 7% of their elderly population were unable to read newsprint, and 10% were unable to recognize a friend across the street. The **Melbourne VIP**[10] and **SEE** studies[11] used standardized visual function questionnaires to assess visual disability. Fifteen percent of the VIP population acknowledged difficulty reading a phone number and 4% had trouble recognizing a coin, whereas 12% of the elderly SEE population reported difficulty with two or more visual tasks (excluding driving). A study of the impact of trichiasis on visual disability in Tanzania[12] identified 25% of the population as having difficulty with visual tasks (excluding subsistence activities).

More recently, in a study[13] of 9,330 participants from the 1958 British Birth Cohort (age 44/45 at time of study) 0.9% reported impaired vision-related quality of life, defined as a summary score >2 on the Vision-related Quality of Life Core Measure 1 (VCM1),[14] indicating more than a little concern about vision. In a nationwide survey of French households (n = 17,000),[15] 2.04% were classified as blind or with low vision. The classification was based on self-reported difficulty reading newsprint, recognizing faces at a distance, or filling out cheques or forms without assistance.

In addition to self-reported visual disability, two population-based studies used measured task performance to determine the prevalence of low vision. The EPESE study[9] measured participants' ability to read type of various sizes. Five percent of their participants were unable to read 10pt type, which is slightly larger than newsprint. In the SEE study[16] 10% of the participants could not read newsprint-sized text faster than 60 words/minute (moderate fluency) and 3% could not read ten words/minute (excluding the illiterate).

Comparisons of self-reported disability with measured performance leads to some interesting discrepancies. In the EPESE study, 46% of those who said they were unable to read newsprint demonstrated that they could read 7pt type (smaller than most newsprint). The large discrepancy may indicate that there was something unusual about the functional vision test. This seems likely as 35% of participants who were legally blind by USA standards (acuity less than 20/200) were still able to read the small print. However, discrepancies between performance and self-report may also be informative. The SEE study[17] found that 11% of participants who reported no difficulty reading a newspaper were unable to read fluently when tested in the clinic. The discrepant group had visual acuities intermediate between those who read fluently and those who acknowledged difficulty and read slowly. The authors suggest that the discrepant group are in a transitional state of pre-clinical disability during which people may successfully compensate for a functional decline and not perceive that they are disabled.

Table 12.1 *Population-based studies of low vision*

Study	Sample size	Age range	Location	Definition	Prevalence %
Rand Health Insurance[6]	6,000	14–61	California, USA	SR difficulty reading newsprint	20
Home Interview Survey[7]	100,000	All ages	USA	SR difficulty reading newsprint	2
				SR difficulty seeing	5
Lighthouse Survey[8]	1,219	45 and older	USA	SR difficulty reading newsprint, recognizing nearby face; poor or very poor vision	9
EPESE[9]	5,335	71 and older	3 Centres, USA	SR difficulty recognising face at a distance; other trouble seeing	8
				SR difficulty reading newsprint	7
VIP[10]	508	40 and older	Melbourne, Australia	PBT unable to read 10pt type	5
				SR difficulty identifying coin	4
SEE[11]	2,520	65–84	Maryland, USA	SR difficulty reading telephone number	15
				SR difficulty with two or more visual tasks	12
				PBT reading newsprint (60 words/minute)	10
Trichiasis Study[12]	3,064	40 and older	Kongwa, Tanzania	SR difficulty with various village activities because of vision	25
1958 British Birth Cohort Study[13]	9,330	44/45	Great Britain	SR concern about vision on VCM1 (14)	1
French Household Survey[15]	17,000	All ages	France	SR difficulty reading newsprint, recognizing faces at a distance, or filling out forms	2

SR: self-report.
PBT: performance-based test.

12.3   THE RELATIONSHIP BETWEEN VISUAL IMPAIRMENT AND LOW VISION

Although it is the premise of this chapter that low vision cannot be equated with visual impairment, obviously the two are closely related. People who are visually impaired are more likely to have difficulty with visual tasks. If we can pin down the relationship between impairment and disability then we can better use the rich epidemiological data on visual impairment. It is now well established that difficulty with some everyday tasks can be predicted from clinical measures of visual function. The best example is reading. For high contrast, well-spaced text, the primary visual limitation on reading speed is letter size. Thus, acuity is an excellent predictor of the letter size required for fluent reading. Most definitions of visual impairment include an acuity cut-off; hence we would expect them to be closely related to a visual disability that is defined by reading difficulty. The 6/18 cut-off adopted by the WHO is based on the acuity required for reading newsprint. One may argue that the cut-off is too high — 6/18 acuity may be sufficient for occasional spot reading but will not support fluent reading of newsprint-sized text[18] — but the principle is reasonable. The USA definition of visual impairment (20/40 or 6/12) is based, in part, on standards for obtaining a driving licence and this is related, in turn, to legibility of road signs. However important reading may be, it is not the only determinant of visual disability. The ability to see well enough to recognize faces and objects and to navigate independently will have important consequences for social interaction, recreation, education and employment. Difficulty with these tasks may be more closely related to domains of visual function other than acuity, such as visual field or contrast sensitivity. Many definitions of visual impairment include a visual field component. However, there exist few population-based data on the relationship between visual field loss and task difficulty.

12.3.1   Contrast sensitivity

On the other hand, the role of contrast sensitivity has received a great deal of attention in recent years. Unlike visual acuity, which evaluates the eye's ability to resolve fine detail at high contrast, contrast sensitivity is a measure of the difference between the light and dark portions of an image required to detect or recognize it. Contrast sensitivity was originally developed as a research tool, and for theoretical reasons most investigators used grating patterns consisting of alternating light and dark bars that have a sinusoidal luminance profile. Sine-wave gratings vary in spatial frequency (bar width) and contrast. By measuring the lowest detectable contrast across a wide range of spatial frequencies, one derives a contrast sensitivity function. The highest frequency sine-wave grating (narrowest bars) that one can distinguish from a uniform field is a measure of visual acuity. Traditional methods for measuring contrast sensitivity require relatively expensive and sophisticated equipment, typically a computer-controlled video display, and employ time-consuming psychophysical procedures. Several contrast sensitivity tests have been developed for clinical use. These include plate tests with photographically reproduced sine-wave gratings and various low contrast optotype tests. There is considerable controversy about the necessity to measure contrast sensitivity at several spatial frequencies using sine-wave gratings or whether a single global measure of contrast sensitivity is adequate for clinical purposes.[19] Changes near the peak of the function are more important predictors of reading performance in people with low vision than subtle irregularities in the curve, and tests using large letters are ideal for measuring the relevant aspects of contrast sensitivity.[19]

While there is no accepted definition of visual impairment based on contrast sensitivity, recent data could be used to develop such a standard. The SEE study[20] measured various visual functions including contrast sensitivity and visual acuity in a population-based sample of 2,500 American adults aged 65 to 84. Visual disability was assessed with the **Activities of Daily Vision Scale (ADVS)**.[21] Figure 12.1a shows the relationship between visual acuity and ADVS score. If we accept an acuity below 6/12 (approximately 0.5 **logMAR**) as meeting the criterion for disability, then this corresponds to an ADVS score of 60 or less. Figure 12.1b shows the relationship between contrast sensitivity

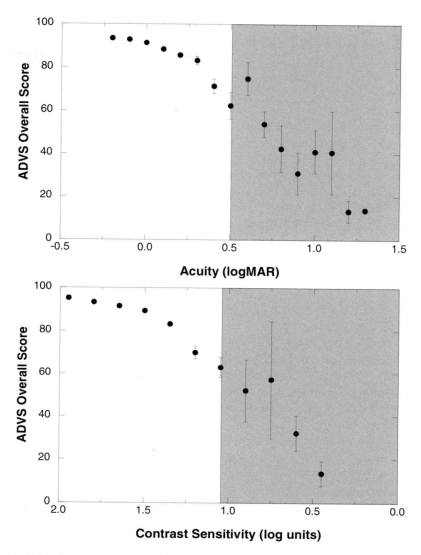

Figure 12.1a+b   *Relationship between visual function and self reported visual disability from the Salisbury Eye Evaluation Study.[11]* **Top Panel:** *Overall score on the Activities of Daily Vision Scale[21] is plotted versus distance acuity on a logMAR scale. Vertical error bars indicate ± 1 SD. In some cases, the errors bars are smaller than the data point. Hatched area indicates visual acuity scores that meet the WHO definition for low vision (acuity worse than 6/18).* **Bottom Panel:** *Overall ADVS score is plotted versus contrast sensitivity for letters on a log contrast scale. Vertical error bars indicate ± 1 SD. Hatched area indicates contrast sensitivities that correspond to levels of visual disability comparable to those in hatched area of top panel*

and ADVS. A score of 60 or less corresponds to contrast sensitivity score less than approximately 1.0 log units (0.6 log units or about four times lower than normal). According to this reasoning, a person with a contrast sensitivity of 1.0 would be as disabled as a person with an acuity of 6/18. A similar method could be used to derive cut-offs for other measures of visual function such as visual field or glare sensitivity; however, these measures are not as closely related to the types of disability as assessed by the ADVS.

We have used a different method to derive definitions of acuity and contrast sensitivity impairment from measured task performance.[16] From the

SEE data we concluded that there was no evidence of a threshold acuity or contrast sensitivity below which a sharp decrement in reading performance could be observed. Instead, there was a gradual decline in task performance with deteriorating visual function. Therefore, we arbitrarily defined a reading disability as a speed more than one standard deviation below the population mean. This corresponds to fewer than 90 words/minute for newsprint, which agrees with a generally accepted cut-off for fluent reading.[18] We then determined the level of visual acuity below which more than half of the affected population would be disabled in terms of reading. The same procedure was followed for other tasks and for determining disabling levels of contrast sensitivity loss. The levels differed for each visual task. For climbing a well-illuminated flight of stairs, visual acuity had to be worse than 1.0 logMAR (6/60) or contrast sensitivity had to be worse than 0.9 log units before 50% of the affected population were disabled. For face recognition the values were 0.3 logMAR (6/12) or 1.3 log contrast sensitivity and for reading newsprint the values were 0.2 logMAR (6/9) or 1.4 log contrast sensitivity.

Ocular conditions that reduce contrast sensitivity often affect visual acuity as well. However, the two measures of visual function are not entirely superfluous, both contributing independently to the risk of visual disability.[11,22] Applying the method based on self-report to the Salisbury population, the prevalence of low vision increases from 2.5% using the acuity cut-off alone to 3% by also including subjects with poor contrast sensitivity. Even after other potentially confounding factors such as age and gender have been taken into account, the addition of a contrast sensitivity criterion increases the estimated prevalence of low vision by about 20%.

It is important to remember that any definition of low vision based solely on visual impairment will miss some individuals who have difficulties with visual tasks for reasons that are not captured by the vision tests used to define impairment. In the SEE study, 12% of the participants who had normal acuity and contrast sensitivity reported difficulty with at least two visual activities. Another example is the Tanzania trichiasis study[12] where the presence of trichiasis doubled the number of tasks reported difficult by women even in the absence of visual acuity loss. Conversely, the presence of visual impairment does not guarantee that the person will be disabled. Almost 35% of the SEE participants with acuity or contrast sensitivity impairment reported no difficulty with visual tasks and in the 1958 British Birth Cohort Study 97% of those with severe visual impairment (presenting acuity worse than 6/60) reported little or no concern about vision-related quality of life.[13]

12.4   CAUSES OF LOW VISION

Much of the research on low vision disregards the underlying causes of the visual disability. From the viewpoint of the low-vision service provider, it makes little difference whether the low-vision patient suffers from macular degeneration or cone dystrophy, glaucoma or optic neuritis. What does matter is how the disease has affected visual function. Thus, there are few epidemiological data on the causes of low vision (as opposed to visual impairment). Nevertheless, it is informative to compare the limited data that are available with the extensive data on the causes of visual impairment.

There have been three large studies that reported the causes of low vision for patients referred for low-vision rehabilitation.[b,23,24] The USA and UK studies are limited to data from single low-vision clinics. The Canadian study gathered information from throughout an entire province, making it more representative of the population than do the other two studies. The data, shown in Fig. 12.2, indicate that approximately half of low-vision referrals are for patients with **AMD**. Other eye diseases each account for 10% or fewer referrals.

Epidemiological studies in developed countries have produced a fairly consistent picture of the causes of visual impairment. Some of these data are summarized in Fig. 12.3, which illustrates the major causes of visual impairment from six published studies.[3,25–29]

---

[b] Habel A. Primary causes of vision impairment in 1,000 consecutive patients seen at the Wilmer Low Vision Clinic. Unpublished data.

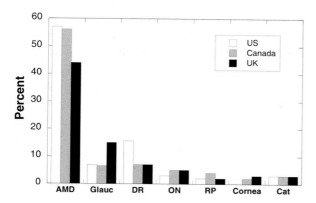

Figure 12.2 The distribution of primary causes of vision loss for three studies of low-vision referral patterns (AMD = age-related macular degeneration; Glauc = primary open-angle glaucoma; DR = diabetic retinopathy; ON = optic neuropathathies; RP = Retinitis Pigmentosa; Cat = cataract.)

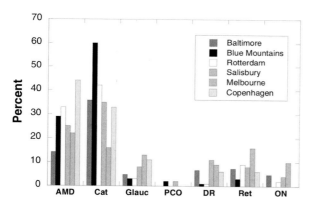

Figure 12.3 The distribution of primary causes of visual impairment from six population-based studies (AMD = age-related macular degeneration; Cat = cataract; Glauc = primary open-angle glaucoma; PCO = posterior capsular pacification; DR = diabetic retinopathy; Ret = other retinal diseases; ON = optic neuropathathies.)

As the prevalence of visual impairment increases dramatically with advancing age, most of these studies concentrate on older age groups. For all six studies cataract and AMD are the leading causes of visual impairment. Glaucoma is also a major contributor in the two US studies, where it accounted for a significant proportion of the visual impairments in African American participants.

A comparison of Figs. 12.2 and 12.3 reveals a consistent over-representation of patients with AMD and under-representation of patients with

cataract among those referred for low-vision services. There are several possible reasons for this. First, the visual impairment resulting from cataract is usually reversible with surgery. According to one study[30] half of those with vision-limiting cataract elect not to have surgery in the two years following diagnosis. Nevertheless, few are referred for vision rehabilitation, and, were they to be referred, many low-vision practitioners would prefer not to treat them until all reasonable medical alternatives had been investigated. A second reason may be that macular degeneration affects central vision, while some of the other common conditions, like glaucoma, initially affect peripheral vision. A drop in central vision is more quickly noticed by the patient and may be more detrimental to everyday visual activities than is true of peripheral involvement. Third, the emphasis of many low-vision services is on providing appropriate magnification. Magnification is effective for problems with poor resolution in central vision, but has little value for addressing peripheral vision problems caused by restricted fields.

The predominance of AMD patients in the low-vision clinic is reflected in the chief complaints of those referred for rehabilitation. In a sample of 1,000 consecutive patients seen at a USA hospital-based clinic, 78% listed reading as one of their chief complaints, while other activities, such as recognizing faces or watching television, were noted by fewer than 15% of patients. Figure 12.4 compares the distribution of vision problems in clinic patients with self-reported vision disability in the SEE study.[11] In contrast to the clinic data, only 43% of visually impaired participants singled out difficulty reading newsprint while approximately 35% reported difficulty viewing television and driving, and 25–30% reported difficulty recognizing faces, navigating steps or writing. These observations reinforce the notion that AMD patients with reading difficulty are over-represented in published surveys of low-vision clinics compared with their prevalence in the community.

12.5 LOW-VISION REHABILITATION

It is important to emphasize that the vast majority of visually impaired people retain some useful vision. Fewer than 10% are totally blind, and over 75% can

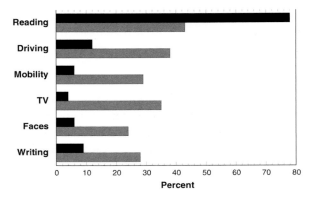

Figure 12.4 Major complaints of low-vision patients referred to a US hospital-based low-vision service (darker bars) and visually disabled participants in a US population-based study of the impact of vision loss on disability (lighter bars)

read newspaper headlines, according to a UK survey.[31] Nevertheless, visual impairment is among the most disabling of medical conditions, i.e. more disabling than other chronic conditions except diabetes and cancer in older adults.[32] Visual impairment is strongly associated with dependency in daily activities, reduced physical activity, social isolation and depression, especially in older individuals. According to one study, the quality of life of low-vision patients was comparable to those with congestive heart failure or clinical depression.[33]

Through the 1950s, visual rehabilitation was dominated by the sight-saving philosophy. According to this view, the use of eyes with partial sight will hasten their deterioration. Although the perpetuation of this philosophy has lead to some beneficial outcomes, such as the development of large print books and special educational programmes for visually impaired children, it also interfered with the establishment and acceptance of low-vision rehabilitation. Even today, many optometrists and ophthalmologists view visual rehabilitation as a service worthy of little attention. This is all the more surprising given that the majority of those who are visually impaired — other than those with cataract — cannot have their vision restored by current medical or surgical treatment.

Low-vision rehabilitation services are provided by practitioners with a wide range of training and in a variety of settings. Educators, social workers,

occupational therapists, opticians, even the local pharmacist may dispense **low-vision assistive devices** (**LVAs**) or provide low-vision rehabilitation services. But most of low-vision rehabilitation is the responsibility of ophthalmologists and optometrists, especially the latter. The majority of low-vision consultations are provided at clinics in eye hospitals or schools of optometry, although some of the largest providers are at specialized agencies like the Lighthouse in New York.

There have been few systematic studies of the provision of low-vision services. The Royal National Institute for the Blind sponsored a survey of low-vision services throughout the UK.[31] Questionnaires were sent to over 2,500 potential providers. Of the 1,900 respondents, 41% provide no low-vision service and 26% just sell LVAs. Only 33% provide services in addition to LVA dispensing. More troublesome are the data on the geographical distribution of services. As expected, there is a concentration of low-vision services in urban centres. Not only is there a wide geographical variation in the availability of low-vision services, but some areas with the highest prevalence of low vision are also the most poorly served.

Throughout most of Western Europe and Canada, low-vision services are at least partly state-funded. The cost of the low-vision exam and prescribed LVAs are subsidized. Until recently, low-vision services in the USA were privately funded except when they were directly related to education or employment, or for military veterans who were eligible for an extensive range of low-vision services. As the vast majority of people with low vision are of retirement age, this meant that most low-vision services in the USA were not publicly funded. There has been a gradual change over the past decade whereby low-vision services have become eligible for Medicare insurance funding. However there is still no coverage for prescribed LVAs. Elsewhere in the industrialized world, low-vision services are well established and state-supported in Australia, Japan and Israel. In some countries, governmental support is funnelled through a private agency such as the Royal New Zealand Foundation for the Blind. Eligibility for publicly funded low-vision rehabilitation is usually determined by level of visual acuity or visual field. Thus, eligibility is based on visual impairment rather than visual disability.

Just as the availability and funding of services varies widely throughout the world, so does the level or type of service offered. Some low-vision services consist of nothing more than a tray of magnifiers from which the patient makes a selection by trial and error. Although disparaged by professionals, the 'cafeteria style' services are the only locally available option for many patients. At the other extreme are the residential low-vision rehabilitation services such as the Blind Rehabilitation Centers run by the US Department of Veterans' Affairs. Eligible veterans receive up to eight weeks of inpatient rehabilitation, covering use of LVAs, orientation and mobility training, manual skills and living skills. The most common type of service is the hospital or optometry school clinic where the patient has a one- to two-hour consultation that includes a needs assessment, detailed low-vision refraction, prescription of LVAs and minimal training with selected devices. This basic level of service may be augmented by additional referrals for counselling, orientation and mobility training, daily living skills training, or further LVA instruction.

A popular alternative to the basic clinic rehabilitation model is an integrated multidisciplinary service referred to as the 'Swedish model'. The team may include an ophthalmologist, optometrist, low-vision therapist, orientation and mobility instructor, educator, and counsellor. The team develops a comprehensive rehabilitation programme administered by the low-vision therapist. Extensive training is a major focus of the Swedish model. The comprehensive multidisciplinary approach has been adopted in other European countries, Israel, and Australia, and is also widely promoted in the USA. However, the high costs of such a programme and limited funding have restricted its implementation. In addition, there is not a consensus regarding the level of services required to achieve the goals of low-vision rehabilitation.

12.5.1   Effectiveness

Data on effectiveness of low-vision rehabilitation are limited.[34] Surveys of patient satisfaction following vision rehabilitation have produced conflicting results, ranging from 90% reporting that the service was sufficient to meet their needs, to 50% reporting dissatisfaction. Without solid evidence as to the benefits of vision rehabilitation, it is difficult to argue for the expansion of rehabilitation services. Despite the substantial number of people with visual impairment there have been only a few, mostly small, controlled trials of vision rehabilitation. The majority of these trials found rehabilitation to be effective but most were limited to older low-vision patients, especially those with AMD.[35]

The largest trial of vision rehabilitation to date was a recent study of enhanced versus conventional low-vision services.[36] Two-hundred and twenty-five patients with AMD were randomly assigned to one of three groups: conventional hospital-based vision rehabilitation, the conventional service plus three home visits by a trained rehabilitation officer, or the conventional service plus home visits by a volunteer community care worker. The third group was included as a control for the additional social contact by the rehabilitation officer. There was a wide range of outcome measures but, contrary to expectations, there was no benefit observed for the enhanced intervention group on any of the outcome measures. A trial involving 126 patients seen in outpatient clinics run by the US Department of Veterans' Affairs[37] demonstrated substantial improvement in self-reported visual functioning following ten hours of rehabilitation. Low-vision patients enrolled in a health-promotion programme[38] (n = 62) maintained independence in activities of daily living better than a control group (n = 69) despite a decline in general health in both groups. In a study of 154 patients with AMD[39] those who viewed an educational and motivational video exhibited better knowledge of their condition and were more likely to use books on tape than those who did not. And finally, a study of 96 patients with low vision from various causes[c] reported less difficulty with everyday visual tasks following a single visit to an optometry-led low-vision clinic

---

[c] Pearce E, Crossland M, Rubin G. The efficacy of low-vision device training in a hospital-based low-vision service. *Br J Ophthalmol*; in press.

than before. There is almost no evidence from controlled trials on the effectiveness of vision rehabilitation for children or adults of working age.

A question of primary interest to policy planners is how extensive does the rehabilitation service have to be? Is a one- or two-session consultation sufficient or do patients need to be seen on multiple occasions by a multidisciplinary team? Evidence from one small study in Sweden[40] suggests that low-vision patients with AMD require intensive training over the course of multiple sessions to make effective use of prescribed LVAs. However, a subsequent study in the UK[36] found that multiple consultations did not improve the effectiveness of the rehabilitation for patients with AMD. Another study found that there was no additional benefit from added low-vision device training as compared with a single visit to an optometrist-based low-vision service. Overall, the evidence for the effectiveness of various models of vision rehabilitation is not strong. Larger trials are required and the diverse causes of visual impairment need to be considered. In addition, there is continued concern about the best way to measure effectiveness.[41] Should it be based on the performance of study participants (e.g. measured reading speed), self-reported difficulty with everyday tasks (e.g. the Massof Activity Inventory)[42] or a combination of both? Even less evidence is available for the effectiveness of non-optometric low-vision interventions such as orientation and mobility training.[43]

12.5.2 Evidence for use of low-vision aids

Similarly, there are wide discrepancies in the reported use of prescribed low-vision aids, such as magnifiers. Some studies report that 80% to 90% of patients find the devices useful for everyday activities, while others indicate that the majority of patients stop using the devices within 18 months. There are many published studies on the benefits of particular LVAs, but most of these are based on patient preference.

The average cost of ready-made optical LVAs for near-vision tasks (hand-held, and stand- or spectacle-mounted magnifiers) is less than Sterling £50 (about US$70). Custom-made devices and aids for distance tasks can cost Sterling £100–£300 (about US$150–$460). However, many patients who require high magnification and enhanced contrast might benefit from electronic LVAs if they were readily available. One of the first high-tech LVAs was the closed circuit TV magnifier, introduced in the 1960s. In recent years there has been a rapid increase in the number and complexity of high-tech LVAs. Publicly funded low-vision services are reluctant to prescribe high-tech LVAs, as their cost, typically more than US$2,000 (about Sterling £1,300), is a drain on already scarce resources. In addition, high-tech LVAs require more extensive training for them to be used successfully. The cost of additional training is another disincentive to prescribing them. Again, there are few data on the effectiveness of high-tech LVAs as compared with conventional optical devices. One study[44] compared user preferences for a high-tech autofocus telescope with conventional low-vision telescopes. Although the participants preferred the autofocus instrument, the conventional devices provided better resolution and field of view, two of the most important design specifications for telescopic LVAs.

12.6   GLOBAL ISSUES

The picture presented so far of a low-vision population that is predominately elderly, with difficulty in reading because of AMD, and with access (albeit limited) to a wide range of low-vision rehabilitation services, ignores the majority of those throughout the world who have low vision. Worldwide data on low vision are scarce, but statistics compiled by the World Health Organization[45] indicate that there are about 161 million visually impaired people worldwide, 37 million of whom meet the WHO definition for blindness (acuity worse than 3/60) and 124 million of whom are moderately to severely impaired (acuity less than 6/18 to 3/60) (see Chapter 1). The leading cause of bilateral blindness worldwide is cataract, which accounts for almost half of all blindness in developing nations compared with less than 5% in established market economies. Other diseases such as trachoma, onchocerciasis and visual impairment due to corneal opacity, including vitamin A deficiency, account for a substantial proportion of those with low vision in developing nations in Africa, Asia, and the Middle East. As much of the vision loss is preventable or treatable, the main emphasis of the international eye care community is rightly focused on improving access to treatment rather than rehabilitation.

There are many obstacles to providing low-vision services in developing nations. Some countries lack the infrastructure for visual rehabilitation, having concentrated instead on services for the blind. India, for example, with an enormous burden of low vision due to cataract, has a long history of providing education and rehabilitation services for the blind. But only recently has India begun to train practitioners for low-vision services and to develop local resources for LVAs. China, with an estimated ten million visually impaired people,[46] has had to rely on either imported LVAs or locally produced devices made of optical glass which are more expensive and less well suited to LVA design than modern plastics. Latin America is faced with a bimodal distribution of people with low vision: young people affected by congenital disorders, ROP and parasitic diseases, particularly toxoplasmosis, and the elderly affected by cataract and AMD. Government services are aimed primarily at the blind while those with low vision must depend on scarce university-based services and private agencies. Low-vision services are available in few parts of Africa.[47] Recent efforts have included the training of low-vision therapists following a Swedish model, and the work of Christoffel-Blindenmission of Germany and Sight Savers of Great Britain to develop low-vision services and set up local manufacturing of LVAs. But for these efforts to have the maximum benefit, more epidemiological research is needed on the types of visual disability that most affect those with ocular disorders and the relative effectiveness of different models of low-vision care and LVAs.

12.7   FUTURE RESEARCH NEEDS

In contrast to the extensive epidemiological data on visual impairment, there are major gaps in our understanding of visual disability (low vision). As in all areas of rehabilitation, the relationship between impairment and disability is not simple. Current estimates of visual impairment, based almost exclusively on visual acuity criteria, miss important components of vision loss that can lead to difficulty with everyday tasks. On the other hand, some of those who are deemed visually impaired appear to manage everyday tasks without difficulty and would not be considered to have low vision. There are many types of low-vision rehabilitation services that compete for scarce resources. Yet there are few studies of their effectiveness on which to base healthcare policy decisions. It is hoped that as we become more aware of the distinction between visual impairment and low vision, the gaps in our knowledge will diminish. It is important to stress that there is virtually no information on the epidemiology of low vision in less industrialized countries, and imperative that additional resources and research be devoted to these problems in these areas as they bear the major part of the worldwide burden of visual disability.

REFERENCES

1. World Health Organization. *International Classification of Impairments, Disabilities, and Handicaps: a Manual of Classification Relating to the Consequences of Disease.* Geneva: WHO; 1980.

2. World Health Organization. *International Classification of Functioning, Disability and Health (ICF).* Geneva: WHO; 2001.

3. Munoz B, West SK, Rubin GS, *et al.* Causes of blindness and visual impairment in a population of older Americans: the Salisbury Eye Evaluation Study. *Arch Ophthalmol* 2000; 118:819–825.

4. Munoz B, West SK, Rodriguez J, *et al.* Blindness, visual impairment and the problem of uncorrected refractive error in a Mexican-American population: Proyecto VER. *Invest Ophthalmol Vis Sci* 2002; 43: 608–614.

5. Wong TY, Chong EW, Wong WL, *et al.* Prevalence and causes of low vision and blindness in an urban Malay population: the Singapore Malay Eye Study. *Arch Ophthalmol* 2008; 126:1091–1099.

6. Rubenstein RS, Lohr KN, Brook RH, *et al*. *Conceptualization and Measurement of Physiologic Health for Adults: Vision Impairments*. Santa Monica, CA: The Rand Corporation; 1982.

7. Kirchner C, Peterson R. *The Latest Data on Visual Disability from NCHS*. New York: American Foundation for the Blind; 1985.

8. Lighthouse International, Louis Harris and Associates. *The Lighthouse National Survey on Vision Loss*. New York: Lighthouse International; 1995.

9. Salive ME, Guralnik J, Christen W, *et al*. Functional blindness and visual impairment in older adults from three communities. *Ophthalmology* 1992; 99: 1840–1847.

10. Weih L, McCarty CA, Taylor HR. Functional implications of vision impairment. *Clin Exp Ophthalmol* 2000; 28:153–155.

11. Rubin GS, Bandeen-Roche K, Huang GH, *et al*. The association of multiple visual impairments with self-reported visual disability: SEE project. *Invest Ophthalmol Vis Sci* 2001; 42:64–72.

12. Frick KD, Melia BM, Buhrmann RR, *et el*. Trichiasis and disability in a trachoma-endemic area of Tanzania. *Arch Ophthalmol* 2001; 119:1839–1844.

13. Rahi JS, Cumberland PM, Peckham CS. Visual impairment and vision-related quality of life in working-age adults: findings in the 1958 British birth cohort. *Ophthalmology* 2009; 116:270–274.

14. Frost NA, Sparrow JM, Hopper CD, *et al*. Reliability of the VCM1 Questionnaire when administered by post and by telephone. *Ophthalmic Epidemiol* 2001; 8:1–11.

15. Brezin AP, Lafuma A, Fagnani F, *et al*. Prevalence and burden of self-reported blindness, low vision, and visual impairment in the French community: a nation-wide survey. *Arch Ophthalmol* 2005; 123:1117–1124.

16. West SK, Rubin GS, Broman AT, *et al*. How does visual impairment affect performance on tasks of everyday life? The SEE Project. Salisbury Eye Evaluation. *Arch Ophthalmol* 2002; 120:774–780.

17. Friedman SM, Munoz B, Rubin GS, *et al*. Characteristics of discrepancies between self-reported visual function and measured reading speed. Salisbury Eye Evaluation Project Team. *Invest Ophthalmol Vis Sci* 1999; 40:858–864.

18. Leat SJ, Legge G, Bullimore D. What is low vision? A re-evaluation of definitions. *Optom Vis Sci* 1999; 76:198–211.

19. Rubin GS, Legge GE. Psychophysics of reading. VI. The role of contrast in low vision. *Vision Res* 1989; 29:79–91.

20. West SK, Muñoz B, Rubin GS, *et al*. Function and visual impairment in a population-based study of older adults: SEE Project. *Invest Ophthalmol Vis Sci* 1997; 38:72–82.

21. Mangione CM, Phillips RS, Seddon JM, *et al*. Development of the 'Activities of Daily Vision Scale': a measure of visual functional status. *Medical Care* 1992; 30:1111–1126.

22. Brabyn J, Schneck M, Haegerstrom-Portnoy G, *et al*. The Smith-Kettlewell Institute (SKI) longitudinal study of vision function and its impact among the elderly: an overview. *Optom Vis Sci* 2001; 78:264–269.

23. Leat SJ, Rumney NJ. The experience of a university-based low vision clinic. *Ophthalmic Physiol Opt* 1990; 10:8–15.

24. Elliot DB, Trukolo-Ilic M, Strong JG, *et al*. Demographic characteristics of the vision-disabled elderly. *Invest Ophthalmol Vis Sci* 1997; 38:2566–2575.

25. Rahmani B, Tielsch JM, Katz J, *et al*. The cause-specific prevalence of visual impairment in an urban population. The Baltimore Eye Survey. *Ophthalmology* 1996; 103:1721–1726.

26. Attebo K, Mitchell P, Smith W. Visual acuity and the causes of visual loss in Australia. The Blue Mountains Eye Study. *Ophthalmology* 1996; 103: 357–364.

27. Klaver CC, Wolfs RC, Vingerling JR, *et al*. Age-specific prevalence and causes of blindness and visual impairment in an older population: the Rotterdam Study. *Arch Ophthalmol* 1998; 116:653–658.

28. Buch H, Vinding T, Nielsen NV. Prevalence and causes of visual impairment according to World Health Organization and United States criteria in an aged, urban Scandinavian population: the Copenhagen City Eye Study. *Ophthalmology* 2001; 108:2347–2357.

29. VanNewkirk MR, Weih L, McCarty CA, *et al*. Cause-specific prevalence of bilateral visual impairment in Victoria, Australia: the Visual Impairment Project. *Ophthalmology* 2001; 108:960–967.

30. Orr P, Barron Y, Schein OD, *et al*. Eye care utilization by older Americans: the SEE Project. Salisbury Eye Evaluation. *Ophthalmology* 1999; 106:904–909.

31. Ryan B, Culham L. *Fragmented vision. Survey of low vision services in the UK*. London: Royal National

Institute for the Blind and Moorfields Eye Hospital NHS Trust; 1999.

32. Verbrugge LM, Patrick DL. Seven chronic conditions: their impact on US adults' activity levels and use of medical services. *Am J Public Health* 1995; 85:173–182.

33. Brody BL, Williams RA, Thomas RG, *et al*. Age-related macular degeneration: a randomized clinical trial of a self- management intervention. *Ann Behav Med* 1999; 21:322–329.

34. Rubin G. Vision rehabilitation. In: Wormald R, Smeeth L, Henshaw K, (eds). *Evidence-Based Ophthalmology*. London: BMJ Books; 2004: pp. 395–399.

35. Hooper P, Jutai JW, Strong G, *et al*. Age-related macular degeneration and low-vision rehabilitation: a systematic review. *Can J Ophthalmol* 2008; 43:180–187.

36. Russell W, Harper R, Reeves B, *et al*. Randomised controlled trial of an integrated versus an optometric low vision rehabilitation service for patients with age-related macular degeneration: study design and methodology. *Ophthalmic Physiol Opt* 2001; 21:36–44.

37. Stelmack JA, Tang XC, Reda DJ, *et al*. Outcomes of the Veterans Affairs Low Vision Intervention Trial (LOVIT). *Arch Ophthalmol* 2008; 126:608–617.

38. Eklund K, Sjostrand J, Dahlin-Ivanoff S. A randomized controlled trial of a health-promotion programme and its effect on ADL dependence and self-reported health problems for the elderly visually impaired. *Scand J Occup Ther* 2008; 15:68–74.

39. Goldstein RB, Dugan E, Trachtenberg F, *et al*. The impact of a video intervention on the use of low vision assistive devices. *Optom Vis Sci* 2007; 84:208–217.

40. Nilsson UL. Visual rehabilitation with and without educational training in the use of optical aids and residual vision. A prospective study of patients with advanced age-related macular degeneration. *Clin Vision Sci* 1990; 6:3–10.

41. Reeves BC, Harper RA, Russell WB. Enhanced low vision rehabilitation for people with age related macular degeneration: a randomised controlled trial. *Br J Ophthalmol* 2004; 88:1443–1449.

42. Massof RW, Hsu CT, Baker FH, *et al*. Visual disability variables. I: the importance and difficulty of activity goals for a sample of low-vision patients. *Arch Phys Med Rehabil* 2005; 86:946–953.

43. Virgili G, Rubin G. Orientation and mobility training for adults with low vision. *Cochrane Database Syst Rev* 2006; 3:CD003925.

44. Greene HA, Pekar J, Brilliant R, *et al*. The Ocutech Vision Enhancing System (VES): utilization and preference study. *J Am Optom Assoc* 1991; 62:19–26.

45. Resnikoff S, Pascolini D, Etya'ale D, *et al*. Global data on visua impairment in the year 2002. *Bull World Health Organ* 2004; 82:844–851.

46. Johnston A, Goodrich GL. Vision rehabilitation services in Asia, the Pacific, and the Middle East. In: Goodrich GL, (ed). *The Lighthouse Handbook on Vision Impairment and Vision Rehabilitation*. New York: Oxford University Press; 2000: pp. 733–50.

47. Backman O. Vision Rehabilitation services in Europe and Africa. In: Silverstone B, Lang MA, Rosenthal BP, *et al*. (eds). *The Lighthouse Book on Vision Impairment and Vision Rehabilitation*. New York: Oxford University Press; 2000: pp. 751–61.

13

Glaucoma

PAUL FOSTER AND HARRY QUIGLEY

13.1	Definition	241
13.2	Classification	243
13.3	Prevalence	245
13.4	Geographical distribution of primary glaucoma	248
13.5	Incidence	251
13.6	Risk factors for primary glaucoma	253

13.7	Genetics of glaucoma	257
13.8	Clinical trials informing glaucoma management	258
13.9	Possibilities for screening	259
13.10	Summary of epidemiological research priorities	261
	References	261

13.1 DEFINITION

The estimated prevalence and incidence of any condition depend on the criteria used to define the disease. A clear definition is similarly essential for epidemiological studies of risk factors. As a result of the difficulties experienced with determining the presence or absence of glaucoma in population-based prevalence surveys, ophthalmic epidemiologists with an interest in glaucoma met at the **International Society for Geographic and Epidemiologic Ophthalmology (ISGEO)** congress in Amsterdam in 1998, to arrive at a proposed definition and classification for the glaucomas.[1] Glaucoma was defined by this group as an optic neuropathy, characterized by specific structural findings in the optic disc, and particular functional deficits in automated visual field testing. This concept of 'end organ damage' provides a uniform definition across the different mechanisms by which glaucoma is caused.

Glaucoma was formerly regarded solely as the result of an abnormally high **intraocular pressure (IOP)**. A number of prevalence surveys (described below) showed that, in some populations, the majority of those with open-angle glaucoma have IOP that is typically within the normal range ($\leq$ mean IOP ± 2 SDs). These observations have influenced the development of theories on the aetiology of glaucomatous optic neuropathy, and have removed the artificial dichotomy inherent in past use of the term 'normal tension glaucoma'. Although IOP is an important risk factor for glaucoma, it is no longer regarded as a defining characteristic of the disease. Studies of glaucoma should treat IOP as a continuous variable in risk factor or clinical studies, without the use of arbitrary and potentially counterproductive dividing lines.

13.1.1 Structural features of glaucomatous optic neuropathy

The features that differentiate glaucomatous damage from other causes of optic neuropathy are the result of loss of neural tissue, and posterior bowing of the connective tissue that comprises the lamina cribrosa.[2] These changes result in the excavated appearance of the disc (Plate 13.1). The **vertical cup–disc ratio (VCDR)** has proved to be a simple, relatively robust, index of glaucomatous loss of the neuroretinal rim. VCDR is usually expressed in units of 0.1 (from 0 to 1.0) with median values within many populations of 0.3 to 0.4. In using VCDR to differentiate between normal and disease status, it is necessary to specify the value which indicates the boundary between the two states. Invoking the statistical convention that a probability of less than 5% represents significant deviation from 'normal', and assuming this 5% split equally between higher and lower values (i.e. 2.5% of the values are abnormally large) the 97.5th percentile for the VCDRs of the normal population represents the 'upper limit of normal'. The 2.5% lying above this can be regarded as statistically different, and potentially diseased. However, if this were the only criterion for diagnosing disease, 2.5% of the normal population would be categorized as diseased. This is clearly not appropriate. By requiring that this anatomical abnormality occurring by chance in less than 2.5% of normal people (a VCDR ≥ 97.5th percentile) must be present in combination with another abnormal feature of glaucoma, the diagnosis is made statistically more secure.

The logical choice of this 'additional feature' is a functional deficit in vision — a visual field abnormality (see below). The 97.5th percentile for the VCDR may vary to some extent between different populations, but from the evidence available so far, a figure of 0.7 applies in all ethnic groups.[3] Variation in optic disc size will lead to interindividual variation.[4] However, some people are unable to complete a visual field test because of impaired vision. Thus, to include this group, structural criteria alone at a more stringent level were adopted, i.e. the 99.5th percentile of VCDR was taken as indicative of glaucoma. The 99.5th percentile for VCDR varies between 0.7 and 0.85 in different data sets, but > 0.8 has been proposed as the standard figure. Similar conventions were applied to asymmetry between the VCDRs of the two eyes, when the 97.5th percentile of the distribution of the differences is approximately 0.2, the 99.5th percentile is 0.3. The inclusion of the asymmetry criterion, and the option of using a

reduction of the neuroretinal rim width to < 0.1 of disc diameter, in large part mitigate the effect of variation of disc size: small discs may not meet the first VCDR criterion but be classified as abnormal on the basis of asymmetry or neuroretinal rimwidth assessment. It should be noted that, given a normal visual field, none of these features alone would suffice to confirm a diagnosis of glaucoma.

13.1.2 Functional damage

By common consensus,[1] either an abnormal glaucoma hemifield test, or a reproducible cluster of three points on a Zeiss–Humphrey Field Analyzer plot (threshold programme, 24-2 test pattern) abnormal at the 5% level and of typical glaucomatous distribution, is the threshold at which a field abnormality is considered proven. If the performance at each point is independent of the others (which it is not), this situation would occur by chance in 1/10,000 people. Combining this (a psychophysical defect) with an anatomical abnormality makes a diagnosis of glaucoma by chance so improbable as to be negligible in studies of thousands of people. There should be no alternative explanation for the field deficit (for example, a retinal vein occlusion or area of chorioretinal scarring). This test strategy is the basis for most ophthalmological research in the fields of glaucoma epidemiology and clinical trials of management.

13.1.3 Levels of evidence

According to the ISGEO definitional structure, glaucomatous nerve damage is present when an eye has both structural changes and a visual field defect meeting the above criteria. However, in any population-based study there will be some individuals in whom a visual field test cannot be satisfactorily performed, and others in whom the optic nerve head cannot be visualized. It is therefore suggested that cases of glaucoma would be defined according to three levels of evidence (Table 13.1). This classification is hierarchical. If possible, the disease status is determined by level 1 evidence. If this is proven to be absent (i.e. the disc criteria are met, but the

Table 13.1 *Levels of evidence for diagnosis of glaucoma in cross-sectional surveys*

Level	Evidence
1	The highest level of evidence requires optic disc abnormalities (VCDR or VCDR asymmetry > 97.5th percentile of the normal population) plus a visual field defect compatible with glaucoma.
2	A severely damaged disc (VCDR > 99.5th percentile of the normal population) would be sufficient if a reliable visual field test were not obtainable.
3	If optic disc not visualized, an IOP exceeding the 99.5th percentile of normal or evidence of previous filtering surgery.

IOP — intraocular pressure; VCDR — vertical cup–disc ratio

visual field is normal), the disease is absent. However, if disease status according to level 1 criteria cannot be determined, the case is evaluated on level 2 (disc only) criteria. If the media are opaque, and the disc be seen adequately, level 3 criteria (poor vision and raised IOP, or a poor vision and a history of glaucoma surgery) may be used.

Indeed, reflecting the problems in the requirement that both structural and functional abnormalities be used as the defining characteristics of glaucoma, clinical trials frequently report cases that progress on the basis of either structural or functional criteria. Even in clinical trials spanning years of follow-up of patients with primary open-angle glaucoma (POAG), numbers with progression in both structural and functional characteristics are invariably small, which reflects the slowly progressive nature of this disease in most cases.

13.2   CLASSIFICATION

There exist many approaches to classification. The most widely used employs the concept of primary and secondary disease. '**Primary**' implies unknown aetiology, whereas '**secondary**' denotes glaucoma developing as a consequence of another, recognizable ocular, regional or systemic disease. Primary cases are typically bilateral but asymmetrical, while secondary disease is largely unilateral. However, with the advance of the study of the genetics of

glaucoma, the molecular pathology associated with around 5% of all cases of primary open-angle glaucoma can be attributed to genetic factors. Hence, the label of 'primary' glaucoma is more usefully regarded as indicating the absence of another clinically recognised disease process (see Genetics, Section 13.8 below).

The division between **infantile** (manifesting within the first year of life), **juvenile** (developing prior to the onset of secondary sexual characteristics) and **adult** is useful in identifying cases with similar modes of presentation, prognosis and need for treatment. These distinctions have both clinical and public health significance, since the likelihood of surgical intervention is greater in younger patients, and in general, both the surgery and the rehabilitation are more complex, costly and challenging.

13.2.1   The importance of gonioscopy

It was well into the 20th century before early models of the gonioscope allowed ophthalmologists to examine the angle between corneal endothelium and the root of the iris, the area containing the trabecular meshwork, which provides access to the outflow route draining aqueous humour from the eye. They recognized that in some glaucomatous eyes the angle of the anterior chamber appeared obstructed, while in others it was open. In 1938, Otto Barkan of San Francisco proposed that glaucoma be divided into one type with a deep anterior chamber and an open angle, and a second type with a shallow anterior chamber. Closed angles were thought to form an anatomical obstruction to aqueous outflow responsible for a rise in intraocular pressure.[5]

Barkan suggested the terms 'wide-angle' and 'narrow-angle', which subsequently became the **open-angle** and **closed-angle** (or angle-closure) glaucomas. This division is important because the two types differ in geographical distribution, risk factors and management. Unfortunately, many published papers on the prevalence and distribution of glaucoma have failed to make the distinction clearly.

Gonioscopic examination is a dynamic process, and its interpretation depends on the pressure applied to the gonio-lens and the level of illumination. It requires considerable skill and experience. Several systems for describing the angle are in use, typically estimating the width, and representing this by a number. The most widely used are the Shaffer and the Spaeth systems, the latter having a more detailed grading of three features: the level of iris insertion, the angular width and the profile of the peripheral iris.[6] None of the currently used systems has been shown by longitudinal study to accurately predict the development of angle-closure glaucoma in those with narrow appearing angles.

At present gonioscopic grading is a subjective procedure. The introduction of imaging techniques, such as **ultrasound biomicroscopy (UBM)** and **anterior segment optical coherence tomography (AS-OCT)**, offers an alternative to clinical techniques, such as gonioscopy, in the assessment of the width of the drainage angle. UBM, in particular, offers an insight into the mechanisms responsible for closure of the angle. However, this comes at the expense of a time-consuming, messy and rather unpleasant examination. AS-OCT offers a more user-friendly alternative approach. Questions remain to be answered about the reason for discrepancies between AS-OCT and gonioscopy.[7] It is possible that AS-OCT is a superior method of identifying irido-trabecular contact. It is also possible that the calibration of the OCT device leads to erroneous image processing in some cases. This remains to be resolved. The appearance of the angle is now known to depend critically on the pupil size and, hence, on lighting conditions and age, and this may explain the variability seen in past studies that utilized any of the subjective or objective methods.

13.2.2 Primary angle-closure and narrow angles

Individuals with either raised IOP or **peripheral anterior synechiae (PAS)** as a consequence of primary irido-trabecular contact, but without damage to the optic nerve head, are classified as having **primary angle-closure (PAC)**. Primary angle-closure glaucoma is diagnosed when these features are combined with structural and functional damage to the optic nerve. If there is iridotrabecular contact, but no pathological features (increased IOP, abnormal disc or field, and no evidence of PAS), the condition is termed **primary angle-closure suspect (PACS)** (Table 13.2).[1] Those with such evidence that their narrow angle has caused initial disorder are called PAC, while those combining narrow angle and glaucomatous damage are denoted **primary angle-closure glaucoma (PACG)**. This does not imply that persons with PAC do not require treatment, but differentiates between those with and without visual dysfunction resulting from glaucomatous optic neuropathy. Symptoms are a poor guide to the presence of angle-closure disease. Although the 'classic' constellation of symptoms of discomfort, redness, and blurring of vision do occur in some cases (used to identify intermittent angle-closure), these symptoms also occur quite often in people with no evidence of angle-closure.[8] Consequently, classifications of angle-closure disease that describe the symptomatology of the condition are too non-specific to be helpful. At all stages of disease, physical signs are a better guide to diagnosis of angle-closure.

Table 13.2 *Classification of primary angle-closure*

Classification	Definition
1	Primary angle-closure suspect (PACS, occludable angle). An eye in which appositional contact between the peripheral iris and posterior trabecular meshwork is considered possible. In epidemiological studies this has most often been defined as an angle in which >270° of the posterior (pigmented) trabecular meshwork cannot be seen.
2	Primary angle-closure (PAC). An eye with an occludable drainage angle and features indicating that trabecular obstruction by the peripheral iris has occurred, such as peripheral anterior synechiae, elevated IOP, iris whorling (distortion of the radially orientated iris fibres), 'glaucomflecken' lens opacities, or excessive pigment deposition on the trabecular surface. The eye does not have glaucomatous optic nerve damage. Those who have had acute attacks without residual optic nerve damage are included here.
3	Primary angle-closure glaucoma (PACG). PAC together with evidence of glaucomatous optic neuropathy.

IOP — intraocular pressure

13.2.3   Primary open-angle glaucoma

Primary open-angle glaucoma (POAG) is present in a person in whom at least one eye has optic nerve damage, meeting any of the three levels of evidence (Table 13.1) without evidence of angle-closure on gonioscopy, and with no identifiable cause to which the glaucoma is secondary.

13.2.4   Secondary glaucoma

Secondary glaucoma typically results when ocular disorders cause IOP to rise significantly above the normal. As in primary glaucoma, the condition is defined by a combination of structural and functional defects of the optic nerve that are indistinguishable from POAG and PACG. However, secondary glaucoma is more often unilateral, rapidly progressive and visually destructive, causing a high rate of uniocular blindness, even in countries with access to advanced medical care. The pathological processes that produce the profound IOP rise (e.g. trauma, uveitis, and neovascularization), damage other ocular structures in addition to retinal ganglion cells and their axons. Many eyes with secondary glaucoma have opaque media, which preclude optic disc and visual field examinations. Their glaucoma is defined by any of the three levels of evidence previously described (Table 13.1).

Opinions differ as to whether people with glaucoma associated with pigment dispersion syndrome or exfoliation syndrome should be classified as primary open-angle glaucoma or as secondary. In the presentation of prevalence and geographical distribution below, they are classified as secondary glaucoma for studies that denoted them separately.

13.2.5   Infantile glaucoma (see Chapter 14f)

Congenital glaucoma develops in early life. This is typically regarded as meaning an onset within the first year of life. However, physical signs may take longer to manifest. Any case of glaucoma in the under-fives, should be regarded as probably congenital until proven otherwise. Despite its relative rarity (1/10,000 births in industrialized nations, 1/1,000 birth in nations with high rates of consanguineous marriage), congenital glaucoma is important because of the years of life affected if there is significant loss of vision. The intensity and complexity (and hence the cost) of treatment, and the relatively poor prognosis are other unfortunate features of this condition. Specialized surgical techniques and intensive, multidisciplinary after-care are needed if vision is to be retained. Genetic causes for congenital glaucoma are increasingly being recognised. Overall, the risk of a second child being affected is far greater than random chance. While it is logical to counsel parents regarding this risk, no study has evaluated the optimal approach to this highly culture-dependent interaction.

13.3   PREVALENCE

13.3.1   Prevalence of glaucoma

The first survey of glaucoma prevalence in a defined population carried out to 'modern standards' was conducted by Hollows and Graham in the Rhondda Valley, South Wales, UK. The key advance compared with previous population studies was placing the emphasis of a diagnosis of glaucoma on the structural characteristics of the optic nerve, combined with abnormalities of the visual field. IOP was not used as a defining feature of the disease.[9] Since then, there have been many population-based studies of prevalence of glaucoma (Table 13.3). Until the introduction of the ISGEO criteria for diagnosis of glaucoma in epidemiological research, there was considerable variability in the criteria used to identify cases. Additional problems with varying methodology and overall data quality have led to significant problems with making meaningful comparisons between studies of glaucoma prevalence. Wolfs and colleagues used the diagnostic criteria employed in different studies of glaucoma prevalence (Baltimore, Barbados, Beaver Dam, Blue Mountains, Egna-Neumarkt, Framingham,

Table 13.3 *Glaucoma prevalence surveys by racial groups*

Racial Group (%)	Year of publication	Location	Age range	PACG (%)	POAG (%)	Secondary glaucoma	Reference
African	2000	Kongwa, Tanzania	40+	0.59	3.1	0.15[a]	[11]
	2002	Hlabisa, South Africa	40+	0.1	2.7	1.7	[12]
African origin	1969	Jamaica	35–74	Nil	1.4	0.35	[13]
	1989	St Lucia	30+	Nil[a]	8.8	A few[b]	[14]
	1991	Baltimore, MD, USA	40+	0.67[c]	4.74[d]	1.42[c]	[15]
	1994	Barbados	40–84	Not stated	7.1[c]	Not stated	[16]
East Asian and Asian origin	1973	Umanaq, Greenland	>40	4.8	1.26	1.00	[17]
	1987	Alaska, USA	40+	2.65	0.24	Nil	[18]
	1988	Alaska, USA	40+	3.8	Nil	Not stated	[19]
	1989	Beijing, China	40+	1.4	0.03	Not stated	[20]
	1991	Japan	40+	0.34	2.62	0.48	[21]
	1996	Taiwan	40+	3.0	Not stated	Not stated	[22]
	1996	Hövsgöl, Mongolia	40+	1.4	0.5	0.3	[23]
	2000	Singapore	40–79	1.14	1.79	0.57[f]	[24]
Indian	1999	Hyderabad, India	30+	0.71[d]	1.62[d]	0.21	[25,26]
			40+	1.08[d]	2.56[d]	0.11	
European origin	1966	Ferndale, Wales, UK	40–74	0.09	0.43	0.26	[9]
	1980	Framingham, MA, USA	52–85	Not stated	1.9	Not stated	[27]
	1981	Dalby, Sweden	55–69	Nil	0.86	0.34	[28]
	1991	Middle Norway	65+	Not stated	3.37	4.97[g]	[29]
	1991	Baltimore, MD, USA	40+	0.31[c]	1.29[d]	0.68[c]	[15]
	1992	Beaver Dam, WI, USA	43–84	0.04	2.1	Not stated	[30]
	1994	Roscommon, Ireland	50+	0.09	1.88	0.41	[31]
	1994	Rotterdam, Netherlands	55+	Nil	1.1	Nil	[32]
	1996	Blue Mountains, Australia	49+	0.27	3.0	0.15	[33]
	1997	Ponza, Italy	40+	0.97	2.51	0.29	[34]
	1998	Egna-Neumarkt, Italy	40+	0.6	2.0[h]	0.3	[35]
	1998	Melbourne, Australia	40+	0.1	1.7	0.2	[36]
Hispanic mixed origin	2001	Tucson+Nogales, AZ, USA	40+	0.1	1.97	0.02	[37]
	1993	Mamre, South Africa	40+	2.3	1.5	0.81	[38]

[a] Further 0.34% 'undetermined' not listed here; [b] personal communication, J. Martone; [c] personal communication, J. Tielsch; [d] adjusted rate; [e] other glaucoma (not specified) 0.7%; [f] further two cases (0.16%) 'unclassifiable'; [g] includes patients with exfoliation syndrome; [h] definition of POAG included exfoliation glaucoma. PACG, primary angle-closure glaucoma; POAG, primary open-angle glaucoma.

Melbourne, Ponza and Rotterdam), and applied them to the same dataset (the Rotterdam Eye Study). This showed that solely by varying the diagnostic criteria, the calculated prevalence varied tenfold.[3] This powerfully underlines the importance of using standardized definitions in the comparison of glaucoma prevalence, and in assessing the impact of risk factors.

A major step forwards in identifying underlying differences in glaucoma prevalence came with the publication of pooled-data analyses of glaucoma prevalence data in 1996 and 2006 by Quigley and colleagues.[10] Data from glaucoma prevalence studies were included if the study met criteria relating to sampling strategy, response rate, and minimum standards of examination methodology. In the 2006 paper, 2,158 publications were considered. Of this number, 34 were included in the model. Key findings were that by 2010, 60 million people are affected by glaucomatous optic neuropathy

Table 13.4 *Number of persons with OAG and ACG combined, 2010[10]*

World region	Total glaucoma	lower CL	upper CL	Total pop > 40	Ratio glaucoma to pop > 40 (%)	lower CL (%)	upper CL (%)
China	15,782,196	11,114,702	23,640,340	593,278,000	2.66	1.87	3.98
Europe	12,064,740	8,910,048	16,475,405	541,993,000	2.23	1.64	3.04
India	11,944,896	9,443,597	15,447,556	468,426,000	2.55	2.02	3.30
Africa	6,458,023	5,227,245	7,979,655	149,408,000	4.32	3.50	5.34
LatAmer	5,677,158	3,252,201	10,035,372	169,215,000	3.35	1.92	5.93
SE Asia	4,257,620	2,990,848	6,432,503	178,899,000	2.38	1.67	3.60
Japan	2,662,446	2,278,345	3,154,376	72,007,000	3.70	3.16	4.38
MidEast	1,618,718	1,171,439	2,268,907	110,094,000	1.47	1.06	2.06
World	60,465,796	44,388,425	85,434,114	2,283,320,000	2.65	1.94	3.74

(Table 13.4). Three quarters of these people (74%) have open-angle glaucoma (OAG) (Table 13.5 and Fig. 13.1). Women are disproportionately strongly affected, comprising 55% of OAG, 70% of ACG and 59% of all glaucoma. In line with the number of people living in different regions, Asians are the numerically largest group affected, constituting 47% of the total with all types of glaucoma, and 87% of PACG in the world (Table 13.6 and Fig. 13.2). The absolute number of people affected is projected to rise in line with increasing longevity worldwide. By 2020, it is expected that the number of people affected by glaucoma will have risen to 80 million (i.e. an increase of 25% in a decade). Numerically, this rise will have the greatest impact in the large, rapidly industrialising nations of Asia: China and India.[10]

> The relative prevalence rates of POAG and PACG vary markedly between populations.
> PACG is much more common in Chinese people (1.5% in people aged > 50 years) than in Europeans, of whom around 0.25% are affected.
> The Japanese have the highest rates of glaucoma occurring within the statistically normal range of IOP for their population. One large study concluded that 92% of open-angle glaucoma occurred with IOP =/< 21 mmHg.[39]
> The prevalence rates of POAG in white Europeans, Americans and Australians are similar when the figures are age-adjusted. Prevalence of POAG in white subjects in the Baltimore, Beaver Dam, Roscommon and Rotterdam studies showed close agreement

Table 13.5 *Number of persons with OAG, 2010[10]*

	Total OAG	lower CL	upper CL	% World OAG
Europe	10,693,335	7,599,188	15,040,703	23.9%
China	8,309,001	6,695,433	10,423,439	18.6%
India	8,211,276	6,812,711	9,937,413	18.4%
Africa	6,212,179	4,992,103	7,722,626	13.9%
LatAmer	5,354,354	2,943,534	9,697,792	12.0%
Japan	2,383,802	2,106,534	2,697,623	5.3%
SE Asia	2,116,036	1,744,523	2,580,354	4.7%
MidEast	1,440,849	1,001,315	2,082,944	3.2%
World	44,720,832	33,895,340	60,182,894	

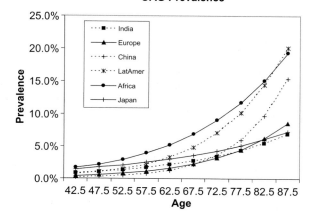

Figure 13.1 *Prevalence of OAG in major ethnic groups[10]*

The prevalence model data showing age-specific prevalence of open-angle glaucoma (OAG) for the six major ethnic groups among whom high quality studies have been performed. Prevalence is highest among the African and Latin American groups.

Table 13.6 *Number of persons with ACG, 2010*[10]

	Total ACG	lower CL	upper CL	% World ACG
China	7,473,195	4,419,269	13,216,902	47.5
India	3,733,620	2,630,886	5,510,142	23.7
SE Asia	2,141,584	1,246,325	3,852,149	13.6
Europe	1,371,405	1,310,861	1,434,702	8.7
LatAmer	322,804	308,667	337,581	2.1
Japan	278,643	171,811	456,753	1.8
Africa	245,844	235,143	257,029	1.6
MidEast	177,869	170,124	185,964	1.1
World	15,744,965	10,493,085	25,251,221	

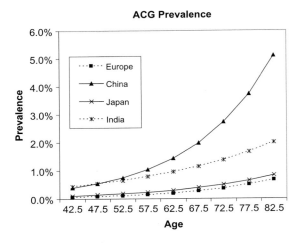

Figure 13.2 *Prevalence of ACG in major ethnic groups*[10]
Prevalence model data for the age-specific prevalence of angle-closure glaucoma (ACG), highest in the China group, second highest among Japanese, and lowest in European and Indian groups.

when age-adjusted to the population of Ponza Island, (2.51, 2.72, 2.82 and 3.06%, respectively) compared with 2.51% (Table 13.3).[34]

➤ Black populations in the Caribbean, East Africa, and the USA have a higher prevalence of POAG than those of European or Asian origin (see Section 13.4).

➤ Data on the prevalence of secondary glaucoma are sparse, poor and vary considerably. The highest rates may reflect particular local circumstances; for example, high frequency of exfoliation syndrome (Norway)[29] or trauma (Mamre, South Africa, where all eight patients identified with secondary glaucoma experienced posttraumatic iris recession).[38] Secondary glaucoma

accounts for approximately 10–15% of all glaucomatous disease in the community.

13.3.2   Prevalence of blindness resulting from glaucoma

Although few surveys report the proportion of glaucoma patients who were blind, the published values vary from none (Dalby, Sweden), through 7.3% (Roscommon, Ireland), 11% (Kongwa, Tanzania), 14% (Singapore), 15% (Mamre, South Africa) to 22% (Hlabisa, South Africa). The 2006 Quigley and Broman study of number of people with glaucoma worldwide described previously also projected the number of people blinded.[40] They calculated that by 2010, 4.5 million people would be blind from OAG, and 3.9 million blind from ACG. By 2020 these figures are set to rise to 5.9 and 5.3 million respectively. Thylefors and Négrel approached the same question by summarizing all available blindness prevalence surveys for which cause-specific data were given. It is interesting that the calculated number of those bilaterally blind from glaucoma is similar to the number derived from glaucoma prevalence surveys available at around the same time.[41,42]

Data from Asia show that PACG and secondary glaucoma cause a greater proportion of blindness than POAG (Fig. 13.3). The key difference between PACG and secondary glaucoma is that the most aggressive forms of secondary glaucoma (uveitic and neovascular) typically lead to severe visual loss in one eye only. In contrast, PACG appears to be a more potent cause of bilateral vision loss. Unlike the leading cause of blindness (cataract), blindness from glaucoma is medically and surgically irreversible.[10]

13.4   GEOGRAPHICAL DISTRIBUTION OF PRIMARY GLAUCOMA

The differences in prevalence rates and predominant types of glaucoma in different populations and geographical areas that are evident in Table 13.3 are intriguing. In Africa, the predominant form of glaucoma is POAG. Among African Americans

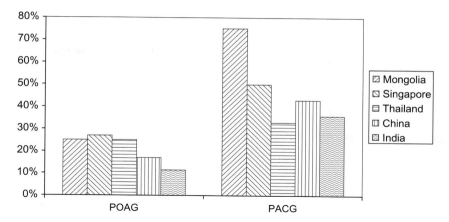

Figure 13.3 *Graph of proportion of blindness from PACG versus POAG. Proportion of uniocular or binocular blindness from open-angle glaucoma and angle-closure glaucoma in five population-based studies in Asia*

living on the Eastern Seaboard of the US, age-adjusted prevalence rates of POAG were four to five times higher as compared with Americans of European origin.[15] The highest prevalence rates for POAG so far reported anywhere are in the black populations of the Caribbean, particularly St Lucia[14] and Barbados.[16] A few population-based surveys focusing on the prevalence and causes of glaucoma in Africans have been published. In addition to the recent results from Kongwa, Tanzania,[11] two surveys were carried out in South Africa, one in a rural Zulu population (Hlabisa),[12] and the other in a mixed urban population (Temba).[43] These three surveys were conducted with similar random sampling methods and contemporary definitions of glaucoma. The prevalence rates of POAG have been adjusted for age and sex by Rotchford to the population of Barbados and compared also with St Lucia and African Americans in Baltimore (Table 13.7).[43] The prevalence rates of POAG in the three populations in Africa itself, which all belong to the Bantu language family, are remarkably similar. The fact that the age-specific prevalence of African-derived persons in Africa and the USA are more similar to each other than to European or Asian populations, despite huge differences in diet, environment, culture and visual experiences, speaks strongly for genetic predispositions that remain to be elucidated.

POAG is also the most prevalent form of glaucoma among European people (Table 13.3).[9,44]

Table 13.7 *Prevalence rates of primary open-angle glaucoma (POAG) in African and African-derived populations*

Location	Sample size (recruitment %)	Cases of POAG	Crude	Prevalence adjusted
St Lucia	1300 (87)	132	10.2 (8.6–11.9)	10.0
Barbados	4498 (84)	302	7.0 (6.3–7.8)	7.3
Baltimore	2395 (84)	100	4.2 (3.0–5.0)	4.4
Tanzania	3268 (90)	100	3.1 (2.5–3.8)	3.6
Temba	839 (75)	31	3.7 (2.5–5.3)	3.5
Hlabisa	1005 (90)	28	2.8 (1.8–4.2)	3.2

A study of prevalence of open angle glaucoma in an older urban Greek population (using non-standardized definitions) reported a similar rate of OAG found in other population-based studies of European people. However, 30% of all OAG was seen in eyes with exfoliation syndrome.[45] Exfoliation syndrome is extremely rare among Chinese people.[46] Data on Chinese people living in urban centres (Singapore and Guangzhou) also indicate similar rates of OAG as those seen in Europeans.[24] A recent population-based study in Tajimi City in Japan confirmed previous data regarding the remarkable difference in glaucoma epidemiology between Japanese people and that seen in almost every other population globally. The prevalence of OAG was 2.62%, with the majority (1.92%) occurring in people with screening pressures of ≤ 21 mmHg. The mean corneal thickness in cases of OAG was similar in people with glaucoma and those without.[39]

The study of glaucoma in South Asia has revealed interesting differences in prevalence between urban and rural areas. POAG in rural Bangladesh occurs in 2.1% of people aged 40 years and older (all subsequent figures apply to this age group).[47] In rural southern India, two studies of populations recorded strikingly similar rates of POAG 1.6% and 1.7% respectively.[48,49] Of people with POAG, 93% had not been previously diagnosed, and one fifth were blind in one or both eyes from glaucoma.[49] In a corresponding urban population (Chennai) POAG prevalence was significantly higher than in the rural area (3.5% versus 1.6%, P < 0.0001).[50] An earlier study of POAG prevalence in urban Hyderabad, also in southern India, gave a relatively high prevalence rate of POAG (2.65%).[26]

Evidence suggests that angle-closure glaucoma occurs in Africans and African-derived persons at rates similar to those found in European-derived persons. Angle-closure glaucoma was identified in 0.6% of black people in Baltimore, USA.[a] In Johannesburg, South Africa, angle-closure was almost as frequent in blacks as in whites living in the same area, although angle-closure was chronic (i.e. asymptomatic) in 66% of black people, compared with 33% in white people. The proportion of glaucoma cases in this clinic series diagnosed with angle-closure was 20% in whites and 17% of black people.[51] Clearly, these proportions may reflect some degree of response bias, with a higher proportion of people with symptomatic angle-closure presenting for medical care as compared with smaller numbers with asymptomatic angle-closure and earlier stages of open-angle glaucoma.

Although the age ranges varied, the prevalence rates of ACG in Wales[9] and Ireland[31] were approximately uniform at 0.1% (10% of the prevalence of OAG). No case of ACG was found in Sweden[28] or Rotterdam.[32] However, the Rotterdam study group did report that 2.2% of the population they examined (aged 55 years and older) had narrow drainage angles, and this rate was twice as high (4.4%) among women. A recent study from

Northern Italy reported a prevalence of angle-closure of 0.6% in people aged 40 years and older.[35] The prevalence of primary angle-closure glaucoma among white people in the Baltimore Eye Study was 0.4% in the same age group.[a] More population-based data from Europe and North America would help to clarify the size of the problem.

Angle-closure glaucoma is more common among the people of Asia than in Africans or Europeans. There is variation in the prevalence in different geographical areas. The highest prevalence rates recorded are from prevalence surveys among the Inuit (Eskimos), with 2.7% and 3.8% of the population affected aged 40 years and older in Alaska,[18,19] 2.9% in the North West Territories of Canada,[40] 3.0% in Labrador[52] and 5.0% in Uummannaq, north-western Greenland.[17]

In India, the population-based study from urban Hyderabad found that cases of POAG outnumbered those of PACG by approximately 2.5 to 1.[26,53] Two more recent population-based studies, both conducted in the southern state of Tamil Nadu, examined glaucoma prevalence in people aged 40 years and older. The first study involved 5,150 people living in the regions surrounding Aravind Eye Hospital. Glaucoma was diagnosed on the basis of structural optic neuropathy with a corresponding visual field defect. PACG was found in 0.5%.[49] The later study in and around the state capital of Chennai used the ISGEO classification system for diagnosing glaucoma. They examined 3,850 people and identified PACG in 32 (0.88%). Only five people (14.7%) had been previously diagnosed with glaucoma, of whom one had undergone glaucoma surgery and two had been diagnosed to have open-angle glaucoma. Prevalence of PACG and PACS were similar in the urban and rural populations. The disease was typically asymptomatic.[54]

From studies of East Asian people aged 40 years and older, PACG rates appear relatively uniform at around 0.6–0.8%.[55,56] In a mainland Chinese population aged 50+ years, He reported a prevalence of 1.5%.[57] Fewer data are available for South East Asians. Previous clinic-based reports of extremely high rates of acute angle-closure in Burma have been lent credence by a report of 2.5% of people aged 40 years and older in rural central Myanmar having PACG, typically associated with acute

---

[a] Tielsch, personal communication 1998.

disease,[58] while in a sub-urban region of Bangkok, PACG was detected in only 0.9% of people aged 50 years and older.[59]

13.5 INCIDENCE

13.5.1 Incidence of POAG (Table 13.8)

To report observed incidence, investigators must conduct a cross-sectional examination of a population, and then a re-examination of the same population after an interval of a number of years. The number of new cases in this time period divided by the total population at risk gives a cumulative incidence. An Australian study and the Barbados Eye Study have also derived five-year incidence figures for POAG. In the predominantly white population of Melbourne in Australia, the overall incidence of definite OAG was 0.5%, probable and definite OAG 1.1%. The incidence of OAG increased significantly as age increased. The incidence of definite OAG increases from 0% of participants aged 40 to 49 years to 4.1% of participants aged ≤ 80 years.[60] Among members of the Barbados Eye Study, the nine-year incidence of definite OAG was 4.4%, or an average of 0.5%/year. Incidence greatly increased with age from 2.2% at ages 40–49 years to 7.9% at ages 70 years or older. The conclusion drawn from this result was that incidence of OAG is markedly higher in black Barbadians than in people of European ancestry.[61] The total number

of new cases on which estimates are based is relatively small, and the extrapolation to other populations is not assured. An alternative to deriving incidence figures from direct observation within a longitudinal study is the use of prevalence data to calculate incidence rates.[62] Using this method, Broman et al. estimated the incidence of OAG in four different racial groups (Fig. 13.4).[64]

Because of the size of the study required and the difficulty and expense of directly observing a cohort over several years, indirect measures or estimates of incidence have been used. Leske and colleagues devised a formula for estimating incidence from age-specific prevalence rates, and applied this method to the data from Ferndale, Wales, and Framingham, Massachusetts, USA.[62] An alternative approach in Olmsted County, Minnesota, USA, gave an incidence of OAG by a retrospective analysis of the medical records of residents known to the health care system.[63] The figures from Sweden may be higher than those from the USA because of presumed greater prevalence of exfoliation glaucoma in Scandinavians, though there exists no standard criterion for this syndrome, and few studies have attempted to categorize POAG subjects into those with and without exfoliation. The method used in Olmsted County (effectively the 'demand incidence') is likely to underestimate considerably the actual number of new cases (Table 13.8).

Using a mathematical approach first published by Quigley and Vitale,[40] Broman et al. derived estimates of incidence of POAG from the data of several population-based prevalence surveys,

Table 13.8 *Incidence of primary open-angle glaucoma (POAG)*

Location	Date of publication	Method	Age (years)	Ethnic group	Annual incidence (%)	Ref.
Sweden	1981	Re-examination	55+	European	0.22	28
Framingham MA, USA	1983	Calculated from age-specific prevalence rates	55 / 75	White American	0.04 / 0.20	62
Sweden	1984	Hospital records	55+	European	0.32[a]	66
Sweden	1989	Re-examination, after two different time periods	55+	European	0.24[a] / 0.19[a]	69
Olmstead County, MN, USA	2001	Medical records; age-adjusted to USA	All	White American white population	0.0145 (95% CI 0.0118–0.0172)	63
Barbados	2001	Re-examination	40+	African Caribbean	0.55[b]	70

[a] Includes capsular glaucoma. [b] Estimated annual incidence from four-year risk of 2.2% (95% CI 1.7–2.8).

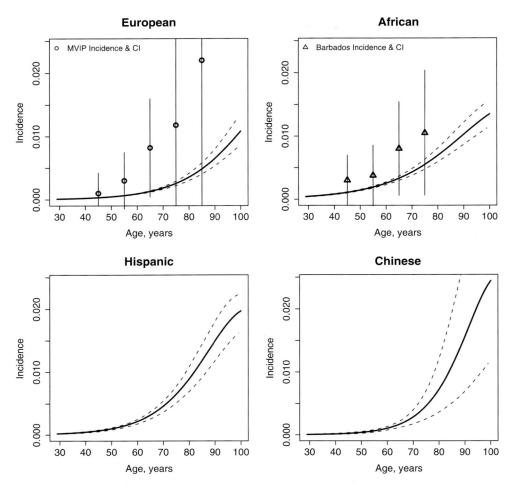

Figure 13.4 *Age-specific incidence by ethnicity. Incidence estimates (solid lines) for OAG in four ethnicities generated from age-specific prevalences. The 95% CI for our estimates (dashed lines) overlap the data from two individual direct measurements of incidence in population surveys (circles and flags, mean and 95% CI). These are the Melbourne VIP study (shown in European-derived curve, top left) and the Barbados Eye Study data (shown in African-derived curve, top right)*

comprising nearly 1,000 persons with POAG.[64] This approach gives incidence estimates for European, African, Chinese and Hispanic groups, and its findings are generally in agreement in the first two ethnicities with the actual measurements from Australian and the Caribbean. Minassian and colleagues[65] found that this approach, as well as an alternative model by Tuck and Crick, gave similar results. In the USA the cumulative probability of POAG in white persons is 4.2% (95% CI 3.01–5.01%), so that approximately 4,200 persons of an initial cohort of 100,000 would develop OAG at some point of their lifetimes. For black people, more than twice as many would be affected

by OAG (cumulative probability 10.3%, or around 10,300 of 100,000 persons). In England and Wales the number of new cases (five-year cumulative incidences) in the elderly population (65 years and older) were 71,146 and 94,485, determined by the Tuck–Crick and Quigley–Vitale methods respectively.

13.5.2 Incidence of PACG and PAC (Table 13.9)

The incidence of angle-closure was estimated by Alsbirk, although this classification is not directly

Table 13.9 *Incidence of primary angle-closure*

Location	Date of publication	Method	Age (years)	Ethnic group	Annual incidence per 100,000 (95% CI)	Ref.
Sweden	1984	Hospital records	40+	European	6.0	66
Singapore	1997	Notification by all ophthalmologists of symptomatic cases of PAC	30+	Chinese (91.5%) and non-Chinese	12.2 (10.5–13.9)	67
Singapore	2000	Hospital discharge Diagnosis of 'PACG'	30+	Chinese	12.2 (10.5–13.7)	68
				Malays	6.0 (4.9–7.3)	
				Indians	6.3 (5.1–7.6)	

comparable with modern conventions of disease definition. Subsequently, longitudinal studies of cases with anatomically narrow angles (PACS) and primary angle-closure (PAC) cases, identified in a population-based study in southern India (Vellore), give incidence rates for PAC and PACG in people with the preceding categories of disease. For PACS converting to PAC, the rate was 22% over five years. Of eleven people who developed PAC seven were synechial, and four appositional. All cases were bilateral PACS. Only one person among a normal 110 progressed to PAC. There was no significant difference in axial length, anterior chamber depth, or lens thickness as between those who progressed and those who did not. None of the patients developed optic disc or field damage attributable to angle-closure.[71] The same group studied progression from PAC to PACG. Eight people (28.5%) had progressed to PACG, two of seven with appositional, and six of 21 with synechial closure. All were advised to have laser peripheral iridotomy (LPI) in 1995; one of the nine (11%) who underwent LPI progressed compared with seven of the 19 (37%) who refused LPI. Four of those originally diagnosed with appositional closure developed peripheral anterior synechiae. None developed acute PACG or blindness due to glaucoma. No feature predicting progression was identified.[72]

In Singapore, Seah and colleagues set up a case registry system in which all local ophthalmologists recorded over one year new cases with symptoms and signs of **acute angle-closure (AAC)**.[67] In the ISGEO classification, those suffering acute symptomatic attacks are classified as PAC unless optic nerve damage is demonstrated. This gave an overall estimate for Chinese citizens of the country, but the

numbers were too small for a separate incidence rate for Malays and Indians to be calculated. A further study was undertaken in Singapore over five years to estimate the rates of hospital admissions with a discharge diagnosis of 'primary angle-closure glaucoma'.[68] Clearly, each of these methods would only capture the minority of PACG patients who are symptomatic with either painfully high IOP or severe vision loss. In the 1997 Singapore nationwide study the incidence of acute angle-closure was 12.2/100,000 per annum. The relative risk of AAC in Singaporeans of Chinese descent compared with Malays, Indians and other groups was 2.8 (95% CI, 1.7–4.7).[67] The relative risk for women was 2.4 (95% CI, 1.8–3.4). For men and women aged 60 years and older, compared with the 30- to 59-year-old age group, the relative risk was 9.1 (95% CI, 6.7–12.3). The incidence rates calculated from hospital discharge data in Singapore were remarkably similar: 11.1/100,000 per annum; Chinese at 12.2 per 100,000, almost twice that for Malays and Indians (6.0/100,000 per annum and 6.3/100,000 per annum respectively).[68]

Hospital episode statistics from both Taiwan and the UK show a decline in acute PAC rates over a period of increasing cataract surgical activity. The authors suggest that the change in hospital episodes associated with angle-closure may be linked to higher cataract surgery rates.[73,74]

13.6 RISK FACTORS FOR PRIMARY GLAUCOMA

Risk factors are attributes of a person or of their environment that increase likelihood of disease.

Some risk factors are immutable (genes), whereas others are variable, and even amenable to change through therapy or behavioural modification. The understanding of risk factors provides clues to causation, but the complexity of most disorders typically frustrates direct, simple cause and effect linkage. Every person with a complex disease may not have the same group of constituent risk factors as others with the same apparent phenotype. Risk factors that are strongly associated with disease but that are infrequent in the population will contribute little to the overall public health picture of a disease; their attributable risk will be low.

13.6.1 Primary open-angle glaucoma

Risk factors for POAG may be divided into those linked to the onset of disease, those associated with progressive worsening in already established disease, and even those associated with response to therapy.[75]

Some risk factors are fixed for the individual: age, ethnicity, and gender. For POAG, incidence (and prevalence) rise exponentially with age in every population studied.[40] While some children and young adults occasionally exhibit POAG, the prevalence is below 0.1% in most populations under the age of 30 years, but rises to as much as 10% or more amongst the elderly. As described in detail above, there are up to four times more cases of POAG in people of African origin than for most other world populations. This feature is shared by East Africans and African-Americans, pointing to a strong genetic basis that transcends environmental influences. Hispanic populations experience a more pronounced increase of POAG rates with age; their prevalence at the age of 40 years is similar to that seen in Europeans, but at age 70 years close to that of Africans.[37] Chinese and other Asian persons have a POAG prevalence similar to that of Europeans (the specific genetic information available on POAG is summarized in Section 13.8). There is no clear gender bias for POAG. Some individual prevalence surveys have found greater prevalence in men or women, but because of the low prevalence, such studies often have fewer than 100 affected persons and are not decisive.

Another group of risk factors associated with the development of POAG are actual signs of damage to the eye caused by incipient disease that is below the threshold for defining its onset. These include larger VCDR, presence of atrophy of the nerve fibre layer leading to the optic disk, small haemorrhages in the retina at the disc, and de-pigmented, crescent-shaped zones around the disk. While initial damage may lead to further injury, prevalence data do not confirm this.

Eyes with high degrees of refractive error (high myopia and hyperopia) are more likely to have POAG. It has been speculated that these eyes have different anatomic configurations in their key portions relevant to POAG, but the precise causative linkages are not delineated. In both the Baltimore and Blue Mountains Eye surveys,[76] there was a weak association between POAG and larger diameter of the optic nerve head (disk). This would be predicted by biomechanical considerations, as a larger opening in the eye wall would be more susceptible to deformation under the influence of IOP. An additional risk factor that may be classified as 'biomechanical' is the increased risk associated with having a thin central corneal thickness, as detected first in the **Ocular Hypertension Treatment Study (OHTS)**. In fact, further studies in this area have shown that the physiological responsiveness of the cornea, as tested by air-puff tonometry's hysteresis measure, is even more strongly associated with both incidence and progression of POAG than is static anatomical thickness.[77]

As discussed above, elevated IOP is a consistent risk factor, although POAG can occur at any IOP; there is no specific IOP level that defines the disease. The higher the IOP, the more likely POAG is to occur, and the more likely it is to deteriorate progressively.[78] The development of POAG rises exponentially with IOP level without any 'breakpoint'. The transition from the 'normal' IOP in a population to the level considered elevated does not distinguish those below and above this zone from each other in a major way. The term 'normal-pressure glaucoma' does not represent a clearly distinct form of open angle glaucoma, and it is now recognized that a substantial minority of POAG occurs at normal levels of IOP. A causative linkage between IOP and POAG has been firmly established by the additional fact that lowering of IOP decreases onset or progression of disease (see Section 13.8), and by the production of a disease identical with human glaucoma using increasing IOP in animal models.

A variety of vascular functions have been linked to POAG. High blood pressure was thought to be a direct risk factor, but this relationship has been shown to be more complex. As persons in prevalence surveys with glaucoma were studied, it became clear that younger persons with hypertension were less likely to have POAG, whereas older hypertensive patients were at greater risk. This suggests that the duration of hypertension is an important modifier of the effect of blood pressure on POAG. Furthermore, low blood pressure is more closely associated with presence of POAG than high blood pressure. POAG incidence and prevalence are dramatically increased when mean blood pressure is near enough to the level of IOP that their difference (blood pressure minus IOP = perfusion pressure) falls below a certain level.[79]

Diabetes mellitus was linked in the past to POAG, but is not associated with either incidence or prevalence of POAG.[80] This is particularly intriguing, as it is documented that persons with diabetes in general have higher IOP than persons without diabetes. As such, they should be at greater risk for POAG, and the fact that this is not the case suggests that there may be some protective features of diabetes. An apparently protective effect of diabetes in early POAG was recently detected in a longitudinal clinical trial.[81]

A variety of tests of blood flow in the retina, optic nerve head and blood vessels that feed the eye are found to be abnormal in glaucomatous eyes. While this may indicate that poor nutritional blood flow or its autoregulation are contributing features in glaucoma, it is equally likely that the retinal ganglion cell (RGC) loss in glaucoma is associated with a compensatory decrease in blood flow. Further research is needed to determine, therefore, whether the measured decreases in blood flow are cause or effect. It is likely that poor vascular autoregulation does contribute to glaucoma damage because systemic symptoms of poor blood flow, such as migraine

and vasospasm on exposure to cold temperatures, have been implicated in glaucoma injury. One major clinical trial has recently determined that women with histories of migraine phenomena are more likely to undergo glaucoma progression.[82] This is one of the only documented risk factors for progression, along with IOP level and perfusion.

Certain features of lifestyle, including cigarette smoking, alcohol consumption and exposure to sunlight, and their consequences, are known to be associated with other eye diseases but are not risk factors for glaucoma. However, aerobic exercise appears to lower IOP and is therefore probably beneficial. An interesting finding among Barbadian persons with glaucoma is the association of leaner body mass with POAG. Other studies have not found that either low or high body mass index is related to POAG.

Other risk factors include exposure to corticosteroid agents in oral, inhaled or topical forms. It is well known that increase in IOP occurs in susceptible individuals after exogenous delivery of steroid medication.

13.6.2 Primary angle-closure glaucoma

The risk of an eye developing PAC depends on anatomic characteristics: smaller eye and narrower anterior chamber, as well as physiological factors that are increasingly recognized as necessary see below. Other factors include being of Monogoloid origin, older age, female, having a family history, and having hypermetropia. Few persons with narrow angles will develop a disease, so that dynamic features of the iris and choroid play key roles in the production of disease, especially as regards its most dramatic events.

The relevant dimensions of the anterior chamber are thought to be under strong genetic control, but may be modified by climatic and other environmental factors. Anterior chamber depth shows significant geographical variation that, some believe, mirrors the distribution of angle-closure (shallower **anterior chamber depth (ACD)** associated with higher rates of disease). However, this theory has been disputed.[83] Within a given population, people with PAC and PACG have shallower ACD, as compared with age- and sex-matched members of the same population without disease. For example, Inuits with ACG had ACDs 0.5 mm shallower than those not affected (1.7–1.9 mm compared with 2.2–2.4 mm).[84] In Mongolia, the PAC and PACG cases were statistically more likely to be amongst the lowest ACD for each age group (Fig. 13.5).[85]

Primary angle-closure is often associated with relatively high resistance to aqueous humour movement through the iris-lens channel, the narrow passage shaped like a flat doughnut through which fluid moves from the posterior to the anterior chamber. In predisposed eyes, and under particularly unfavourable physiological conditions, resistance for aqueous movement through the pupil can be so high that the pressure gradient generated across the iris causes it to bow forward ('balloon') to touch the trabecular meshwork. This interferes with the outflow of aqueous from the anterior chamber. While a variety of features contribute to this pathological resistance in the iris-lens channel, making a hole in the iris, however small, relieves the problem.

Acute, symptomatic episodes of angle-closure occur more frequently when the pupil is in its mid-dilated position. As a result, agents that dilate the pupil can participate in causing angle-closure, as do activities carried out in dim light. However, few eyes with narrow angles by gonioscopy develop measurable IOP elevation in dim light. Recent research has demonstrated that there are additional, dynamic factors playing a role in causing angle-closure. One of these is the fact that the iris is a sponge-like tissue that gains and loses extracellular water as the pupil constricts and dilates. In fact, in normal eyes the iris loses half of its volume when the pupil diameter dilates from 3 mm to 7 mm. Imaging of iris cross-sectional area by anterior segment optical coherence tomography (AS-OCT) shows that eyes with PAC and PACG lose less iris volume on pupil dilation than do non-angle-closure eyes.[86] In the extreme situation, i.e. acute symptomatic attacks, eyes lack this feature entirely, and their irises lose no volume on dilation, leaving them more bulky to block the trabecular meshwork.[87]

Since pupil block of aqueous is a primary mechanism, eyes after laser iridotomy would be expected to have angles that appear more open by gonioscopic evaluation. For 65–80% of eyes, this is the case. However, between 18–35% remain narrow despite

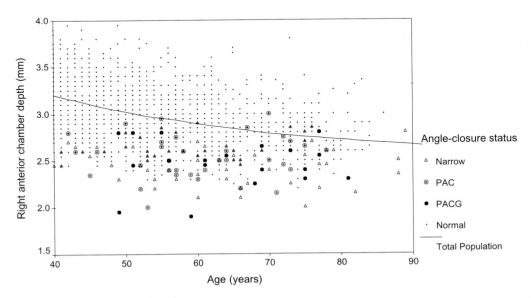

Figure 13.5 *Distribution of true optical anterior chamber depth (ACD) by age. Solid line represents estimated lowess (sic) curve for mean age-specific ACD. Triangles are cases of suspected primary angle-closure; double open circles, primary angle-closure; and solid circles, primary angle-closure glaucoma. Small dots represent the rest of the study population with ACD measurement. (Source of data: Foster PJ, Deverux JG, Baasanhu J, et al.)*

having a patent iridotomy.[88,89] The lack of response in this setting is widely attributed to plateau iris configuration, and seems to relate to the anatomical relation of the iris dilator to the ciliary body epithelium into which it inserts, anchoring the iris through an articulated attachment to the eye wall. Several studies have shown that this configuration does not confer additional risk for long-term development of glaucoma. In a small number of cases of plateau configuration, high IOP occurs with dilation of the pupil, and are designated plateau iris syndrome.[90]

Recent investigations with both ultrasonic biomicroscopy and AS-OCT have confirmed theoretical hypotheses that expansion of the volume of the choroid contributes to PAC and PACG by moving the lens forward, increasing iris-lens channel resistance.[91] Lucencies (clear zones) that denote small choroidal effusions are now known to contribute to the anatomical risk factors that lead to PACG.[92,93]

13.7   GENETICS OF GLAUCOMA

Population-based surveys indicate that persons with POAG are likely to have affected family members, though, as with any complex disease, the genetics of POAG are likely to be complex. The Rotterdam survey examined all available family members of persons who were found to have POAG,[94] determining that there is a ten times increased risk for a POAG sibling having the disease. Further research is needed in this area for other ethnic groups.

The examination of family history data for POAG shows weaknesses in methodology. Persons who report that family members are affected are frequently shown to be incorrect when the particular individual in question is examined in detail. Furthermore, as 50% of POAG is undiagnosed, family members may not know that they have the disease or may not have communicated this to the **proband**. In addition, studies indicate that family history data are increasingly unreliable (and of lower association with POAG) as the family relationship becomes more distant. In most situations, data on aunts and cousins appears uninformative.

At least five areas of the human genome have been associated with POAG by linkage analysis of affected families. The first gene cloned in the study of primary adult glaucoma was identified in an extended family from Iowa, USA. The gene, on the long arm of chromosome 1, produces a protein named myocilin.[95] Persons with polymorphisms in this gene often develop high IOP in their third decade and have a particularly aggressive form of POAG. The gene product is known to be made by cells of the outflow channels of the eye, providing a rational, causative pathway for its participation in blocking water movement from the eye, and leading to high IOP. Clinic-based information on gene mutation frequency suggests that up to 2% of European-derived persons with POAG exhibit a myocilin mutation. This indicates that alterations in this gene alone would not explain the vast majority of POAG cases.

A second gene is associated with open-angle glaucoma, positioned on the short arm of chromosome 10 (10p14–15). The gene product is the protein optineurin, more often linked with those who exhibit POAG at normal levels of IOP. One group suggested that sequence alterations in optineurin were found in 17% of families with hereditary POAG, but subsequent research has found different attributable risks of variations in this gene. Optineurin's function is not specifically determined, but is expressed in trabecular meshwork, non-pigmented ciliary epithelium, retina and brain.[96] Patients carrying the E50K mutation suffer a more severe course of the disease than do those without.[97]

The third gene so far associated with POAG is WDR 36, residing at 5q22.1. Overall, four mutations were identified in 17 (5.0–6.9%) unrelated POAG subjects, 11 with higher IOP and six with lower IOP-associated glaucoma. WDR36 encodes 951 amino acids and a protein with multiple G-beta WD40 repeats. Gene expression has been observed in lens, iris, sclera, ciliary muscles, ciliary body, trabecular meshwork, retina and optic nerve.[98]

Research on a population database among Icelandic persons has identified polymorphisms in the LOXL1 gene (15q24.1) among > 99% of those with exfoliation syndrome.[99] The product of

LOXL1 catalyses the formation of elastin fibres, found to be a major component of ocular connective tissue. However, these polymorphisms were not significantly associated with exfoliation glaucoma; they are found in more than 80% of normal, non-glaucomatous Icelandic persons. Thus it is clear that additional features — perhaps additional genes — must be mutated to lead to exfoliation glaucoma.

Primary congenital glaucoma is a group of disorders with variable inheritance that is associated with a variety of developmental defects in the anterior eye segment. Mutations in the gene encoding the metabolic enzyme CYP1B1 (2p21) have been linked to congenital glaucoma, as have mutations in the PAX6 gene.[100]

Molecular genetics will surely add greatly to our knowledge of POAG, but it is important to remain realistic about its potential value. There may well be many more mutations in many loci found that relate to POAG, but none of these is likely to be associated with a high proportion of cases. Persons with mutations in loci that are associated with POAG may or may not develop the disease. Whilst the presence of mutations at associated loci will provide information on which persons should be monitored more frequently, environmental influences and multiple gene interactions will make the occurrence of POAG far from certain.

13.8   CLINICAL TRIALS INFORMING GLAUCOMA MANAGEMENT

During the past 15 years, a series of controlled clinical trials has been conducted to determine the performance of medical, laser and surgical therapy for POAG. Prior to these studies, there was a group of longitudinal cohort studies that assessed the rate at which suspects for POAG developed initial visual field injury, and another in which the rate of progressive deterioration in field testing under therapy was measured. Progression to initial loss of visual field occurred in about 1–3% per year of those at risk because of IOP above the normal range. Prevalence data and clinic-based records suggested that a deterioration of field tests occurred in about 4% of treated patients per year of follow-up.

Ultimate legal blindness in both eyes was expected in fewer than 10% of treated persons.

A clinical trial compared surgical treatment of POAG with and without adjunctive injections of 5-Fluorouracil, which alters the wound-healing response, and helps to maintain aqueous outflow following glaucoma surgery. There was a statistically significant benefit with the use of this agent. In a more recent study, newly diagnosed glaucoma patients were randomized to eye drop treatment or surgical trabeculectomy in both eyes (**Collaborative Initial Glaucoma Treatment Study, CIGTS**).[101] After five years, there was no significant difference between the two groups in visual function, although the surgery group had an initial decrease of vision in the first year, and developed more cataracts. Interestingly, the subjects reported, in detailed quality-of-life instruments, that they suffered more side effects from the surgery than from chronic, daily eye drop treatment. The result of this study is in contrast to an earlier, similar clinical trial carried out in the UK.[102] In this study, three groups of initial therapy POAG patients were randomized to treatment with eye drops, to laser treatment or to surgery. While the surgery group reportedly did better, the visual function studies performed in this trial were not sufficient for the outcome to be judged by present standards. In addition, the improved performance of medical treatment in the newer CIGTS study may be attributable to the appearance, since the British study, of eye drops with greater IOP lowering potency and fewer side effects.

Clinical trials, have evaluated whether IOP lowering is truly beneficial in POAG. The most direct demonstration was in the Collaborative Normal Tension Glaucoma Study,[103] in which persons with POAG at IOP in the normal range were randomized either to therapy that lowered IOP or to no therapy. The trial result showed that lowering of IOP reduced the risk of progressive glaucoma damage by a factor of 2 to 3, although there was a greater risk of cataract requiring surgical removal among treated patients. It was of great interest that as many as 40% of POAG patients did not progressively deteriorate in an eight-year follow-up, even if they were not treated. If lower IOP is beneficial for those with POAG at normal IOP, it is even more likely that it will reduce risk for those with higher IOP.

Indeed, the **Advanced Glaucoma Intervention Study (AGIS)**,[104] which compared laser with surgical treatment for those with failed topical therapy, confirmed that the lower the IOP in treated glaucoma, the less likely was progressive decline. The reports of this trial appear to show that both laser and trabeculectomy surgery are effective in slowing POAG, even when it is advanced, although again, the development of cataract at a greater rate appears to be an inevitable consequence of treatment. The AGIS study group has presented some differences among their population stratified by ethnicity (white versus black), but the baseline differences in disease severity and prior treatment were not used as adjustments for these conclusions.

The **Early Manifest Glaucoma Treatment Study (EMGTS)** compared the effect, on the progression of newly detected open-angle glaucoma, of immediately lowering the IOP, versus no treatment or later treatment. Two hundred and fifty-five people aged 50 to 80 years with early glaucoma were identified mainly by population screening. Patients were randomized to either laser trabeculoplasty plus topical betaxolol hydrochloride (n = 29) or to no initial treatment (n = 26). After a median follow-up period of six years, treatment reduced the IOP by 5.1 mmHg. Progression was less frequent, and occurred later in the treatment group than in controls (45% versus 62%, P = 0.007,[105] The authors concluded from the same dataset that each higher mmHg of IOP on follow-up was associated with an approximate 10% increased risk of progression.[106]

The Ocular Hypertension Treatment (OHT) Study enrolled 1,636 participants with no evidence of glaucomatous damage, with an IOP between 24 mmHg and 32 mmHg in one eye, and between 21 mmHg and 32 mmHg in the other eye. They were randomized with either observation or treatment with commercially available topical ocular hypotensive medication. The goal in the medication group was to reduce the IOP by 20% or more, and to reach an IOP of 24 mmHg or less. At 60 months, the cumulative probability of developing POAG was 4.4% in the medication group and 9.5% in the observation group. The authors concluded that this does not imply that all patients with borderline or elevated IOP should receive medication, but that clinicians should consider initiating treatment for individuals with ocular hypertension who are at moderate or high risk for developing POAG.[107] The findings from this study have resulted in considerable debate around the world. With an absolute risk reduction of 5.1%, the Number Needed to Treat in this study was 20 (i.e. need to treat 20 people to prevent one case of early POAG). Some have suggested that this constitutes a strong argument for not treating people with OHT. Recent follow-up of patients in this trial who were initially untreated for several years, and in whom IOP-lowering was then begun, has been interpreted to show that delay in the initiation of treatment did not adversely affect the degree of benefit conferred by therapy.

13.9 POSSIBILITIES FOR SCREENING

To meet the criteria for the introduction of a screening programme (see Chapter 8), proposed screening tests must be valid (high sensitivity and specificity) and reliable, as well as being inexpensive, rapid and acceptable in order to test large numbers of people.

13.9.1 Primary open-angle glaucoma

Two of the tests routinely used in screening for POAG — intraocular pressure and cup–disc ratio — are continuous variables, and there is no cut-off point that discriminates adequately between normal eyes and those affected. Data from the Baltimore Eye Study by Tielsch and others clearly showed that there was no satisfactory combination of sensitivity and specificity for either test (see also Figure 8.2 and Section 8.7.2).[44] The third diagnostic test — detection of a visual field defect — does not become positive with present techniques until nearly 50% of the optic nerve fibres have atrophied (the 'Quigley gap'). It is a subjective test, with problems of reliability. Therefore, at the present time, general population screening for POAG cannot be recommended. The emphasis must be on methods of detection of those cases which already have advanced glaucoma and need urgent treatment.

13.9.2   Primary angle-closure

13.9.2.1   *Screening tests*

The presently available tests aim to detect variations in the dimensions of the anterior chamber that are the predisposing factors for angle-closure. Three tests have been proposed:

➢ The 'oblique flashlight test';
➢ Limbal anterior chamber depth;
➢ Axial anterior chamber depth;

The 'oblique flashlight test'

A small pen-torch or flashlight is held close to the temporal side of the eye in the same plane as the limbus. Depending on the degree of forward curvature of the iris, a greater or smaller area of the iris is illuminated, and the extent of the shadow on the nasal side can be graded. Congdon *et al.* reviewed the use of this test in clinics and population surveys.[108] High sensitivity and specificity were claimed, for example in China. The experience in Mongolia was less encouraging. The challenge is to standardize the size of the light source, the exact position and plane in which it is held, and how to record the size of the shadow.

Limbal anterior chamber depth (van Herick)

The limbal anterior chamber depth test was first described by van Herick, Shaffer and Schwartz in 1969.[109] The narrow beam of a high-quality slit-lamp is shone at right angles to the peripheral cornea, close to the limbus. The clear optical section through the cornea is then viewed with the biomicroscope offset nasally at an angle of 60°, and the depth of the space between the back of the cornea and the peripheral iris is expressed as a fraction (¼, ½, 1) of the thickness of the cornea. This estimate has been found to correlate well with the width of the angle judged gonioscopically.

Alsbirk and colleagues developed an augmented grading scheme that expresses the ACD as a percentage of corneal thickness (Plate 13.2).[110] In Mongolia the 15% grade yielded sensitivity of 84% and specificity of 86% for detection of occludable angles, while a 5% estimate gave sensitivity of 91% and specificity of 93% for established PACG. There was good inter-observer agreement.

This test is of value for opportunistic screening in a clinic, but the problems of transporting and setting up a high-quality and stable slit-lamp limit its application in rural areas. The test has a theoretical advantage over the measurement of axial ACD in being less likely to miss cases of angle-closure resulting from plateau iris in those populations where this is common.

Axial anterior chamber depth

Angle-chamber depth in the optic axis may be measured by optical pachymetry, using the Haag–Streit attachments; by slit-lamp mounted A-mode ultrasound, or by ultrasound, with the probe hand-held. Devereux *et al.* showed, in two Mongolian populations, that ultrasound with the probe mounted on the tonometer head at the slit-lamp performed with almost the same validity as optical pachymetry, in detecting occludable angle, PAC and PACG; these were judged by gonioscopy, optic disc assessment and visual fields.[85] At appropriate cut-off levels it gave sensitivities of 83% and 86% and specificities of 81% and 84% for occludable angles and PACG, respectively. This measurement is therefore a possible screening test, and could be used with a simple chin-rest and forehead-support and a stabilized mounting for the ultrasound probe, without having to transport a bulky slit-lamp. It could be applied to large numbers of subjects in populations with a high prevalence of angle-closure.

As suggested in 13.2.1, AS-OCT may be an effective and user-friendly method of identifying irido-trabecular contact, and form the basis of a screening test.

13.9.2.2 *Diagnostic tests*

The definitive test is gonioscopy. Actual apposition between iris and trabecular meshwork (irido-trabecular contact, ITC) may cause peripheral anterior synechiae or pigment smearing in the drainage angle. Evidence of this can be seen when manipulative or indentational gonioscopy is used.

With the aim of improving inter-observer reliability, and providing more objective cut-offs for detecting angle-closure, Congdon and associates introduced the concept of biometric gonioscopy.[111] The distance from the iris insertion to Schwalbe's line was measured in all four quadrants using a reticule etched in the slit-lamp eyepiece. This measurement correlated well with conventional gonioscopy by an experienced gonioscopist, and correctly identified occludable angles. There was excellent inter-observer reliability, and the method was readily learned by an inexperienced observer.

The dark-room prone provocative test exploits the conditions under which a susceptible individual is thought to be most likely to develop pupil block. The patient is situated in a dark room, or with both eyes bandaged (so that the pupil becomes partially dilated) and placed lying face down for up to one hour, and then the intraocular pressure rise induced is measured. If positive (8 mmHg rise), this test is useful, but a negative test does not exclude the possibility of angle-closure, and the test is now not greatly used in epidemiological studies.

As mentioned in Section 13.6.2 above, recent research has indicated that physiological risk factors, such as iris volume loss on dilation and choroidal expansion, are key in producing PAC and PACG. This has led to prospective trials that are evaluating these as risk factors for later development of this disease.

13.9.2.3 *Prevention of progression*

In order to justify the introduction of a screening programme, there must be an established method of treatment, an agreed policy on whom to treat, and the capacity to treat all those picked out by screening, and subsequent diagnosis, as being at risk of angle-closure or further progression of PAC. Nolan followed up the subjects who had been treated with YAG laser peripheral iridotomy for occludable angles, PAC or PACG during two previous surveys in rural areas of Mongolia.[112] All 98.1% (all except three) peripheral iridotomies had remained patent after a period of between one and

three years. The median increase in depth of the drainage angle by gonioscopy was two Shaffer grades, no eyes with PAC had progressed to PACG, and the iridotomy alone was sufficient treatment for half the cases of PACG. Friedman *et al.* have shown that iridotomy in fellow eyes of those with acute attacks of angle-closure (AAC) prevents development of glaucoma injury in more than 95% for six years or more.[113]

13.10 SUMMARY OF EPIDEMIOLOGICAL RESEARCH PRIORITIES

➢ Further glaucoma surveys in specific populations, with establishment of normal values for intraocular pressure, optic disc appearances, and anterior chamber dimensions. This will become particularly important for the age group 80 years and above.
➢ Demonstration in further populations whether laser peripheral iridotomy prevents narrow angles progressing to angle-closure glaucoma with vision loss.
➢ Refinement of screening tests for occludable angles.
➢ Improvement in methods of case-detection of established open-angle glaucoma, including disc imaging and analysis as a possible screening test in the future.
➢ Basic science research to increase understanding of the mechanisms of POAG.

REFERENCES

1. Foster PJ, Buhrmann R, Quigley HA, *et al.* The definition and classification of glaucoma in prevalence surveys. *Br J Ophthalmol* 2002; 86:238–242.
2. Quigley HA, Green WR. The histology of human glaucoma cupping and optic nerve damage: clinicopathologic correlation in 21 eyes. *Ophthalmology* 1979; 86:1803–1830.
3. Wolfs RC, Borger PH, Ramrattan RS, *et al.* Changing views on open-angle glaucoma: definitions and prevalences. The Rotterdam Study. *Invest Ophthalmol Vis Sci* 2000; 41:3309–3321.

4. Crowston JG, Hopley CR, Healey PR, *et al.* The effect of optic disc diameter on vertical cup to disc ratio percentiles in a population based cohort: the Blue Mountains Eye Study. *Br J Ophthalmol* 2004; 88:766–770.

5. Barkan O. Glaucoma: classification, causes and surgical control. Results of microgonioscopic research. *Am J Ophthalmol* 1938; 21:1099–1117.

6. Spaeth GL. The normal development of the human anterior chamber angle: a new system of descriptive grading. *Trans Ophthalmol Soc UK* 1971; 91: 709–739.

7. Nolan WP, See JL, Chew PT, *et al.* Detection of primary angle-closure using anterior segment optical coherence tomography in Asian eyes. *Ophthalmology* 2007; 114:33–39.

8. Ong EL, Baasanhu J, Nolan W, *et al.* The utility of symptoms in identification of primary angle-closure in a high-risk population. *Ophthalmology* 2008; 115:2024–2029.

9. Hollows FC, Graham PA. Intra-ocular pressure, glaucoma, and glaucoma suspects in a defined population. *Br J Ophthalmol* 1966; 50:570–586.

10. Quigley HA, Broman AT. The number of people with glaucoma worldwide in 2010 and 2020. *Br J Ophthalmol* 2006; 90:262–267.

11. Buhrmann RR, Quigley HA, Barron Y, *et al.* Prevalence of glaucoma in a rural East African population. *Invest Ophthalmol Vis Sci* 2000; 41:40–48.

12. Rotchford AP, Johnson GJ. Glaucoma in Zulus: a population-based cross-sectional survey in a rural district in South Africa. *Arch Ophthalmol* 2002; 120:471–478.

13. Wallace J, Lovell HG. Glaucoma and intraocular pressure in Jamaica. *Am J Ophthalmol* 1969; 67:93–100.

14. Mason RP, Kosoko O, Wilson MR, *et al.* National survey of the prevalence and risk factors of glaucoma in St Lucia, West Indies. Part I. Prevalence findings. *Ophthalmology* 1989; 96: 1363–1368.

15. Tielsch JM, Sommer A, Katz J, *et al.* Racial variations in the prevalence of primary open-angle glaucoma. The Baltimore Eye Survey. *JAMA* 1991; 266:369–374.

16. Leske MC, Connell AM, Schachat AP, *et al.* The Barbados Eye Study. Prevalence of open angle glaucoma. *Arch Ophthalmol* 1994; 112:821–829.

17. Alsbirk PH. Angle-closure glaucoma surveys in Greenland Eskimos. A preliminary report. *Can J Ophthalmol* 1973; 8:260–264.

18. Arkell SM, Lightman DA, Sommer A, *et al.* The prevalence of glaucoma among Eskimos of North-west Alaska. *Arch Ophthalmol* 1987; 105: 482–485.

19. Van Rens GH, Arkell SM, Charlton W, *et al.* Primary angle-closure glaucoma among Alaskan Eskimos. *Doc Ophthalmol* 1988; 70:265–276.

20. Hu Z ZZDF. An epidemiological investigation of glaucoma in Beijing and Shun-yi County. *Chin J Ophthalmol* 1989; 25:115–118.

21. Shiose Y, Kitazawa Y, Tsukahara S, *et al.* Epidemiology of glaucoma in Japan — a nationwide glaucoma survey. *Jpn J Ophthalmol* 1991; 35:133–155.

22. Congdon NG, Quigley HA, Hung PT, *et al.* Screening techniques for angle-closure glaucoma in rural Taiwan. *Acta Ophthalmol Scand* 1996; 74:113–119.

23. Foster PJ, Baasanhu J, Alsbirk PH, *et al.* Glaucoma in Mongolia. A population-based survey in Hovsgol province, northern Mongolia. *Arch Ophthalmol* 1996; 114:1235–1241.

24. Foster PJ, Oen FT, Machin D, *et al.* The prevalence of glaucoma in Chinese residents of Singapore: a cross-sectional population survey of the Tanjong Pagar district. *Arch Ophthalmol* 2000; 118:1105–1111.

25. Dandona L, Dandona R, Mandal P, *et al.* Angle-closure glaucoma in an urban population in southern India. The Andhra Pradesh eye disease study. *Ophthalmology* 2000; 107:1710–1716.

26. Dandona L, Dandona R, Srinivas M, *et al.* Open-angle glaucoma in an urban population in southern India: the Andhra Pradesh eye disease study. *Ophthalmology* 2000; 107:1702–1709.

27. Leibowitz HM, Krueger DE, Maunder LR, *et al.* The Framingham Eye Study monograph: An ophthalmological and epidemiological study of cataract, glaucoma, diabetic retinopathy, macular degeneration, and visual acuity in a general population of 2,631 adults, 1973–1975. *Surv Ophthalmol* 1980;24:335–610.

28. Bengtsson B. The prevalence of glaucoma. *Br J Ophthalmol* 1981; 65:46–49.

29. Ringvold A, Blika S, Elsas T, *et al.* The middle-Norway eye-screening study. II. Prevalence of

simple and capsular glaucoma. *Acta Ophthalmol (Copenh)* 1991; 69:273–280.

30. Klein BE, Klein R, Sponsel WE, *et al*. Prevalence of glaucoma. The Beaver Dam Eye Study. *Ophthalmology* 1992; 99:1499–1504.

31. Coffey M, Reidy A, Wormald R, *et al*. Prevalence of glaucoma in the west of Ireland. *Br J Ophthalmol* 1993; 77:17–21.

32. Dielemans I, Vingerling JR, Wolfs RC, *et al*. The prevalence of primary open-angle glaucoma in a population-based study in The Netherlands. The Rotterdam Study. *Ophthalmology* 1994; 101: 1851–1855.

33. Mitchell P, Smith W, Attebo K, *et al*. Prevalence of open-angle glaucoma in Australia. The Blue Mountains Eye Study. *Ophthalmology* 1996; 103:1661–1669.

34. Cedrone C, Culasso F, Cesareo M, *et al*. Prevalence of glaucoma in Ponza, Italy: a comparison with other studies. *Ophthalmic Epidemiol* 1997; 4:59–72.

35. Bonomi L, Marchini G, Marraffa M, *et al*. Prevalence of glaucoma and intraocular pressure distribution in a defined population. The Egna–Neumarkt Study. *Ophthalmology* 1998; 105:209–215.

36. Wensor MD, McCarty CA, Stanislavsky YL, *et al*. The prevalence of glaucoma in the Melbourne Visual Impairment Project. *Ophthalmology* 1998; 105:733–739.

37. Quigley HA, West SK, Rodriguez J, *et al*. The prevalence of glaucoma in a population-based study of Hispanic subjects: Proyecto VER. *Arch Ophthalmol* 2001; 119:1819–1826.

38. Salmon JF, Mermoud A, Ivey A, *et al*. The prevalence of primary angle-closure glaucoma and open angle glaucoma in Mamre, Western Cape, South Africa. *Arch Ophthalmol* 1993; 111:1263–1269.

39. Iwase A, Suzuki Y, Araie M, *et al*. The prevalence of primary open-angle glaucoma in Japanese: the Tajimi Study. *Ophthalmology* 2004; 111: 1641–1648.

40. Quigley HA, Vitale S. Models of open-angle glaucoma prevalence and incidence in the United States. *Invest Ophthalmol Vis Sci* 1997; 38:83–91.

41. Quigley HA. Number of people with glaucoma worldwide. *Br J Ophthalmol* 1996; 80:389–393.

42. Thylefors B, Negrel AD. The global impact of glaucoma. *Bull World Health Organ* 1994; 72:323–326.

43. Rotchford AP, Kirwan JF, Muller MA, *et al*. Temba glaucoma study: a population-based cross-sectional survey in urban South Africa. *Ophthalmology* 2003; 110:376–382.

44. Tielsch JM, Katz J, Singh K, *et al*. A population-based evaluation of glaucoma screening: the Baltimore Eye Survey. *Am J Epidemiol* 1991; 134: 1102–1110.

45. Topouzis F, Wilson MR, Harris A, *et al*. Prevalence of open-angle glaucoma in Greece: the Thessaloniki Eye Study. *Am J Ophthalmol* 2007; 144:511–519.

46. Foster PJ, Aung T, Nolan WP, *et al*. Defining 'occludable' angles in population surveys: drainage angle width, peripheral anterior synechiae, and glaucomatous optic neuropathy in east Asian people. *Br J Ophthalmol* 2004; 88:486–490.

47. Rahman MM, Rahman N, Foster PJ, *et al*. The prevalence of glaucoma in Bangladesh: a population based survey in Dhaka division. *Br J Ophthalmol* 2004; 88:1493–1497.

48. Vijaya L, George R, Paul PG, *et al*. Prevalence of open-angle glaucoma in a rural south Indian population. *Invest Ophthalmol Vis Sci* 2005; 46:4461–4467.

49. Ramakrishnan R, Nirmalan PK, Krishnadas R, *et al*. Glaucoma in a rural population of southern India: the Aravind comprehensive eye survey. *Ophthalmology* 2003; 110:1484–1490.

50. Vijaya L, George R, Baskaran M, *et al*. Prevalence of primary open-angle glaucoma in an urban south Indian population and comparison with a rural population. The Chennai Glaucoma Study. *Ophthalmology* 2008; 115:648–654.

51. Luntz MH. Primary angle-closure glaucoma in urbanized South African caucasoid and negroid communities. *Br J Ophthalmol* 1973; 57:445–456.

52. Johnson GJ, Green JS, Paterson GD, *et al*. Survey of ophthalmic conditions in a Labrador community: II. Ocular disease. *Can J Ophthalmol* 1984; 19: 224–233.

53. Dandona L, Dandona R, Mandal P, *et al*. Angle-closure glaucoma in an urban population in southern India. The Andhra Pradesh eye disease study. *Ophthalmology* 2000; 107:1710–1716.

54. Vijaya L, George R, Arvind H, *et al*. Prevalence of primary angle-closure disease in an urban south Indian population and comparison with a rural population. The Chennai Glaucoma Study. *Ophthalmology* 2008; 115:655–660.

55. Foster PJ, Johnson GJ. Glaucoma in China: how big is the problem? *Br J Ophthalmol* 2001; 85:1277–1282.

56. Yamamoto T, Iwase A, Araie M, *et al*. The Tajimi Study report 2: prevalence of primary angle-closure and secondary glaucoma in a Japanese population. *Ophthalmology* 2005; 112:1661–1669.

57. He M, Foster PJ, Ge J, *et al*. Prevalence and clinical characteristics of glaucoma in adult Chinese: a population-based study in Liwan District, Guangzhou. *Invest Ophthalmol Vis Sci* 2006; 47:2782–2788.

58. Casson RJ, Newland HS, Muecke J, *et al*. Prevalence of glaucoma in rural Myanmar: the Meiktila Eye Study. *Br J Ophthalmol* 2007; 91:710–714.

59. Bourne RR, Sukudom P, Foster PJ, *et al*. Prevalence of glaucoma in Thailand: a population based survey in Rom Klao District, Bangkok. *Br J Ophthalmol* 2003; 87:1069–1074.

60. Mukesh BN, McCarty CA, Rait JL, *et al*. Five-year incidence of open-angle glaucoma: the visual impairment project. *Ophthalmology* 2002; 109:1047–1051.

61. Leske MC, Wu SY, Honkanen R, *et al*. Nine-year incidence of open-angle glaucoma in the Barbados Eye Studies. *Ophthalmology* 2007; 114:1058–1064.

62. Leske MC, Ederer F, Podgor M. Estimating incidence from age-specific prevalence in glaucoma. *Am J Epidemiol* 1981; 113:606–613.

63. Schoff EO, Hattenhauer MG, Ing HH, *et al*. Estimated incidence of open-angle glaucoma in Olmsted County, Minnesota. *Ophthalmology* 2001; 108:882–886.

64. Broman AT, Quigley HA, West SK, *et al*. Estimating the rate of progressive visual field damage in those with open-angle glaucoma, from cross-sectional data. *Invest Ophthalmol Vis Sci* 2008; 49:66–76.

65. Minassian DC, Reidy A, Coffey M, *et al*. Utility of predictive equations for estimating the prevalence and incidence of primary open angle glaucoma in the UK. *Br J Ophthalmol* 2000; 84:1159–1161.

66. Lindblom B, Thorburn W. Observed incidence of glaucoma in Halsingland, Sweden. *Acta Ophthalmol (Copenh)* 1984; 62:217–222.

67. Seah SK, Foster PJ, Chew PT, *et al*. Incidence of acute primary angle-closure glaucoma in Singapore. An island-wide survey. *Arch Ophthalmol* 1997; 115:1436–1440.

68. Wong TY, Foster PJ, Seah SK, *et al*. Rates of hospital admissions for primary angle-closure glaucoma among Chinese, Malays, and Indians in Singapore. *Br J Ophthalmol* 2000; 84:990–992.

69. Bengtsson BO. Incidence of manifest glaucoma. *Br J Ophthalmol* 1989; 73:483–487.

70. Leske MC, Connell AM, Wu SY, *et al*. Incidence of open-angle glaucoma: the Barbados Eye Studies. The Barbados Eye Studies Group. *Arch Ophthalmol* 2001; 119:89–95.

71. Thomas R, George R, Parikh R, *et al*. Five-year risk of progression of primary angle-closure suspects to primary angle-closure: a population based study. *Br J Ophthalmol* 2003; 87:450–454.

72. Thomas R, Parikh R, Muliyil J, *et al*. Five-year risk of progression of primary angle-closure to primary angle-closure glaucoma: a population-based study. *Acta Ophthalmol Scand* 2003; 81:480–485.

73. Hu CC, Lin HC, Chen CS, *et al*. Reduction in admissions of patients with acute primary angle-closure occurring in conjunction with a rise in cataract surgery in Taiwan. *Acta Ophthalmol* 2008; 86:440–445.

74. Keenan TD, Salmon JF, Yeates D, *et al*. Trends in rates of primary angle-closure glaucoma and cataract surgery in England from 1968 to 2004. *J Glaucoma* 2009; 18:201–205.

75. Boland MV, Quigley HA. Risk factors and open-angle glaucoma: classification and application. *J Glaucoma* 2007; 16:406–418.

76. Healey PR, Mitchell P. Optic disk size in open-angle glaucoma: the Blue Mountains Eye Study. *Am J Ophthalmol* 1999; 128:515–517.

77. Congdon NG, Broman AT, Bandeen-Roche K, *et al*. Central corneal thickness and corneal hysteresis associated with glaucoma damage. *Am J Ophthalmol* 2006; 141:868–875.

78. Cartwright MJ, Anderson DR. Correlation of asymmetric damage with asymmetric intraocular pressure in normal-tension glaucoma (low-tension glaucoma). *Arch Ophthalmol* 1988; 106: 898–900.

79. Tielsch JM, Katz J, Sommer A, *et al*. Hypertension, perfusion pressure, and primary open-angle glaucoma. A population-based assessment. *Arch Ophthalmol* 1995; 113:216–221.

80. Tielsch JM, Katz J, Quigley HA, *et al*. Diabetes, intraocular pressure, and primary open-angle glaucoma in the Baltimore Eye Survey. *Ophthalmology* 1995; 102:48–53.

81. Quigley HA. Can diabetes be good for glaucoma? Why can't we believe our own eyes (or data)? *Arch Ophthalmol* 2009; 127:227–229.

82. Drance S, Anderson DR, Schulzer M. Risk factors for progression of visual field abnormalities in normal-tension glaucoma. *Am J Ophthalmol* 2001; 131: 699–708.

83. Congdon NG, Youlin Q, Quigley H, *et al.* Biometry and primary angle-closure glaucoma among Chinese, white, and black populations. *Ophthalmology* 1997; 104:1489–1495.

84. Alsbirk PH. Early detection of primary angle-closure glaucoma. Limbal and axial chamber depth screening in a high risk population (Greenland Eskimos). *Acta Ophthalmol (Copenh)* 1988; 66:556–564.

85. Devereux JG, Foster PJ, Baasanhu J, *et al.* Anterior chamber depth measurement as a screening tool for primary angle-closure glaucoma in an East Asian population. *Arch Ophthalmol* 2000; 118:257–263.

86. Quigley HA, Silver DM, Friedman DS, *et al.* Iris cross-sectional area decreases with pupil dilation and its dynamic behaviour is a risk factor in angle-closure. *J Glaucoma* 2009; 18:173–179.

87. Aptel F, Denis P. Optical coherence tomography quantitative analysis of iris volume changes after pharmacologic mydriasis. *Ophthalmology* 2010; 117:3–10.

88. Quigley HA. Long-term follow-up of laser iridotomy. *Ophthalmology* 1981; 88:218–224.

89. He M, Friedman DS, Ge J, *et al.* Laser peripheral iridotomy in primary angle-closure suspects: biometric and gonioscopic outcomes: the Liwan Eye Study. *Ophthalmology* 2007; 114:494–500.

90. Wand M, Grant WM, Simmons RJ *et al.* Plateau iris syndrome. *Trans Sect Ophthalmol Am Acad Ophthalmol Otolaryngol* 1977; 83:122–130.

91. Quigley HA. Angle-closure glaucoma — simpler answers to complex mechanisms. LXVI Edward Jackson Memorial Lecture. *Am J Ophthalmol* 2009; 148:657–669.

92. Sakai H, Morine-Shinjyo S, Shinzato M, *et al.* Uveal effusion in primary angle-closure glaucoma. *Ophthalmology* 2005; 112:413–419.

93. Kumar RS, Quek D, Lee KY, *et al.* Confirmation of the presence of uveal effusion in Asian eyes with primary angle-closure glaucoma: an ultrasound biomicroscopy study. *Arch Ophthalmol* 2008; 126: 1647–1651.

94. Wolfs RC, Klaver CC, Ramrattan RS, *et al.* Genetic risk of primary open-angle glaucoma. Population-based familial aggregation study. *Arch Ophthalmol* 1998; 116:1640–1645.

95. Stone EM, Fingert JH, Alward WL, *et al.* Identification of a gene that causes primary open angle glaucoma. *Science* 1997; 275:668–670.

96. Rezaie T, Child A, Hitchings R, *et al.* Adult-onset primary open-angle glaucoma caused by mutations in optineurin. *Science* 2002; 295:1077–1079.

97. Aung T, Rezaie T, Okada K, *et al.* Clinical features and course of patients with glaucoma with the E50K mutation in the optineurin gene. *Invest Ophthalmol Vis Sci* 2005; 46:2816–2822.

98. Monemi S, Spaeth G, DaSilva A, *et al.* Identification of a novel adult-onset primary open-angle glaucoma (POAG) gene on 5q22.1. *Hum Mol Genet* 2005; 14:725–733.

99. Thorleifsson G, Magnusson KP, Sulem P, *et al.* Common sequence variants in the LOXL1 gene confer susceptibility to exfoliation glaucoma. *Science* 2007; 317:1397–1400.

100. Stoilov I, Akarsu AN, Sarfarazi M. Identification of three different truncating mutations in cytochrome P4501B1 (CYP1B1) as the principal cause of primary congenital glaucoma (Buphthalmos) in families linked to the GLC3A locus on chromosome 2p21. *Hum Mol Genet* 1997; 6:641–647.

101. Lichter PR, Musch DC, Gillespie BW, *et al.* Interim clinical outcomes in the Collaborative Initial Glaucoma Treatment Study comparing initial treatment randomized to medications or surgery. *Ophthalmology* 2001; 108:1943–1953.

102. Migdal C, Gregory W, Hitchings R. Long-term functional outcome after early surgery compared with laser and medicine in open-angle glaucoma. *Ophthalmology* 1994; 101:1651–1656.

103. Comparison of glaucomatous progression between untreated patients with normal-tension glaucoma and patients with therapeutically reduced intraocular pressures. Collaborative Normal–Tension Glaucoma Study Group. *Am J Ophthalmol* 1998; 126: 487–497.

104. The AGIS Investigators. The Advanced Glaucoma Intervention Study (AGIS): 7. The relationship between control of intraocular pressure and visual field deterioration. *Am J Ophthalmol* 2000; 130: 429–440.

105. Heijl A, Leske MC, Bengtsson B, *et al.* Reduction of intraocular pressure and glaucoma progression: results from the Early Manifest Glaucoma Trial. *Arch Ophthalmol* 2002; 120:1268–1279.

106. Leske MC, Heijl A, Hussein M, *et al.* Factors for glaucoma progression and the effect of treatment: the early manifest glaucoma trial. *Arch Ophthalmol* 2003; 121:48–56.

107. Kass MA, Heuer DK, Higginbotham EJ, *et al.* The Ocular Hypertension Treatment Study: a randomized trial determines that topical ocular hypotensive medication delays or prevents the onset of primary open-angle glaucoma. *Arch Ophthalmol* 2002; 120:701–713.

108. Congdon N, Wang F, Tielsch JM. Issues in the epidemiology and population-based screening of primary angle-closure glaucoma. *Surv Ophthalmol* 1992; 36:411–423.

109. van Herick W, Shaffer RN, Schwartz A. Estimation of width of angle of anterior chamber. Incidence and significance of the narrow angle. *Am J Ophthalmol* 1969; 68:626–629.

110. Foster PJ, Devereux JG, Alsbirk PH, *et al.* Detection of gonioscopically occludable angles and primary angle-closure glaucoma by estimation of limbal chamber depth in Asians: modified grading scheme. *Br J Ophthalmol* 2000; 84:186–192.

111. Congdon NG, Spaeth GL, Augsburger J, *et al.* A proposed simple method for measurement in the anterior chamber angle: biometric gonioscopy. *Ophthalmology* 1999; 106:2161–2167.

112. Nolan WP, Foster PJ, Devereux JG, *et al.* YAG laser iridotomy treatment for primary angle-closure in east Asian eyes. *Br J Ophthalmol* 2000; 84: 1255–1259.

113. Friedman DS, Chew PTK, Gazzard G, *et al.* Long-term outcomes in fellow eyes after acute primary angle-closure in the contra-lateral eye. *Ophthalmology* 2006; 113:1087–1091.

14

Visual impairment and blindness in children

14a   Magnitude and causes   269
14b   Vitamin A deficiency disorders   291
14c   Ophthalmia neonatorum   317
14d   Corneal disease in children   323

14e   Cataract in children   331
14f   Glaucoma in children   341
14g   Retinopathy of prematurity   353

14   EDITORS' NOTE

In this edition of the book, the epidemiology of the major blinding eye diseases of childhood are presented as separate sections in one chapter. The first section gives an overview of the prevalence, magnitude and causes of visual impairment and blindness in children, highlighting the regional variation and some of the methodological challenges. The next three sections cover the major preventable causes, and the last three sections are concerned with the major treatable causes. The sections have been written by experts in their respective fields.

14a

Magnitude and causes

CLARE GILBERT AND JUGNOO RAHI

14a.1	Introduction	269	14a.7	Time trends for the major causes of blindness in children	282
14a.2	Definition of childhood and categories of visual loss	270	14a.8	Prevalence and causes of functional low vision in children	284
14a.3	Prevalence and magnitude of childhood blindness and visual impairment	273	14a.9	Avoidable causes of blindness in children	285
14a.4	Magnitude of blindness in children and change over the last decade	277	14a.10	Summary and future areas of research	285
14a.5	Incidence of blindness in children	278		References	285
14a.6	Causes of blindness in children	281			

14a.1 INTRODUCTION

Visual loss in childhood has implications for all aspects of the child's development.[1] It poses educational, occupational and social challenges, with affected children being at risk of behavioural, psychological and emotional difficulties, impaired self-esteem and poorer social integration.[2] A high proportion of visually impaired children — half or more in industrialized countries — have other motor, sensory or cognitive impairments.[3] Many visually impaired children have chronic disorders that are not amenable to ophthalmic treatment but require visual rehabilitation, educational support and/or developmental interventions. Thus the impact of visual impairment in childhood at an individual level is considerable. The impact can extend beyond the affected child to siblings, parents and other family members, although research about this, especially from developing countries, is sparse. Studies in the USA demonstrate that having a disabled child increases the likelihood of parents divorcing or living apart, of the mother not going out to work, of the father working shorter hours and of the parents having lower rates of social participation. Positive impacts include a greater awareness of inner strengths, enhanced family cohesion and broadened horizons.[4]

The control of blindness in children remains one of the main priorities of the World Health Organization's (WHO) **VISION 2020 The Right to Sight** initiative for a number of reasons. First, the number of 'blind years' resulting from blindness in children is more than double the number of 'blind years' attributable to cataract in adults. Second, the causes of blindness in children are very different from the causes of blindness in adults, and strategies to combat blindness in adults will not work for the control of blindness in children. Third, unlike in adults, a delay in treatment for some causes can lead to **amblyopia**. There is, therefore, a level of urgency about managing eye diseases in children. Fourth, children's eyes are not like small adult eyes — they respond differently to treatment, and specific expertise, equipment and training is required.

14a.1.1 Challenges of epidemiological studies of childhood visual disability

There are particular difficulties in undertaking epidemiological research on visual impairment in childhood. First, although the same categories of visual loss can be applied to infants and children as to adults, measuring visual function in children, particularly those under the age of five and those with additional disabilities, can be very difficult and time-consuming. In addition, although many disorders are present from early childhood, visual maturation is not complete until much later. Second, most visually impairing disorders of childhood are individually rare, necessitating large studies, which are difficult and expensive to undertake.

Third, many of the blinding disorders of childhood currently lack robust definitions or classification systems, or classification, systems are being changed or modified in light of phenotype/genotype correlations (for example, see Section 14d on corneal dystrophies). Fourth, important outcomes can only be reliably determined through long-term follow up, which is difficult to achieve. And finally, there are a number of ethical considerations about children's participation in research, especially in trials, that are the subject of ongoing debate, which do not arise with adult subjects able to consent to participate themselves.[5] These potential obstacles partly account for the limited epidemiological research and will be expanded upon below.

14a.2 DEFINITION OF CHILDHOOD AND CATEGORIES OF VISUAL LOSS

Childhood is defined by **UNICEF** as the period of life before 16 years of age. Blindness is defined according to the WHO's categories of visual impairment as a corrected visual acuity in the better eye of <3/60, or a constricted visual field of <10° from the point of central fixation. Visual impairment is defined as a corrected acuity of <6/18 in the better eye. A further category of visual loss, which has been termed 'functional low vision', is used to identify children and adults who might benefit from assessment for low-vision services. The definition excludes those with treatable causes of visual loss and is defined as follows: 'a person with low vision is an individual, who after refraction and medical or surgical treatment, has a best corrected visual acuity of <6/18 to light perception in the better eye, but who uses, or has the potential to use, vision for the planning and/or execution of a task'.[6] (See Chapter 12, Section 12.3.)

14a.2.1 Visual development and measuring visual function in children

The visual system is relatively immature at birth, and maturation depends on both structural and functional changes. The various visual functions mature at different rates, being rapid in the first year of life; adult levels of some functions are achieved only in late childhood.[7] Thus it can be difficult to predict final visual outcome in young children with visual defects.

When assessing the ability of a child to see it is important to be aware of visual development and age-specific visual norms. For example, normally sighted babies should blink to a flash from birth but may not fix on and follow a face at around half a metre until three months of age, and may not blink to a threat until five months of age.[8]

Assessment of different visual functions is fundamental to the management of eye disease in children. A variety of visual functions, such as visual fields, contrast sensitivity, and binocularity are all relevant to overall function, and age-specific 'normal' ranges have been reported for many of these.[9] Nevertheless, distance visual acuity remains the most frequently measured visual function in clinical practice and epidemiological research.

Distance visual acuity

Visual acuity can usually be measured in older children (i.e. aged five years and above) using standard optotypes or **Early Treatment Diabetic Retinopathy Study** (**ETDRS**) type charts. **LogMAR** charts are now the gold standard acuity chart and are being increasingly used in paediatric clinics. Charts are also available for use at three metres, and many countries have Snellen charts using local scripts or alphabets. However, these tests require levels of comprehension and concentration, educational development and verbal skills that a young child or a child with additional disabilities may not possess. The Snellen E chart requires motor skills, co-ordination and a sense of orientation, and most children aged four to five years old or above can comply with this method, whatever their cultural background.

Cultural-sensitive visual acuity tests for younger children, or those with additional impairments, include use of pictures (e.g. Allen cards, Kays pictures), matching tests (e.g. LH symbols; Sonksen Silver test; Sheridan–Gardiner test; Cambridge cards), or forced choice preferential looking techniques (e.g. Teller acuity cards; Cardiff cards — both of which require age-specific and setting-specific norms for reliable interpretation). Many of these methods have been modified to include elements of crowding, to improve detection of visual acuity loss from amblyopia and the use of such cards should be encouraged (e.g. Glasgow acuity cards; isolated surrounded HOTV optotypes). Other advantages of tests such as LH symbols and HOTV are that they have fewer symbols than a standard Snellen chart, and in the case of HOTV, all symbols are reversible, enabling the use of mirrors to obtain appropriate testing distances when physical space is limited.

(*Continued*)

(*Continued*)

Measuring acuity in infants, or in children with other disabilities, is challenging and time consuming.[10] Many of the methods employed do not measure acuity, but can be used to determine whether an infant is totally blind or not (e.g. observation of visually evoked reflexes such as head turn towards a light and blink reflex; maintenance of fixation while the child is being rotated; observation of eye and head movements in response to small, moving targets). Forced choice preferential looking tests are often used with infants, and visually evoked potentials (e.g. pattern reversal VEPs) can be used to gauge levels of visual function in broader terms, but the latter require skilled electrophysiologists to undertake and interpret the findings.

Many of the tests mentioned above require a distraction-free environment and trained personnel to give reliable information. Cardiff cards and the Cambridge cards have been evaluated in young children during population-based studies in the Gambia and Ghana, but in both instances the logistical difficulties of obtaining a distraction-free environment made the tests unworkable. However, these optotype tests are used in standard clinical practice in many other settings and can be used in facility-based studies.

In order to obtain reliable information on visual acuity in young children it is often necessary to repeat the assessment on different occasions, as the child may not be able to concentrate or cooperate well enough for a one-off test to give meaningful results. These factors have to be borne in mind when interpreting the childhood blindness prevalence data, particularly data obtained from population-based surveys where the Snellen E chart was usually the method used for all ages. To date, none of the methods that would be appropriate for measuring visual acuity in the under-five-year age group have been stringently evaluated and validated in a field setting. It is not known whether

(*Continued*)

(Continued)

they can be performed by trained field workers, or whether the equipment is robust enough to withstand testing in the field, or whether the methods give valid results in different cultures or in communities that may have high levels of illiteracy.

Near visual acuity

Assessment of near visual acuity is often overlooked in clinical practice and in research but is critically important because the young child's visual world is near. As with distance acuity, older children can be tested using near acuity charts, or E charts if they are too young to read or know the alphabet. Matching tests can be used for younger children.

Visual fields

Knowledge of visual fields can be uniquely important to making a diagnosis, predicting prognosis, monitoring therapy and assessing outcomes in diverse contexts. It is particularly relevant in the management of children with retinal dystrophies, glaucoma, optic neuropathy/neuritis, intracranial tumours, or raised intracranial pressure, as well as those on drugs with potential ocular toxicity, such as the antiepileptic drug vigabatrin. However, reliably assessing the visual fields of children is challenging, as evidenced by the numerous and diverse techniques proposed (e.g. static and kinetic perimetry).[11] Normative data have been reported for some of these. Nevertheless, there remain differing views regarding optimal perimetric strategies in children. Further work is required to evaluate different approaches.

Colour vision and contrast sensitivity

Older children can comply with standard tests for adults and tests suitable for younger children are being developed, e.g. the 'Hiding Heidi' contrast sensitivity test.[12]

14a.2.2   Patient-reported outcome measures

Clinical parameters, such as visual acuity or visual fields, have traditionally been the main outcomes in clinical practice and research. However, although these objective clinical outcomes describe the level of impairment, they do not characterize either the functioning (overall functional visual status) or the disability (consequent disadvantage) experienced.[13] This is partly because they cannot capture variation in functional adaptation between individuals to the same level of visual loss. There is increasing interest in developing objective measures of overall function that assess vision-dependent functional abilities in relation to social contact, mobility, sustained near-tasks and tasks of daily living.[14] These would be important outcomes in clinical practice and research, as alternatives or in addition to clinical outcomes. Equally, children's perspectives of the consequences of their visual loss and of their treatment have not been widely investigated. To address this, generic paediatric health status and health-related quality of life instruments have been used in some studies of children with ophthalmic disease. However, it is widely recognized that vision-specific subjective outcome measures, such as paediatric vision-related quality of life tools, would be of value in prioritizing, planning and allocating resources, and in the evaluation of interventions in health, education and social services.[15]

In ophthalmic literature, concepts of functional vision and vision-related quality of life have often been used interchangeably, with instruments being developed to assess in broad terms the 'impact' of vision loss on an individual.[16] However, there is a distinction between these two concepts. Functional vision should be considered as the child's ability to perform a task or activity that requires vision,[17] whilst vision-related quality of life is the child's view of the gap between his/her current experiences and his/her expectations as a result of the visually impairing disorder and its therapy, and affecting his/her physical, emotional, psychological, cognitive and social functioning.[14–15,18]

There is an extensive range of functional vision/visual function and vision-related quality of life instruments for use with adults with eye disease or visual impairment.[19–22] However, only two patient-based measures have been reported to date for the assessment of functional vision in children and young people: the **Children's Functional Vision Questionnaire (CVFQ)**[23–24] and the **LV Prasad–Functional Vision Questionnaire (LVP–FVQ)**.[17] The development of the CVFQ and the LVP–FVQ was drawn mostly from the perspectives of care-givers and the professionals rather than being grounded in children's own experiences. In addition, the CVFQ uses items adapted from a variety of existing developmental tests and adult functional vision instruments,[21] and is designed for proxy (typically a parent) rather than self-completion. The LVP–FVQ was developed specifically for children in the developing world and some items have limited applicability to industrialized country settings.

There are many methodological difficulties in this field. The development of psychometrically robust instruments that children and young people can use for self-reporting, is best addressed through a multidisciplinary approach.

14a.3 PREVALENCE AND MAGNITUDE OF CHILDHOOD BLINDNESS AND VISUAL IMPAIRMENT

14a.3.1 Prevalence data

Possible sources of data on the frequency and causes of blindness and visual impairment, together with their challenges and limitations are given in Table 14a.1. From this it will become clear that the 'gold standard' cross-sectional prevalence survey has many challenges when applied to visual impairment and blindness in children, and other sources of data are required.

Table 14a.2 summarizes the data that have been published since 1990, and Table 14a.3 shows data from the eight standardized, population-based surveys of refractive errors in children. Only surveys which had a sample size of at least 2,500 children were included, as estimates from smaller studies will have extremely wide confidence intervals. As will be seen, most of the data from industrialized countries come from national or local blind registers, while

data from other regions have come from a variety of sources, including cross-sectional prevalence surveys. An important limitation of registration data is that not all eligible children are registered for a variety of reasons,[25] and the register is not usually 'live', i.e. children's names are not removed if they die, or have sight-restoring procedures. Several studies have used the key informant method,[26–27] and several have attempted to identify all blind children within a defined population using multiple methods of ascertainment.[28–30] In addition to the use of different methods, studies also differ in relation to the definition of blindness and the age group; however, studies are becoming more standardized and hence comparable. In virtually all the studies visual acuity was measured using optotypes, but most publications do not report how young children were tested, which is an important limitation in the description of the methodology. In studies using the key informant method and others using multiple approaches to ascertainment, where the denominator was an estimate, derived by extrapolating census data, any inaccuracies in the denominator can have a major impact on the blindness prevalence estimate.

As anticipated, prevalence estimates obtained from the Established Market Economies are far lower than estimates from Sub-Saharan Africa. The higher prevalence in poorer countries is likely to reflect a higher incidence of some conditions as well as poorer access to services which restore visual function.

14a.3.2 Relationship between blindness prevalence and mortality rates in children under five years old

Earlier reviews of childhood prevalence data suggested that the prevalence of blindness in children was associated with **under-five mortality rates (U5MR)**.[31] To assess whether this association still holds true, the prevalence data in Table 14a.2 were plotted against the U5MR for the year five years prior to the study (Fig. 14a.1). This time point was chosen so that the U5MR used related to the central five years of the 15 years of childhood (see Table 14a.2, heading marked 'Relevant U5MR').

Table 14a.1 Advantages and limitations of different sources of epidemiological data in relation to childhood visual impairment and blindness

Method/source of data	Measure(s)	Advantages	Disadvantages/challenges
Prevalence and causes of visual impairment and blindness:			
Population-based cross-sectional surveys specifically designed to assess visual loss in children	Prevalence of blindness, visual impairment and/or low vision. Causes if sample large enough	Gold standard method	Many, both technical and practical: • A very large sample size is needed to give precise estimates (30,000), and 40,000–60,000 for reliable data on causes • Enumeration has to be meticulous to ensure that children not enumerated are not included • Response rates likely to be low (at school; disabled children away from home, etc.) • Measuring visual acuity in the field, and in young children very challenging • Needs a two-stage process so logistically difficult • Clinical team who confirm the impairment and examine children to determine the cause need equipment and high levels of expertise • Very time-consuming • Very expensive
Population-based cross-sectional survey designed for other purposes, e.g. vitamin A deficiency; refractive errors	Prevalence of blindness, visual impairment and/or low vision. Causes if sample large enough	May provide some data; shared costs	• As above, and • May lead to an imprecise estimate, as sample size not determined for visual impairment • May miss children with causes that are not obvious, i.e. posterior segment pathology
Community based rehabilitation (CBR) programmes for the blind	Prevalence of blindness, visual impairment and/or low vision. Causes if sample large enough	Data collected while identifying blind individuals	Unreliable data likely on the: • Denominator, as this is usually an estimate • Numerator, as children who have some residual vision may not be included in the programme i.e. < 3/60 to hand movements • Causes data may be unreliable as children not always examined by an ophthalmologist
Key informant method[27]	Prevalence of blindness, visual impairment and/or low vision. Causes if sample large enough	Quick Inexpensive Leaves trained 'case finders' in the community	• Denominator is an estimate • Not all cases will be ascertained, so prevalence is an underestimate: potential for bias
'Piggy backing' onto other surveys, e.g. RAABs	Prevalence of blindness, visual impairment and/or low vision. Causes if sample large enough	Cheaper than designing a survey just for children	• Sample size usually low so estimates have wide confidence intervals • Selection bias as sampling strategy will be for the primary outcome and not for blindness/visual impairment in children
National census data collected by house to house visits	Prevalence from self-reported data. No data on causes	Costs of data collection included in census data collection	• Relies on self report, which is subjective and likely to overestimate prevalence • Census staff may not be adequately trained

(Continued)

Table 14a.1 (Continued)

Method/source of data	Measure(s)	Advantages	Disadvantages/challenges
Specific population-based health surveillance studies	Prevalence and causes data	Can provide reliable data	Requires a highly organized health system with high population coverage
Questionnaires such as the ten-question questionnaire[27]	Prevalence data	Quick to administer by field workers	Questionnaires can have high sensitivity and specificity for some disabling disorders, but their validity is low for hearing and visual loss[47]
Incidence and causes of visual impairment and blindness:			
Blindness registers	Incidence and causes, if a standard classification used, e.g. ICD-10	Can provide accurate data	• Requires well-organized health systems and a limited number of service providers • Not all individuals eligible will be registered unless this is a statutory requirement. This particularly applies to children
Active surveillance	Incidence and causes	Can provide accurate data	• Requires well-organized health systems and a limited number of service providers • Under-ascertainment likely even in the best circumstances
Incidence of specific conditions:			
Disease specific/anomaly registers[49]	Incidence of the specific conditions regardless of functional impact	Can provide accurate data	• Do not take account of functional impact, e.g. anomaly registers include microphthalmos and isolated iris coloboma regardless of visual acuity • Under-reporting is common[48] • Misdiagnosis can occur as children often examined and registered by non-specialists
Causes of visual impairment blindness and low vision:			
Hospital-based studies	Causes only	Easy to do	Selection bias: treatable causes tend to be over-represented
Examination of children enrolled in special education	Causes only	Quick and a large number of children can be examined quickly	Selection bias likely

Table 14a.2 Childhood blindness prevalence data published since 1990, by World Bank region

Region/country	Year of study	Source of data	Sample size	Blindness definition	Age group	Prev./1,000	Relevant U5MR Year	U5MR
Established Market Economies:								
Canada[50]	2006	Local register	NR	<3/60	0–19	0.00	2001	9
Ireland[51]	2004	Multiple	NR	<3/60	0–15	0.50	1999	7
Denmark[52]	1993	Register	NR	<3/60	0–15	0.41	1988	10
Finland[52]	1993	Register	NR	<3/60	0–15	0.15	1988	7
Iceland[52]	1993	Register	NR	<3/60	0–15	0.19	1988	7
Norway[52]	1993	Register	NR	<3/60	0–15	0.15	1988	10
Middle East Crescent:								
Iran[53]	2008	KIM	136,000 E	<6/60	0–15	0.40	2003	45
Oman[54]	2002	Survey all ages	6,208	<3/60	0–14	0.80	1997	17
Israel[55]	2000	Register	NR	ND	0–18	0.45	1995	8
China:								
China[56]	2004	Survey	60 124	ND	0–6	0.33	2000	38
China[57]	2008	Survey	17,699	<3/60	3–6	0.28	2003	39
India:								
India[58]	1996–2000	Survey	2,861	<6/60	0–15	1.05	1995	103
India[59]	2008	HtH survey	13,421	<3/60	0–15	1.06	2003	101
India[60]	2002	Survey	10,605	<3/60	0–15	0.62	1997	103
India[61]	1995–97	Survey	5,342	<3/60	0–19	0.75	1992	119
India[62]	1996	CBR	113,514 E	<3/60	0–15	0.95	1991	119
India[63]	2007	KIM	63,030 E	<6/60	0–15	0.62	2002	93
Other Asia and Islands:								
Malaysia[64]	1996	Survey	8,504	<3/60	0–19	0.82	1991	19
Bangladesh[PC]	2002	KIM	NA	<6/60	0–15	0.78	1997	118
Mongolia[28]	1999–2000	Multiple	339,657 E	<6/60	0–15	0.19	1995	121
Fiji[29]	2007–07	Multiple	133,000 E	<6/60	0–15	0.36	2002	22
Sub-Saharan Africa:								
Ethiopia[65]	2006	Survey	16,820	<3/60	0–15	1.00	2001	172
Sudan[66]	2003	HH cluster	29,048	<6/60	0–15	1.38	1998	112
Malawi[67]	2008	KIM	43,000 E	<3/60	0–15	0.90	2003	183
Ghana[68]	2005	KIM	23,000 E	<6/60	0–15	0.74	2000	100
Tanzania[30]	2009	Multiple	95,040 E	<3/60	0–15	0.17	2004	165

NA = not applicable; NR = not relevant; ND = no data; HtH = house-to-house; KIM = Key Informant Method; HH = household; E = estimate; CBR = Community Based Rehabilitation; PC = Muhit MA, personal communication.

Table 14a.3 *Prevalence data derived from the Refractive Error surveys of Children[69]*

Country	Year	Sample size	Blindness definition (corrected)	Age group	Prev./1,000	Relevant U5MR Year	U5MR
S Africa[70]	2002	4,890	≤ 6/60	5–15	0.20	1995	65
China rural[71]	1998	5,884	≤ 6/60	5–15	0.20	1991	38
China urban[72]	2003	4,364	≤ 6/60	5–15	0.00	1996	38
India rural[73]	2001	4,082	≤ 6/60	7–15	1.30	1994	119
India urban[74]	2001	6,527	≤ 6/60	5–15	0.46	1994	119
Malaysia[75]	2003	4,634	≤ 6/60	7–15	0.00	1996	15
Nepal[76]	1998	5,067	≤ 6/60	5–15	1.50	1991	117
Chile[77]	1998	5,303	≤ 6/60	5–15	0.6	1991	17

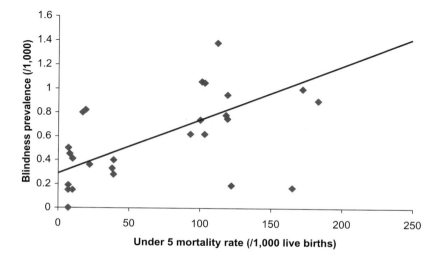

Figure 14a.1 *Plot of blindness prevalence (/1,000) against under-five mortality rate (U5MR) relevant to the date of the study*

Note: Linear regression line excludes data points from the two studies with unexpectedly low prevalence estimates, Mongolia and Tanzania.

The available data are suggestive of a linear relationship between the prevalence of blindness in children and U5MRs. The higher blindness prevalence in poorer countries with high U5MRs almost certainly reflects poorer access to primary healthcare and specific services for children with treatable disease, as well as exposure to environmental risk factors that do not occur in affluent regions but which cause both blindness in children and child deaths, e.g. **vitamin A deficiency disorders (VADD)**, measles, meningitis, tumours, congenital rubella syndrome etc. Indeed, U5MRs are now being used as a proxy to indicate whether communities of children are at risk of VADD at levels of public health significance.[32]

14a.4 MAGNITUDE OF BLINDNESS IN CHILDREN AND CHANGE OVER THE LAST DECADE

The association between U5MR and blindness prevalence in children can be used to estimate the prevalence of blindness (Table 14a.4). The magnitude of blindness in children can then be estimated by country, region and globally, by applying the rel-

Table 14a.4 *Using under five mortality rates to estimate the prevalence of blindness in children*

Under-five mortality rate per 1000 live births	Estimate of prevalence per 1,000 children
0–19	0.3
20–39	0.4
40–59	0.5
60–79	0.6
80–99	0.7
100–119	0.8
120–139	0.9
140–159	1.0
160–179	1.1
180–199	1.2
200–219	1.3
220–239	1.4
240+	1.5

evant prevalence estimate to the child population in each country. This process assumes that U5MRs are uniform across any particular country, which is unlikely. In India there is a five-fold difference in U5MR between Kerala and Uttar Pradesh, and there are also likely to be rural/urban differences. In 1999 the estimate was that there were 1.4 million blind children in the world[33] and this figure has been revised down to 1.26 million in 2010 (a 10% reduction over the last ten years) (Table 14a.5 and Fig. 14a.2). In China, Other Asia and Islands, the Established Market Economies and Former Socialist economies, Latin America and the Caribbean, there has been a reduction in the estimated number of children who are blind despite the child population remaining relatively stable (Table 14a.5). In the Middle East Crescent and India there has not been much change and sub-Saharan Africa is the only region where the number of children who are blind is estimated to have increased over the last ten years. This is, in part, explained by a 5.4% growth in the child population, but more notably, this is a region where the U5MRs have actually increased in some countries over the last decade, on account of the direct and indirect impact of the HIV/AIDS epidemic.[34]

In developing countries a much higher proportion of the population are children than in affluent regions, which means that the actual number of blind children in a total population of ten million can vary by a factor of x10, from an estimate of 600 per million in established market economies to 6,000 per million total population in the poorest countries of Africa (Fig. 14a.3).

14a.5   INCIDENCE OF BLINDNESS IN CHILDREN

There are few sources of data on the incidence of childhood visual impairment in any region of the world. A particular challenge in estimating and monitoring the cause-specific incidence of visual impairment in children is that any one disorder will be uncommon. Registers of the blind and population-based surveillance can both be used to identify eligible cases. A study of severe visual impairment and blindness in the UK (British Childhood Visual Impairment Study), in which newly diagnosed children were identified through the national active surveillance schemes in ophthalmology (British Ophthalmological Surveillance Unit) and paediatrics (British Paediatric Surveillance Unit) has been undertaken.[3] Four-hundred and thirty-nine children were newly diagnosed over the course of one year, of whom 336 (77%) had additional non-ophthalmic conditions. The total annual incidence (95% CI) was highest in the first year of life, being 4.0 (3.6 to 4.5) per 10,000 with a cumulative incidence by 16 years of 5.9 (5.3 to 6.5) per 10,000. Incidence varied with presence of non-ophthalmic conditions, birth weight and ethnicity.

Registers exist in many industrialized countries and have traditionally been used to monitor incidence. However, most rely on voluntary notification and, as not all eligible children will be registered for a variety of reasons, registers can provide only minimum estimates of incidence. The following registration data are available for the following countries: UK (in one region), children aged 0–12 years between 1984 and 1998, 4.0/10,000 live births;[35] Israel, children aged 0–4 years in 1999, 0.7/10,000 population;[36] Kuwait, individuals aged 0–20 years between 2000 and 2004, 0.56/10,000 person years;[37] and Scandinavian registers give an estimated incidence of blindness of 0.8/10,000 children/year.

Table 14a.5 *Estimates of the number of children who are blind and changes between 1999 and 2010 estimates*

	1999 estimate		2010 estimate		% change between 1999 and 2010	
	Child pop (millions)	Blind children	Child pop (millions)	Blind children	In child population	In estimates of blind children
Lower in 2010 than 1999:						
China	340	210,000	340	116,000	0%	−44.8%
Other Asia and Islands	260	220,000	266	136,000	−2.3%	−38.2%
EME + FSE	248	90,000	244	70,000	−1.6%	−22.2%
Latin America & Caribbean	170	100,000	170	71,000	0%	−29.0%
Not much change:						
Middle East Crescent	240	190,000	241	168,000	+0.4%	−11.6%
India	350	270,000	345	280,000	−1.4%	+ 3.7%
Higher in 2010 than 1999:						
Sub-Saharan Africa	260	320,000	274	419,000	+5.4%	+30.9%
TOTAL:	**1,868**	**1,400,000**	**1,880**	**1,260,000**	**+0.6%**	**−10%**

EME + FSE: Date for the Established Market Economies and Former Socialist Economies have been combined as some countries changed region between 1999 and 2010.

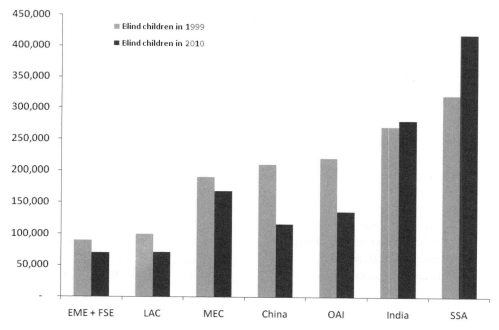

Figure 14a.2 *Estimates of the number of blind children in 1999 and 2010, by World Bank region*

EME = Established Market Economies; FSE = Former Socialist Economies. These regions have been combined as some countries were re-designated between 1999 and 2010. MEC = Middle East Crescent; LAC = Latin America and Caribbean; OAI = Other Asia and Islands; SSA = Sub-Saharan Africa.

There are no comparable incidence data from developing countries. Earlier estimates indicated that approximately 500,000 children became blind worldwide each year, the majority of whom lived in developing countries.[33] However, these estimates were derived more than 20 years ago when VADD and measles were major causes of corneal blindness in children as well as important cause of child mortality.

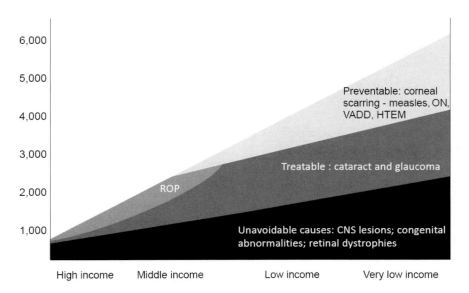

Figure 14a.3 *Schematic representation of the magnitude and causes of blindness in children, by level of socio-economic development*

ROP = retinopathy of prematurity; ON = ophthalmia neonatorum; VADD = vitamin A deficiency disorders; HTEM = harmful traditional eye medicines; CNS = central nervous system.

Given the improved coverage with measles immunization (see Section 14d) and high-dose vitamin A supplementation it is likely that this figure is now much lower.[38]

Broad trends in incidence and prevalence may also be examined through referrals to multidisciplinary teams serving geographically defined populations, but again these are likely to underestimate rates. Modifications have been proposed to improve the routine collection, recording and collation of data about disability in child health systems in industrialized countries. Both approaches would improve the ability to monitor the frequency and causes of visual disability within defined child populations using routinely collected data.

Inclusion of a standardized minimum dataset about visual impairment in longitudinal studies of children with other disabilities has also been advocated. Finally, birth cohort studies allow estimation of cumulative incidence (lifetime risk) of various eye diseases, as well as prevalence. As it is difficult to derive reliable estimates of disease frequency (incidence or prevalence) from any single source, the use of multiple sources, wherever possible, is advocated.

14a.5.1   Mortality in blind children

Many of the blinding conditions of childhood are associated with a high mortality rate; in developing countries these include measles, VADD, meningitis, cerebral tumours and retinoblastoma; in middle and high income countries children who are blind as a consequence of preterm birth, neuro-developmental disorders, head injuries, and chromosomal and metabolic conditions, are likely to have higher mortality rates than children who are not blind. In countries where VADD is a significant public health problem it is thought that over 50% of children die within one to two years of becoming blind, if they are not given supplements.[39]

The following mortality rates have been reported from industrialized countries: 10% within a year of diagnosis of blindness (UK surveillance study);[3] 13% of a Swedish cohort born between 1962–1976 died before reaching adulthood;[40] and 19% of all visually impaired children on a UK disability register died over a 15-year period, with over half dying before the age of five years.[35] To investigate this further, a large cohort of blind children would have to be identified and followed, and the mortality rate in this group compared with the mortality rate in a control group of sighted children. Given the high mortality rate, prevalence data almost certainly markedly underestimate the magnitude of the problem of blindness in children.

14a.6 CAUSES OF BLINDNESS IN CHILDREN

14a.6.1 Sources of data

In industrialized countries information on the causes of blindness in children can be obtained from blind registration data. However, this source is subject to information and selection bias for the following reasons. First, observer bias is likely as many different ophthalmologists will have examined and registered the child, and although the International Classification of Diseases is usually used to code causes, children with the same condition may not always be coded in exactly the same way. Selection bias is also likely, as in most countries (the exception being some Scandinavian countries) not all eligible children are registered. If the causes of blindness in registered children are different from those in children who are not registered, the data will not be representative of the total population of blind children; for example, if children with multiple disabilities (who often have central nervous system (CNS) causes of blindness) are less likely to be registered, the causes will be biased in favour of conditions that are not associated with additional handicap, such as retinal dystrophies and other genetic diseases that give rise to isolated visual impairment.

In developing countries, where registers of the blind are not available, information on the major causes can be obtained from **CBR** programmes, and studies using the **Key Informant Method** (**KIM**). Population-based prevalence surveys or cohort studies would provide the most accurate data on the causes of visual impairment in childhood. However, as childhood blindness is rare and the causes vary widely (see below) a very large sample would be required to provide meaningful data (approximately 60,000 children). The British birth cohort studies, which followed up large numbers of children, identified only a few blind children; this would not give representative data. To date no similar study has been conducted in a developing country.

Examination of children enrolled in special education programmes has several advantages, the main one being that a relatively large number of blind children can be examined by one observer using standard methods in a relatively short period of time. However, this source of data is also subject to selection bias because children in schools for the blind do not represent the total number of children who are blind in a population for the following reasons:

➢ Most schools are in urban centres and parents living in isolated rural areas may not know of the school, or may not wish to send their child so far away.
➢ Cultural beliefs relating to the explanation of disease may make parents reluctant to seek medical help, and the child remains unidentified.
➢ In countries with low levels of school attendance, educating a child who is blind may not be a high priority — this may apply more to girls than to boys.
➢ Special education services usually do not cater for pre-school-age children or those with additional handicaps.
➢ Some of the causes of blindness are associated with a high mortality rate (i.e. VADD and measles), and only the survivors will be in special education.

The degree to which selection bias alters the information obtained from blind school studies is difficult to quantify, as the degree of bias is likely to vary from place to place and over time. However, data on causes of blindness in children have been collected from CBR programmes, and from Key Informant studies in Bangladesh[26] and Mongolia,[28] and these data were compared with the findings obtained from examining children in blind schools in the same geographical area. After taking differences in age distribution into account (community-based surveys will include pre-school-age children), the findings are broadly comparable. One important difference observed in these two studies is that children with lesions of the central nervous system are under-represented in blind school studies. Likely explanations are that these children often have other handicaps, which render them ineligible for admission to special education, and in rural communities they are likely to have a high mortality rate.

Hospital studies are another possible source of information on causes of blindness in children in developing countries, but again, these data are likely to be biased in favour of treatable conditions and children whose parents have access to healthcare.

14a.6.2   Classification of the causes of blindness in children

The WHO has developed a system for classifying the causes of blindness in children[41] (available from http://www.cehjournal.org/files/s0801.html). There are two different ways of classifying the causes of visual loss in each child: the first is a descriptive, anatomical classification (Table 14a.6) and the second depends on the time of onset of the condition leading to visual loss. For each child, a main anatomical site and underlying cause should be determined for each eye, and one site and cause selected for the child. Advantages of the descriptive classification are that information can be collected on every child on the basis of clinical examination and the results of visual function tests. However, these data are not as useful as aetiological data for planning control strategies. Reliably ascertaining the time of onset of the condition leading to visual loss can be very difficult, particularly in developing countries where medical records may not be available, the history not always clear, and where there are limited facilities for investigation.

14a.6.3   Regional variation in the causes of blindness in children

Data from a variety of sources are presented in Table 14a.6. Most of the data from developing countries have been obtained by examining children in schools for the blind, while those from industrialized countries come mainly from registers of the blind. Over the last ten years or so, data have been published on over 17,500 children, the majority of whom were blind or severely visually impaired. Most of the data have been collected using the WHO classification system and so can be compared.

The data show that the causes of blindness in children vary widely from region to region, with lesions of the central nervous system predominating in the Established Market Economies. In the UK Surveillance Study, prenatal aetiological factors affected 61% (268) of children, with perinatal/neonatal and childhood factors each affecting 18%.[3] In the middle income countries of Latin America, the Former Socialist Economies and the Middle East crescent, conditions of the retina predominate. In some of these middle income countries **retinopathy of prematurity (ROP)** is the single commonest cause[42] whereas in the Middle East Crescent retinal dystrophies are the commonest cause. In India congenital abnormalities which affect the whole eye, such as microphthalmos, are important causes whereas in the Other Asia and Islands region disorders of the lens, mainly un-operated cataract but also amblyopia following delayed surgery are also important causes. In Sub-Saharan Africa corneal scarring is still a frequent cause of blindness in children, due principally to measles, VADD, the use of traditional eye medicines and ophthalmia neonatorum.

The underlying aetiology could not be determined in all regions with any degree of certainty in a relatively high proportion of the children examined.

There are insufficient data on the causes of blindness (i.e. from only 21 countries over the last decade) to estimate the number of children who are blind globally, by cause. But there is no reason to believe that the pattern of causes illustrated in Fig. 14a.3 have changed over the last decade.

14a.7   TIME TRENDS FOR THE MAJOR CAUSES OF BLINDNESS IN CHILDREN

Accurate evaluation of trends can only be determined from reliable population-based data which provide information on the incidence of disease. As outlined above, this information is largely lacking for childhood blindness at the moment,

Table 14a.6 Causes of blindness in children by World Bank region

Country	Year	Source	Definition	Sample	WHO C	1	%	2	%	3	%	4	%
Established Market Economics:													
UK[25]	2010	Register - L	Eligible	256	No	CNS	51	Retina	30	Uvea	7	Whole eye	6
UK[78]	2008	Register - N	Eligible	328	No	CNS	38	Others	20				
Scotland[79]	2004	Register - L	Eligible	30	No	CNS	47	Retina	20				
US[80]	2007	Register - L	Eligible	2,155	No	CNS	33	Retina	27	Whole globe	5	Unknown	5
Sweden[81]	1997	Multiple	<3/60	579	No	CNS	57	Retina	33	Whole globe	5	Lens	3
Hong Kong[82]	2005	BSS	<6/60	82	Yes	Retina	48	CNS	17	Glaucoma	12	Cornea	7
Former Socialist Economies:													
Poland[83]	2001	MS	NS	3,000	No	Optic atrophy	22	ROP	19	Lens	14	Myopia	12
Latin American and Caribbean:													
Brazil[84]	2007	LV clinic	<6/24	3,210	Yes	Retina	45	Glaucoma	11	CNS	8	Whole globe	4
Middle East Crescent:													
Iran[85]	2005	BSS	<6/18*	362	No	Retina	51	Lens	14	Optic atrophy	10	Cornea	9
Turkey[86]	2004	Hospital	<6/18	148	Yes	Retina	25	Lens	23	Optic nerve	11	Cornea	2
Saudi Arabia[87]	2006	BSS	<6/60	247	No	Retina	62	Glaucoma	14	Optic atrophy	12	Other	12
China/India:													
India[88]	2006	BSS	<6/60	1,778	Yes	Whole globe	41	Cornea	22	Retina	11	Lens	6
India[89]	2008	BSS	<6/60	258	Yes	Cornea	36	Whole globe	32	Lens	11	Retina	6
India[90]	2009	BSS	<6/60	891	Yes	Whole globe	41	Retina	20	Lens	14	Cornea	14
Other Asia and Islands:													
Malaysia[91]	2002	BSS	<6/60	332	Yes	Lens	22	Retina	21	Whole eye	17	Cornea	15
Nepal[92]	2009	BSS	<6/60*	285	Yes	Cornea	36	Retina	20	Whole globe	13	lens	13
Myanmar[93]	2009	BSS	<6/60	202	Yes	Cornea	44	Whole globe	21	Lens	14	Retina	7
Indonesia[94]	2007	BSS	<6/60*	477	Yes	Whole globe	36	Retina	19	Cornea	16	Lens	16
Bangladesh[95]	2007	KIM/other	<6/60	1,935	Yes	Lens	33	cornea	27	Whole globe	13	Retina	13
Sub-Saharan Africa:													
Kenya[45]	2009	BSS	<6/60	182	Yes	Retina	16	Optic nerve	13	Cornea	16	Whole globe	13
Malawi[45]	2009	BSS	<6/60	178	Yes	Cornea	23	Whole globe	20	Lens	12	R error	10
Uganda[45]	2009	BSS	<6/60	149	Yes	Retina	22	Cornea	20	Optic nerve	16	Lens	15
Tanzania[45]	2009	BSS	<6/60	192	Yes	Cornea	35	Whole globe	18	Retina	15	Lens	14
Ethiopia[96]	2003	BSS	<6/60	295	Yes	Cornea	62	Optic nerve	10	Lens	10	Uvea	9
Total:				17,551									

*includes a few children with mild or severe visual impairment who were not analyzed separately.

and accurate cause-specific population-based data are also unavailable. Such information could be obtained from large cohort studies, or from comprehensive, accurately kept live registers, or from ongoing active surveillance. Data from Canada suggest that post-natal acquired causes of childhood blindness in children aged 0–19 years have declined from 0.6/10,000 to 0.2/10,000 over the past 30 years;[43] whilst in Saudi Arabia genetic diseases have become more frequent than corneal scarring. However, comparing the proportion of childhood blindness from different causes at different times can give misleading interpretations, as the denominator is not population-based; for example, if the proportion of children blind from one cause changes from 25% at one point in time to 50% at another point in time, this could either be the result of a higher incidence of the cause of interest, or a lower incidence of other causes.

There is historical evidence that the major causes of childhood blindness have changed over time in European countries; for example, in many European countries ophthalmia neonatorum (conjunctivitis of the newborn, often caused by infection with *Neisseria gonorrhoea*) was reported to be one of the commonest causes of blindness around 1900. During the late 1940s and 1950s there was an 'epidemic' of ROP in the USA and to a lesser extent in Western Europe, which occurred because of the introduction of intensive neonatal care services with oxygen supplementation and increased survival of premature babies. During this period almost 50% of childhood blindness was attributable to ROP.

Over the past four decades, inherited retinal dystrophies, albinism, congenital ocular anomalies and ROP have increased among newly registered blind children in England and Wales, while cataract and optic atrophy have decreased. Similar trends have been reported from other industrialized countries. The interpretation of these trends is not straightforward as they are influenced by changes in case ascertainment and registration practices as well as by the availability of effective treatment for different disorders.

Data that might suggest changing trends over time from other parts of the world are even more difficult to obtain, but there is evidence that ROP is emerging as an important cause in countries with moderate levels of socio-economic development, and in urban centres of newly industrializing countries.[44] However, the higher proportion of blindness attributable to ROP in these countries may equally well be explained by a lower incidence of other causes. There is anecdotal evidence that improved measles immunization coverage rates and the extensive programmes to reduce childhood mortality from VADD are reducing the incidence of corneal ulceration from these preventable causes, but reliable data to back this up are difficult to obtain.[45] Monitoring the impact of improved vitamin A status and measles immunization would require comprehensive surveillance of communities of children, with identification of all blind children and examination to determine the underlying cause.

14a.8 PREVALENCE AND CAUSES OF FUNCTIONAL LOW VISION IN CHILDREN

Some data are available on the prevalence and causes of **functional low vision (FLV)** from eight population-based studies of refractive error in children that were undertaken in India (×2), China (×2), Chile, Nepal, Malaysia and South Africa.[46] Using the same protocol developed by the National Eye Institute of the USA, 4,082 to 6,527 children aged five (or seven) to 15 years of age were examined at each site. Uncorrected and presenting distance visual acuities were successfully measured with retro-illuminated logMAR E charts in 91–99.9% of children; cycloplegic autorefraction was performed, and best corrected acuities assessed. All children were examined by an ophthalmologist and a cause of visual loss assigned to eyes with uncorrected acuity ≤6/12. A total of 39,555 children were examined and the prevalence of FLV ranged from 0.65 to 2.75/1,000 children, with wide confidence intervals. The overall prevalence was 1.52/1,000 children (95% CI 1.16–1.95). FLV was significantly associated with age (OR 1.13 for each year, p = 0.01), and parental education was protective (OR 0.75 for each of five levels of education, p = 0.017). Retinal lesions and amblyopia were the commonest causes.

14a.9 AVOIDABLE CAUSES OF BLINDNESS IN CHILDREN

Data collected using the WHO/PBL Eye Examination Form for Children with Blindness and Low Vision suggest that in many countries a high proportion of children in special education are blind from conditions that are entirely preventable (i.e. are amenable to primary prevention). These include corneal scarring from vitamin A deficiency disorder, measles infection, ophthalmia neonatorum and the use of harmful traditional eye medicines. Other conditions, such as cataract, glaucoma and corneal ulceration, if diagnosed early and the child referred to centres with the necessary expertise and facilities, can be treated to prevent or minimize visual loss (i.e. are amenable to secondary prevention). Sight can sometimes also be restored through surgery to children with congenital cataract and corneal scarring (i.e. tertiary prevention). The term 'avoidable blindness' is used to encompass causes that can be prevented or treated. Overall 30–73% of the children included in blind school studies had avoidable causes of visual loss. In the UK Surveillance Study only 25% of children had disorders that were potentially preventable or treatable, with current knowledge.

14a.10 SUMMARY AND FUTURE AREAS OF RESEARCH

The epidemiology of childhood blindness is an interesting and challenging field of research, not only because it involves an age group that is difficult to study, but also because the case definition encompasses a range of conditions and diseases. Unlike adult blindness there appears to be marked regional variation in the major causes of blindness, reflecting the wide variation in the main risk factors in different geographical locations and populations. Risk factors can vary over time as a result of changes in levels of socio-economic development and healthcare provision, which are reflected in the changing patterns of childhood blindness over time.

➢ It will be vital to continue to monitor the major avoidable causes and prevalence of blindness in children, through further studies that are designed specifically for children. These must use appropriate and reliable methods to ascertain eligible children, and ensure large enough sample sizes for meaningful analysis.

➢ Further work is also required on assessing the most appropriate methods of measuring visual acuity in a field setting.

➢ Finally, there is a need for follow-up studies to determine the developmental, social and educational outcomes of affected children; the uptake and outcomes of accessing services; and also the mortality rates. These studies will better inform planning of services.

REFERENCES

1. Tadic V, Pring L, Dale N. Attentional processes in young children with congenital visual impairment. *Br J Dev Psychol* 2009; 27:311–330.

2. Jan JE. Chapter 15. The visually impaired child and family. In *Paediatric Ophthalmology and Strabismus*, 3rd Edition. Taylor D, Hoyt CS (eds). London: Elsevier Saunders; 2005.

3. Rahi JS, Cable N. Severe visual impairment and blindness in children in the UK. *Lancet* 2003; 362:1359–1365.

4. Reichman NE, Corman H, Noonan K. Impact of child disability on the family. *Matern Child Health J* 2008; 12:679–683.

5. Davidson AJ, O'Brien M. Ethics and medical research in children. *Paediatr Anaesth* 2009; 19:994–1004.

6. World Health Organization. *Management of Low Vision in Children*. WHO/PBL/93.27: Geneva: WHO; 1992.

7. Adams DL. Chapter 2. Normal and abnormal visual development. In *Paediatric Opthalmology and Strabismus,* 3rd Edition. Taylor D, Hoyt CS (eds). London: Elsevier Saunders; 2005.

8. Balyeroju A, Bowman R, Gilbert C, *et al.* Managing eye health in young children. *Community Eye Health J* 2010; 23:4–11.

9. Moller HU. Chapter 5. Milestones and normative data. In *Paediatric Ophthalmology and Strabismus,* 3rd Edition. Taylor DT, Hoyt CS (eds). London: Elsevier Saunders; 2005.

10. Day SH, DA S. Chapter 9. History, examination and further investigation. In *Paediatric Ophthalmology and Strabismus,* 3rd Edition. Taylor D, Hoyt CS (eds). London: Elsevier Saunders; 2005.

11. Verriest G. Visual field in childhood. *Bull Soc Belge Ophtalmol* 1982; 202:41–58.

12. Leat SJ, Wegmann D. Clinical testing of contrast sensitivity in children: age-related norms and validity. *Optom Vis Sc* 2004; 81:245–254.

13. World Health Organization. *International Classification of Functioning, Disability and Health.* Geneva: WHO; 2001.

14. Calman KC. Quality of life in cancer patients — an hypothesis. *J Med Ethics* 1984; 10:124–127.

15. WHOQOL Group. Development of the WHOQOL: Rationale and current status. *Int J Men Health* 1994; 23:24–56.

16. Massof RW, Rubin GS. Visual function assessment questionnaires. *Surv Ophthalmol* 2001; 45: 531–548.

17. Gothwal VK, Lovie-Kitchin JE, Nutheti R. The development of the LV Prasad-Functional Vision Questionnaire: a measure of functional vision performance of visually impaired children. *Invest Ophthalmol Vis Sci* 2003; 44:4131–4139.

18. Eiser C, Vance YH, Seamark D. The development of a theoretically driven generic measure of quality of life for children aged 6–12 years: a preliminary report. *Child Care Health Dev* 2000; 26: 445–456.

19. Frost NA, Sparrow JM, Durant JS, *et al.* Development of a questionnaire for measurement of vision-related quality of life. *Ophthalmic Epidemiol* 1998; 5:185–210.

20. Haymes SA, Johnston AW, Heyes AD. The development of the Melbourne low-vision ADL index: a measure of vision disability. *Invest Ophthalmol Vis Sci* 2001; 42:1215–1225.

21. Mangione CM, Lee PP, Gutierrez PR, *et al.* Development of the 25-item National Eye Institute Visual Function Questionnaire. *Arch Ophthalmol* 2001; 119:1050–1058.

22. Mangione CM, Phillips RS, Seddon JM, *et al.* Development of the 'Activities of Daily Vision Scale'. A measure of visual functional status. *Med Care* 1992; 30:1111–1126.

23. Birch EE, Cheng CS, Felius J. Validity and reliability of the Children's Visual Function Questionnaire (CVFQ). *J AAPOS* 2007; 11:473–479.

24. Felius J, Stager DR Sr, Berry PM, *et al.* Development of an instrument to assess vision-related quality of life in young children. *Am J Ophthalmol* 2004; 138:362–372.

25. Durnian JM, Cheeseman R, Kumar A, *et al.* Childhood sight impairment: a 10-year picture. *Eye* 2010; 24:112–117.

26. Muhit MA, Shah SP, Gilbert CE, *et al.* The key informant method: a novel means of ascertaining blind children in Bangladesh. *Br J Ophthalmol* 2007; 91:995–999.

27. Muhit MA. Finding children who are blind. *Community Eye Health J* 2007; 20:30–31.

28. Bulgan T, Gilbert CE. Prevalence and causes of severe visual impairment and blindness in children in Mongolia. *Ophthalmic Epidemiol* 2002; 9: 271–281.

29. Cama AT, Sikivou BT, Keeffe JE. Childhood vision impairment in Fiji. *Arch Ophthalmol* 2010; in press.

30. Shirima S, Lewallen S, Kabona G, *et al.* Estimating numbers of blind children for planning services: findings in Kilimanjaro, Tanzania. *Br J Ophthalmol* 2009; 93:1560–1562.

31. Gilbert C, Foster A. Childhood blindness in the context of VISION 2020 — the Right to Sight. *Bull World Health Organ* 2001; 79:227–232.

32. Sommer A, Davidson FR. Assessment and control of vitamin A deficiency: the Annecy Accords. *J Nutr* 2002; 132:2845S–2850S.

33. World Health Organization. *Preventing blindness in children.* WHO/PBL/0077. Geneva: WHO; 2000.

34. Chopra M, Daviaud E, Pattinson R, *et al.* Saving the lives of South Africa's mothers, babies, and children: can the health system deliver? *Lancet* 2009; 374:835–846.

35. Bodeau-Livinec F, Surman G, Kaminski M, *et al.* Recent trends in visual impairment and blindness in the UK. *Arch Dis Child* 2007; 92:1099–1104.

36. Farber MD. National Registry for the Blind in Israel: estimation of prevalence and incidence rates and causes of blindness. *Ophthalmic Epidemiol* 2003; 10:267–277.

37. Al-Merjan JI, Pandova MG, Al-Ghanim M, *et al.* Registered blindness and low vision in Kuwait. *Ophthalmic Epidemiol* 2005; 12:251–257.

38. UNICEF. *State of the World's Children 2009.* Maternal and Newborn Health. New York; 2009.

39. Cohen N, Rahman H, Sprague J, *et al.* Prevalence and determinants of nutritional blindness in Bangladeshi children. *World Health Stat Q* 1985; 38:317–330.

40. Blohme J, Tornqvist K. Visually impaired Swedish children. The 1980 cohort study — aspects on mortality. *Acta Ophthalmol Scand* 2000; 78:560–565.

41. Gilbert C, Foster A, Negrel AD, *et al.* Childhood blindness: a new form for recording causes of visual loss in children. *Bull World Health Organ* 1993; 71:485–489.

42. Gilbert C, Fielder A, Gordillo L, *et al.* Characteristics of infants with severe retinopathy of prematurity in countries with low, moderate, and high levels of development: implications for screening programs. *Pediatrics* 2005; 115:e518–525.

43. Robinson GC, Jan JE. Acquired ocular visual impairment in children. 1960–1989. *Am J Dis Child* 1993; 147:325–328.

44. Gilbert C. Retinopathy of prematurity: a global perspective of the epidemics, population of babies at risk and implications for control. *Early Hum Dev* 2008; 84:77–82.

45. Njuguna M, Msukwa G, Shilio B, *et al.* Causes of severe visual impairment and blindness in children in schools for the blind in eastern Africa: changes in the last 14 years. *Ophthalmic Epidemiol* 2009; 16:151–155.

46. Gilbert CE, Ellwein LB. Prevalence and causes of functional low vision in school-age children: results from standardized population surveys in Asia, Africa, and Latin America. *Invest Ophthalmol Vis Sci* 2008; 49:877–881.

47. Zaman SS, Khan NZ, Islam S, *et al.* Validity of the 'Ten Questions' for screening serious childhood disability: results from urban Bangladesh. *Int J Epidemiol* 1990; 19:613–620.

48. Durkin MS, Davidson LL, Desai P, *et al.* Validity of the ten questions screened for childhood disability: results from population-based studies in Bangladesh, Jamaica, and Pakistan. *Epidemiology* 1994; 5:283–289.

49. Rahi JS, Botting B. Ascertainment of children with congenital cataract through the National Congenital Anomaly System in England and Wales. *Br J Ophthalmol* 2001; 85:1049–1051.

50. Maberley DA, Hollands H, Chuo J, *et al.* The prevalence of low vision and blindness in Canada. *Eye* 2006; 20:341–346.

51. Khan RI, O'Keefe M, Kenny D, *et al.* Changing pattern of childhood blindness. *Ir Med J* 2007; 100:458–461.

52. Riise R. Nordic registers of visually impaired children. *Scand J Soc Med* 1993; 21:66–68.

53. Razavi H, Kuper H, Rezvan F, *et al.* Prevalence and causes of severe visual impairment and blindness among children in the Lorestan province of Iran, using the key informant method. *Ophthalmic Epidemiol* 2010; 17:95–102.

54. Khandekar R, Mohammed AJ, Negrel AD, *et al.* The prevalence and causes of blindness in the Sultanate of Oman: the Oman Eye Study (OES). *Br J Ophthalmol* 2002; 86:957–962.

55. Merrick J, Bergwerk K, Morad M, *et al.* Blindness in adolescents in Israel. *Int J Adolesc Med Health* 2004; 16:79–81.

56. Fu P, Yang L, Bo SY, *et al.* A national survey on low vision and blindness of 0–6-year-old children in China [Article in Chinese]. *Zhonghua Yi Xue Za Zhi* 2004; 84:1545–1548.

57. Lu Q, Zheng Y, Sun B, *et al.* A population-based study of visual impairment among pre-school children in Beijing: the Beijing study of visual impairment in children. *Am J Ophthalmol* 2009; 147:1075–1081.

58. Dandona L, Dandona R, Srinivas M, *et al.* Blindness in the Indian state of Andhra Pradesh. *Invest Ophthalmol Vis Sci* 2001; 42:908–916.

59. Dorairaj SK, Bandrakalli P, Shetty C, *et al.* Childhood blindness in a rural population of southern India: prevalence and etiology. *Ophthalmic Epidemiol* 2008; 15:176–182.

60. Nirmalan PK, Vijayalakshmi P, Sheeladevi S, *et al.* The Kariapatti pediatric eye evaluation project: baseline ophthalmic data of children aged 15 years or younger in Southern India. *Am J Ophthalmol* 2003; 136:703–709.

61. Thulasiraj RD, Nirmalan PK, Ramakrishnan R, *et al.* Blindness and vision impairment in a rural south Indian population: the Aravind Comprehensive Eye Survey. *Ophthalmology* 2003; 110:1491–1498.

62. Dandona L, Williams JD, Williams BC, *et al.* Population-based assessment of childhood

blindness in southern India. *Arch Ophthalmol* 1998; 116:545–546.

63. Parkar TH. Evaluating the role of Anganwadi workers as key informants to identify blind children in Pune, India. *Community Eye Health J* 2007; 20:72.

64. Zainal M, Ismail SM, Ropilah AR, *et al.* Prevalence of blindness and low vision in Malaysian population: results from the National Eye Survey 1996. *Br J Ophthalmol* 2002; 86:951–956.

65. Berhane Y, Worku A. *National Survey of Blindness, Low Vision and Trachoma in Ethiopia.* Ethiopian Public Health Association, Addis Ababa, Ethiopia; 2006.

66. Zeidan Z, Hashim K, Muhit MA, *et al.* Prevalence and causes of childhood blindness in camps for displaced persons in Khartoum: results of a household survey. *East Mediterr Health J* 2007; 13:580–585.

67. Kalua K, Patel D, Muhit M, *et al.* Productivity of key informants for identifying blind children: evidence from a pilot study in Malawi. *Eye* 2009; 23:7–9.

68. Boye T. Validating the key informant method in detecting blind children in Ghana. *Community Eye Health J* 2005; 18:130–134.

69. Negrel AD, Maul E, Pokharel GP, *et al.* Refractive error study in children: sampling and measurement methods for a multi-country survey. *Am J Ophthalmol* 2000; 129:421–426.

70. Naidoo KS, Raghunandan A, Mashige KP, *et al.* Refractive error and visual impairment in African children in South Africa. *Invest Ophthalmol Vis Sci* 2003; 44:3764–3770.

71. Zhao J, Pan X, Sui R, *et al.* Refractive Error Study in Children: results from Shunyi District, China. *Am J Ophthalmol* 2000; 129:427–435.

72. He M, Zeng J, Liu Y, *et al.* Refractive error and visual impairment in urban children in southern China. *Invest Ophthalmol Vis Sci* 2004; 45:793–799.

73. Dandona R, Dandona L, Srinivas M, *et al.* Refractive error in children in a rural population in India. *Invest Ophthalmol Vis Sci* 2002; 43:615–622.

74. Murthy GV, Gupta SK, Ellwein LB, *et al.* Refractive error in children in an urban population in New Delhi. *Invest Ophthalmol Vis Sci* 2002; 43:623–631.

75. Goh PP, Abqariyah Y, Pokharel GP, *et al.* Refractive error and visual impairment in school-age children in Gombak District, Malaysia. *Ophthalmology* 2005; 112:678–685.

76. Pokharel GP, Negrel AD, Munoz SR, *et al.* Refractive error study in children: results from Mechi Zone, Nepal. *Am J Ophthalmol* 2000; 129:436–444.

77. Maul E, Barroso S, Munoz SR, *et al.* Refractive error study in children: results from La Florida, Chile. *Am J Ophthalmol* 2000; 129:445–454.

78. Bunce C, Wormald R. Causes of blind certifications in England and Wales: April 1999–March 2000. *Eye* 2008; 22:905–911.

79. Bamashmus MA, Matlhaga B, Dutton GN. Causes of blindness and visual impairment in the West of Scotland. *Eye* 2004; 18:257–261.

80. Hatton DD, Schwietz E, Boyer B, *et al.* Babies Count: the national registry for children with visual impairments, birth to three years. *J AAPOS* 2007; 11:351–355.

81. Blohme J, Tornqvist K. Visual impairment in Swedish children. III. Diagnoses. *Acta Ophthalmol Scand* 1997; 75:681–687.

82. Fan DS, Lai TY, Cheung EY, *et al.* Causes of childhood blindness in a school for the visually impaired in Hong Kong. *Hong Kong Med J* 2005; 11:85–89.

83. Seroczynska M, Prost ME, Medrun J, *et al.* The causes of childhood blindness and visual impairment in Poland. *Klin Oczna* 2001; 103:117–120.

84. Haddad MA, Sei M, Sampaio MW, *et al.* Causes of visual impairment in children: a study of 3,210 cases. *J Pediatr Ophthalmol Strabismus* 2007; 44:232–240.

85. Mirdehghan SA, Dehghan MH, Mohammadpour M, *et al.* Causes of severe visual impairment and blindness in schools for visually handicapped children in Iran. *Br J Ophthalmol* 2005; 89:612–614.

86. Cetin E, Yaman A, Berk AT. Etiology of childhood blindness in Izmir, Turkey. *Eur J Ophthalmol* 2004; 14:531–537.

87. Kotb AA, Hammouda EF, Tabbara KF. Childhood blindness at a school for the blind in Riyadh, Saudi Arabia. *Ophthalmic Epidemiol* 2006; 13:1–5.

88. Gogate P, Deshpande M, Sudrik S, *et al.* Changing pattern of childhood blindness in Maharashtra, India. *Br J Ophthalmol.* 2007; 91:8–12.

89. Bhattacharjee H, Das K, Borah RR, *et al.* Causes of childhood blindness in the northeastern states of India. *Indian J Ophthalmol* 2008; 56:495–499.

90. Gogate P, Kishore H, Dole K, *et al.* The pattern of childhood blindness in Karnataka, South India. *Ophthalmic Epidemiol* 2009; 16:212–217.

91. Reddy SC, Tan BC. Causes of childhood blindness in Malaysia: results from a national study of blind school students. *Int Ophthalmol* 2001; 24: 53–59.

92. Kansakar I, Thapa HB, Salma KC, *et al*. Causes of vision impairment and assessment of need for low vision services for students of blind schools in Nepal. *Kathmandu Univ Med J (KUMJ)* 2009; 7:44–49.

93. Muecke J, Hammerton M, Aung YY, *et al*. A survey of visual impairment and blindness in children attending seven schools for the blind in Myanmar. *Ophthalmic Epidemiol* 2009; 16:370–377.

94. Sitorus RS, Abidin MS, Prihartono J. Causes and temporal trends of childhood blindness in Indonesia: study at schools for the blind in Java. *Br J Ophthalmol* 2007; 91:1109–1113.

95. Muhit MA, Shah SP, Gilbert CE, *et al*. Causes of severe visual impairment and blindness in Bangladesh: a study of 1935 children. *Br J Ophthalmol* 2007; 91:1000–1004.

96. Kello AB, Gilbert C. Causes of severe visual impairment and blindness in children in schools for the blind in Ethiopia. *Br J Ophthalmol* 2003; 87: 526–530.

14b

Vitamin A deficiency disorders

KEITH WEST JR AND ALFRED SOMMER[a]

14b.1	Introduction	291
14b.2	Historical context	292
14b.3	Dietary sources of vitamin A	293
14b.4	Vitamin A absorption and metabolism	296
14b.5	VADD and their health consequences	297
14b.6	Epidemiology of vitamin A deficiency disorders	302
14b.7	Prevention	307
14b.8	Conclusions	310
	References	310

14b.1 INTRODUCTION

Vitamin A deficiency is a major nutritional concern throughout the developing world. Corneal xerophthalmia resulting from vitamin A deficiency is well known to ophthalmologists, nutritionists and epidemiologists as a leading cause of preventable paediatric blindness. Corneal lesions of xerophthalmia, however, represent the 'tip' of the vitamin A deficiency 'iceberg', with milder stages of xerophthalmia (night blindness and conjunctival xerosis accompanied by 'Bitot's spots') posing a smaller ocular risk but being far more prevalent. Indeed, ocular manifestations of xerophthalmia represent only a small fraction of the total burden of vitamin A deficiency among young children. Milder stages of vitamin A deficiency, before any clinical evidence of eye disease, can also depress

growth, disturb haematopoiesis, disrupt epithelial barrier function, impair immunity and increase severity of infection and consequent mortality.[1] These and other physiological and health consequences of vitamin A deficiency are now collectively known as '**vitamin A deficiency disorders**', or **VADD**.[2-4]

Vitamin A deficiency disorders extend beyond early childhood into adolescent years and adulthood. Mild xerophthalmia has often been reported in older children and adults during national surveys and, in recent years, maternal night blindness during pregnancy has become a well-described condition in a number of populations[5-7] associated with increased risks of maternal[8,9] and infant[10] morbidity and mortality. Maternal and early infant deficiency even has serious consequences for organogenesis, particularly the lung.[11] Xerophthalmia, at any age, is unique among VADD in that, owing to its specificity, the ocular stages serve both as clinical indicators and

---

[a] Donald S McLaren also was an author for the chapter on VADD in prior editions, upon which this revision is based.

health consequences of deficiency. Vitamin A deficiency disorders result from tissue depletion of retinol, which can be reflected by a range of biochemical indicator values. While infection may exacerbate vitamin A deficiency (and vice versa), virtually the entire population burden of vitamin A deficiency in the developing world can be traced to chronic dietary inadequacy of vitamin A. The concept of vitamin A deficiency and associated disorders is depicted in Fig. 14b.1.

Most of what is known about the epidemiology, treatment and prevention of VADD has been learned from observational and intervention studies in children and women of child-bearing age, with biological plausibility of causal pathways provided by laboratory animal experiments over the past century. Drawing on this wealth of - evidence, this chapter reviews the health consequences of vitamin A deficiency, including their extent, severity and epidemiology, concentrating on xerophthalmia, morbidity and mortality among the highest risk groups — young children and women of reproductive age. It evaluates the effectiveness of current approaches to prevent VADD, which include direct supplementation, food fortification and other food-based strategies. The condition is now much less common than it once was, thanks to a global

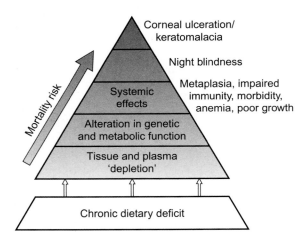

Figure 14b.1 *A diet chronically low in vitamin A causes vitamin A deficiency, reflected by a gradient of health consequences collectively called vitamin A deficiency disorders or VADD.[7] Reproduced with permission from West KP. Extent of vitamin A deficiency among preschool children and women of reproductive age.*

intervention programme largely spearheaded by UNICEF and underwritten by Canada. Any perturbations to socio-economic advancement can, however, lead to its rapid re-emergence.

14b.2   HISTORICAL CONTEXT

Contrary to what has been repeatedly copied from textbook to textbook, it is unclear whether xerophthalmia was an important disease in ancient times. Extracts of liver were undoubtedly prescribed by the Egyptians, Chinese and later the Greeks and Romans for eye disease, as they were for many other diseases. The Egyptian medical papyrus Ebers 351 has no word that could be translated as night blindness,[12,13] but even today, local terms for what is clearly night blindness do not always include an obvious term either.

Corneal destruction was first described by the French physician Guillemeau, in 1585. Reports of keratomalacia (softening of the cornea) in young children were increasingly filed by physicians working in Africa, Latin America, Asia and Europe from the 18th to the early 20th centuries,[13] commonly linking the condition to poor, starch-based diets, and implicating one or more missing dietary factors. Approximately 90 years ago, McCollum and Davis,[15] and shortly thereafter Osborne and Mendel,[16] discovered 'fat-soluble (vitamin) A', linking its deficiency in rats to poor growth, increased infection, ocular lesions and death. Soon after, the Danish paediatrician Bloch attributed the eye lesions of xerophthalmia, poor growth and morbidity, observed among orphans during World War I to a gruel-based diet that was lacking whole milk or butter and, therefore, McCollum's fat-soluble factor A. Bloch identified the vitamin A deficiency syndrome as 'dystrophia alipogenetica'.[17] By the late 1930s, a number of studies had made clear the links between vitamin A deficiency and risk of infection in groups of children and adults,[18] including women during pregnancy.[19]

Although great advances occurred throughout the 1940s and 1950s in understanding the role of vitamin A deficiency as a cause of xerophthalmia, poor growth and infection,[20,21] the 'public health era' of vitamin A deficiency was not ushered in until the global endemic of xerophthalmia was first exposed by a multi-country assessment by Oomen, McLaren and Escapini in 1964,[22] where some 43 countries were reported to have significant vitamin A deficiency among pre-school children. Over the past four decades, this list has become a register of countries at risk, updated periodically by the World Health Organization (WHO) as new data become available; it informs public health and nutrition sectors around the world of the current state of vitamin A deficiency (Fig. 14b.2).[7,23–27]

14b.3 DIETARY SOURCES OF VITAMIN A

Vitamin A is an essential dietary nutrient in humans, meaning that it is indispensable for life and must be provided by diet, either as preformed retinol or as provitamin A carotenoids. However, given that animals need vitamin A but cannot synthesize it, all naturally formed vitamin A ultimately derives from plant biosynthesis of provitamin A carotenoids that, once ingested, are split into molecules of retinol, absorbed and utilized or stored.

14b.3.1 Foods with provitamin A carotenoids

Fifty to sixty of some 500 naturally occurring carotenoids known to exist can be bioconverted to vitamin A in mammals.[28] β-carotene is by far the most ubiquitous carotenoid precursor of vitamin A. Rich sources of the provitamin include dark green leafy vegetables, carrots, red palm oil and ripe yellow fruit such as mango and papaya. Historically, it was assumed, for purposes of estimating dietary equivalence, that β-carotene from vegetables and fruits was bioconverted to preformed vitamin A at a ratio of 6:1, because of inefficiencies of carotenoid digestion, uptake, cleavage and utilization. Other provitamin A carotenoids, such as α-carotene and β-crypto-xanthin, have been assumed to be half, or even less, as efficient as β-carotene in their

bioconversion to retinol.[29] Recent studies, however, have revealed the bioconversion of β-carotene from vegetables and fruits to retinol to be half, or even less, as efficient as previously thought, especially from dark green leaves.[30,31] The lower absorptive efficiency has been attributed to several factors, including plant food matrices that must be digested to free carotenoid for enzyme action in the gut.[32,33] As a result, it is now accepted that 12 μg of dietary β-carotene and 24 μg of other provitamin A carotenoids from a mixed diet are required to obtain the bioactivity of 1 μg of preformed retinol, called a **retinol activity equivalent (RAE)**.[34]

The revision in bioconversion efficiency of food-based carotenoids has provided several new insights:

➢ The global food supply, considered by the Food and Agriculture Organization in 1979–1981 to have supplied an average of 720μg of retinol equivalents per capita, of which 500 retinol equivalents (~70%) were thought to derive from 3,000 μg of β-carotene (using a ratio of 6:1),[28] is now understood to have supplied a total activity of only 470 retinol equivalents, with only slightly more than half obtained from vegetables and fruit.

➢ In many developing countries of Asia and Africa, where 80% or more of the total food supply of vitamin A has been thought to derive from provitamin A carotenoid-rich vegetables and fruits,[1,29] the amount of bioactive vitamin A in such food systems is ~40% lower than previous estimates.

➢ Although an ample intake of provitamin A-containing foods clearly protects against xerophthalmia,[1] it is also now evident that young children may have difficulty meeting their vitamin A requirements solely through a vegetarian diet.

➢ These changes in equivalence have helped solve a long-standing paradox as to why vitamin A deficiency is globally pervasive and why it persists as a public health problem amid seemingly bountiful supplies of dark green leaves and other provitamin A foods.[35]

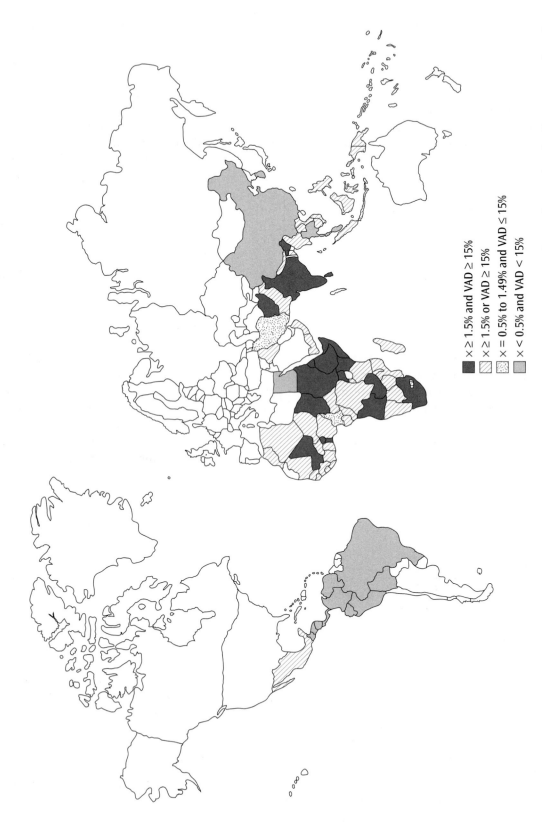

Figure 14b.2 *Distribution of countries by prevalence of vitamin A deficiency (VAD) and xerophthalmia (X) as of 2002.[7] Reproduced with permission from the Journal of Nutrition © J Nutr. American Society for Nutritional Sciences.*

Legend:

- X ≥ 1.5% and VAD ≥ 15%
- X ≥ 1.5% or VAD ≥ 15%
- X = 0.5% to 1.49% and VAD ≤ 15%
- X < 0.5% and VAD < 15%

14b.3.2   Foods with preformed vitamin A

Most dietary preformed vitamin A is present in food as retinyl esters. Food sources of preformed vitamin A include animal liver, fish liver oils, egg, cheese and whole milk. These sources constitute a relatively small proportion of the total vitamin A activity in the food supply of many developing countries, particularly in rural Asia and Africa.[29] In industrialized countries, fortified foods provide a major dietary source of preformed vitamin A. To date, fortification has been successfully implemented in only a small number of developing countries.

14b.3.3   Dietary reference intakes

Amounts of dietary vitamin A, from provitamin and preformed food sources, needed to sustain normal health of individuals and populations have recently been revised by the Institute of Medicine in the USA to reflect new definitions of requirement based on evidence of bioavailability. The **Recommended Dietary Allowance (RDA)** has been redefined as the amount of a nutrient that is 'sufficient to meet the daily nutrient requirement of most individuals in a specific life-stage and gender group'. The RDA is a statistical estimate, being set at 2 SD above the **Estimated Average Requirement (EAR),** considered to be that level of nutrient intake needed to prevent deficiency, as defined by a functional indicator of nutrient status (dark adaptation testing for vitamin A), in half of all individuals in a life-stage and gender group. Where data are lacking for setting an estimated average requirement and RDA, an 'adequate intake' has been proposed by the Institute of Medicine based on observed intakes that are presumably sufficient to maintain normal status; for example, an adequate intake has been set for vitamin A intake based on levels of vitamin A consumed through breast milk in healthy infant populations.[34] Finally, a Tolerable Upper Intake Level represents a routine, daily level of intake of a nutrient that can, with high probability, be biologically tolerated within a population.[36] Estimates of these various Dietary Reference Intakes for vitamin A are provided in Table 14b.1. While considerable variation can be found in RDA estimation around the world, this new system provides a standard logic and approach for evidence-based derivation of dietary requirements across different populations.

Table 14b.1 *Dietary reference intakes for vitamin A (μg RAE[a])*[34]

Age Years	EAR				RDA				UL			
	Male	Female			Male	Female			Male	Female		
		NP[e]	Preg	Lact		NP	Preg	Lact		NP	Preg	Lact
≤ 0.5	b	b							600			
0.5–1	b	b							600			
1–3	210	210			300	300			600			
4–8	275	275			400	400			900			
9–13	445	420			600	600			1,700			
14–18	630	485	630	880	900	700	750	1,200	2,800	2,800	2,800	2,800
≥ 19	625	500	550	900	900	700	770	1,300	3,000	3,000	3,000	3,000

[a]1 *mg* Retinol Activity Equivalent: = 1 *mg* of all-*trans*-retinol, 12 *mg* of all-*trans*-b-carotene, 24 *mg* of other provitamin A carotenoids, 3.33 IU of vitamin A activity.
[b]No EAR has been set for infants. Adequate intakes of 400 *mg* and 600 *mg* RAE have been established for infants £ 0.5 (£ 6 months) and 0.5–1.0 (6–11 months) years of age.
EAR = estimated average requirement; RDA = recommended dietary allowance; UL = tolerable upper intake level; NP = non-pregnant; Preg = pregnant; Lact = lactating.

14b.4   *Vitamin A Absorption and Metabolism*

Vitamin A esters consumed in food are hydrolyzed to retinol, which, along with carotenoids, becomes dispersed with other dietary lipids and bile salts to form mixed micelles. These micelles transport vitamin A and carotenoids to the brush border of intestinal mucosal cells for uptake. Retinol uptake is efficient (>80%), probably facilitated by cellular retinol-binding protein, whereas carotenoids appear to diffuse passively into the intestinal mucosa with half the absorptive efficiency of retinol. Absorptive efficiency of carotenoids decreases with increased intakes.[37] Within the enterocyte, retinol is re-esterified, whereas β-carotene is first cleaved, degraded to retinal and then further reduced to retinol. A small proportion of β-carotene is absorbed intact and transported into circulation associated with lipoproteins. In the enterocyte, retinol is esterified before being incorporated into chylomicrons, which become hydrolyzed during transport, leaving retinol-rich remnants to deliver the nutrient to the liver. More than 90% of the vitamin A in the body is stored in the liver, mostly as ester in stellate cells.[38] Prior to hepatic release, retinyl esters are hydrolyzed to retinal, which binds with its carrier **(retinol-binding protein (RBP))** and another protein, transthyretin (formerly prealbumin). Holo-RBP transports retinol to peripheral tissues, where transfer into target cells occurs via cell-surface receptors.

In the cell, retinol and other vitamin A intermediates are transported by retinoid carrier proteins. **Retinoic acids (RA),** most notably all-*trans* RA and 9-*cis* RA, are transported into the nucleus by a cellular RA-binding protein. Within the nucleus, RA moieties bind non-covalently to at least one RA receptor belonging to either of two distinct families of receptors that regulate gene transcription. The two families, known as RARs and RXRs, are each members of a large and complex superfamily of steroid–thyroid–retinoid hormone nuclear receptors. Each family of receptors comprises three different types (α, β and γ), each of which has multiple subtypes. Both all-*trans* RA and 9-*cis* RA bind to RARs, while RXRs are specifically induced by 9-*cis* RA.[38] These ligand-dependent receptors bind to RA response elements, consisting of short sequences of deoxyribonucleic acid (DNA) located near target genes whose expression may be either retinoid-activated or suppressed. All cells examined express one or more RA receptors, giving insight into the pleiotropy of vitamin A that governs processes of embryogenesis, morphogenesis, and differential expression of (a) epithelial cells lining the eye, respiratory, gastro-intestinal and other tracts and ducts of the body, and (b) pluripotent stem cells that commit themselves to haemopoietic, osteoid and immune lineages and systems.[39,40] This breadth of regulatory control also provides biological plausibility for the protean nature of health effects observed with depleted vitamin A nutrition.

More completely understood is the unique and fundamental role of vitamin A in vision where, in the retina of the eye, the vitamin enables photoreceptor cells to absorb and transfer energy from light. This single event, under vitamin A control, produces a structural change in photopigments that initiates the entire visual cascade (phototransduction). Vitamin A aldehyde (11-*cis* retinal and its derivatives) performs this function by acting as a chromophore that attaches to apoproteins (opsins) located in the outer segment of rod and cone photoreceptor cells. Three (iodopsins) are located in cones and are responsible for colour and daytime vision. The fourth (rhodopsin or 'visual purple') resides in rods and mediates mono-chromatic vision under low illumination.[41] The visual pigments are examples of a large group of G-proteins, which link a wide variety of receptors to various effector systems; in this case these are ion channels.

While retinal serves as the visual chromophore for photopigments, its function in the

(*Continued*)

(Continued)

visual cycle is best described in relation to rhodopsin because of the greater abundance of this pigment, its ease of isolation[42] and its clinical relevance in vitamin A deficiency.

Briefly, in the eye all-*trans*-retinol, circulating as holo-RBP, is delivered to the **retinal pigment epithelium (RPE)** via the choriocapillaris, where it undergoes enzymatic oxidation to 11-*cis*-retinal. The molecule leaves the RPE and is transported through the extracellular (interphoto-receptor cell) matrix by an interstitial retinoid binding protein into the outer segment of the rod photoreceptor cell, where it combines with membrane-bound opsin to form a purplish visual pigment, rhodopsin.[37] The initial step in vision occurs when 11-*cis*-retinal is isomerized to all-*trans*-retinal in response to light, producing a conformational change that activates rhodopsin (to meta-rhodopsin). Transducin, a G-protein also located on the disk membrane that is bound to the opsin moiety, interacts with 3',5' cyclic-guanosine monophosphate (cGMP) phosphodiesterase. On activation, this enzyme catalyzes cGMP to 5'cGMP, an event that leads to a decreased concentration of cGMP, a cytoplasmic molecule that serves as gatekeeper for ion channels located in the rod outer segment membrane. Reduction of intracellular cGMP leads to closure of ion channels, a change in membrane potential (hyperpolarization) associated with reduced influx of Na^+ (and Ca^{2+}) ions, and a cascade of amplified signals that traverse the photoreceptor to stimulate neuronal transmission along the optic nerve to the brain.[41]

Once 11-*cis*-retinal is photoisomerized to all-*trans* retinal, it is reduced to all-*trans*-retinol by nicotinamide adenine dinucleotide phosphate in a reaction that is catalyzed by retinol dehydrogenase. The sequence of reactions is known as 'bleaching', owing to colour changes that occur in the visual pigment, as rhodopsin (purple) is converted to meta-rhodopsin (yellow) and then separated to opsin and retinol (clear) moieties.[42] Subsequently, 11-*cis*-retinal must be regenerated for vitamin A to continue to be recycled for use in this visual system. Reconversion takes place only in the RPE. This requires that all-*trans*-retinol diffuse out of the rod outer segment and be transported back to the RPE by interphotoreceptor retinol-binding protein, where it undergoes esterification, isomerization, reduction to 11-*cis*-retinol and oxidation back to 11-*cis*-retinal for further recycling. Modern, detailed descriptions of the role of vitamin A in vision are available.[41-44]

14b.5   VADD AND THEIR HEALTH CONSEQUENCES

Health consequences of vitamin A deficiency include those that are highly specific, such as the ocular manifestations of xerophthalmia,[45] as well as those of a more general nature, such as infection, anaemia, poor growth, poor development of the lungs and other organs, and mortality.[4] Only xerophthalmia, morbidity resulting from infection, and mortality are discussed here.

14b.5.1   Xerophthalmia

Excellent, detailed reviews of the clinico-histopathology of all stages of xerophthalmia exist,[1,45-48] allowing this chapter to emphasize key clinical manifestations of epidemiologic relevance. A system for classifying the clinical stages of xerophthalmia, revised by WHO in 1982, remains in widespread use today (Table 14b.2).[24,45]

Night blindness (XN), the earliest and most common ocular manifestation of vitamin A deficiency, results from rod photoreceptor dysfunction in the retina, which impairs vision under conditions of low illumination. Night blindness is most readily assessed by a careful history of guarded

Table 14b.2 *World Health Organization classification and minimum prevalence criteria for paediatric xerophthalmia[a] and maternal vitamin A deficiency as a public health problem[3]*

Definition (code)	Minimum prevalence (%)
Night blindness (XN)	
Children 2–5 years	1.0
Pregnant women	5.0
Conjunctival xerosis (X1A)	—
Bitot's spots (X1B)	0.5
Corneal xerosis (X2)	
Corneal ulceration/keratomalacia < 1/3 of surface (X3A)	} 0.01
Corneal ulceration/keratomalacia ≥ 1/3 of surface (X3B)	
Xerophthalmic corneal scar (XS)	0.05
Xerophthalmic fundus (XF)	—
Serum retinol < 0.70 μmol/L	15.0
Abnormal CIC/RDR/MRDR	20.0[b]

[a]All stages refer to pre-school children except where noted.
[b]Provisional cut-offs above which community interventions may be warranted.
CIC, conjunctival impression cytology; RDR, relative dose response; MRDR, modified RDR.

Table 14b.3 *Current IVACG[a] recommendations for vitamin A treatment and prevention[4,53,138]*

Age	Oral treatment at diagnosis (IU)[b]	Prevention dosage (IU)	Frequency
< 6 months	50,000	50,000	3 times, 1 month apart[c]
6–12 months	100,000	100,000	Every 4–6 months
≥ 1 year	200,000	200,000	Every 4–6 months
Women	200,000[d]	400,000[e]	6 weeks after delivery

[a]International Vitamin A Consultative Group.
[b]Treat all cases of xerophthalmia and measles with the same age-specific dosage the next day and again 1–4 weeks later.
[c]This dose may be most efficacious when given at birth. Alternatively, give 25,000 or 50,000 IU at each diphtheria-pertussis-polio visit at 6, 10 and 14 weeks of age.
[d]For women of reproductive age, give 200,000 IU only for corneal xerophthalmia; for milder eye signs (night blindness or Bitot's spots) give women 10,000 IU per day or 25,000 IU per week for ≥ 4 weeks.
[e]As two doses of 200,000 IU 3 1 day apart.

behaviour in the evening or twilight.[45] Groups at highest risk for developing night blindness are pre-school-aged children (> 1 year of age; younger children do not engage in activities that readily permit recognition of this disability) and adult women during the latter half of pregnancy, when nutritional demands of gestation are high. Night-blind children[49,50] and pregnant women[6] typically exhibit low-to-deficient serum retinol concentrations as compared with controls with normal night vision. A parental history of night blindness can be reliably obtained for young children, especially in cultures where a specific term already exists (like

'chicken blindness' in Indonesian). A reliable history of maternal night blindness can be elicited for pregnancies that ended as live births during the previous three years, allowing use of such a history in nutritional and demographic surveys.[51,52] Prevalence rates of 1% and 5% represent public health minima in pre-school children and pregnant women, respectively (Table 14b.2).[4] Night blindness in children usually responds within 48 hours of initiating standard 200,000 IU vitamin A treatment orally (Table 14b.3). The recommended treatment for pregnant women with XN is an oral dose of either 10,000 IU per day or

25,000 IU weekly over a four-week period or longer,[45] motivated by the desire to minimize risk of foetal toxicity. However, this treatment regimen remains untested. In a recent field trial in Nepal, a weekly prophylactic dose of ~25,000 IU given prior to and during pregnancy failed to prevent night blindness in roughly one third of cases,[6] suggesting a need to evaluate the efficacy of this treatment.

Conjunctival xerosis (X1A) represents early keratinizing metaplasia of the epithelium with losses of mucus-secreting goblet cells that are required to maintain a normal bulbar surface. The lesion does not affect vision. Still relevant is the classic clinical description of the dry, irregular appearance of a xerotic conjunctiva resembling 'sandbanks at the receding tide' as the tear film is allowed to drain from the ocular surface.[53] Advanced xerosis may cause **Bitot's spots (X1B)** to form (Plate 14b.1); they are composed of patches of desquamated keratinized epithelium, often mixed with Gram-negative, saprophytic bacilli and other microbes. A Bitot's spot may be bubbly, cheesy or foamy in appearance, small or large, round to triangular in shape, nearly always occurring temporal to the limbus in both eyes. Nasal lesions may appear in advanced deficiency.[46,47] Pre-school children with X1B typically have low serum retinol concentration. The minimum prevalence of X1B considered to be of public health importance is 0.5% (Table 14b.2). Standard treatment with 200,000 IU vitamin A on two consecutive days (Table 14b.3) initiates a clinical response within several days, although a cure may require weeks to months.[45] Bitot's spots may persist in older pre-school and school-aged children and adults in the presence of normal circulating retinol concentrations; this is believed to reflect non-responsive metaplasia *in situ*.[1]

Corneal xerophthalmia is a medical emergency. **Xerosis of the cornea (X2)** (Plate 14b.2) appears as a bilateral, granular, hazy and lustreless condition that often starts on the inferior surface before spreading across the cornea, likened in appearance to the skin of an orange (*peau d'orange*) on handlight examination.[47] Stromal oedema is a universal finding in corneal xerosis. Thick keratinized plaques can form on the corneal surface, usually in the interpalpebral zone. A fully reversible condition, corneal

xerosis can rapidly advance to ulceration and keratomalacia in the absence of immediate vitamin A and other supportive therapies (Table 14b.3).

Corneal ulceration (X3A) (see Plate 14d.5), presents as a small, oval, 'punched-out' defect, often forming on the inferior, peripheral surface of the cornea. Typically, only one ulcer occurs in an affected eye, accompanied by conjunctival injection and, less often, hypopyon (pus in the anterior chamber). Ulcers may be shallow or sufficiently deep to perforate Descemet's membrane. The iris may plug the perforated ulcer, which can limit the loss of ocular content and visual loss when healed.[47] Vitamin A treatment is efficacious, resulting, in the event of an attached iris,[45,47,48] in a healed, scarred cornea or adherent leukoma.

Keratomalacia (softening of the cornea) (Plate 14b.3) involves full-thickness necrosis of the cornea, presenting as a raised, opaque, yellow-grey lesion. Usually one eye is more involved than the other. Prompt treatment of keratomalacia, and ulceration involving less than one third of the cornea (**X3A**), usually spares the central pupillary zone and vision. Ulceration and generalized necrosis involving one third or more of the cornea (**X3B**) usually result in perforation, loss of ocular content, a shrunken globe and blindness. Occasionally, the eye may protrude, but not perforate, resulting in (a blinding) staphyloma. Vitamin A and supportive treatment may spare the less affected eye and the life of the child.[45]

Active corneal xerophthalmia is both rare and of short duration in the community. Extremely high case fatalities give rise to a low prevalence of survivors with scarred corneas; a very low prevalence, 0.01%, is therefore indicative of a serious public health problem (Table 14b.2).

Xerophthalmic **corneal scarring (XS)** is a potentially blinding consequence of healed ulceration and kerato-malacia, with the type, location, shape, extent and density of scar determining the level of remaining useful vision.[45] Mild scars such as nebulas and peripheral leukomas permit sight, whereas dense central leukoma, descemetocele and staphyloma are sequelae responsible for childhood blindness resulting from vitamin A deficiency. Corneal scars attributable to previous vitamin A deficiency (XS) should be distinguished from those of other causes, such as trauma or infection, by careful analysis of the patient's (or parent's) history. Since mortality among children blinded by vitamin A deficiency is extremely high (estimated at 90% to 95% for those not receiving urgent therapy) few will be found in blindness prevalence surveys, so that the importance of vitamin A deficiency as a cause of childhood blindness is grossly underestimated.

14b.5.2   Infection

Vitamin A deficiency and infection engage in a 'vicious cycle', as one leads to increased severity of the other.[21] One way in which vitamin A deficiency may weaken host resistance to infection is by compromising the integrity and 'barrier' function of epithelial linings.[1] Beyond affecting conjunctival and corneal surfaces, progressive vitamin A depletion induces metaplasia throughout most, if not all, epithelial linings of the body. Respiratory epithelium undergoes loss of mucociliated cells[54] and keratinizing squamous metaplasia.[55,56] These lesions could increase the risk of infection by impairing microbial clearance, thereby promoting their colonization and potential for invasion. Supporting this notion, bacterial (*Klebsiella pneumoniae*) adherence to nasopharyngeal cells has been observed to increase with severity of xerophthalmia eye signs in Indian preschool children.[57] In two- to six-month-old South Indian infants, high potency vitamin A supplementation appeared to reduce colonization of *Streptococcus pneumoniae* bacteria in nasopharyngeal secretions.[58] Vitamin A deficiency has long been known to induce squamous metaplasia and keratinization of the genitourinary tract and glandular ducts,[59] processes which may, in part, give rise to increased risk of urinary tract infection, as has been observed in mildly xerophthalmic children (78%) compared with controls (17%).[60] Intestinal epithelium does not keratinize, but undergoes losses in intestinal brush border and goblet cells,[61] impaired cell turnover[62] and alterations in mucosal immunity,[63] which may weaken gut defences against infection.

Vitamin A deficiency also impairs aspects of innate, cell-mediated and humoral immunity. These functions directly relate to the ability of vitamin A (primarily all-*trans*-retinoic acid) genetically to regulate differentiation and proliferation. Notwithstanding variation by species, tissue specificity and experimental design, animals depleted in vitamin A often exhibit thymic, splenic and lymphoid atrophy, decreased lymphopoiesis and lymphocyte proliferative responses, altered lymphocyte ratios (especially of **CD4+** and **CD8+** cells) and trafficking patterns, impaired natural killer cell cytotoxicity, macrophage activation and certain T-cell-dependent antibody responses to antigen.[63,64] Vitamin A supplementation usually restores observed defects to control levels. Immune defects seen in animals can also be observed in children. Vitamin A-deficient rats, for example, show depressed primary and secondary antibody responses to viral and bacterial antigenic challenge, including exposure to *Clostridium tetani*.[39] Similarly, young Indonesian children with mild-to-moderate vitamin A deficiency were found to express abnormal proportions of circulating **T-cells**[65] and depressed **immunoglobulin (IgG)** responses specific to tetanus toxoid,[66,67] that returned to normal following vitamin A supplementation. Treating cases of severe measles with vitamin A has, in addition to lowering morbidity and mortality,[68,69,70] led to increases in lymphocyte counts and measles IgG antibody concentrations.[71] Malaria infection and immunoglobulin responses are more severe in experimentally vitamin A-deficient versus vitamin A-replete animals, with similarities beginning to be revealed in children infected with *Plasmodium falciparum* malaria.[72]

14b.5.3   Childhood morbidity and mortality

Xerophthalmic children are more like to have diarrhoea, respiratory infection and other febrile illnesses than children of apparently normal vitamin A status.[1,73–76] Prospective studies show that the association is bidirectional. Mildly xerophthalmic children have a higher risk of incident lower respiratory infection[50,77] and diarrhoea[50] than non-xerophthalmic children. Conversely, children appear to be at greater risk of developing xerophthalmia following episodes of diarrhoea or respiratory infection relative to children remaining disease-free.[78] Also, measles has long been known to increase risk of keratomalacia in malnourished populations.[46,79] Both causal directions are biologically plausible, given that (a) vitamin A deficiency can compromise host defences; and (b) infection can deplete vitamin A nutrition through marked increases in tissue utilization and urinary losses of the vitamin.[80,81] In addition, serum retinol concentration can be depressed during the acute phase of illness, probably as a result of increased metabolism as well as reduced hepatic synthesis and release of holo-retinol binding protein into circulation.[82]

While incidence of disease may be affected, the weight of evidence points toward vitamin A-deficiency increasing the severity of infectious illness, and that supplementation or treatment with vitamin A can reduce such severity. Certain illnesses appear more responsive to vitamin A than others. Specifically, vitamin A supplementation has been consistently shown to reduce the severity, duration and complication rates associated with diarrhoea and dysentery.[83–88] In Papua New Guinea high-potency vitamin A prophylaxis in the community reduced severity of falciparum malaria measured by clinic attack rates, rates of spleen enlargement and parasite density.[72] High-potency vitamin A treatment has been shown to reduce rates of complications[68] and case fatality from severe measles by 40 to 60%,[69,70,89–91] making vitamin A an important adjunct to any therapeutic regimen for this disease. Paradoxically, however, vitamin A therapy has consistently failed to improve health outcomes (incidence, duration, severity or mortality) associated with non-measles-related pneumonia or acute lower respiratory infections.[92] In a few instances, trials have reported increased frequency and severity of respiratory symptoms with vitamin A therapy.[88,93] Some studies have observed increased rates of respiratory or diarrhoeal infections in better-nourished children given vitamin A,[87,88] explanations for which are lacking at present.

Despite variation in disease-specific outcome indices, meta-analyses of effects from large, community-based trials involving more than 150,000 children across Southern Asia[94–98] and Africa[99,100] have concluded that increasing vitamin A intake in pre-school children over six months of age,

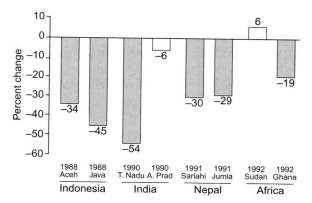

Figure 14b.3 *Effect of vitamin A supplementation on pre-school child mortality from eight trials in Southern Asia and Africa. T. Nadu, Tamil Nadu; A. Prad., Andhra Pradesh. Gray bars denote statistical significance (P < 0.05). (Reproduced with permission from the American Journal of Clinical Nutrition © AMJ Clin Nutr. American Society for Clinical Nutrition.)*

via direct supplementation or food fortification, can reduce mortality from all causes by 23–30% in populations where vitamin A deficiency exists (Fig. 14b.3).[90,91,101] In Asian populations with very high infant mortality, and in two of the three trials, with very poor vitamin A status,[102–104] vitamin A supplementation before six months of age has demonstrated little benefit, except when given within the first two or three days of life. Findings related to mortality have provided a powerful public health impetus to preventing paediatric vitamin A deficiency as a means of enhancing child survival throughout the developing world, which in turn has reduced the risk of xerophthalmia and blindness.

14b.5.4   Maternal morbidity and mortality

Maternal vitamin A deficiency has recently been recognized as a major public health problem that can increase risk of morbidity and mortality of women in relation to pregnancy. In Nepal, night-blind pregnant women were more likely to be vitamin A deficient, anaemic, wasted (by measures of arm circumference and body mass index), and to report symptoms of diarrhoea or dysentery and urinary or reproductive tract infections than non-night blind controls.[6] Despite the disappearance of night blindness shortly after parturition, cases remained four times more likely to have died during pregnancy and through the first two years postpartum than non-cases (3,600 versus 900 deaths per 100,000 pregnancies).[9]

The causality of association between maternal vitamin A deficiency and mortality related to pregnancy has been tested to date in three settings: Nepal,[8] Bangladesh[105] and Ghana.[106] In the first of these trials, in Nepal, night blindness was prevalent among pregnant women and maternal mortality was high. Women were randomized (by community) to receive a supplement of vitamin A (7000 μg retinol equivalents), β-carotene (42 mg) or placebo each week for over three years. From the time of pregnancy ascertainment (usually at around four months' gestation) through 12 weeks postpartum, mothers assigned to receive vitamin A or β-carotene died from all causes at rates that were 60% (P < 0.04) and 51% (P < 0.01) those of placebo controls. The protective effect was consistent during pregnancy through 12 weeks after termination of pregnancy (Fig. 14b.4). Combining the effects of both nutrients yielded a relative risk of 0.56, equivalent to a 44% reduction in pregnancy-related mortality.[8] Virtually all the excess

mortality occurred among night-blind women in the placebo arm.[9] By contrast, maternal mortality in the placebo arms in the Asian and African studies was only half to one third that of Nepal. Vitamin A supplementation had no discernible impact on mortality in either of these two populations.

Vitamin A supplementation appeared modestly to reduce the burden of third-trimester and postpartum infectious morbidity in Nepal,[107] while β-carotene supplementation seemed to enhance antioxidant status of women.[108] Causes of death most responsive to the intervention could not be precisely determined. Based on findings among night-blind women in this population,[107] reports of previous trials showing effects of vitamin A on puerperal sepsis[19,109] and other types of analyses,[110] plausible mechanisms are the effects of vitamin A or β-carotene supplementation on infection, haemorrhage, anaemia and hypertension-related causes of death.

14b.6 EPIDEMIOLOGY OF VITAMIN A DEFICIENCY DISORDERS

The epidemiology of VADD can be characterized in terms of its extent and severity across different populations, its distribution by person, place and time, and risk factors that provide guidance for developing and targeting intervention programmes.

14b.6.1 Indicators of vitamin A deficiency

Understanding of the epidemiology of VADD rests, in part, on precise definition of deficiency by specific and responsive indicators.

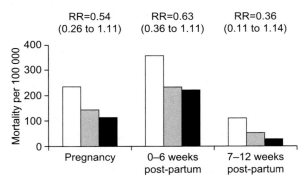

Figure 14b.4 *Effect of weekly vitamin A (gray bars) or β-carotene (black bars) supplementation of Nepalese women on mortality (per 100 000 pregnancies) related to pregnancy among controls (clear bars) stratified by time period. RR, relative risk; (values) are 95% confidence intervals adjusted for design effect. Intent-to-treat RR, both supplements combined, 0.56(0.37–0.84).[7] (Reproduced with permission from RE Black and K Fleischer Michaelsen, Public Health Issues in Infant and Child Nutrition. Lippincott Williams & Wilkins, 2002.)*

Xerophthalmia

Clinical stages of xerophthalmia serve as highly specific indicators of moderate to severe vitamin A deficiency. The original 1976 WHO classification system for active stages of xerophthalmia in young children, ranging from night blindness (XN) through keratomalacia (X3B), and corneal scarring (XS) representing sequelae of previous severe disease,[23] continues to be used.[45] Cut-offs to define the public health importance of xerophthalmia have been modified slightly over the past 25 years and, at times, the sub-stages of corneal ulceration and keratomalacia (X3A and X3B) have been combined to report the joint prevalence of these rare lesions. The WHO classification system of xerophthalmia with accepted minimum prevalence cut-offs for defining public health significance is presented in Table 14b.2. Conjunctival xerosis (X1A), whilst a valid stage of xerophthalmia, is difficult to diagnose reproducibly, and is not recommended for estimating prevalence. **Xerophthalmic fundus (XF)** is another stage of the classification system, but is little used owing to its difficulty in ascertainment, rarity and uncertain significance. The use of maternal night blindness (during the most recent pregnancy yielding a live birth, or especially during the third trimester) is gaining widespread use both for individual and community assessment, with a prevalence $\geq 5\%$ considered to represent a public health problem.[4,51,52]

Biochemical indicators

Biochemical indicators represent tissue concentrations of vitamin A in circulation in the liver (where >90% of all vitamin A is stored), in the total body, or in breast milk,[111] which also serves as a proxy for intake by breast-fed infants.[112] The concentration of retinol in blood is under homeostatic control over a broad range of hepatic stores, and reflects these stores only when they are very low (5 μg/g fresh liver) or very high (hundreds of μg/g of liver in hypervitaminosis A).[113] This control, coupled with the tendency for **serum retinol (SROL)** also to decrease with its carrier protein (RBP) during acute infection, chronic inflammation or severe protein-energy malnutrition, renders this measure unreliable for assessing individual status. However, frequency distributions of SROL concentration are informative in assessing and comparing status of populations. Concentrations below 0.35 μmol/L (10 μg/dl) represent severe deficiency and values between 0.35 and 0.69 μmol/L (10–19 μg/dl) reflect low or deficient status in children. Because SROL distributions tend to rise with age, values below 1.05 μmol/L (30 μg/dl) reflect low-to-deficient status in adults, such as women of reproductive age.[7] Dried blood-spot retinol, obtained on filter paper following a finger prick, represents a promising new field technique for assessing circulating vitamin A concentration by high pressure liquid chromatography, with reported R^2 values of 0.77 to 0.95 when compared with serum retinol concentrations obtained by venous draw, and analyzed by high pressure liquid chromatography.[114,115]

Liver storage adequacy of vitamin A is indirectly assessed through use of the **relative dose response (RDR)** or its modification (**MRDR**).[116,117] The tests are based on a principle that release of RBP from the liver depends on availability of vitamin A from dietary or endogenous sources. Apo-RBP accumulates in the liver during deficiency. After ingestion of an oral test dose of vitamin A (450–1,000 μg retinyl ester), retinol bound to RBP (holo-RBP) in circulation should rise above baseline levels (after five hours) only when endogenous liver retinol concentrations are initially inadequate. The RDR (%) is calculated as:

$$\int RDR = \frac{(5 \text{ hour SROL} - \text{baseline SROL})}{5 \text{ hour SROL}} \times 100$$

An RDR of 20% or higher suggests inadequate liver reserves. In the MRDR test, **3, 4-didehydroretinol (DR)**, naturally found in very low levels in circulation, is used as a ligand for apo-RBP release. No baseline concentration is, therefore, required. A single oral dose of DR is given (100 μg/kg body weight), followed by a single blood sample taken ~ five hours later to determine both retinol and DR concentrations. The molar ratio of serum DR/SROL is calculated: a value of >0.06 is considered abnormal.

All biochemical indicators require expensive equipment and highly trained staff, and blood sampling may have associated problems of inconvenience, infection and non-compliance. Different conditions under which these have been run suggest alternative, ideal cut-offs.

Functional indicators

Common tests of 'function' that have public health application include cytohistological status, by **conjunctival impression cytology (CIC)**, and dark adaptation. Both are considered to be indicators of early or mild deficiency, but theoretically would be expected to reveal abnormal change following decline in tissue vitamin A concentration.

The validity of CIC draws on the role of vitamin A in maintaining a normal, mucus-secreting conjunctival surface, and the fact that keratinizing metaplasia occurs in vitamin A deficiency. This non-invasive technique involves briefly applying a small strip[118] or disk[119] of cellulose acetate filter paper to the inferotemporal aspect of the bulbar conjunctiva of both eyes. After fixing specimens, adherent epithelial cells, goblet cells and mucin are stained with hematoxylin and periodic acid–Schiff reagent, and examined for evidence of loss and keratinization by light microscopy. A modification, **impression cytology with transfer**, or **ICT**, involves immediately impressing harvested cells onto a glass slide. Specimens are classified as normal (adequate numbers of normal epithelial and goblet cells and mucin spots) or abnormal, which may be graded according to severity of loss of goblet cells and mucin and keratinization of epithelial cells. The prevalence of CIC abnormality is directly associated with severity of vitamin A deficiency measured by joint clinico-biochemical indicators.[1] Population prevalence figures for vitamin A deficiency obtained by CIC or ICT generally approximate to those obtained by evaluating distributions of serum retinol below a cut-off of 0.70 μmol/l (20 μg/dl). Although considered a valid functional indicator of vitamin A status, its use under field conditions has proved unpredictable, suggesting that CIC may be unreliable for monitoring changes in population status over time.

Measurement of dark adaptation represents a non-invasive way for assessing early changes in vitamin A-dependent rod photoreceptor function, prior to clinical appearance of night blindness. New, relatively portable techniques have been developed to permit assessment of scotopic vision under controlled field conditions. Impaired status can be inferred, based on either a delayed time to reach a dark-adapted state or a raised light stimulus threshold.[1]

Experience has been gained in field studies with a scotopic vision test that determines the minimum light intensity required to constrict the pupil in a partially dark-adapted individual; this is now largely automated and computer-controlled.[120] The test is based on evidence that the readily observable, afferent pupillary reflex (constriction) to a light stimulus occurs near the visual threshold. Subjects undergo binocular partial bleaching with a flash followed by ten minutes of partial dark adaptation. As light intensity is increased in the test eye, the consensual pupillary response in the other eye is detected: the higher the score (setting) the higher the visual threshold, the less sensitive the rods, and the more abnormal the subject's status. Pupillary scores have been shown to be negatively associated with serum retinol concentrations in Indonesian[121] and Indian[122] children, and among pregnant women in Nepal,[123] with further testing under way in several other countries.

14b.6.2   Extent of vitamin A deficiency

Estimates of the global burden of vitamin A deficiency are fraught with error, particularly as global control programmes have dramatically reduced the severity and prevalence.[4,26] A review in 2002, drawing on previous work from new population and programme coverage data, suggests there are 127 million pre-school vitamin A-deficient children (SROL < 0.70 μmol/L or abnormal CIC) in the developing world.[7] Estimates of cases of xerophthalmia in pre-school children in recent decades have varied from five million in South and South East Asia in the early 1980s[124] to 13 million globally in the early 1990s.[125] The latter figure was reduced by WHO in 1995 to 2.8 million,[2,3] possibly reflecting combinations of improved data, and effects of more widespread vitamin A programme activity. Subsequent estimates are slightly higher: 3.3 million in the late 1990s[26] and 4.4 million most recently,[7] with approximately 40–45% of all vitamin A-deficient and xerophthalmic children residing in South and South East Asia. Provisional estimates suggest there are, each year, nearly 20 million pregnant women with low vitamin A status (serum or breast milk ROL < 1.05 μmol/L), of whom seven million are deficient (<0.70 μmol/L) and six million are night blind. Approximately 45% of all pregnant women with low-to-deficient vitamin A status live in South and South East Asia.[7]

14b.6.3 Location (geographical clustering) of vitamin A deficiency

Mild xerophthalmia has been found to cluster by province within high-risk countries,[1] by village and especially within households. Population surveys in Malawi, Zambia, Nepal and Indonesia have consistently shown the presence of one case to predict a two-fold higher risk of xerophthalmia among other children in the same village.[126] Correlated risk in the community is likely to stem from shared dietary and socio-economic causes: for example, children with xerophthalmia in Aceh, Indonesia, were more likely to come from poorer villages than their age- (but not village-) matched controls.[127] Pre-school children have been reported to be 7–13 times more likely to have, or to develop xerophthalmia if another sibling is affected, compared with children in households with no history of xerophthalmia. In one Asian setting, the diets of older and younger siblings were correlated, reflecting persistent dietary habits across sibling ages, both with respect to foods that were high (r = 0.14–0.66) and low (r = 0.22–0.45) in vitamin A (Table 14b.4).[128] Clustering of deficiency means that index cases 'carry' information to permit resources to be targeted for prevention. For example, siblings of a xerophthalmic child should be given vitamin A, the household diet should be evaluated as regards adequacy, mothers should be counselled on child (and maternal) feeding behaviour, and the community should be

Table 14b.4 *Correlations in reported frequency of current consumption of selected food items between household siblings in rural Nepal (n = 67 sibling pairs[a])*[128]

Food items	Spearman's rank correlation	P-value
Preformed vitamin A sources		
Meat (with liver)	0.38	< 0.002
Fish	0.39	< 0.002
Animal milk	0.66	< 0.001
Other breast milk	0.50	< 0.001
Eggs	0.53	< 0.001
Carotenoid sources		
Mango	0.54	< 0.001
DGLV	0.33	< 0.010
Papaya	0.14	0.270
Low vitamin A foods		
Sweet potato (white)	0.44	< 0.001
Rice and dal	0.42	< 0.001
Other vegetables	0.25	< 0.050
Watery rice and dal mix	0.45	< 0.001
Unleavened wheat bread	0.20	0.100
Honey	0.24	< 0.050
Banana	0.22	< 0.080

[a]Only younger siblings age > 24 months at time of interview used.
DGLV = dark green leafy vegetables.

targeted for food-based or direct supplementation programmes.

14b.6.4   Person (target groups)

The prevalence of mild xerophthalmia (XN and X1B) has been consistently observed to rise with age, from the second year of life throughout the pre-school years.[1,2] In parts of Southern Asia, rates of xerophthalmia continue to rise into the school-aged pre-adolescent years, although the proportion of cases with severe, potentially blinding disease and high mortality are clustered among young children, 0 to five years of age.[1] Boys tend to exhibit higher prevalence rates of mild xerophthalmia but gender differences tend to disappear at more severe, corneal stages of eye disease.[47] Poverty is a root cause of food insecurity and resulting VADD, so that reliable local indicators of low socio-economic status are usually associated with a 1.5 to three times higher risk of xerophthalmia in children. However, low predictive value (often ≤12%) limits the usefulness of socio-economic status indicators for targeting high-risk individuals and households in deficient regions.[1]

Nutritional stresses of pregnancy and lactation appear to increase the risk of VADD among reproductively active women, with prevalence rates of night blindness of ~10% among malnourished populations.[51]

14b.6.5   Time (periodicity)

Incidence of xerophthalmia, and presumably other VADD, can vary by season; for example, in areas of South Asia young children are more prone to develop Bitot's spots and night blindness during the pre-monsoon months of May to mid-July, i.e. a late dry-season period accompanied by a rise in vitamin A-stressing infectious diseases (measles and diarrhoea). Contributing to this peak may be generally low body vitamin A stores following a typical growth spurt that occurs in early winter (December–March) after the rice harvest.[1,129] The 'mango season' may play an important role in ending the seasonal peak in xerophthalmia in West Bengal (Fig. 14b.5). Knowledge of periodicity can help time supplementation programmes so that high-potency vitamin A can be distributed just prior to seasonal peaks in risk.

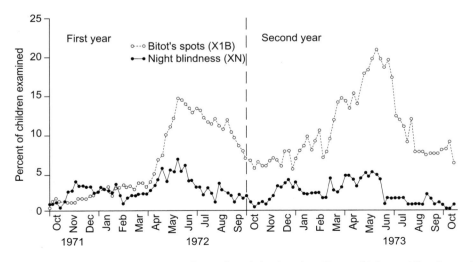

Figure 14b.5 *Seasonality of X1B (open dots) and XN (closed dots) in the village of Ichang, West Bengal, over 2 consecutive years. (Reproduced with permission from the American Journal of Clinical Nutrition, © AMJ Clin Nutr. American Society of Clinical Nutrition.)*

14b.6.6 Dietary risk factors

Vitamin A deficiency becomes a public health problem when large groups of individuals eat a diet chronically lacking in adequate vitamin A to meet normal needs for growth, vision, the demands of pregnancy and lactation, and for resisting infection. Given that newborn babies, even in well-nourished societies, have low hepatic stores of vitamin A,[130] breast feeding provides a first opportunity to supply the growing infant with a reliable, daily source of highly bio-available, preformed vitamin A.[131] In rural populations of Africa,[132] South Asia[74,133,134] and South East Asia[135] breast-fed children have been found to be 10–35% as likely as weaned peers of the same age to have xerophthalmia (odds ratios from 0.10 to 0.35) during the fourth year of life.[1] Risk related to complementary feeding, however, may start even earlier in infancy; for example, in Malawi, pre-school-aged children with XN or X1B were reported to have started taking porridge a month earlier than controls (three versus four months of age), possibly also setting into motion a shorter period of partial breast feeding than practices by non-xerophthalmic peers.[132] In rural India, an early peak in the incidence of keratomalacia among infants <6 months of age has long been evident, and ascribed to being abruptly weaned from the breast.[123,136] Where no protective effect of (partial) breast feeding has been observed, routine consumption of preformed vitamin A and carotenoid-rich foods (e.g. ripe mango, papaya, cooked greens, egg) is associated with consider-able protection of children from xerophthalmia, reflected by protective odds ratios of 0.15 to 0.30.[127]

In the later pre-school years, frequent intake of cooked dark green leaves, yellow sweet potatoes and carrots, and dairy products minimizes risk of xerophthalmia in a dose response manner.[1,135] These foods protect women of reproductive age as well.[6] In recent years, investigations have focused on risks of VADD associated with household eating behaviours. In rural Nepal, pre-schoolers sharing a plate with another family member were more likely to eat greater amounts of green leafy vegetables, fruits, meat, fish and dairy products than children eating alone. Those with a confirmed history of xerophthalmia (having been treated previously) were less likely to eat vitamin A-rich foods, reflecting neglect of the quality of a child's diet, and 70% more likely to share a meal plate with an older male (>15 years of age). In comparison, children from lower risk households (where there was no child with xerophthalmia) were 40% more likely to share a plate with another female.[137]

14b.7 PREVENTION

While formidable in extent and consequence, vitamin A deficiency is readily preventable. Three major preventive strategies exist for improving vitamin A intake and status in high risk populations: (1) periodic, high-potency vitamin A supplementation and food-based approaches that include (2) fortifying food items with vitamin A, and (3) increasing local availability and consumption of food sources of provitamin A carotenoids and preformed vitamin A.[138] The three approaches can be complementary, with respect to their programme and performance characteristics. Choice of strategy depends on numerous factors, including the extent and severity of VADD, age of the population at risk (e.g. young children, pregnant women), agricultural capacity, the local food culture and adequacy of the food production, processing and marketing system, capability of the health service delivery infrastructure, transport, and personnel costs and so forth. Determined political will is essential for the success of any programme.

14b.7.1 Vitamin A supplementation

Periodic delivery of large oral doses of vitamin A in an oily base, either in capsular or syrup form, is the most widely practised strategy to prevent and control VADD among school-aged children. Prophylactic efficacy of high-dose vitamin A delivery is based on the principle that a large amount of preformed vitamin A ester given orally is efficiently absorbed, stored in the liver, and then time-released into the circulation to meet tissue needs for the vitamin over a period of several months. First suggested in 1964,[139] semi-annual, community-based, high-potency vitamin A distribution is now known to be ~90% effective in preventing xerophthalmia and its blinding sequelae,[140] ~30% effective in reducing all-cause mortality[1] but only ~15% effective in preventing low serum retinol in a sustained way[7] among pre-school-aged children in chronically undernourished populations. The oral vitamin A prophylaxis schedule recommended by the **IVACG** is shown in Table 14b.3. Supplement safety has been established when given in recommended dosages for age. Infants <6 months of age receiving 50,000 IU have been shown to be 2–10 times more likely than controls to develop a transient, bulging fontanelle, which largely subsides within 48 hours without further sequelae. Among older infants and pre-school-aged children, receipt of dosages of 100,000 IU and 200,000 IU has been associated with twice and 4–7 times higher risks, respectively, and very transient side effects of nausea, vomiting, headache or diarrhoea.[1] With adequate effort to inform both programme staff and recipient populations of minor side effects, these rarely interfere with achieving adequate distribution coverage.

UNICEF distributes annually between 400 and 600 million 200,000 IU (60,000 μg RAE) vitamin A capsules to developing country governments for use in prevention and treatment programmes.[b] Each costs ~US$0.02, although delivery-related costs have been estimated to be roughly 10–15 times this amount.[140] Nevertheless, vitamin A supplementation is accepted as one of the most cost-effective strategies available for reducing early childhood mortality.[141] Supplements can be restricted to the treatment of xerophthalmia and other high-risk medical conditions, or can be expanded to cover an increasing proportion of high-risk children through community-based distribution. High community coverage rates (> 80%) have been observed when supplements are delivered during nationally orchestrated, semi-annual campaigns,[142] which are likely to be most effective when timed to precede any expected seasonal peak in deficiency. Over 50 countries now

report vitamin A supplement coverage rates of over 80%.[143] Challenges to sustaining high vitamin A coverage relate to assuring adequate and timely availability of supplement supplies, effective supervision and adequate evaluation and documentation of programme performance.

It is advised that women living in endemic areas of vitamin A deficiency receive 400,000 IU (two capsules) within the six weeks following childbirth (to minimize risk of intake during a subsequent periconceptual period) as a means to improve maternal stores to support lactation and, therefore, infant intake via breast milk. Few countries practise this guideline and currently no other recommendation exists for more general vitamin A prophylaxis of women of reproductive age as a means to reduce risk of maternal night blindness or possible pregnancy-related mortality, nor has its benefit been widely demonstrated.

14b.7.2   Food fortification

The goal of food fortification is to provide a fraction of a day's nutritional requirement by adding one or more nutrients (in this case vitamin A) to food 'vehicles' that are widely consumed by a targeted, at-risk population. The amount of nutrient added should be sufficient to improve, or help maintain, adequate nutritional status when the food is consumed in normal-to-low amounts on a regular basis, without posing a risk of toxicity to chronic 'over-consumers'. Where few fortification possibilities exist, the goal should be to provide at least 30–50% of a day's requirement; where multiple options exist, 10–25% of requirement may suffice. Decisions on which food vehicles to fortify depend on many factors. These include:

➢ Purchasing patterns of fortifiable foods in target populations.
➢ Usual intake distributions of possible potential vehicles, especially among groups whose intake of the food item may be routinely low (to estimate efficacy) and high (to assess risk).
➢ Stability of a fortified vehicle under ambient production, transport, marketing, storage and

---

[b] W Schultink, UNICEF, personal communication, 2002.

consumption conditions with respect to nutrient retention, colour, flavour and other organoleptic properties (all of which affect acceptability).

➤ Demonstrated impact of fortification with respect to indicators of status or health.

➤ Estimated cost of fortification relative to the existing price of the product and its substitutes in the market.

➤ Capacity of a local food industry to fortify a food in accordance with quality control standards, with central processing by few facilities preferred to large numbers of fortification facilities.

In addition, the success of fortification depends on other factors, such as the existence of a cooperative and capable private food industry, coupled with enabling yet firm government legislation that sets, monitors and enforces standards for quality control, product packaging, labelling and advertising of fortified products. With the exception of food aid, experience has shown that, ultimately, the consumer must pay for fortified foods in the market place to sustain this strategy.

Food fortification has been extensively practised for decades in industrialized countries as a means to ensure dietary micronutrient adequacy; for example, ready-to-eat cereals are second only to carrots as the leading food source of vitamin A in the USA. In developing countries, a variety of food vehicles have been fortified, including sugar, monosodium glutamate (a common flavour-enhancing agent), grain products, dried milk powder and other dairy foods, margarine, edible oils and special formulae.[1] Of these, the most extensive national experience to date has been gained with sugar fortification, especially in Guatemala over the past 25 years,[144] where vitamin A-fortified sugar clearly shifted the distribution of serum retinol in the population towards adequacy,[145,146] and continues to provide an estimated half day's allowance of vitamin A to young children.[147] Sugar is now fortified with vitamin A in several Latin American countries and this method has begun to be implemented elsewhere, including Zambia and the Philippines.

Experience with monosodium glutamate in the Philippines[148] and Indonesia[149] has amply demonstrated the ability of such a food item, when fortified with vitamin A, to affect favourably status, growth and survival of children.[1] More recently, vitamin A status has been shown to improve in children consuming vitamin A-fortified products such as non-refrigerated margarine[150] and wheat-flour buns[151] compared with controls receiving unfortified products. Many other opportunities for fortification are arising as food production systems become more able to fortify and penetrate markets of poor economic sectors with semi-processed foods. The Manila Forum 2000[152] gave momentum to this preventive strategy for the future. The greatest obstacle remains the relative poverty of the highest-risk populations and the rarity with which they purchase 'processed' products that are amenable to fortification.

14b.7.3   Dietary improvement

Enhancing the nutritional quality of the diet in high-risk populations, especially among children and women of reproductive age, is a fundamental goal to prevent vitamin A and other nutrient deficiencies. The strategy builds on extant agricultural and horticultural capabilities by season and location, food transport and marketing systems, socio-economic and cultural determinants of food security, preferences and dietary access within households as well as numerous other influences. Approaches that can effect dietary change may include combined efforts to increase seasonal or year-round availability of local food sources of preformed vitamin A (e.g. through animal husbandry leading to increased milk production, poultry and egg production) and provitamin A carotenoids (e.g. enhancing vegetable and fruit production through home, school and community gardens or improved solar drying).[153] Low-cost horticultural extension and market pricing subsidies may be important mechanisms in ensuring continuous market access to nutritious foods throughout the year by rural families of low socio-economic means. Both aspects of improving family access to food economic return should be important messages to convey in promotion of home gardening.[154] Recent horticultural breeding practices have dramatically increased β-carotene content of a variety of local foods, including bananas and sweet potatoes, while genetic engineering has developed a number of new food items with enhanced provitamin A activity, particularly 'golden rice'.

Where household access to a balanced diet generally exists, nutrition education, adapted to local cultural norms, should stress the importance of sustained, wholesome feeding practices in safeguarding the health, growth and development of children, and the health of mother and child during periods of pregnancy and lactation. A variety of community-organized, social marketing techniques may be employed to develop and convey educational messages aimed at increasing intakes of, especially, provitamin A carotenoid food sources by young children and mothers.[155] Ethnographic data and epidemiologic patterns of risk associated with vitamin A deficiency should guide the content of nutrition education messages. However, much work remains to be accomplished with respect to developing, implementing and evaluating the effectiveness and costs of dietary diversification strategies in improving vitamin A status and health and survival outcomes related to preventing vitamin A deficiency.

14b.8   CONCLUSIONS

Over the past 30 years, governments have dramatically reduced the threats of xerophthalmia and blindness from vitamin A deficiency, largely because of their interest in improving vitamin A status as an effective child survival strategy. But reduced prevalence of xerophthalmia should not be taken as evidence that these programmes can now be abandoned. Rather, one needs evidence that the vitamin A status of the highest-risk population has truly moved into a safe, normal zone, with evidence that it will not fall back, with disastrous consequences, once these programmes are withdrawn or challenged by financial or food crises.

REFERENCES

1. Sommer A, West KP Jr. *Vitamin A Deficiency: Health, Survival, and Vision.* New York: Oxford University Press; 1996.

2. McLaren DS, Frigg M. *Sight and Life Manual on Vitamin A Deficiency Disorders (VADD),* 1st Edition. Basel: Task Force Sight and Life; 1997.

3. IVACG Statement. *The Annecy Accords to Assess and Control Vitamin A Deficiency: Summary and Clarifications.* Washington, DC: International Vitamin A Consultative Group; 2002.

4. Sommer A, Davidson FR. Assessment and control of vitamin A deficiency: the Annecy accords. *J Nutr* 2002; 132:2845S–2850S.

5. Katz J, Khatry SK, West KP Jr, *et al.* Night blindness is prevalent during pregnancy and lactation in rural Nepal. *J Nutr* 1995; 125:2122–2127.

6. Christian P, West KP, Jr., Khatry SK, *et al.* Night blindness of pregnancy in rural Nepal — nutritional and health risks. *Int J Epidemiol* 1998; 27:231–237.

7. West KP, Jr., Extent of vitamin A deficiency among preschool children and women of reproductive age. *J Nutr* 2002; 132:2857S–2866S.

8. West KP, Jr., Katz J, Khatry SK, *et al.* and the NNIPS-2 Study Group. Double blind, cluster randomized trial of low dose supplementation with vitamin A or β-carotene on mortality related to pregnancy in Nepal. *Br Med J* 1999; 318: 570–575.

9. Christian P, West KP, Jr., Khatry SK, *et al.* Night blindness during pregnancy and subsequent mortality among women in Nepal: effects of vitamin A and β-carotene supplementation. *Am J Epidemiol* 2000; 152:542–547.

10. Christian P, West KP, Jr., Khatry SK, *et al.* Maternal night blindness increases risk of infant mortality in the first 6 months of life in Nepal. *J Nutr* 2001; 131:1510–1512.

11. Checkley W, West KP, Wise RA, *et al.* Maternal vitamin A supplementation and lung function in offspring. *N Engl J Med* 2010; 362:1784–1794.

12. Nunn JF. *Ancient Egyptian Medicine.* London: British Museum; 1996.

13. McLaren DS. *Towards the Conquest of Vitamin A Deficiency Disorders.* Basel: Task Force Sight and Light; 1999.

14. McLaren DS. *Nutritional Ophthalmology.* London: Academic Press; 1980.

15. McCollum EV, Davis M. The necessity of certain lipins in the diet during growth. *J Biol Chem* 1913; 15:167–175.

16. Osborne TB, Mendel LB. The influence of butterfat on growth. *J Biol Chem* 1913; 16:423–437.

17. Bloch CE. Clinical investigation of xerophthalmia and dystrophy in infants and young children (xerophthalmia et dystropia alipogenetica). *J Hygiene* 1921; 19:283–304.

18. Semba RD. Vitamin A as 'anti-infective' therapy, 1920–1940. *J Nutr* 1999; 129:783–791.

19. Green HN, Pindar D, Davis G, *et al.* Diet as a prophylactic agent against puerperal sepsis. *Br Med J* 1931; 2:595–598.

20. Moore T. *Vitamin A*. Amsterdam: Elsevier Publishing Co; 1957.

21. Scrimshaw NS, Taylor CE, Gordon JE. *Interactions of Nutrition and Infection*. Geneva: WHO; 1968.

22. Oomen HAPC, McLaren DS, Escapini H. Epidemiology and public health aspects of hypovitaminosis A. A global survey on xerophthalmia. *Trop Geogr Med* 1964; 4:271–315.

23. World Health Organization. *Vitamin A Deficiency and Xerophthalmia*. Technical Report Series 590. Report of a Joint WHO/USAID Meeting. Geneva: WHO; 1976.

24. World Health Organization. *Control of Vitamin A Deficiency and Xerophthalmia*. Technical Report Series 672. Report of a Joint WHO/UNICEF/USAID/Helen Keller International/IVACG Meeting. Geneva: WHO; 1982.

25. World Health Organization. *The Global Prevalence of Vitamin A Deficiency*. Micronutrient Deficiency Information System (MDIS) Working Paper 2, WHO/NUT/95.3. Geneva: WHO; 1995.

26. Micronutrient Initiative. *Progress in Controlling Vitamin A Deficiency*. Ottawa, Canada: the Micronutrient Initiative, The United Nations Children's Fund. Tulane University; 1998.

27. Mason JB, Lotfi M, Dalmiya N, *et al.* *The Micronutrient Report. Current Progress and Trends in the Control of Vitamin A, Iodine, and Iron Deficiencies.* Ontario: the Micronutrient Initiative; 2001.

28. Bendich A, Olson JA. Biological actions of carotenoids. *FASEB J* 1989; 3:1927–1932.

29. FAO/WHO Expert Consultation. Requirements of vitamin A, iron, folate and vitamin B12. *FAO Food and Nutrition Series* 1988; 23:16–32.

30. De Pee S, West CE, Muhilal, *et al.* Lack of improvement in vitamin A status with increased consumption of dark-green leafy vegetables. *Lancet* 1995; 346:75–81.

31. De Pee S, West CE, Permaesih D, *et al.* Orange fruit is more effective than are dark-green, leafy vegetables in increasing serum concentrations of retinol and β-carotene in schoolchildren in Indonesia. *Am J Clin Nutr* 1998; 68:1058–1067.

32. West CE, Castenmiller JJ. Quantification of the 'SLAMENGHI' factors for carotenoid bioavailability and bioconversion. *Int J Vit Nutr Res* 1998; 68:371–377.

33. West C. Meeting requirements for vitamin A. *Nutr Rev* 2000; 58:341–345.

34. Institute of Medicine. *Dietary Reference Intakes for Vitamin A, Vitamin K, Arsenic, Boron, Chromium, Copper, Iodine, Iron, Manganese, Molybdenum, Nickel, Silicon, Vanadium, and Zinc*. Washington, DC: National Academy Press; 2001.

35. Olson JA. Needs and sources of carotenoids and vitamin A. *Nutr Rev* 1994; 52:67–73.

36. Anonymous. Dietary reference intakes. *Nutr Rev* 1997; 55:319–326.

37. Olson JA. Vitamin A. In: Ziegler EE, Frier LJ, Jr. (eds). *Present Knowledge in Nutrition*. Washington, DC: ILSI Press; 1996. pp. 109–119.

38. Kastner P, Chambon P, Leid M. Role of nuclear acid receptors in the regulation of gene expression. In: Blomhoff R (ed) *Vitamin A in Health and Disease*. New York: Marcel Dekker; 1994.

39. Ross AC, Hammerling UG. Retinoids and the immune system. In: Sporn MB. Roberts AB, Goodsman DS (eds). *The Retinoids: Biology, Chemistry, and Medicine*. New York: Raven Press Ltd; 1994. pp. 521–543.

40. Blomhoff HK, Smeland EB. Role of retinoids in normal hematopoiesis and the immune system. In: Blomhoff R (ed). *Vitamin A in Health and Disease*. New York: Marcel Dekker; 1994.

41. Oyster CW. *The Human Eye — Structure and Function*. Sunderland, MA: Sinauer Associates Inc; 1999. pp. 545–594.

42. Saari JC. Retinoids in photosensitive systems. In: Sporn MB. Roberts AB, Goodman DS (eds). *The Retinoids: Biology, Chemistry, and Medicine*. New York: Raven Press Ltd; 1994. pp. 351–385.

43. Rando RR. Retinoid isomerization reactions in the visual system. In: Blomhoff R (ed) *Vitamin A in Health and Disease*. New York: Marcel Dekker; 1994.

44. Pepperberg DR, Crouch RK. An illuminating new step in visual pigment regeneration. *Lancet* 2001; 358:2098–2099.

45. Sommer A. *Vitamin A Deficiency and its Consequences. A Field Guide to Detection and Control*, 3rd Edition. Geneva: WHO; 1995.

46. McLaren DS. History of vitamin A deficiency and xerophthalmia. In: Cox FEG (ed). *The Wellcome Trust Illustrated History of Tropical Diseases*. London: Wellcome Trust; 1996. pp. 378–385.

47. Sommer A. *Nutritional Blindness: Xerophthalmia and Keratomalacia*. New York: Oxford University Press; 1982.

48. Wittpenn JR, Sommer A. Clinical aspects of vitamin A deficiency. In: Bauernfiend JC (ed). *Vitamin A Deficiency and its Control*. Orlando: Academic Press; 1986. pp. 177–206.

49. Sommer A, Hussaini G, Muhilal, *et al*. History of night blindness: a simple tool for screening. *Am J Clin Nutr* 1980; 33:887–891.

50. Sommer A, Katz J, Tarwotjo I. Increased risk of respiratory disease and diarrhoea in children with preexisting mild vitamin A deficiency. *Am J Clin Nutr* 1984; 40:1090–1095.

51. Christian P. Maternal night blindness: a new indicator of vitamin A deficiency. IVACG Statement. Washington DC: International vitamin A Consultative Group (IVACG); 2002.

52. Christian P. Recommendations for indicators: night blindness during pregnancy — a simple tool to assess vitamin A deficiency in a population. *J Nutr* 2002; 132:2884S–2888S.

53. McLaren DS, Oomen HAPC, Escapini H. Ocular manifestations of vitamin A deficiency in man. *Bull World Health Organ* 1966; 34:257–361.

54. Stofft E, Biesalski HK, Zschaebitz A, *et al*. Morphological changes in the tracheal epithelium of guinea pigs in conditions of 'marginal' vitamin A deficiency. *Int J Vit Nutr Res* 1992; 62:134–142.

55. McDowell EM, Keenan KP, Huang M. Restoration of mucociliary tracheal epithelium following deprivation of vitamin A. *Virchows Arch (Cell Pathol)* 1984; 45:221–240.

56. Lancillotti F, Darwiche N, Celli G, *et al*. Retinoid status and the control of keratin expression and adhesion during the histogenesis of squamous metaplasia of tracheal epithelium. *Cancer Res* 1992; 52:6144–6152.

57. Chandra RK. Increased bacterial binding to respiratory epithelial cells in vitamin A deficiency. *Br Med J* 1988; 297:834–835.

58. Coles CL, Rahmathullah L, Kanungo R, *et al*. Vitamin A supplementation at birth delays pneumococcal colonization in South Indian infants. *J Nutr* 2001; 131:255–261.

59. Wolbach SB, Howe PR. Tissue changes following deprivation of fat-soluble A vitamin. *J Exp Med* 1925; 42:753–777.

60. Brown KH, Gaffar A, Alamgir SM. Xerophthalmia, protein-calorie malnutrition, and infections in children. *J Pediatr* 1979; 95:651–656.

61. Rojanapo W, Lamb AJ, Olson JA. The prevalence, metabolism and migration of goblet cells in rat intestine following the induction of rapid, synchronous vitamin A deficiency. *J Nutr* 1980; 110:178–188.

62. Zile M, Bunge EC, Deluca HF. Effect of vitamin A deficiency on intestinal cell proliferation in the rat. *J Nutr* 1977; 107:552–560.

63. Semba RD. Vitamin A, immunity, and infection. *Clin Infect Dis* 1994; 19:489–499.

64. Ross AC. The relationship between immunocompetence and vitamin A status. In: Sommer A, West KP, Jr. *Vitamin A Deficiency: Health, Survival, and Vision*. New York: Oxford University Press; 1996. pp. 252–273.

65. Semba RD, Muhilal, Ward BJ, *et al*. Abnormal T-cell subset proportions in vitamin-A-deficient children. *Lancet* 1993; 341:5–8.

66. Semba RD, Muhilal, Scott AL, *et al*. Depressed immune response to tetanus in children with vitamin A deficiency. *J Nutr* 1992; 122:101–107.

67. Semba RD, Muhilal, Scott AL, *et al*. Effect of vitamin A supplementation on immunoglobulin G subclass responses to tetanus toxoid in children. *Clin Diagn Lab Immunol* 1994; 1:172–175.

68. Coutsoudis A, Broughton M, Coovadia HM. Vitamin A supplementation reduces measles morbidity in young African children: a randomized, placebo-controlled, double-blind trial. *Am J Clin Nutr* 1991; 54:890–895.

69. Hussey GD, Klein M. A randomized, controlled trial of vitamin A in children with severe measles. *N Engl J Med* 1990; 323:160–164.

70. Barclay AJG, Foster A, Sommer A. Vitamin A supplements and mortality related to measles: a

randomized clinical trial. *Br Med J* 1987; 29: 294–296.

71. Coutsoudis A, Kiepiela P, Coovadia HM, *et al.* Vitamin A supplementation enhances specific IgG antibody levels and total lymphocyte numbers while improving morbidity in measles. *Pediatr Infect Dis J* 1992; 11:203–209.

72. Shankar AH, Genton B, Semba RD, *et al.* Effect of vitamin A supplementation on morbidity due to Plasmodium falciparum in young children in Papua New Guinea: a randomized trial. *Lancet* 1999; 354:203–209.

73. Ramalingaswami V. Nutritional diarrhoea due to vitamin A deficiency. *Ind J Med Sci* 1948; 2:665–674.

74. Khatry SK, West KP, Jr., Katz J, *et al.* and the Sarlahi Study Group. Epidemiology of xerophthalmia in Nepal. A pattern of household poverty, childhood illness, and mortality. *Arch Ophthalmol* 1995; 113:425–429.

75. Tielsch JM, West KP, Jr., Katz J, *et al.* Prevalence and severity of xerophthalmia in southern Malawi. *Am J Epidemiol* 1986; 124:561–568.

76. Bloem MW, Wedel M, Egger RJ, *et al.* Mild vitamin A deficiency and risk of respiratory tract diseases and diarrhoea in preschool and school children in northeastern Thailand. *Am J Epidemiol* 1990; 131:332–339.

77. Milton RC, Reddy V, Naidu AN. Mild vitamin A deficiency and childhood morbidity — an Indian experience. *Am J Clin Nutr* 1987; 46:827–829.

78. Sommer A, Tarwotjo I, Katz J. Increased risk of xerophthalmia following diarrhoea and respiratory disease. *Am J Clin Nutr* 1987; 45:977–980.

79. Foster A, Sommer A. Corneal ulceration, measles, and childhood blindness in Tanzania. *Br J Ophthalmol* 1987; 71:331–343.

80. Alvarez JO, Salazar-Lindo E, Kohatsu J, *et al.* Urinary excretion of retinol in children with acute diarrhoea. *Am J Clin Nutr* 1995; 61: 1273–1276.

81. Stephensen CB, Alvarez JO, Kohatsu J, *et al.* Vitamin A is excreted in the urine during acute infection. *Am J Clin Nutr* 1994; 60: 388–392.

82. Filteau SM. Vitamin A and the acute-phase response. *Nutrition* 1999; 15:326–328.

83. Biswas R, Biswas AB, Manna B, *et al.* Effect of vitamin A supplementation on diarrhoea and acute respiratory tract infection in children. *Eur J Epidemiol* 1994; 10:57–61.

84. Barreto ML, Santos LMP, Assis AMO, *et al.* Effect of vitamin A supplementation on diarrhoea and acute lower-respiratory-tract infections in young children in Brazil. *Lancet* 1994; 344:228–231.

85. Walser BL, Lima AAM, Guerrant RL. Effects of high-dose oral vitamin A on diarrhoeal episodes among children with persistent diarrhoea in a northeast Brazilian community. *Am J Trop Med Hyg* 1996; 54:582–585.

86. Hossain S, Biswas R, Kabir I, *et al.* Single dose vitamin A treatment in acute shigellosis in Bangladeshi children: randomized double blind controlled trial. *Br Med J* 1998; 316:422–426.

87. Sempertegui F, Estrella B, Camaniero V, *et al.* The beneficial effects of weekly low-dose vitamin A supplementation on acute lower respiratory infections and diarrhoea in Ecuadorian children. *Pediatrics* 1999; 104:e1.

88. Fawzi WW, Mbize R, Spiegelman D, *et al.* Vitamin A supplements and diarrhoeal and respiratory tract infections among children in Dar es Salaam, Tanzania. *J Pediatr* 2000; 137:660–667.

89. Ellison JB. Intensive vitamin therapy in measles. *Br Med J* 1932; 2:708–710.

90. Fawzi WW, Chalmers TC, Herrera G, *et al.* Vitamin A supplementation and child mortality. A meta-analysis. *JAMA* 1993; 269:898–903.

91. Glasziou PP, Mackerras DEM. Vitamin A supplementation in infectious diseases: a meta-analysis. *Br Med J* 1993; 306:366–370.

92. Vitamin A and Pneumonia Working Group. Potential interventions for the prevention of childhood pneumonia in developing countries: a meta-analysis of data from field trials to assess the impact of vitamin A supplementation on pneumonia morbidity and mortality. *Bull World Health Organ* 1995; 73:609–619.

93. Stephensen CB, Franchi LM, Hernandez H, *et al.* Adverse effects of high-dose vitamin A supplements in children hospitalized with pneumonia. *Pediatrics* 1998; 101:1–8.

94. Sommer A, Tarwotjo I, Djunaedi E, *et al.* and the Aceh Study Group. Impact of vitamin A supplementation on childhood mortality: a randomized controlled community trial. *Lancet* 1986; 1:1169–1173.

95. West KP, Pokhrel RP, Katz J, *et al.* Efficacy of vitamin A in reducing preschool child mortality in Nepal. *Lancet* 1991; 338:67–71.

96. Rahmathullah L, Underwood BA, Thulasiraj RD, *et al.* Reduced mortality among children in southern India receiving a small weekly dose of vitamin A. *N Engl J Med* 1990; 323:929–935.

97. Daulaire NM, Starbuck ES, Houston RM, *et al.* Childhood mortality after a high dose of vitamin A in a high risk population. *Br Med J* 1992; 304:207–210.

98. Vijayaraghavan K, Radhaiah G, Prakasam B, *et al.* Effect of a massive dose of vitamin A on morbidity and mortality in Indian children. *Lancet* 1990; 336:1342–1345.

99. Ghana VAST Study Team. Vitamin A supplementation in northern Ghana: effects on clinic attendances, hospital admissions, and child mortality. *Lancet* 1993; 342:7–12.

100. Herrera MG, Nestel P, El Amin A, *et al.* Vitamin A supplementation and child survival. *Lancet* 1992; 340:267–271.

101. Beaton GH, Martorell R, Aronson KJ, *et al. Effectiveness of Vitamin A Supplementation in the Control of Young Child Morbidity and Mortality in Developing Countries.* ACC/SCN State-of-the-Art Series. Nutrition Policy Discussion Paper No. 13. Geneva: WHO; 1993.

102. Tielsch JM, Rahmathullah L, Thulasiraj RD, *et al.* Newborn vitamin A dosing reduces the case fatality but not incidence of common childhood morbidities in South India. *J Nutr* 2007; 137: 2470–2474.

103. Klemm RD, Labrique AB, Christian P, *et al.* Newborn vitamin A supplementation reduced infant mortality in rural Bangladesh. *Pediatrics* 2008; 122:e242–e250.

104. Humphrey JH, Agoestina T, Wu L, *et al.* Impact of neonatal vitamin A supplementation on infant morbidity and mortality. *J Pediatr* 1996; 128:489–496.

105. West KP, Jr., Christian P, Katz J, Labrique A, Klemm R, Sommer A. Effect of vitamin A supplementation on maternal survival. *Lancet* 2010; 376:873–874.

106. Kirkwood BR, Hurt L, Amenga-Etego S, *et al.* The ObaapaVitA Trial Team. Effect of vitamin A supplementation in women of reproductive age on maternal survival in Ghana (ObaapaVitA): a cluster-randomised, placebo-controlled trial. *Lancet* 2010; 375:1640–1649.

107. Christian P, West KP, Jr., Khatry SK, *et al.* Vitamin A or β-carotene supplementation reduces symptoms of illness in pregnant and lactating Nepali women. *J Nutr* 2000; 130:2675–2682.

108. Yamini S, West KP, Jr., Wu L, *et al.* Circulating levels of retinal, tocopherol and carotenoid in Nepali pregnant and postpartum women following long-term β-carotene and vitamin A supplementation. *Eur J Clin Nutr* 2001; 55:252–259.

109. Hakimi M, Dibley MJ, Suryono A, *et al.* Impact of vitamin A and zinc supplements on maternal postpartum infections in rural central Java, Indonesia. International Vitamin A Consultative Group Meeting. Durban, South Africa: IVACG; 1999.

110. Faizel H, Pittrof R. Vitamin A and causes of maternal mortality: association and biological plausibility. *Pub Health Nutr* 2000; 3:321–327.

111. International Vitamin A Consultative Group (IVACG). *A Brief Guide to Current Methods of Assessing Vitamin A Status.* Washington, DC: The Nutrition Foundation; 1993.

112. Stoltzfus RJ, Underwood BA. Breast-milk vitamin A as an indicator of the vitamin A status of women and infants. *Bull World Health Org* 1995; 73:703–711.

113. Olson JA. Serum levels of vitamin A and carotenoids as reflectors of nutritional status. *J Natl Cancer I* 1984; 73:1439–1444.

114. Craft NE, Bulux J, Valdez C, *et al.* Retinol concentrations in capillary dried blood spots from healthy volunteers: method validation. *Am J Clin Nutr* 2000; 72:450–454.

115. Craft NE, Haitema T, Brindle LK, *et al.* Retinol analysis in dried blood spots by HPLC. *J Nutr* 2000; 130:882–885.

116. Tanumihardjo SA. The relative dose-response assay. In: *A Brief Guide to Current Methods of Assessing Vitamin A Status.* A report by the International Vitamin A Consultative Group (IVACG). Washington, DC: The Nutrition Foundation; 1993. pp. 12–13.

117. Tanumihardjo SA. The modified relative dose-response assay. In: *A Brief Guide to Current Methods of Assessing Vitamin A Status.* A report by the International Vitamin A Consultative Group (IVACG). Washington, DC: The Nutrition Foundation; 1993. pp. 14–15.

118. Natadisastra G, Wittpenn JR, West KP, Jr., *et al.* Impression cytology for detection of vitamin A deficiency. *Arch Ophthalmol* 1987; 105: 1224–1228.

119. Keenum DG, Semba RD, Wirasasmita S, *et al.* Assessment of vitamin A status by a disk applicator for conjunctival impression. *Arch Ophthalmol* 1990; 108:1436–1441.

120. Labrique AB, West KP, Jr., Christian P, *et al.* An advanced portable dark Adaptometer for assessing functional vitamin A deficiency. Poster. 19th International Congress of Nutrition (ICN), October 4–9, 2009. Bangkok, Thailand.

121. Congdon N, Sommer A, Severns M, *et al.* Pupillary and visual thresholds in young children as an index of population vitamin A status. *Am J Clin Nutr* 1995; 61:1076–1082.

122. Sanchez AM, Congdon NG, Sommer A, *et al.* Pupillary threshold as an index of population vitamin A status among children in India. *Am J Clin Nutr* 1997; 65:61–66.

123. Congdon N, Dreyfuss M, Christian P, *et al.* Dark adaptation thresholds as an indicator of vitamin A status among pregnant and lactating women in Nepal. *Am J Clin Nutr* 2000; 72: 1004–1009.

124. Sommer A, Tarwotjo I, Hussaini G, *et al.* Incidence, prevalence and scale of blinding malnutrition. *Lancet* 1981; 1:1407–1408.

125. World Health Organization. *National Strategies for Overcoming Micronutrient Malnutrition.* Forty-fifth World Health Assembly, WHO A45/17. Geneva: WHO; 1992.

126. Katz J, Zeger SL, West KP, Jr., *et al.* Clustering of xerophthalmia within households and villages. *Int J Epidemiol* 1993; 22:709–715.

127. Mele L, West KP, Jr., Kusdiono, *et al.* and the Aceh Study Group. Nutritional and household risk factors for xerophthalmia in Aceh, Indonesia: a case-control study. *Am J Clin Nutr* 1991; 53:1460–1465.

128. Gittelsohn J, Shankar AV, West KP, Jr., *et al.* Infant feeding practices reflect antecedent risk of xerophthalmia in Nepali children. *Eur J Clin Nutr* 1997; 51:484–490.

129. Sinha DP, Bang FB. The effect of massive doses of vitamin A on the signs of vitamin A deficiency in preschool children. *Am J Clin Nutr* 1976; 29:110–115.

130. Olson JA, Gunning DB, Tilton RA. Liver concentrations of vitamin A and carotenoids, as a function of age and other parameters, of American children who died of various causes. *Am J Clin Nutr* 1984; 39:903–910.

131. Wallingford JC, Underwood BA. Vitamin A deficiency in pregnancy, lactation, and the nursing child. In: Bauernfeind JC (ed). *Vitamin A Deficiency and its Control.* Orlando: Academic Press; 1986. pp. 101–152.

132. West KP, Jr., Chirambo MC, Katz J, *et al.* the Malawi Survey Group. Breastfeeding, weaning patterns and the risk of xerophthalmia in southern Malawi. *Am J Clin Nutr* 1986; 44:690–697.

133. McLaren DS. A study of factors underlying the special incidence of keratomalacia in Oriya children in the Phulbani and Ganjam Districts of Orissa, India. *J Trop Pediatr* 1956; 2:135–140.

134. Mahalanabis D. Breast feeding and vitamin A deficiency among children attending a diarrhoea treatment center in Bangladesh: a case-control study. *Br Med J* 1991; 303:493–496.

135. Tarwotjo I, Sommer A, Soegiharto T, *et al.* Dietary practices and xerophthalmia among Indonesian children. *Am J Clin Nutr* 1982; 35:574–581.

136. Rahmathullah L, Paul Raj MS, Chandravathi TS. Aetiology of severe vitamin A deficiency. *Natl Med J India* 1997; 10:62–64.

137. Shankar AV, Gittelsohn J, West KP, Jr., *et al.* Eating from a shared plate affects food consumption in vitamin A-deficient Nepali children. *J Nutr* 1998; 128:1127–1133.

138. World Health Organization. *Vitamin A Supplements: a Guide to their use in the Treatment and Prevention of Vitamin A Deficiency and Xerophthalmia*, 2nd edition. WHO/UNICEF/IVACG Task Force. Geneva: WHO; 1997.

139. McLaren DS. Xerophthalmia: a neglected problem. *Nutr Rev* 1964; 22:289.

140. West KP, Jr., Sommer A. Delivery of oral doses of vitamin A to prevent vitamin A deficiency and nutritional blindness: a state of the art review. Nutrition Policy Discussion Paper No. 2. Geneva: Administrative Committee on Coordination — Subcommittee on Nutrition of the United Nations; 1987.

141. World Development Report 1993. *Investing in Health.* New York: Oxford University Press; 1993.

142. Bloem MW, Hye A, Wijnroks M, *et al.* The role of universal distribution of vitamin A capsules in combating vitamin A deficiency in Bangladesh. *Am J Epidemiol* 1995; 142:843–855.

143. UNICEF. *State of the World's Children: Special Edition.* United Nations Children's Fund (UNICEF); November 2009.

144. Arroyave G, Aguilar JR, Flores M, *et al. Evaluation of Sugar Fortification with Vitamin A at the National Level.* Washington DC: Pan American Health Organization; 1979.

145. Arroyave G, Mejia LA, Aguilar JR. The effect of vitamin A fortification of sugar on the serum vitamin A levels of preschool Guatemalan children: a longitudinal evaluation. *Am J Clin Nutr* 1981; 34:41–49.

146. Pineda O. Fortification of sugar with vitamin A. *Nutriview* 1993; 2:6–7.

147. Krause VM, Delisle H, Solomons NW. Fortified foods contribute one half of recommended vitamin A intake in poor urban Guatemalan toddlers. *J Nutr* 1998; 128:860–864.

148. Solon F, Fernandez TL, Latham MC, *et al.* An evaluation of strategies to control vitamin A deficiency in the Philippines. *Am J Clin Nutr* 1979; 32:1445–1453.

149. Muhilal, Permeisih D, Idjradinata YR, *et al.* Vitamin A-fortified monosodium glutamate and health, growth, and survival of children: a controlled field trial. *Am J Clin Nutr* 1988; 48:1271–1276.

150. Solon FS, Solon MS, Mehansho H, *et al.* Evaluation of the effect of vitamin A-fortified margarine on the vitamin A status of preschool Filipino children. *Eur J Clin Nutr* 1996; 50:720–723.

151. Solon FS, Klemm RDW, Sanchez L, *et al.* Efficacy of a vitamin A-fortified wheat-flour bun on the vitamin A status of Filipino schoolchildren. *Am J Clin Nutr* 2000; 72:738–744.

152. Manila Forum 2000: Strategies to fortify essential foods in Asia and the Pacific. *Proceedings of a Forum on Food Fortification Policy for Protecting Populations in Asia and the Pacific from Mineral and Vitamin Deficiencies, 21–24 February 2000.* Manila: Asian Development Bank; 2000.

153. West KP, Jr., Darnton-Hill I. Vitamin A deficiency. In: Semba RD and Bloem MW (eds). *Nutrition and Health in Developing Countries.* Totowa, NJ: Humana Press; 2001. pp. 267–306.

154. Horton S. The Economics of Nutritional Interventions. In: Semba RD and Bloem MW (eds). *Nutrition and Health in Developing Countries.* Totowa, NJ: Humana Press; 2001. pp. 507–521.

155. Smitasiri S, Attig G, Dhanamitta S. Participatory action for nutrition education: social marketing vitamin A-rich foods in Thailand. *Ecol Food Nutr* 1992; 28:199–210.

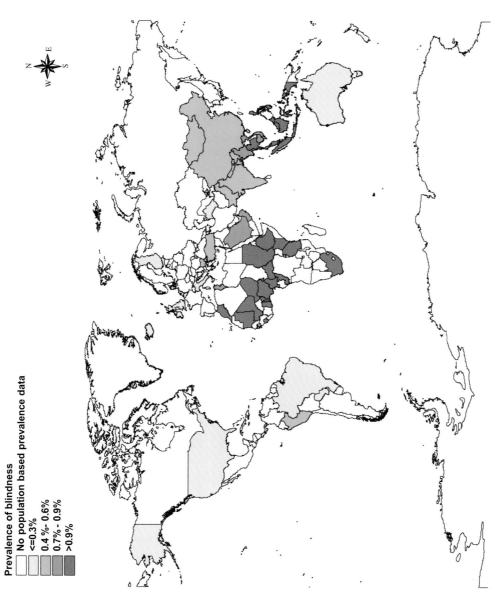

Plate 1.1 *WHO estimated prevalence of blindness (all ages) for each sub-region, applied to each country in which a survey has been done which contributed to the estimates (data, with permission, from Resnikoff S, Pascolini D, Etya'ale D, et al., Bull World Health Organ 2004; 82:844–851. Map: Sarah Polack).*

Prevalence of blindness
- No population based prevalence data
- <=0.3%
- 0.4 %- 0.6%
- 0.7% - 0.9%
- >0.9%

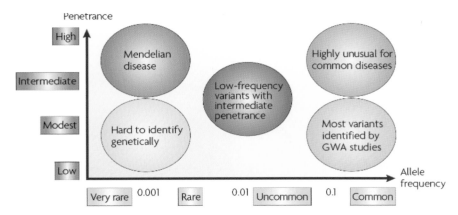

Plate 6.1 *Genetic mutations for Mendelian diseases, which are rare but highly penetrant and of strong effect, have been discovered by linkage analysis. Genome-wide association studies (GWAS) have identified common variants for common diseases, often of modest effect size, and significant genetic variance remains unexplained. However, a proportion of this 'missing heritability' will be attributable to low-frequency variants with intermediate penetrance effects, which have been difficult to identify. New resequencing technologies, allied to large-scale association testing, and other variants, such as copy number (CNV) studies, may help identify these variants. Those rare variants of small effect are likely to remain elusive. (With permission of Nature Publishing Group. McCarthy MI, et al.[16] Genome-wide association studies for complex traits: consensus, uncertainty, and challenges. Nat Rev Genet 2008; 9:356–369).*

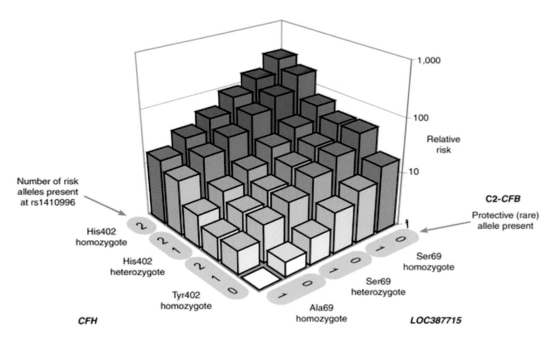

Plate 6.2 *Relative risk plotted as a function of the genetic load of the five variants that influence risk of AMD. Knowledge of five SNP variants (two in the CFH gene, Y402H and rs1410996, one A69S in LOC387715 and two relatively rare variants are observed in the C2 and BF genes) allowed Seddon's group[32] to calculate that individuals with all five high-risk alleles have a lifetime risk of 50% of developing AMD, while those with all low-risk alleles have less than 1% risk. (With permission of Nature Publishing Group. Maller J, et al.[32] Common variation in three genes, including a noncoding variant in CFH, strongly influences risk of age-related macular degeneration. Nat Genet. 2006; 38:1055–1059).*

Standard photographs for the World Health Organization Programme for the Prevention of Blindness and Deafness (WHO/PBD) simplified cataract grading system. (WHO Cataract Grading Group. A simplified cataract grading system. WHO/PBL/01.81. Geneva: World Health Organization; 2002; Thylefors B, Chylack JR LT, Konyama K, *et al*. A simplified cataract grading system. The WHO Cataract Group. Ophthalmic Epidemiol 2002; 9:83–95.)

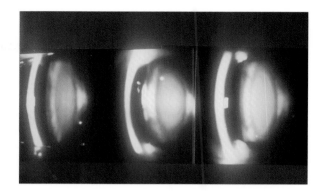

Plate 10.1 *Nuclear standards 1, 2 and 3 (significant, moderately advanced and very advanced nuclear cataract formation, respectively)*

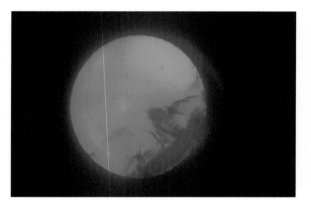

Plate 10.2 *Standard photograph for early cortical cataract (COR). Sharply-defined anterior and posterior cortical opacities, seen on retro-illumination at the slit-lamp, are assessed*

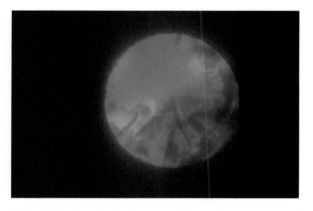

Plate 10.3 *Standard photograph for advanced cortical cataract (COR). Dispersed cortical opacities are aggregated in order to grade extent in terms of 'eighths' of the circumference*

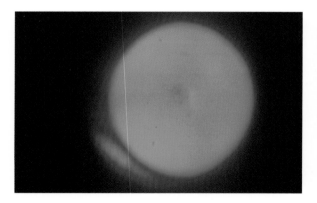

Plate 10.4 *Standard retro-illumination photograph of pure early posterior subcapsular cataract (PSC). PSC is graded according to the vertical extent in millimetres*

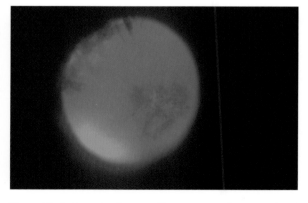

Plate 10.5 *Standard retro-illumination photograph of complex (more advanced) posterior subcapsular cataract (PSC) showing paracentral disc of cataract and a lacy pattern of opacification*

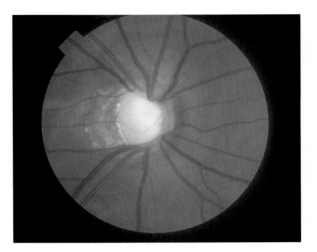

Plate 13.1 *Optic neuropathy characteristic of glaucoma, with severe cupping and peripapillary atrophy.*

Photograph: PJ Foster

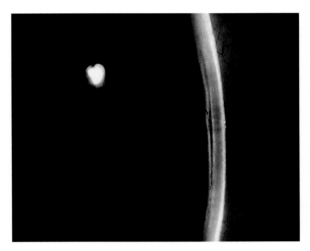

Plate 13.2 *Modified grading scheme for the van Herick test: the space between the endothelium and the iris was estimated in this case to be 15% of the corneal thickness.*[110]

Photograph: PJ Foster

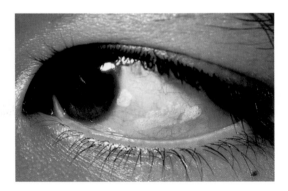

Plate 14b.1 *Vitamin A deficiency; X1B, Bitot's spots*

Photograph: DS Mclaren

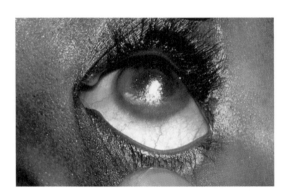

Plate 14b.2 *Vitamin A deficiency; X2, corneal xerosis*

Photograph: GJ Johnson

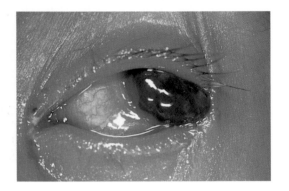

Plate 14b.3 *Vitamin A deficiency; X3B, keratomalacia*

Photograph: S Franken

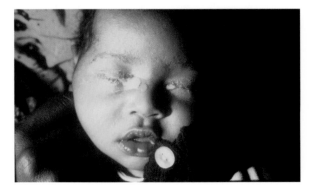

Plate 14c.1 *Ophthalmia Neonatorum due to Neisseria gonorrhoeae*

Photograph: The late JDC Anderson

Plate 14d.1–14d.6 *Images of measles-related corneal ulceration*

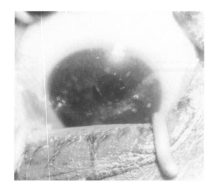

Plate 14d.1 *Punctate keratitis*
Photograph: Allen Foster

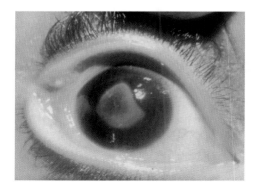

Plate 14d.2 *More extensive measles keratoconjunctivitis*
Photograph: Allen Foster

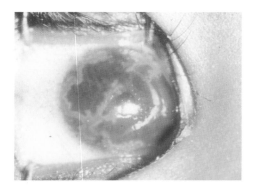

Plate 14d.3 *Herpes simplex keratoconjunctivitis*
Photograph: Allen Foster

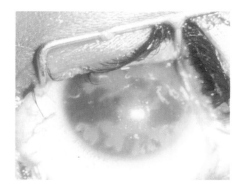

Plate 14d.4 *Herpes simplex keratoconjunctivitis*
Photograph: Allen Foster

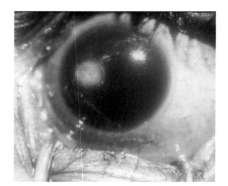

Plate 14d.5 *Xerophthalmia: X3A corneal ulceration from acute vitamin A deficiency secondary to measles*
Photograph: Allen Foster

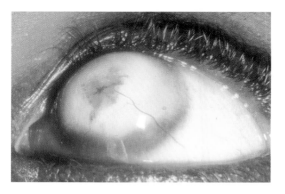

Plate 14d.6 *Corneal scarring following perforating corneal ulceration associated with measles infection*
Photograph: Clare Gilbert

Immunization coverage with measles-containing vaccines in infants, 2009

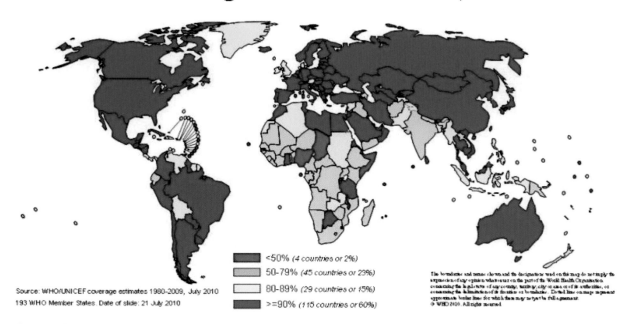

- <50% *(4 countries or 2%)*
- 50-79% *(45 countries or 23%)*
- 80-89% *(29 countries or 15%)*
- >=90% *(115 countries or 60%)*

Source: WHO/UNICEF coverage estimates 1980-2009, July 2010
193 WHO Member States. Date of slide: 21 July 2010

Plate 14d.7 *Immunization coverage with measles-containing vaccines, WHO 2009*

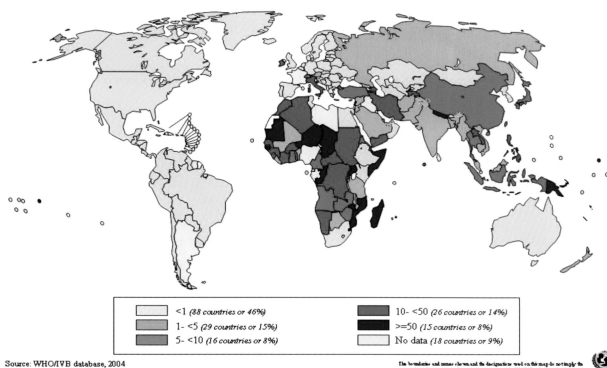

- <1 *(88 countries or 46%)*
- 1- <5 *(29 countries or 15%)*
- 5- <10 *(16 countries or 8%)*
- 10- <50 *(26 countries or 14%)*
- >=50 *(15 countries or 8%)*
- No data *(18 countries or 9%)*

Source: WHO/IVB database, 2004

Plate 14d.8 *Measles incidence/100,000 population, WHO 2003*

Plates 14e.1–14e.4 Morphology of childhood cataract

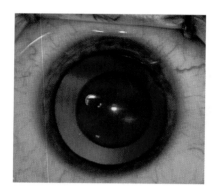

Plate 14e.1 *Lamellar cataract*
Photograph: ME Wilson

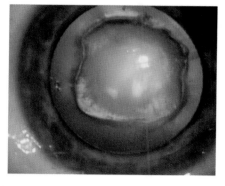

Plate 14e.2 *Foetal nuclear cataract. A dense white foetal nuclear cataract spreading into the surrounding cortex*
Photograph: ME Wilson

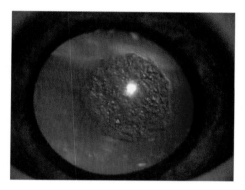

Plate 14e.3 *Posterior lentiglobus cataract in a 4-year-old child*
Photograph: ME Wilson

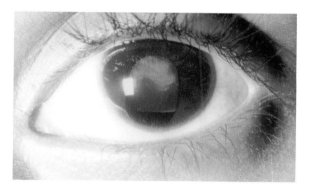

Plate 14e.4 *Eye of child with coloboma of iris and localised lens opacities*
Photograph: CE Gilbert

Plates 14f.1–14f.2 *Examples of childhood glaucoma*

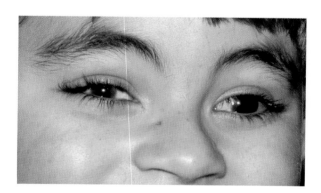

Plate 14f.1 *Aphakic glaucoma with left buphthalmos following congenital cataract surgery*
Photograph: M Papadopoulos

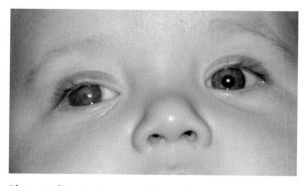

Plate 14f.2 *Right corneal haze from stromal oedema due to elevated intraocular pressure*
Photograph: M Papadopoulos

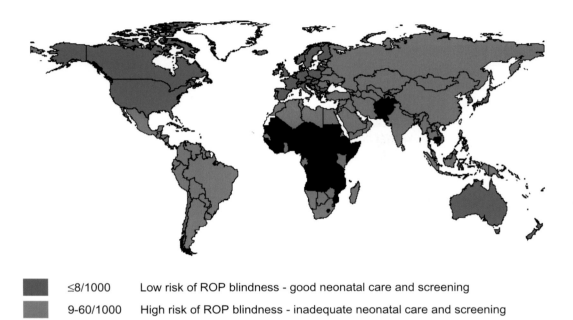

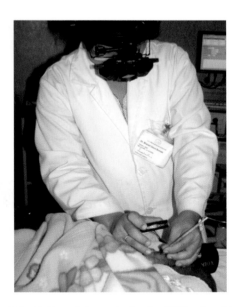

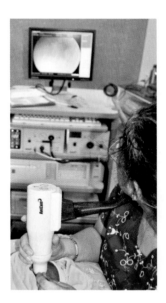

	≤8/1000	Low risk of ROP blindness - good neonatal care and screening
	9-60/1000	High risk of ROP blindness - inadequate neonatal care and screening
	≤61/1000	Low risk of ROP blindness - neonatal care not well developed

Plate 14g.1 *Probable distribution of blindness in children due to retinopathy of prematurity in 2011, using infant mortality rates as a proxy indicator. (Map: Jyoti Shah)*

Plate 14g.2 *Examining a baby for ROP using binocular indirect ophthalmoscopy*

Plate 14g.3 *Examining for ROP using a hand-held contact digital imaging (Retcam)*

Plates 14g.4–14g.9 *Stages of Retinopathy Prematurity*

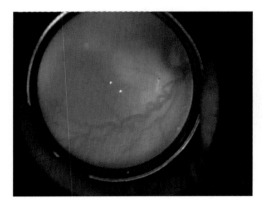

Plate 14g.4 *Plus disease as seen by indirect ophthalmoscopy*
Photograph: S Jalali

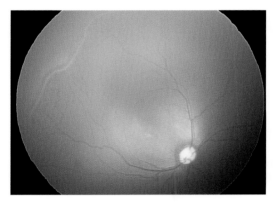

Plate 14g.5 *Stage 2 ROP (ridge) in zone 2. RetCam image*
Photograph: A Ells

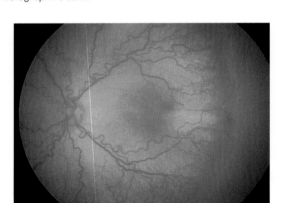

Plate 14g.6 *Stage 3 with marked plus disease in posterior zone 2. RetCam image*
Photograph: A Ells

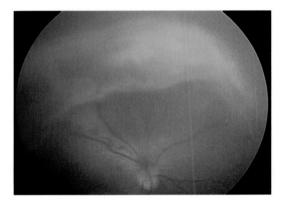

Plate 14g.7 *Stage 4 with subtotal retina detachment. RetCam image*
Photograph: R Azad

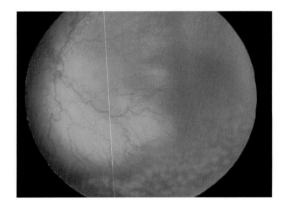

Plate 14g.8 *Near-confluent laser anterior to the ridge*
Photograph: A Ells

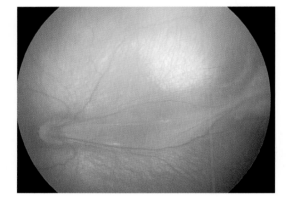

Plate 14g.9 *Stage 4B ROP (subtotal retinal detachment) with a macula fold*
Photograph: A Ells

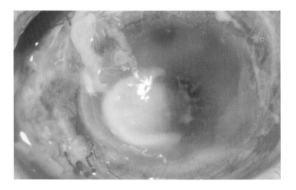

Plate 16a.1 *Corneal ulcer due to Pseudomonas sp., with immune ring and hypopyon*

Photograph: JP Whitcher

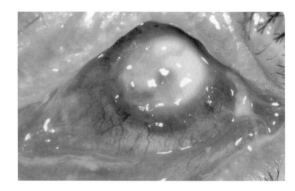

Plate 16a.2 *Ulcer due to Streptococcus pneumoniae, leaving peripheral cornea clear*

Photograph: JP Whitcher

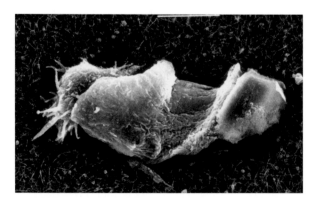

Plate 16a.3 *Corneal ulcer due to Moraxella sp., with stromal necrosis, and hypopyon containing a hyphaema*

Photograph: JP Whitcher

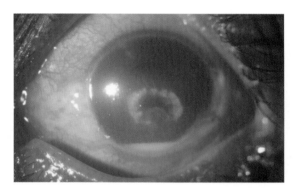

Plate 16a.4 *Indolent fungal corneal ulcer, with satellite lesions around the original infiltrate, hypopyon, and a fibrin plaque on the endothelium*

Photograph: JP Whitcher

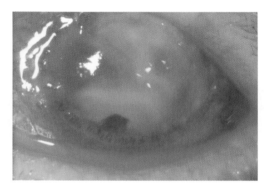

Plate 16c.1 *Photograph of an excysting amoeba*

Photograph: L McLaughlin-Borlace

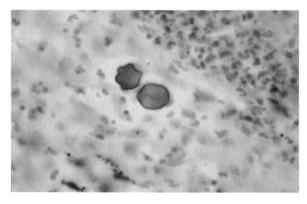

Plate 16c.2 *Histology from a corneal biopsy demonstrating intrastromal cysts of acanthamoeba*

Photograph: JKG Dart

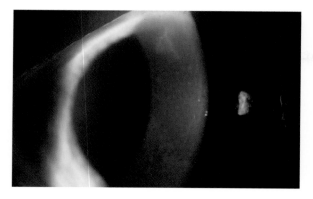

Plate 16c.3 *Radial keratoneuritis in early acanthamoeba keratitis.*

Photograph: JKG Dart

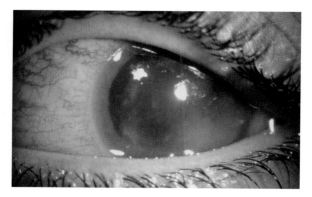

Plate 16c.4 *Early acanthamoeba keratitis with diffuse infiltrates*

Photograph: JKG Dart

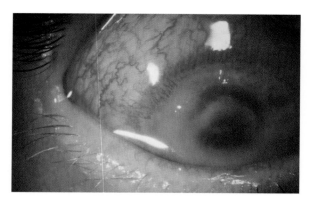

Plate 16c.5 *Severe scleritis and a ring abscess with advanced acanthamoeba keratitis*

Photograph: JKD Dart

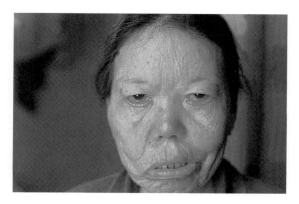

Plate 16d.1 *Ocular complications of leprosy; lagophthalmos*

Photograph: P Courtright

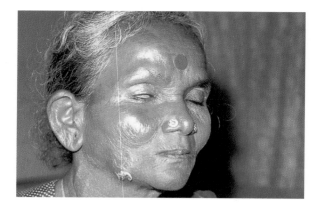

Plate 16d.2 *Ocular complication of leprosy: acute onset of lagophthalmos of the right eye due to Type 1 reaction, in the presence of a malar skin patch on the same side*

Photograph: M Hogeweg

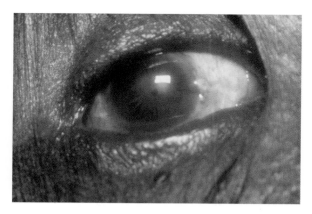

Plate 16d.3 *Complication of leprosy: chronic uveitis, with extreme constriction of the pupil*

Photograph: M Hogeweg

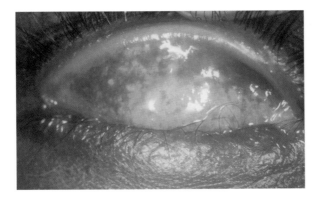

Plate 16e.1 *Vernal keratoconjunctivitis. Diffuse papillary hypertrophy of conjunctiva over the upper tarsal plate*
Photograph: S Franken

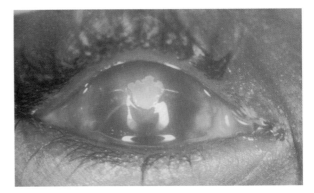

Plate 16e.2 *Vernal keratoconjunctivitis with 'shield ulcer' of cornea*
Photograph: S Franken

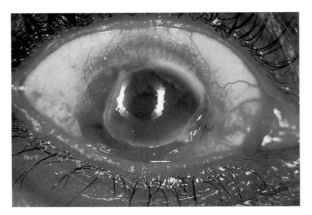

Plate 16f.1 *Mooren's ulcer, early stage*
Photograph: S Franken

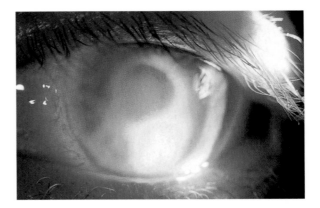

Plate 16g.1 *Climatic droplet keratophathy, Grade 3*
Photograph: GJ Johnson

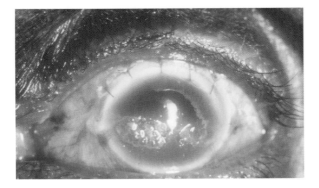

Plate 16g.2 *Climatic droplet keratopathy, Grade 4*
Photograph: GJ Johnson

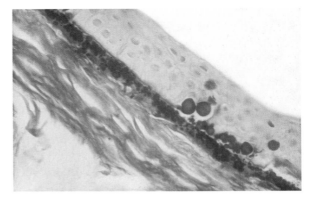

Plate 16g.3 *Histology of climatic droplet keratopathy in lamellar keratectomy specimen (Martius-Scarlet-Blue stain, collagen blue, spheroidal deposits orange)*
Photograph: GJ Johnson

Plates 17.1–17.5 Clinical features of trachoma, illustrated by the stages of the World Health Organization Simplified Trachoma Grading System. (Thylefors B, Dawson C, Jones BR, et al. A simple system for the assessment of trachoma and its complications. *Bull World Health Organ* 1987; 65:477–483.

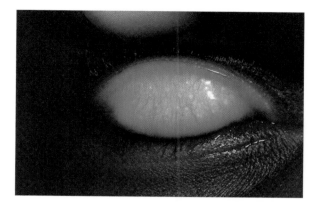

Plate 17.1 *Simplified trachoma grading: TF (follicles)*
Photograph: SK West

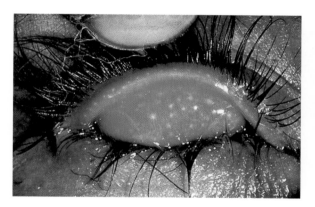

Plate 17.2 *Simplified trachoma grading: TI (intense inflammation) plus TF (follicles)*
Photograph: GJ Johnson

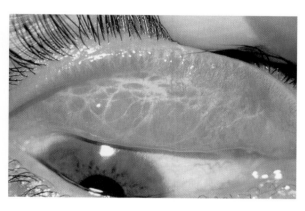

Plate 17.3 *Simplified trachoma grading: TS (scarring)*
Photograph: HR Taylor

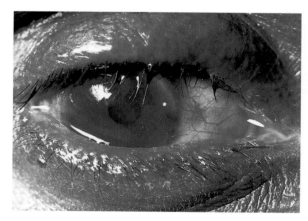

Plate 17.4 *Simplified trachoma grading: TT (trichiasis)*
Photograph: the late JDC Anderson

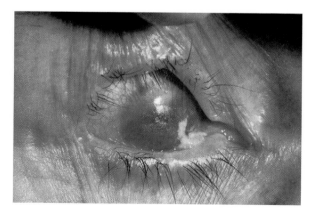

Plate 17.5 *Simplified trachoma grading: CO (corneal opacity) and TT (trichiasis)*
Photograph: A Foster

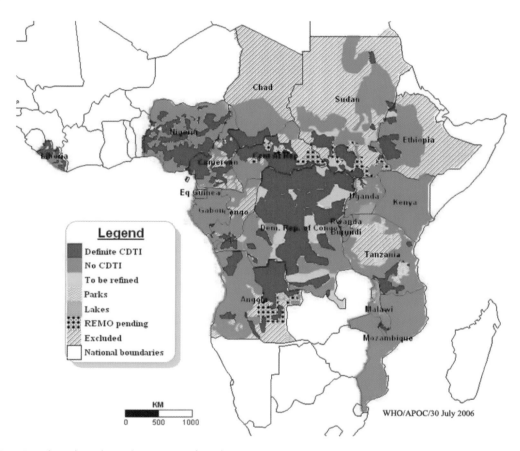

Plate 18.1 *Rapid epidemiological mapping of onchocerciasis (REMO) in countries covered by African Programme for Onchocerciasis Control (APOC), 2006. CDTI — community-directed treatment with ivermectin (by permission of APOC).*

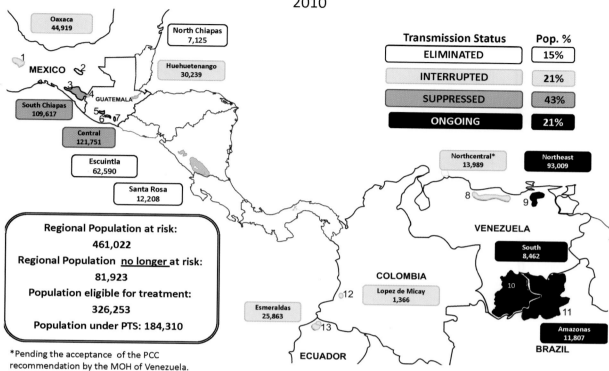

Geographic distribution and transmission status of the 13 foci of the Americas 2010

Transmission Status	Pop. %
ELIMINATED	15%
INTERRUPTED	21%
SUPPRESSED	43%
ONGOING	21%

Oaxaca
44,919

North Chiapas
7,125

MEXICO

Huehuetenango
30,239

GUATEMALA

South Chiapas
109,617

Central
121,751

Escuintla
62,590

Santa Rosa
12,208

Northcentral*
13,989

Northeast
93,009

VENEZUELA

South
8,462

COLOMBIA

Lopez de Micay
1,366

Esmeraldas
25,863

Amazonas
11,807

BRAZIL

ECUADOR

Regional Population at risk:
461,022
Regional Population no longer at risk:
81,923
Population eligible for treatment:
326,253
Population under PTS: 184,310

*Pending the acceptance of the PCC recommendation by the MOH of Venezuela.

Plate 18.2 *Progress of Onchocerciasis Elimination Programmes in the Americas (OEPA). Foci under treatment in 2009 (black areas). Blue areas have no transmission and shaded areas are being tested further to ensure that transmission has been interrupted (by permission of OEPA).*

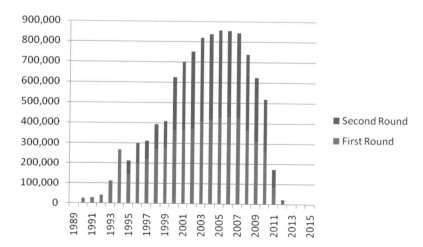

Plate 18.3 *Number of treatments in OEPA countries since 1989 and projected to 2012. Effective scale up of twice yearly treatment began in 2001 and reached satisfactory coverage in 2003. The programme is already scaling down treatment as is shown in the graph*[41]

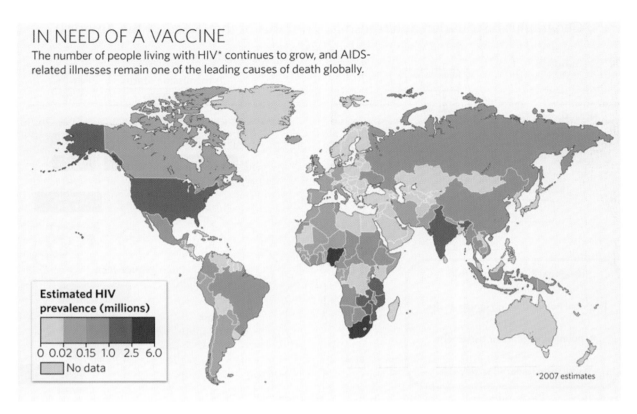

IN NEED OF A VACCINE

The number of people living with HIV* continues to grow, and AIDS-related illnesses remain one of the leading causes of death globally.

Estimated HIV prevalence (millions)

0 0.02 0.15 1.0 2.5 6.0

No data

*2007 estimates

Plate 20.1 *Estimated HIV prevalence (millions), in 2007.* (Reprinted by permission from Macmillan Publishers Ltd. Koff. Accelerating HIV vaccine development. *Nature*, 2010; 464: 161–162).

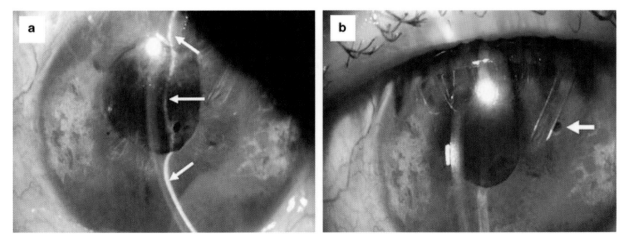

Plate 20.2 a+b *Anterior segment photographs of the left eye: (a) at presentation showing marked AC shallowing, extensive iris/cornea contact (oblique arrows) and bowed fibrin membrane over the posterior chamber IOL (horizontal arrow); (b) after argon laser iridotomy (horizontal arrow), showing a deep chamber and flattened iris and fibrin membrane contours*

Photographs: DA Jabs

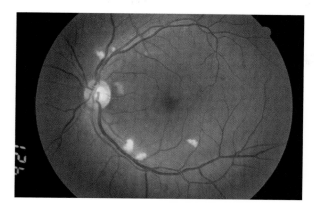

Plate 20.3 *Human immunodeficiency virus retinopathy, manifested by cotton-wool spots and/or dot-blot haemorrhage*

Photograph: DA Jabs

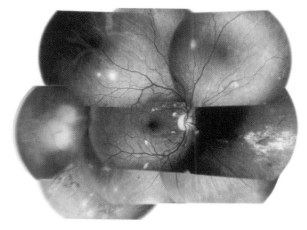

Plate 20.4 *Montage illustrating human immunodeficiency (HIV) virus retinopathy, cytomegalovirus (CMV) retinitis and the acute retinal necrosis (ARN) syndrome. The CMV retinitis lesion is located on the right of the montage. The posteriorly located cotton-wool spots represent HIV retinopathy. The remaining peripheral lesions represent the acute retinal necrosis syndrome. The patient initially presented for evaluation for herpes zoster ophthalmicus*

Photograph: DA Jabs

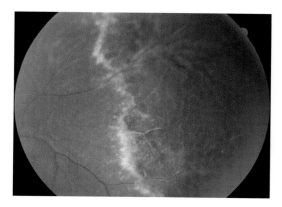

Plate 20.5 *Cytomegalovirus retinitis. Typical findings of full-thickness retinal necrosis and patchy haemorrhage are illustrated. More peripherally located lesions are likely to have a more 'granular' appearance of the retinal necrosis, because the peripheral retina is less thick than in the posterior pole*

Photograph: DA Jabs

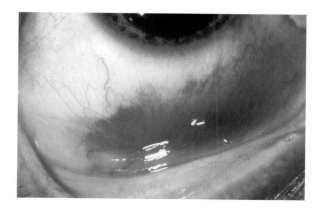

Plate 20.6 *Ocular adnexal Kaposi's sarcoma typically presents as an eyelid lesion, or as a subconjunctival lesion*

Photograph: DA Jabs

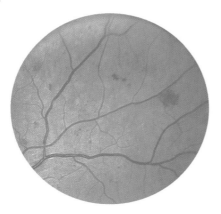

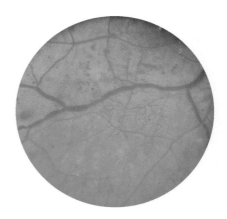

Plate 21.1 *Diabetic retinopathy: non-proliferative.*

Plate 21.2 *Diabetic retinopathy: severe non-proliferative (pre-proliferative)*

(Plates 21.1, 21.2 and 21.5 printed with permission from the Early Treatment Diabetic Retinopathy Study (ETDRS) Manual of Operations 1985, ETDRS Coordinating Centre, Department of Epidemiology and Preventative Medicine, University of Maryland School of Medicine, Baltimore. Available from: National Technical Information Service, 5285 Port Royal Road, Springfield, VA 22161 (accession #PB85223006)).

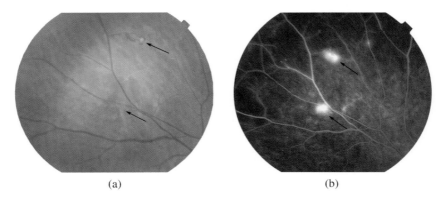

(a)   (b)

Plate 21.3 a+b *Fundus photo with early neovascularization (black arrows). Frame from a companion fluorescein angiogram of the same area of the fundus. The new vessels are leaking, causing a white area in the photograph (see arrow heads)*

Photographs: BE Klein

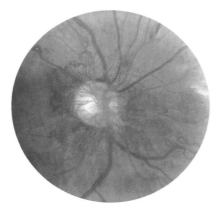

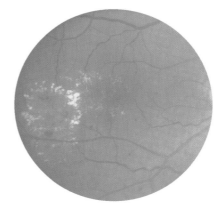

Plate 21.4 *Diabetic retinopathy: proliferative — new vessels at disc*

Photograph: GJ Johnson

Plate 21.5 *Diabetic retinopathy: clinically significant macular oedema, with adjacent hard exudates*

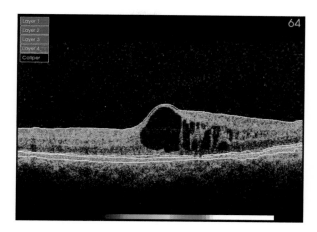

Plate 21.6 *Spectral domain ocular coherence tomography of the macula, demonstrating diabetic macular oedema*

Photograph: BE Klein

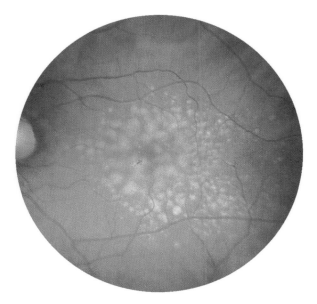

Plate 22.1 *Early age-related macular degeneration; large, soft drusen at macula*

Photograph: S Owens

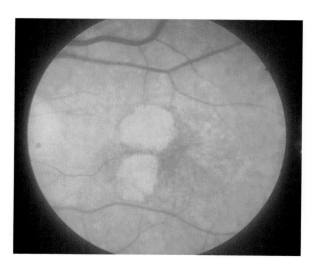

Plate 22.2 *Late age-related macular degeneration; atrophy*

Photograph: AC Bird

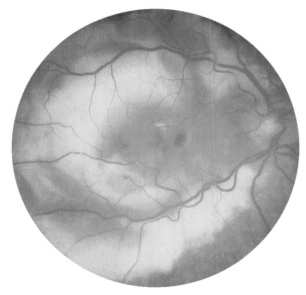

Plate 22.3 *Late age-related macular degeneration; disciform scar*

Photograph: S Owens

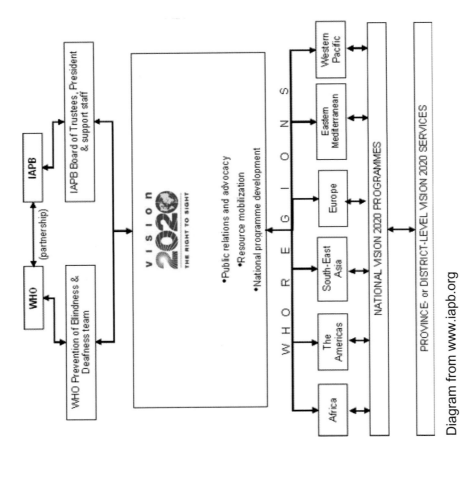

Diagram from www.iapb.org

Plate 24.1 *Organogram of the structure of VISION 2020 and the inter-relationship between WHO and IAPB*

Ophthalmia neonatorum

VOLKER KLAUSS AND ULRICH SCHALLER

14c.1	Definition	317
14c.2	Clinical features and classification	317
14c.3	Prevalence	318
14c.4	Incidence and geographical distribution	319
14c.5	Prevention of ophthalmia neonatorum	319
14c.6	Treatment of established ophthalmia neonatorum	320
14c.7	Community healthcare management	320
14c.8	Epidemiological research priorities	320
	References	320

14c.1 DEFINITION

Ophthalmia neonatorum (ON) is defined as conjunctivitis in an infant less than 28 days old (WHO), due to infection acquired during delivery. The main organisms are *Neisseria gonorrhoeae* and *Chlamydia trachomatis* (Serotypes D–K).

14c.2 CLINICAL FEATURES AND CLASSIFICATION

The time of onset and clinical signs of ON vary according to the different causative agents. Gonococcal ON tends to be more severe and with earlier onset than chlamydial ON.[1] Early involvement of the cornea can be present and may progress rapidly to perforation and endophthalmitis. Gonococcal infection is not limited to the eye but can also involve the respiratory tract, the middle ear, the digestive tract and the vaginal canal of the newborn. The initiation of treatment dramatically changes the course and outcome of the disease, usually with noticeable improvement within 24 hours.

Ophthalmia neonatorum caused by *Chlamydia trachomatis* (serotype D–K) appears later than gonococcal ophthalmia. Inflammatory membranes (pseudomembranes) may appear during the second week of disease. Blinding complications are rare and much slower than in gonococcal ON. Chlamydial infection can also be extra-ocular, leading to pneumonitis, otitis, pharyngeal and rectal colonization.[1]

When it is due to other microbial agents, ON is usually milder. Corneal complications are rare but have been reported in cases of pseudomonal ON. *Herpes simplex* keratoconjunctivitis most often presents in an infant with generalized *Herpes simplex*, and leads to corneal involvement.[2]

Following instillation of silver nitrate drops, chemical conjunctivitis mostly develops within 24 hours. Signs are reddening and swelling of the lids.[1,3,4]

A grading system has been suggested (0 to three for lid redness, lid swelling and discharge, which would lead to a maximum score of 9; corneal changes are not included).[5]

14c.3   PREVALENCE

14c.3.1   Prevalence of ophthalmia neonatorum

The prevalence of **sexually transmitted diseases (STDs)** has been increasing throughout the world over the past decades.[2] A study from a health centre in a multicultural area of Amsterdam reported an increase in the annual number of cases of gonorrhea from four in 1996 to 14 in 2,000 (total cases);[6] the number of chlamydial infections rose from seven to 29 per year (total cases).[6] These infections among pregnant women are particularly important because they cause maternal complications and serious disease, including ophthalmia neonatorum. In industrialized countries ophthalmia neonatorum resulting from infection with *Neisseria gonorrhoeae* (Plate 14c.1) is today rare owing to a lower prevalence in pregnant women (0.1–7%) and because of prophylaxis at birth.[4,5] In Germany alone, between 1,000 and 4,500 pregnant women can be expected to be infected with gonorrhea each year; the prevalence of gonococci in the newborn is put at about 0.1%, but this percentage is clearly reduced by using the Credé method.[5] In developing countries data levels during pregnancy are incomplete, but *N. gonorrhoeae* can be recovered in 4–18% of pregnant women.[2]

About 30% of infants exposed to *N. gonorrhoeae* during birth will develop gonococcal infection of the eye in the absence of prophylaxis; this implies that up to approximately 6% of infants born in some developing countries will develop gonococcal conjunctivitis.[2]

The prevalence of chlamydia is far higher (2–11%) because of increasingly common infections with *Chlamydia trachomatis*. In the USA *C. trachomatis* infection of the genital tract has been found in 2–24% of pregnant women. Between 25% and 50% of neonates exposed to this infection during birth develop chlamydial conjunctivitis, so that 0.5–12% of all newborns may be infected, depending on the population group. A

recent publication reported between 85 to 198 annual cases of ON between 1998 and 2006 in England and Wales.[7] However, the authors suspected that there had been under-notification of ON due to *Chlamydia trachomatis*, and suggested that national studies be undertaken to determine how widespread this problem may be. An Irish study between 2002 and 2006 reported on 51 cases of ON: *C. trachomatis* was cultured in 48 cases and *N. gonorrhoeae* in three cases. This recent increase also of ON caused by *N. gonorroeae* requires a high index of suspicion and prompt treatment.[8]

Data from developing countries are incomplete, but up to 7% of pregnant women have been reported to have chlamydial infections in some populations. However, it is more difficult to determine infection by *C. trachomatis* because reliable laboratory facilities are not available everywhere.[2,4] A recent study from New Delhi, India, found *C. trachomatis* in 18 (31%) of 58 newborns with signs and symptoms of conjunctivitis, as the most common cause of ON.[9]

14c.3.2   Prevalence of blindness from ophthalmia neonatorum

Before 1900, up to 50% of children at schools for the blind had been blinded by ophthalmia neonatorum caused by *N. gonorrhoeae*. Since the introduction of silver nitrate prophylaxis, the number of children affected has been continuously declining in developed countries.[4,10] However, in developing countries data are seldom available on blindness in children under five years old, and on the proportion of cases caused by neonatal conjunctivitis. Figures often indicate a low prevalence of blindness because childhood blindness is associated with high mortality in early childhood (cf. Chapter 14a). Ophthalmia neonatorum is therefore a substantial health problem in developing countries.[2] A report from China showed that the common prevalence of chlamydial infection is clearly correlated with low birth weight and neonatal morbidity.[8] Data from East Africa indicated that ON is responsible for 6% of bilateral corneal ulcers in children, and for an estimate of 5% of childhood blindness.[12] A study from India on 1,318 children in blind schools reports blindness resulting from ON in 10 (0.8%).[13]

14c.4 INCIDENCE AND GEOGRAPHICAL DISTRIBUTION

Incidence depends on the routine use of silver nitrate, or any other prophylaxis at birth, and the prevalence of **sexually transmitted disease (STD)** organisms in pregnant women. With the help of the Credé method the incidence of gonococcal ON has fallen to 0.04% in most industrialized countries.[10] The original application of a 2% solution of silver nitrate was then reduced to 1% solution, which in many countries is still the gold standard to prevent ON. However, the spectrum of organisms has changed since Credé developed this method. In industrialized countries *C. trachomatis* now represents the most frequently sexually transmitted agent.[1,2] The incidence of chlamydial ON ranges from five to 60 cases per 1,000 live births.[4,10] The present authors' data from Munich showed a chlamydial infection in ten out of 15 neonates with ON. *Neisseria gonorrhoeae* could not be isolated.[1]

In contrast, data from Kenya show that *N. gonorrhoeae* can be isolated in 40% of mothers of children with ON. In another study from Kenya 28.5% of mothers showed infection with *C. trachomatis* and 9.5% infection with *N. gonorrhoeae*. Of neonates with clinical signs of conjunctivitis, 28.7% had chlamydial ON and 20.2% gonococcal ON.[4,5] In the United Arab Emirates 81.5% of children with ON showed bacterial or fungal infection, but only 5% of all cases were caused by *C. trachomatis* or *N. gonorrhoeae*.[14]

14c.5 PREVENTION OF OPHTHALMIA NEONATORUM

As in all cases of STD, preventive methods involve behavioural change and the use of barrier contraceptives for primary prevention of ON. Different types of prevention strategies for ON may be suitable, and the choice will depend on the prevalence of the causative STD agents in that population and on financial, laboratory and diagnostic resources.

In most parts of the world, the gold standard to prevent ON is still cleansing of the eyelids immediately after birth followed by instillation of 1% silver nitrate. However, its use in ocular prophylaxis was criticized because it may itself cause chemical conjunctivitis.[3,4,5,7] In several countries silver nitrate was replaced by prophylaxis with erythromycin 0.5% or tetracycline ointment 1% (e.g. in the USA). Antibiotic treatment was also presumed to be effective in preventing chlamydial ophthalmia.[4,5,10]

A different strategy is to abandon a general prophylaxis for ON. Countries like Denmark, Sweden and the UK argued that no substance is 100% effective in preventing ON, and silver nitrate can itself cause a chemical conjunctivitis. Also in these countries the risk of a sight-threatening infection with *N. gonorrhoeae* is extremely low.[10] Interestingly, in some of these countries an increase has been noticed in the incidence of gonococcal ON.[10]

Another strategy is to prevent disease in the mother by treating infection in pregnant women.[4] However, screening for chlamydial infection in pregnant women is not easily implemented, although it is more accessible than it used to be. The timing has to be correct, otherwise re-infection may occur before birth. In developing countries a general screening programme would also be too costly.

Recently, povidone–iodine has been shown to be effective in preventing ON.[3,5] Prophylaxis has to be applied once shortly after birth. For gonococcal ON, prophylaxis with tetracycline or erythromycin ointment, silver nitrate and povidone–iodine eye drops are equally effective. However, strains of *N. gonorrhoeae* with primary resistance against tetracycline have been reported. Silver nitrate is not effective against chlamydial ON. Furthermore, silver nitrate may cause chemical conjunctivitis. Tetracycline or erythromycin ointment and povidone–iodine eye drops are able to prevent chlamydial ON. An ophthalmic solution of 2.5% povidone–iodine provides effective antibacterial prevention in both chlamydial and gonococcal ON, and is a relatively non-toxic agent when placed on the conjunctiva of a newborn.[3] Other advantages are lack of development or any resistance, and the fact that povidone–iodine is also effective against human immunodeficiency virus and *Herpes simplex* virus.

A recent study found also povidone–iodine 2.5 % to be cheaper than topical azithromycin for ophthalmia neonatorum prophylaxis. In Kenya the cost of a 5 ml container is: povidone–iodine $0.10; tetracycline ointment $0.31; erythromycin ointment $0.74; and one dose of silver nitrate $7.30.[10,15] These data suggest povidone–iodine 2.5% to be the ideal antiseptic substance for broad, cheap and safe use to prevent ON in developing countries.

14c.6 TREATMENT OF ESTABLISHED OPHTHALMIA NEONATORUM

Treatment of gonococcal or chlamydial ON requires systemic therapy to ensure that extraocular sites of infection are also treated. In the past, gonococcal ON was treated with crystalline benzyl penicillin G 50,000 units (for full-term normal weight babies) or 20,000 units (for premature or low weight babies) IM twice daily for three days (if susceptible to penicillin). Since so many gonococci are now penicillinase producing, recommended treatment includes a single intramuscular dose of cefotaxime (25–50 mg/kg to a maximum of 125 mg), or similar β-lactamase-stable cephalosporin. Chlamydial ON requires oral erythromycin (50 mg/kg over 24 hours divided into four doses for two to three weeks). Topical therapy is of uncertain outcome, and is not required.[10]

14c.7 COMMUNITY HEALTHCARE MANAGEMENT

Primary prophylaxis against contracting ON would entail the use of barrier contraceptives or having a sole sexual partner. In this context antenatal care must also be improved. The efficacy of cleaning the eyes of the newborn baby at birth and the one-time application of an antiseptic or antibiotic substance has been proven as an effective protection from ON. The early start of treatment for acute conjunctivitis of a newborn following the guidelines from WHO will cure the infection before sight-threatening corneal complications can develop. Therefore, community efforts to prevent corneal blindness from ON should include:[12]

➢ Training of all health workers, including traditional birth attendants, concerning the importance and practice of cleaning the eyes at birth and applying tetracycline/erythromycin eye ointment (or one drop of 1% silver nitrate drops or povidone–iodine 2.5% eye drops).

➢ The provision of 1% tetracycline/erythromycin 0.5% eye ointment or 1% silver nitrate drops, povidone–iodine 2.5% eye drops to health workers and their inclusion in national essential drug lists.

➢ Education of all health workers in the diagnosis of acute conjunctivitis in the newborn and immediate referral of infants with suspected ON to centres able to adequately manage the condition.

14c.8 EPIDEMIOLOGICAL RESEARCH PRIORITIES

Blindness resulting from ophthalmia neonatorum is preventable with proper management. Therefore, primary and secondary prophylaxis should be made available globally to stop this potentially blinding condition. This requires the correct prophylactic regimen based on the prevalence and geographical distribution of ON over time and knowledge of its causative agents. Therefore, prevalence and geographical distribution of ON should be evaluated on a regular basis.

REFERENCES

1. Schaller U, Miño de Kaspar H, Schriever S, *et al.* Ophthalmia neonatorum from Chlamydia trachomatis: quick diagnosis and treatment [Article in German]. *Ophthalmologe* 1997; 94:317–320.

2. World Health Organization. *Conjunctivitis of the newborn.* Geneva: WHO; 1986. pp. 1–7.

3. Isenberg SJ, Apt L, Yoshimori R, *et al.* Povidone–iodine for ophthalmia neonatorum prophylaxis. *Am J Ophthalmol* 1994; 118:701–706.

4. Klauss V, Fransen L. Neonatal ophthalmia in tropical countries. In: Bialasiewicz AA, Schaal KP (eds). *Infectious Disease of the Eye*. London: Butterworth–Heinemann; 1994.

5. Kramer A, Behrens-Baumann W. Prophylactic use of topical anti-infectives in ophthalmology. *Ophthalmologica* 1997; 211:68–76.

6. van Bergen JE. Increased incidence of gonorrhea and Chlamydia trachomatis infections in family practice in southeast Amsterdam, 1996–2000. *Ned Tijdschr Geneeskd* 2001; 145:1691–1693.

7. Pilling R, Long V, Hobson R, *et al*. Ophthalmia neonatorum: a vanishing disease or underreported notification? *Eye* 2009; 23:1879–1880.

8. Quirke M, Cullinane A. Recent trends in chlamydial and gonococcal conjunctivitis among neonates and adults in an Irish hospital. *Int J Infect Dis* 2008; 12:371–373.

9. Kakar S, Bhalla P, Maria A, *et al*. Chlamydia trachomatis causing neonatal conjunctivitis in a tertiary care center. *Indian J Med Microbi* 2010; 28:45–47.

10. Schaller UC, Klauss V. Is Credé's prophylaxis for ophthalmia neonatorum still valid? *Bull WHO* 2001; 79:262–266.

11. Ying C, Wang B, Zheng D. The effect of Chlamydia trachomatis infection in pregnant women on pregnant outcome and neonates. *Zhonghua Fu Chan Ke Za Zhi* 1999; 34:348–450.

12. Foster A, Gilbert C. Community efforts in the reduction of corneal blindness in developing countries. *J Refract Corneal Surg* 1991; 7: 445–448.

13. Rahi JS, Sripathi S, Gilbert CE, *et al*. Childhood blindness in India: Causes in 1318 blind school students in nine states. *Eye* 1995; 9:545–550.

14. Nsanze H, Dawodu A, Usmani A, *et al*. Ophthalmia neonatorum in the United Arab Emirates. *Ann Trop Paediatr* 1996; 16:27–32.

15. Keenan JD, Eckert S, Rutar T. Cost analysis of povidone–iodine for Ophthalmia neonatorum prophylaxis. *Arch Ophthalmol* 2010; 128: 136–137.

14d

Corneal disease in children

CLARE GILBERT

14d.1   Overview   323
14d.2   Congenital abnormalities and   323
        corneal dystrophies
14d.3   Measles infection   325
14d.4   Harmful traditional eye medicines   327

14d.5   Management of corneal ulcers   328
        and scarring in children
14d.6   Implications for future research   329
        needs
        References   329

14d.1   OVERVIEW

Corneal conditions of childhood form a heterogeneous group of conditions. Some are present from birth, due to genetic or chromosomal abnormalities or secondary to intra-uterine conditions, while others are due to acquired conditions in childhood. This section focuses on corneal conditions of childhood which are not covered in other sections (i.e. vitamin A deficiency disorders, Section 14b; ophthalmia neonatorum, Section 14c; congenitally acquired rubella, Section 14e; congenital glaucoma, Section 14f; vernal keratoconjunctivitis, Section 16e). The following conditions will be described: corneal dystrophies; congenital abnormalities, whether due to known or unknown factors operating during pregnancy; and corneal ulceration and scarring following measles infection or the use of harmful traditional eye remedies.

14d.2   CONGENITAL ABNORMALITIES AND CORNEAL DYSTROPHIES

Corneal opacity from birth, from any causes, is rare, affecting approximately 3/100,000 births in Europe.[1]

14d.2.1   Congenital abnormalities

In addition to congenital glaucoma, other corneal conditions present from birth include Peters anomaly and sclerocornea, both of which can be bilateral or unilateral. Both are thought to be due to defects in genes important in eye development such as PAX6, PITX2 and PITX3[2] although many more genes remain to be elucidated.

Conditions secondary to intrauterine events are usually bilateral, and include keratitis secondary to congenital syphilis, congenital rubella syndrome (see Section 14e) and corneal opacities as part of the **foetal alcohol syndrome/disorder (FAS/D)**. Although corneal opacity is not a major feature of FAS/D,[3] the prevalence is far higher in many populations than previously thought. Estimates range from 2–7 per 1,000 children in socio-economically mixed populations in the USA and 2–5% in some other Western countries.[4] Studies of primary school children undertaken in South Africa revealed that almost one in ten children in Northern Cape Province had features of FAS/D.[5] Rates are influenced not only by patterns of alcohol consumption among women of child-bearing age, but also by the presence of genes that might confer susceptibility to the toxic effects of alcohol during development. Indeed the HOX 1.5 gene has been linked to the craniofacial manifestations of FAS.[6] Investigating rates of FAS/D, as with other congenital anomalies, is challenging not only because they are rare but also because rates obtained from anomaly registers are likely to be spuriously low as the milder signs and features of FAS/D (e.g. developmental delay and learning difficulties) will not be picked up through routine surveillance or be detected at a young enough age to be reported to congenital anomaly registers. Registers will, therefore, only reflect the more severe end of the spectrum in terms of phenotype as well as birth prevalence. It is notable that studies reporting higher rates of FAS/D were community-based studies of school children even though the more severely affected children may not have been ascertained as they would not be at school.

14d.2.2   Corneal dystrophies

The term 'corneal dystrophy' embraces a heterogenous group of bilateral, genetically determined, non-inflammatory corneal diseases, many of which only become manifest later in life. Up until very recently corneal dystrophies were classified according to the part of the cornea primarily affected, e.g. the endothelium (e.g. congenital hereditary endothelial dystrophy) or the stroma (e.g. lattice and granular dystrophy). A new classification has recently been developed that better describes the genotype/phenotype correlations.[7] It is based on the layer of the cornea primarily affected (epithelial and subepithelial layers; Bowman's layer; stroma; and those affecting Descemets membrane and the endothelium.[7] Within each anatomical site four categories are described:

Category 1: A well-defined corneal dystrophy in which the gene has been mapped and identified and specific mutations are known.
Category 2: A well-defined corneal dystrophy that has been mapped to one or more specific chromosomal loci, but the gene(s) remains to be identified.
Category 3: A well-defined corneal dystrophy in which the disorder has not yet been mapped to a chromosomal locus.

Category 4: This category is reserved for a suspected new, or previously documented, corneal dystrophy, for which the evidence is not yet convincing.

This classification will not only aid the understanding of the pathogenesis of these conditions but will also assist in both descriptive epidemiological and intervention studies. It might not be fanciful to suggest that a similar classification system could also be applied to congenital anomalies of the whole eye (i.e. anophthalmos, microphthalmos and coloboma), which are important causes of visual impairment and blindness in children, but which are poorly defined and classified.[8]

Keratoconus is the most common corneal dystrophy that occurs in all ethnic groups, and that affects males and females equally.[9] The onset is usually in puberty, and in some the condition progresses to profound visual loss as a result of corneal thinning, protrusion and distortion. Keratoconus used to be defined according to purely clinical criteria, but advances in technology and imaging techniques mean that early stages can now be identified and quantified, and progression closely monitored.[10] The lack of a clear definition probably explains the wide variation in prevalence estimates, which range from 4–600/100,000 population, with most estimates falling in the range of 50 to 230 per 100,000 population.[9] Keratoconus is nearly always isolated but is known to complicate Down's syndrome and connective tissue disorders. There is often a positive family history, and there is emerging evidence that keratoconus has a genetic basis[11] and that genetic factors increase susceptibility in individuals who are atopic. Although pronounced visual loss is unusual during childhood, the results of penetrating keratoplasty are better than for many of the other causes of corneal opacity in children.[12]

Congenital abnormalities of the cornea, corneal dystrophies and FAS/D appear to affect children all over the world. Apart from FAS/D, there are few population-based data for these rare conditions, and it is not known whether they are more frequent in some populations than in others. Variation in prevalence might be expected, particularly for autosomal recessive conditions, as consanguinity is known to increase the risk of recessively inherited disorders[13] and higher rates of visual impairment have been reported among ethnic minorities in the UK.[14]

The following causes of corneal ulceration and scarring occur almost exclusively in developing countries, particularly in Sub-Saharan Africa.

14d.3   MEASLES INFECTION

Measles is one of the most infectious of all diseases, having a basic reproductive number of 15 (i.e. the average number of people infected by one person, if everyone is susceptible). The infection is rare in infants under the age of four months because of the protective effect of maternal antibodies, but has been a leading cause of child mortality in developing countries. Measles-related mortality has a J-shaped distribution, being higher in infants and in older children and adolescents. Over the last decades the number of deaths has fallen dramatically from several million per year to 733,000 in 2000, and to an estimated 164,000 in 2008[15] (Fig. 14d.1). However, some have questioned

these estimates, as they are based on assumptions that the **case fatality ratios (CFRs)**, i.e. the proportion of children with measles who die, have remained relatively stable; but it is known that there are considerable geographical variations, temporal trends and age-specific variation in CFRs.[16] The decline in the number of measles-related deaths is almost certainly due to a combination of better and safer vaccines, improved case management, which includes vitamin A supplementation, as well as improved immunization coverage. After a long period of time without adequate evidence,[17] clinical trials have now shown that prophylactic antibiotics reduce pneumonia and other serious infections.[18]

14d.3.1   Risk factors for severe measles infection and mortality

Measles CFRs are much higher in Sub-Saharan Africa than in industrialized countries. Detailed prospective cohort studies carried out in West Africa, as well as analyses of European data, have suggested that overcrowding (i.e. many people

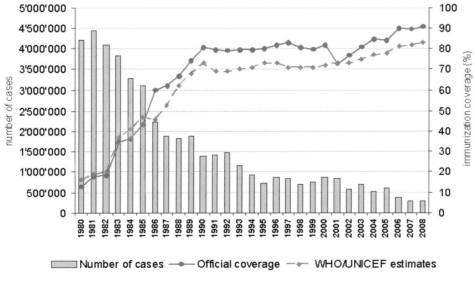

Source: WHO/IVB database, 2009
193 WHO Member States. Data as of September 2009

Date of slide: 21 December 2009   WHO

Figure 14d.1 *Measles: reported cases globally each year and measles immunization coverage (%) between 1980 to 2008*

living together in the same household or institution) is an important risk factor for severe measles infection. This has thrown doubt on the commonly held belief that pre-existing malnutrition was the main risk factor for severe disease and the higher mortality rate in Africa.[19,20] Overcrowding is thought to result in a higher infecting dose of virus in children infected within the household, causing more severe disease and a higher CFR in secondary cases than in index cases (the first case in the household). Overcrowding also causes children to be infected at a younger age, which is also associated with a higher CFR. Measles infection can precipitate a child with borderline liver stores of vitamin A into acute deficiency, leading to keratomalacia and a high risk of mortality.[21] (See Section 14b) Systematic reviews of randomized, placebo-controlled clinical trials of high-dose vitamin A supplementation have shown that two doses significantly reduces measles related mortality.[22] Lack of affordable healthcare facilities in many developing countries also means that the complications (e.g. dehydration and pneumonia) are rarely adequately treated.

14d.3.2   Causes of corneal ulceration following measles infection

Hospital-based studies in Africa have shown that corneal ulceration follows measles infection in 0.75–3.3% of cases. Blind school studies have indicated that up to 81% of cases of corneal scarring followed measles infection, while hospital-based studies of children with corneal ulceration have shown that measles infection preceded the ulcer in 36% of cases. The pathogenesis of corneal scarring following measles infection is complex and multifactorial. The following mechanisms have been implicated: acute vitamin A deficiency disorder leading to corneal ulceration and **keratomalacia**; secondary **Herpes simplex** virus keratitis; secondary bacterial infection; exposure keratitis; measles keratitis; and the use of traditional eye medicines (Plates 14d.1–6). In a hospital-based study of 48 Tanzanian children with corneal ulceration following measles infection, 24 had keratomalacia, ten

had **Herpes simplex** virus keratitis and six measles keratitis, while in eight children the ulceration was attributed to the use of **harmful traditional eye medicines** (HTEM).[23] Case-control studies show that children with measles infection have lower serum vitamin A levels than age- and sex-matched controls. Measles infection depresses cell-mediated and humoral immunity, which may explain the secondary herpetic infection. Traditional eye medicines can cause corneal ulceration from thermal and chemical burns, physical trauma, and by introducing secondary bacterial or fungal infection.

14d.3.3   Measles immunization

The current vaccine uses live attenuated viruses, which requires a cold chain (i.e. storage at +/− 4°C), as the vaccine is sensitive to heat and light. The vaccine has to be injected rather than given orally, which also adds to the cost, complexity, safety and acceptability of programmes. In developing countries the recommended age for immunization has been nine months and not younger because of the neutralizing effect of maternal antibodies. This leaves a window of high risk for infants aged between four and nine months where CFRs are high. Recent trials have shown that an early two-dose regime (at six and again at eight months) increases coverage and provides better protection to infants.[24] An important factor to bear in mind when considering immunization is that not all those infants immunized will develop protective antibodies for a variety of reasons, one of which being that seroconversion rates are estimated to be approximately 85% following a single dose at nine months of age.

Measles is highly contagious, and transmission is influenced by factors such as household size and overcrowding, as well as population density, and hence immunization coverage needs to be high to control the spread of the disease (at least 90% to prevent epidemics). Measles immunization programmes have been introduced as part of the WHO **Expanded Programme of Immunization (EPI)**, which was initiated by the World Health Assembly in 1974. By 1992 available data suggested that measles immunization coverage was 80%, but even at this level it was estimated that in 1991 there were 41 million cases of measles and one million measles-associated deaths. By 2008 all regions except South East Asia had achieved 90% reduction in measles deaths, two years ahead of target (Plate 14d.7). Although the incidence of measles is lower in South East Asia than in Sub-Saharan Africa (Plate 14d.8), and Africa is the continent with the largest number of countries where immunization is below target coverage, the very large populations in South East Asia mean that there were more cases and deaths in this region than in other regions.[25] Despite the excellent progress that has been made there are currently concerns that high coverage may not be maintained on account of inadequate political and financial commitment. Indeed, in the 1990s there was an epidemic of measles in the USA which affected 55,000 people, and there were more than 130 deaths. In 2008 more cases were recorded in Europe and the UK than for decades, partly on account of ill-founded fears about the risk of autism with the use of 'triple vaccine' **MMR** in some parts of the world.[26-27] This has contributed to fears of a resurgence of cases if coverage should fall.[28] While some countries, like India, plan to scale up coverage, other regions are close to eradicating the disease.[29]

The Measles Initiative, which was launched in 2001, is committed to reducing measles deaths globally. The lead organizations, which include the American Red Cross, UNICEF and the United Nations Foundation, work with partners such as the Bill and Melinda Gates Foundation, the Global Alliance for Vaccines and Immunization (GAVII), and the Canadian International Development Organization to provide technical and financial assistance to governments and communities in support of their vaccination campaigns and disease surveillance.[30]

14d.3.4 Impact of measles immunization on corneal ulceration and scarring in children

There is extensive anecdotal evidence that improved measles immunization coverage reduces the number of children presenting to facilities with corneal ulceration, but very little published evidence.[23] A long-term study of children, recruited from community outreach and static facilities in Uganda, showed a decline in the number of corneal cases over time, but not cataract cases.[31] It seems likely that much of this reduction is also due to vitamin A supplementation.

14d.4 HARMFUL TRADITIONAL EYE MEDICINES

Animism, which is still practised in much of Sub-Saharan Africa, is the ancient belief system that natural objects, natural phenomena and the universe itself possess souls; that natural objects have souls that may exist apart from their material bodies; that the soul is the principle of life and health; and that spiritual beings or agencies exist. In animist societies diseases are believed to have very different origins from the understanding by non-animistic communities. For example, underlying causes of ill health may be supernatural (caused by spirits or angered ancestors, or due to breaking of taboos or customs); they may arise as a result of immoral behaviour, conflict or jealousy; or they may be the result of the 'evil eye' or witchcraft. Some conditions are thought to be passed down within the family, and the problem is usually attributed to the female line. Other conditions are attributed to weakness or eating unclean food or to lack of respect towards parents or elders. Given the different ideas surrounding causation it is not surprising that behaviours and remedies, which are based on these concepts, may seem inexplicable to the outsider even though they have an internal cultural logic.

In the absence of allopathic medicine, traditional societies have developed their own systems, many of which are extremely longstanding, to prevent and treat illnesses; e.g. Ayurvedic medicine, which originated in India thousands of years ago. The World Health Organization has defined traditional healing as 'the sum total of all the knowledge and practices, used in diagnosis, prevention and elimination of physical, mental or social imbalance and relying exclusively on practical experience and observation handed down from generation to generation, whether verbally or in writing'.[32] Putting it in an African context: 'Traditional medicine might be considered as solid amalgamation of dynamic medicine know-how and ancestral experience. Traditional African medicine might also be considered to be the sum total of practices, measures, ingredients and procedures of all kinds, whether material or not, which from time immemorial has enabled the African to guard against disease, to alleviate his suffering and to cure himself.'[32]

Traditional remedies can be harmless or harmful. While some are administered on the advice of traditional healers, many are handed down within the family. Benign practices include ritual bathing and dances, and some may actually be beneficial, e.g. direct application of breast milk into the eye, steam baths and inhalations. There is even some evidence that plant extracts added to foods by the Maasai in East Africa may have anti-measles virus activity.[33] However, the use of harmful traditional practices is an important cause of corneal blindness in children, particularly in Sub-Saharan Africa.[34–36] Traditional remedies are often used for measles[37] as the condition is feared, is known to cause blindness, and measles keratitis can cause pronounced photophobia which exacerbates parents' concerns. Traditional remedies can lead to eye damage and blindness through the following mechanisms:

1. Adnexal injuries (e.g. from thermal, acid or alkaline burns and incisions) can lead to secondary infection and exposure keratitis.
2. Exposure keratitis can occur if parents hold open the eyes of their child, a practice believed to prevent blindness following measles in parts of West Africa.
3. Mechanical damage and burns from objects and material inserted into the eye (e.g. toxic sap from plants; twigs and leaves; ground up cowrie shells, and acidic or alkaline liquids).
4. Fungal infection, particularly if plant material is inserted.
5. Bacterial infection (e.g. instillation of urine from someone infected with gonorrhoea; use of breast milk expressed into a contaminated container).

6. Harmless traditional remedies commonly lead to blindness indirectly, as a consequence of delay in seeking more appropriate treatment.

The practice of traditional medicine varies from locality to locality, and the tradition and remedies are often passed down within the family. Some healers develop specific areas of expertise, for example in the area of mental health or herbal remedies. Even in settings where eye care services are available, members of the community will often consult the traditional healer first, or want to discuss decisions having already seen an eye care worker. Traditional healers are respected members of the community who share local beliefs about the causation of disease; they can become important primary eye care workers.[38]

Obtaining reliable population-based data on the importance of harmful traditional eye remedies as a cause of blindness in children is challenging for many reasons but primarily because the signs are diverse and not pathognomonic, and users and communities are often reluctant to acknowledge the use of these remedies.

14d.5 MANAGEMENT OF CORNEAL ULCERS AND SCARRING IN CHILDREN

Correct diagnosis is essential. A history of measles should be sought, and use of traditional medicines enquired after. In countries where vitamin A deficiency is common, all children with corneal ulcers should be treated with high-dose vitamin A (see Section 14b). If there are facilities for laboratory investigation, corneal scrapes should be taken, with gram staining and culture. In many instances treatment will be empirical: a broad-spectrum antibiotic, with an antifungal agent.

14d.5.1 Corneal surgery for corneal opacity in childhood

The only evidence of the benefit of corneal surgery for children with corneal opacities comes from case series, as no clinical trial has been undertaken. The available evidence suggests that **penetrating kerato-plasty (PK)** for children with congenital corneal opacity (e.g. for Peters anomaly) can reduce deprivation amblyopia but the prognosis has to be guarded as there are often additional ocular and/or systemic abnormalities.[39] Outcomes are better for acquired conditions and keratoconus.[12] It needs to be remembered that these case series were all reported from industrialized countries where there are tertiary centres of excellence, high quality corneas for transplantation and where intensive and long-term follow-up is possible. Grafting can preserve the integrity of eyes with acute keratomalacia,[40] but the long-term outcomes of PK for eyes with vascularized corneas is poor. If the corneal periphery is clear, optical iridectomy can restore varying degrees of visual function depending on the extent, timing and duration of the visual deprivation.[41]

14d.6 IMPLICATIONS FOR FUTURE RESEARCH NEEDS

➢ Improved figures are needed for prevalence and incidence of causes of childhood corneal diseases.

➢ Ongoing research is needed into measles virus inhibitors[42] and vaccines that can be given orally and that do not require a cold chain.

➢ More research is needed into the role that traditional healers can play as primary eye care workers, after training.

REFERENCES

1. Bermejo E, Martinez-Frias ML. Congenital eye malformations: clinical-epidemiological analysis of 1,124,654 consecutive births in Spain. *Am J Med Genet* 1998; 75:497–504.

2. Nischal K, Sowden J. Chapter 28. Anterior segment and developmental anomalies. In: Taylor D, Hoyt CS (eds). *Pediatric Ophthalmology and Strabismus*, 3rd Edition. London: Elsevier Saunders; 2005.

3. Stromland K, Pinazo-Duran MD. Ophthalmic involvement in the fetal alcohol syndrome: clinical and animal model studies. *Alcohol Alcoholism* 2002; 37:2–8.

4. May PA, Fiorentino D, Phillip Gossage J, *et al.* Epidemiology of FASD in a province in Italy: Prevalence and characteristics of children in a random sample of schools. *Alcohol Clin Exp Res* 2006; 30:1562–1575.

5. Urban M, Chersich MF, Fourie LA, *et al.* Fetal alcohol syndrome among grade 1 schoolchildren in Northern Cape Province: prevalence and risk factors. *S Afr Med J* 2008; 98:877–882.

6. Johnston MC, Bronsky PT. Animal models for human craniofacial malformations. *J Craniofac Genet Dev Bio* 1991; 11:277–291.

7. Weiss JS, Moller HU, Lisch W, *et al.* The IC3D classification of the corneal dystrophies. *Cornea* 2008; 27:S1–83.

8. Shah SP, Taylor AE, Sowden JC, *et al.* Anophthalmos, microphthalmos and typical coloboma in the UK: a prospective study of incidence and risk. *Invest Ophth Vis Sci*; in press.

9. Krachmer JH, Feder RS, Belin MW. Keratoconus and related noninflammatory corneal thinning disorders. *Surv Ophthalmol* 1984; 28:293–322.

10. Rabinowitz YS. Keratoconus. *Surv Ophthalmol* 1998; 42:297–319.

11. Wang Y, Rabinowitz YS, Rotter JI, *et al.* Genetic epidemiological study of keratoconus: evidence for major gene determination. *Am J Med Genet* 2000; 93:403–409.

12. Patel HY, Ormonde S, Brookes NH, *et al.* The indications and outcome of paediatric corneal transplantation in New Zealand: 1991–2003. *Br J Ophthalmol* 2005; 89:404–408.

13. Woods CG, Cox J, Springell K, *et al.* Quantification of homozygosity in consanguineous individuals with autosomal recessive disease. *Am J Hum Genet* 2006; 78:889–896.

14. Rahi JS, Cable N. Severe visual impairment and blindness in children in the UK. *Lancet* 2003; 362:1359–1365.

15. Global measles mortality, 2000–2008. *Morb Mortal Wkly Rep* 2009; 58:1321–1326.

16. Wolfson LJ, Grais RF, Luquero FJ, *et al.* Estimates of measles case fatality ratios: a comprehensive review of community-based studies. *Int J Epidemiol* 2009; 38:192–205.

17. Chalmers I. Why we need to know whether prophylactic antibiotics can reduce measles-related morbidity. *Pediatrics* 2002; 109:312–315.

18. Kabra SK, Lodha R, Hilton DJ. Antibiotics for preventing complications in children with measles. *Cochrane Db Syst Rev* 2008: CD001477.

19. Aaby P, Bukh J, Lisse IM, *et al.* Severe measles in Sunderland, 1885: a European–African comparison of causes of severe infection. *Int J Epidemiol* 1986; 15:101–107.

20. Aaby P, Coovadia H. Severe measles: a reappraisal of the role of nutrition, overcrowding and virus dose. *Med Hypotheses* 1985; 18:93–112.

21. Sommer A, West K. *Vitamin A Deficiency: Health, Survival and Vision.* Oxford: Oxford University Press; 1996.

22. Huiming Y, Chaomin W, Meng M. Vitamin A for treating measles in children. *Cochrane Db Syst Rev* 2005:CD001479.

23. Foster A, Sommer A. Corneal ulceration, measles, and childhood blindness in Tanzania. *Br J Ophthalmol* 1987; 71:331–343.

24. Garly ML, Martins CL, Bale C, *et al.* Early two-dose measles vaccination schedule in Guinea-Bissau: good protection and coverage in infancy. *Int J Epidemiol* 1999; 28:347–352.

25. Zarocostas J. Measles deaths fell by more than 90% worldwide from 2000 to 2008, except in southern Asia. *Br Med J* 2009; 339:b5362.

26. Eggertson L. Lancet retracts 12-year-old article linking autism to MMR vaccines. *CMAJ* 2010; 182: Epub.2010 Feb 8.

27. Jefferson T, Price D, Demicheli V, *et al.* Unintended events following immunization with MMR: a systematic review. *Vaccine* 2003; 21:3954–3960.

28. Global reductions in measles mortality 2000–2008 and the risk of measles resurgence. *Wkly Epidemiol Rec* 2009; 84:509–516.

29. Moss WJ. Measles control and the prospect of eradication. *Curr Top Microbiol* 2009; 330:173–189.

30. Bradsher CA, Stotts RC, Carter MA, *et al.* The Measles Initiative to control measles in Kenya. *Public Health Nurs* 2007; 24:26–33.

31. Waddell KM. Childhood blindness and low vision in Uganda. *Eye* 1998; 12:184–192.

32. World Health Organization. *The Promotion and Development of Traditional Medicine.* Reports of a WHO meeting. WHO Technical Report Series, no. 662. Geneva; 1978.

33. Parker ME, Chabot S, Ward BJ, *et al.* Traditional dietary additives of the Maasai are antiviral against the measles virus. *J Ethnopharmacol* 2007; 114: 146–152.

34. Courtright P, Lewallen S, Kanjaloti S, *et al.* Traditional eye medicine use among patients with corneal disease in rural Malawi. *Br J Ophthalmol* 1994; 78:810–812.

35. Kello AB, Gilbert C. Causes of severe visual impairment and blindness in children in schools for the blind in Ethiopia. *Br J Ophthalmol* 2003; 87:526–530.

36. Mselle J. Visual impact of using traditional medicine on the injured eye in Africa. *Acta Trop* 1998; 70:185–192.

37. Sonibare MA, Moody JO, Adesanya EO. Use of medicinal plants for the treatment of measles in Nigeria. *J Ethnopharmacol* 2009; 122:268–272.

38. Courtright P. Eye care knowledge and practices among Malawian traditional healers and the development of collaborative blindness prevention programmes. *Soc Sci Med* 1995; 41:1569–1575.

39. Yang LL, Lambert SR, Lynn MJ, *et al.* Surgical management of glaucoma in infants and children with Peters anomaly: long-term structural and functional outcome. *Ophthalmology* 2004; 11:112–117.

40. Vajpayee RB, Vanathi M, Tandon R, *et al.* Keratoplasty for keratomalacia in preschool children. *Br J Ophthalmol* 2003; 87:538–542.

41. Sundaresh K, Jethani J, Vijayalakshmi P. Optical iridectomy in children with corneal opacities. *J AAPOS* 2008; 12:163–165.

42. Plemper RK, Snyder JP. Measles control — can measles virus inhibitors make a difference? *Curr Opin Invest Dr* 2009; 10:811–820.

Cataract in children

EDWARD WILSON AND RUPAL TRIVEDI

14e.1	Introduction	331	14e.6	Surgical management of cataract	336
14e.2	Classification of childhood cataract	331	14e.7	Evidence from clinical trials or other published literature	337
14e.3	Prevalence and incidence	332	14e.8	Suggestions/priorities for future epidemiological research	337
14e.4	Aetiology	333			
14e.5	Preventive and control strategies	335		References	338

14e.1　INTRODUCTION

The term cataract refers to an opacification of the crystalline lens. Cataracts remain one of the most important causes of treatable blindness in children. In 1999 it was estimated that approximately 200,000 children were blind from disorders of the lens, principally unoperated cataract, but also dense **amblyopia** following delayed surgery, complications of surgery or from associated ocular abnormalities.[1] Because of the high prevalence and treatable nature of the condition, it is reasonable to think that an improved approach to the management of childhood cataracts would have a large impact on childhood blindness as a whole.

14e.2　CLASSIFICATION OF CHILDHOOD CATARACT

Childhood cataracts can be classified as congenital, infantile or juvenile, depending on the age of onset. Childhood cataract can also be classified according to aetiology (e.g. traumatic cataract, autosomal dominant cataract etc.) or morphology (lamellar, nuclear, total etc.).[2–4] Non-traumatic total cataracts are not very common in industrialized countries. In a published series of paediatric cataracts from the USA, only four of 199 were classified as total.[3] In the developing countries, total cataracts are seen commonly. In a series from Nepal, most (68.5%, 1804/2633) of the lens opacities were described as total cataract.[5]

Childhood cataracts have different morphological characteristics (Plates 14e.1–3). Anterior polar cataracts are often bilateral, hereditary and visually insignificant. Lamellar cataracts usually develop after birth and involve a layer surrounding the foetal nucleus (Plate 14e.1). They are almost always bilateral. The most common cataract detected in infants is the foetal nuclear cataract (Plate 14e.2). Posterior lentiglobus is mostly unilateral and not associated with microphthalmia (Plate 14e.3). Spontaneous rupture may occur, leading to a total white cortical cataract.[6] An important and varied type of opacity is associated with **persistent foetal vasculature**

(PFV), formally known as PHPV (persistence and hyperplasia of the primary vitreous). With severe PFV, a retrolental membrane is attached to the ciliary processes, pulling them in toward the centre of the pupillary space.

14e.3   PREVALENCE AND INCIDENCE

Several articles have been published that attempt to quantify blindness from childhood cataract. Such studies either describe the frequency of lens opacity irrespective of its impact on vision or report the prevalence of blindness due to lens opacity. Using a standardized classification and coding system, Gilbert and colleagues[7] reported that the lens is responsible for 12% of ocular anatomical abnormalities in children. Cataract-associated vision loss in these children may be caused by a combination of the lens opacity and other associated findings (for example, amblyopia, secondary opacification of the visual axis, residual refractive error).

The prevalence of cataract in childhood has been reported as 0.8 to 13.6/10,000 children (Table 14e.1).[8-19] The Nordic registers of the blind suggest that the prevalence of visual impairment as a result of cataract is 0.6/10,000 children aged 0–17 years.[20] Wirth and co-workers[21] reported an incidence of 2.2 per 10,000. Rahi and colleagues[22] found that the adjusted annual age-specific incidence of new diagnosis of congenital and infantile cataract was highest in the first year of life, being 2.49 per 10,000 children. Adjusted cumulative incidence at five years was 3.18 per 10,000, increasing to 3.46 per 10,000 by 15 years. A Danish study reported overall cumulative risk of childhood cataract as 10.84 per 10,000 children.[23]

Distribution by age and gender

Children with cataract typically present late in developing-world settings.[24,25] Reasons for late presentation include lack of awareness on the part of parents that their child has a treatable condition, and in some countries there is a belief that children who are born blind cannot have their sight restored.[1] There is also a lack of awareness among general physicians, who are often the first point of contact, who tell parents that their child is too young for surgery, or that the cataract needs to mature.

In many developing countries, boys present for cataract surgery much more frequently than girls,[1,5] despite there being no evidence that there are significant gender differences in the incidence.[22,23] Derogative parents in these settings may be more willing to use their scarce resources for healthcare for their sons than for their daughters.[1]

Table 14e.1 *Prevalence of childhood cataract*

Country	Type of study	Number of cataract	Prevalence/10,000	Ref.
USA	National surveillance	214	0.8	James et al.[10]
USA	National surveillance		1.3	Edmonds et al.[11]
USA	Surveillance		2.1	Metropolitan Atlanta Congenital Defects Program[12]
USA	Population-based, comprehensive medical record retrieval	10	3	Holmes et al.[13]
		15 (including possible)	4.5	
USA	National cohort	73	13.6	SanGiovanni et al.[14]
China	Population-based survey	76	3.7	Hu[15]
UK	Cohort	4	3	Stayte[16]
Sweden	Population-based prevalence	2	4	Kohler[17]
Denmark	Population-based prevalence	2	4	Jensen et al.[18]
France	Surveillance	2	2.3	Stoll et al.[19]

Geographical distribution of blindness

The prevalence of blindness from cataracts in children in developing countries is 1–4/10,000, compared with 0.1–0.4/10,000 children in the industrialized world.[8] This is because there is a higher prevalence of cataract itself (may be attributed to **congenital rubella syndrome (CRS)** and consanguinity), clinical services to restore sight or prevent blindness are less well developed in poor countries, and parents may not understand the need for surgery or may not be able to afford the treatment.

Changes in prevalence or distribution with time

The major preventable causes of blindness in children (those causing corneal opacification) are declining in poor countries as a result of large-scale public health interventions and cataract is becoming a relatively more important avoidable cause.[1]

14e.4   AETIOLOGY

The common teaching, now challenged, for many years, has been that roughly one third of childhood cataracts are inherited, one third are associated with other diseases and the remaining third are idiopathic.[3] In a national study that ascertained cases through active surveillance throughout the UK, Rahi et al.[26] reported that no underlying causes or risk factors were identified in 92% of unilateral and 38% of bilateral cases. Over half of bilateral cases were hereditary compared with only 6% of unilateral cases. Prenatal infections and other systemic factors were reported in only 6% of bilateral and 2% of unilateral cases. In a population-based study in Denmark,[27] almost two thirds of the childhood cataracts were of unknown aetiology. A study from India reported that 88.4% of the affected children had non-traumatic cataract and 11.6% had traumatic cataracts. Among non-traumatic cataracts, 7.2% were hereditary, 4.6% were due to congenital rubella syndrome, 15.1% were secondary and 73% were undetermined.[28]

Hereditary cataract and modes of inheritance

Hereditary cataracts are most frequently inherited as **autosomal dominant (AD)** traits, but can also be inherited in an **autosomal recessive (AR)**, or **X-linked** fashion.[29,30] These cataracts are bilateral but may be asymmetric. There can be marked variability between affected family members. There are also a number of rare hereditary syndromes where cataracts are part of a systemic illness. Less commonly, the inheritance may be autosomal recessive. Cataract may be associated with renal and cerebral disease in Lowe oculo-cerebro-renal syndrome, which is X-linked recessive. It is, therefore, important that a paediatrician examine the child to exclude a systemic disorder.

Molecular genetics

In 2008, it was reported that there were 39 genetic loci to which isolated or primary cataracts had been mapped, although the number is constantly increasing.[30] Twenty-six of the 39 mapped loci for isolated congenital or infantile cataracts have been associated with mutations in specific genes. Of the cataract families for whom the mutant gene is known, about half have mutations in crystallins, about a quarter have mutations in gap junction protein connexins, with the remainder divided among the genes for heat shock transcription factor-4, aquaporin-0, and beaded filament structural protein-2. The crystallins are stable water-soluble proteins that are highly expressed in the lens; they make up 90% of the lens proteins and play a key role in maintaining lens transparency. The lens crystallins represent excellent candidate gene targets for inherited cataract. Connexins 46 and 50 are constituents of gap junctions, especially important for nutrition and inter-cellular communication in the avascular lens. Mutations in both connexin 46 and connexin 50 tend to produce phenotypically similar autosomal dominant nuclear and especially zonular pulverulent cataracts.[30] There is often some correlation between the pattern of expression of the mutant protein and the morphology of the resulting cataract. However, as has been mentioned previously, inheritance of the same mutation in different families or even the same mutation within the same family can result in radically different cataract morphologies and severities. This suggests that additional genes or environmental factors often modify the expression of the primary mutation associated with the cataracts. Conversely, cataracts with similar or identical clinical presentations can result from mutations in completely different genes.

Metabolic causes of cataract in children

Childhood lens opacities may have an underlying metabolic cause. Galactosaemia, for example, is a metabolic disorder where galactose, a major component of milk and milk products, cannot be metabolized, giving rise to vomiting and diarrhoea and oil droplet cataracts. Up to 30% of newborn infants with classic galactosaemia develop cataracts in the first few weeks of life, which usually reverse on a galactose-restricted diet. Regular eye examinations are essential as cataract surgery is sometimes necessary when dietary treatment is delayed. Another metabolic disorder is glucose 6-phosphatase dehydrogenase deficiency, which is an X-linked disorder affecting mainly males. Hypoglycaemia from any cause may give rise to lens opacities in a child. Hypocalcaemia may result in cataracts, though these are usually functionally less significant than those secondary to hypoglycaemia.

Cataract associated with other syndromes

There are a large number of chromosomal and dysmorphic syndromes that can be associated with congenital cataracts (e.g. Down's syndrome), and systemic examination is advisable. It is essential that the correct diagnosis is made so that the child is appropriately treated and that parents can receive genetic risk counselling.

Congenital rubella syndrome (CRS)

Congenital rubella syndrome is an important, potentially preventable, cause of congenital cataract in children. The cataracts are usually bilateral, and the children often also have hearing impairment. Rubella infection (German measles) is characterized by rash, fever and lymphadenopathy. It is usually a mild illness that primarily affects young children. The **immunoglobulin G (IgG)** antibody response confers protection against subsequent infection in the majority of instances. The diagnosis of acquired infection is determined by the appearance of rubella-specific **immunoglobulin M (IgM)** antibodies, or a four-fold increase in rubella-specific IgG antibodies in paired sera one–two weeks apart or by detection of rubella RNA directly in clinical specimens.[31] Antibodies can be detected in serum by **enzyme-linked immunosorbent assay (ELISA)**, or in saliva using antibody-capture radioimmunoassay. Rubella infection occurs in epidemics of roughly four-year cycles, depending on the number of susceptible individuals in the population (i.e. the proportion without protective IgG antibodies). Rates of rubella-specific seronegativity (which determines susceptibility) decrease with age. Factors that affect sero-prevalence include population density, geographical location, sex and social class.

Although the acquired disease is mild (and may even be subclinical), if a woman becomes infected during the first trimester of pregnancy the developing foetus can be infected, giving rise to intrauterine death, premature birth, perinatal death and a range of congenital and developmental abnormalities. These include congenital eye disease, deafness, cardiovascular disease, microcephaly and developmental delay (congenital rubella syndrome). When maternal infection occurs during the first ten weeks of gestation 90% of foetuses are affected, which reduces to 3% after 17 weeks of gestation. The presence of CRS can be confirmed by isolation of the virus, by polymerase chain reaction detection of viral RNA,[31] or by detection of rubella-specific IgM in serum or saliva. As maternal rubella-specific IgG crosses the placenta, IgG cannot be used to confirm the diagnosis of CRS as it cannot distinguish previous maternal infection from CRS. Rubella-specific IgM antibodies produced following congenital infection persist for three months after birth in 100% of infants, and for 6–12 months in 62%; detection of congenital infection must therefore be made before one year of age and, ideally, an IgM antibody testing should be performed within the first six months of life.

In an article published in 2003, it was suggested that at least 100,000 infants are born each year with CRS, and this is likely to be a marked underestimate.[32] Despite these large numbers, data are limited on the importance of CRS as a potentially preventable cause of ocular abnormality and blindness in developing countries. A blind-school study in Jamaica in 1988 showed that 39% of children were blind from cataract, and CRS was implicated in almost half of these cases, suggesting that there must have been a recent epidemic of rubella.[33] A prospective hospital-based study of infants presenting to a large eye hospital in southern India used saliva antibody-capture to detect rubella-specific IgM antibodies. In 25/95 (26%) consecutive cases of infants with congenital cataract, CRS was diagnosed.[34] A large blind-school study in India demonstrated that 19.3% of blindness in children aged 4–15 years was the result of cataract and 20.7% was caused by microphthalmos.[35] If a quarter of the cataract blindness was a result of CRS this would mean that approximately 10,000 of the estimated 218,000 blind children in India are blind as a result of CRS.[35]

Iatrogenic cataracts

Iatrogenic cataract is most commonly seen in children who have had total body irradiation for leukaemia, and in children who have had organ transplants and are on long-term systemic steroid therapy. These children are usually older and do well after cataract surgery. Cataracts have been reported after laser treatment for threshold retinopathy of prematurity. Also, cataract may develop after vitrectomy to remove vitreous haemorrhage from birth trauma or to treat retinal detachment.

Secondary cataract

The most common type of secondary cataract is a cataract associated with uveitis seen in conjunction with arthritis (juvenile idiopathic arthritis (JIA)) or as a result of intermediate or posterior uveitis of any cause. The cataract may be as a direct result of intraocular inflammation, or from the use of topical or systemic steroids, which typically cause posterior subcapsular lens opacities. Less frequently, cataract may be seen secondary to an intraocular tumour, foreign body, or chronic retinal detachment.

Traumatic cataract

Cataracts following penetrating or blunt trauma are a common cause of unilateral visual loss in children. Most injuries occur during play or while involved in sports. Reported causes include thorns, firecrackers, sticks, arrows, darts, BB-gun pellets and car airbags. Cataracts caused by blunt trauma classically form stellate- or rosette-shaped posterior axial opacities that may be stable or progressive, whereas penetrating trauma with disruption of lens capsule forms cortical changes that may remain focal if small or may progress rapidly to total cortical opacification.

Idiopathic cataract

The vast majority of non-traumatic unilateral cataracts are 'idiopathic' and bilateral cataracts may also be of unknown aetiology. However, the heredity of some cataracts will not be evident from the history alone and careful examination of the parents and siblings may reveal visually insignificant cataract. Within the context of the overall medical and developmental history and the age of onset of the cataract, a metabolic and genetic work-up may be indicated before an idiopathic aetiology can be declared. Investigations should ideally be undertaken with the input of a developmental paediatrician or clinical geneticist so that a targeted work-up can be done that is customized to the child's history and physical signs.

14e.5 PREVENTIVE AND CONTROL STRATEGIES

Johar and colleagues[28] report that nearly 12% of non-traumatic cataracts are due to potentially preventable causes such as CRS.

Rubella immunization

Strategies of immunization include selective targeting of girls and women of child-bearing age in order to protect this particular population at risk. This strategy does not provide herd immunity, and does not reduce the overall incidence of acquired rubella among children. Another strategy is to immunize male and female infants, to confer herd immunity, and also women of child-bearing age who are seronegative, particularly health workers who come into contact with infants and children with CRS.[36] In the UK, immunization of girls aged 12–13 years was the policy between 1970 and 1988. In 1988 the policy was changed to adopt the **MMR** (mumps, measles, rubella) immunization of all infants, together with selective immunization of seronegative women of child-bearing age identified through antenatal screening.

The question of which immunization strategy to adopt in developing countries needs careful consideration. If immunization coverage rates in infants are high enough to prevent epidemics, but lower than seropositive rates as a result of rubella infection in childhood (i.e. naturally acquired immunity), the proportion of women of child-bearing age who are susceptible can actually increase.[37] In this situation more pregnant females are at risk of acquiring the infection and there is a real danger of an increased incidence of CRS. This has occurred in Panama, and more recently in Greece. Several hospital-based serological studies of women of child-bearing age have been undertaken, showing a range of susceptibilities, but fewer population-based studies have been undertaken. Before planning which immunization strategy to adopt, if any, population-based data on the epidemiology of rubella are required, together with immunization coverage rates among infants.[38]

Other strategies

In children, early detection of cataract is important to avoid lifelong visual impairment. Paediatricians play a key role in early detection of infantile cataract. Red reflex testing is generally used for early detection of cataract. The American Academy of Pediatrics recommends red reflex assessment as a component of the eye evaluation in

the neonatal period and during all subsequent routine health supervision visits.[39] Eyes with a diminished red reflex should be referred to an ophthalmologist. In the case of infants, the referral should be arranged within a reasonably short time. Direct communication with the ophthalmologist or confirmation of an appointment is optimal since families may not understand the importance of timely interventions or be able to navigate the appointment systems. Infants or children in high-risk categories, including relatives of patients with childhood-onset cataract, should not only have red reflex testing performed in the nursery but also be referred to an ophthalmologist who is experienced in carrying out a complete eye examination regardless of the findings of the red reflex testing by the paediatrician.

14e.6   SURGICAL MANAGEMENT OF CATARACT

The aim of paediatric cataract surgery is to provide and maintain a clear visual axis and a focused retinal image. Achieving better visual outcome requires a team approach (involving the patient, the ophthalmologist, parents and other caregivers), and needs to consider visual, economic, psychological, and social issues. We reported that better postoperative visual acuity was associated with bilateral cataract, older age at surgery, and normal interocular axial length difference.[40,41] Amblyopia was the major cause of residual visual deficit. Congdon and colleagues[42] reported that factors predictive of better acuity included receiving an **intraocular lens (IOL)** during surgery and provision of postoperative spectacles. Predictive of worse acuity were amblyopia, postoperative complications, unilateral surgery and being female. The results underscore the importance of surgical training in reducing complications, early intervention before amblyopia can develop, and vigorous treatment if amblyopia is present. Chak and colleagues[43] reported that poor compliance with occlusion was the factor most strongly associated with poorer acuity.

14e.7 EVIDENCE FROM CLINICAL TRIALS OR OTHER PUBLISHED LITERATURE

Only a very few randomized clinical trials have been undertaken for childhood cataract.[44] There are several reasons for this. First, most paediatric ophthalmologists do not see enough cases to give an adequate sample size and so multicentre studies are required. Second, there are ethical issues that apply to studies involving children which do not apply to trials of adults who can give their own consent to be involved. Third, visual and person-related outcome measures are ideally required, which adds complexity and the need for long-term follow-up; and lastly, to design a trial the investigators must have equipoise, i.e. the investigators must believe that there is inadequate evidence demonstrating the superiority of one intervention over another. To date many of the factors that have driven change in technique have come from adult cataract surgery, or new techniques have been introduced to overcome complications (e.g. lensectomy was used extensively to avoid the almost inevitable **posterior capsule opacification (PCO)** associated with very early surgery). Most of the data on the outcomes of surgery for paediatric cataract come from case series which vary in size, and which often do not report unilateral and bilateral cases separately. As with all case series, the findings are subject to a range of different biases.

14e.7.1 Optimum age for surgery for congenital cataract

In the case of a unilateral dense cataract diagnosed at birth, the surgeon can wait until four to six weeks of age.[45] Waiting until this age decreases anaesthesia-related complications and facilitates the surgical procedure. Waiting beyond this time, however, adversely affects visual outcome. In the case of a dense bilateral cataract diagnosed at birth, a good visual outcome can be achieved if the child is operated before the onset of sensory nystagmus. Lambert and co-workers[46] found no loss of prognosis in bilateral cataracts through ten weeks of

age. In these cases, a reasonable option is to perform surgery on the first eye at four to six weeks of age, followed by surgery on the second eye one to two weeks later. For an infant it is important to keep the time interval between the surgeries on each eye to a minimum. When older children develop cataracts after having had normal visual development in infancy, surgical timing is related to the degree of visual deficit caused by the cataract. Since cataract surgery in childhood eliminates the eye's ability to accommodate, surgery for partial or mild to moderately dense cataracts in older children is not done until the loss of accommodation that will result from the surgery can be justified by the degree of improvement in the image quality after surgery.

14e.7.2 Youngest age at which it is safe to insert an IOL

Intraocular lens implantation has become the standard of care for the optical rehabilitation of children with cataract from the toddler age group and up. The use of IOLs in infants, however, remains controversial. The **Infant Aphakic Treatment Study (IATS)** is a multicentre (12 sites), randomized, controlled clinical trial comparing IOL and contact lens treatments after cataract surgery performed in 114 children with unilateral congenital cataract at one to six months of age.[47-48] One-year postoperative results of infants enrolled in IATS suggest that visual outcome was not different between two groups: aphakia treated with contact lens versus primary IOL implantation.[48] Longer-term results are needed and will be provided when the IATS cohort reaches age five years.

14e.8 SUGGESTIONS/PRIORITIES FOR FUTURE EPIDEMIOLOGICAL RESEARCH

➢ Further epidemiological studies are required to describe the incidence, prevalence and causes of childhood cataract in different populations.

➤ Surveillance for congenital rubella syndrome, using cataract as a marker, is also needed in countries that do not have a national policy of rubella immunization but where a relatively high proportion of infants are being immunized.

➤ Further trials are required to assess different elements of the surgical procedure, such as the optimum power IOL for insertion during infancy while the eyes are still rapidly growing, and to assess the role of heparin in preventing posterior capsule opacification.

REFERENCES

1. Gilbert C. Chapter 5. Worldwide causes of blindness in children. In: Wilson ME, Saunders RA, Trivedi RH (eds). *Pediatric Ophthalmology: Current Thought and a Practical Guide*. Heidelberg, Germany: Springer; 2009. pp. 47–60.

2. Amaya L, Taylor D, Russell-Eggitt I, *et al*. The morphology and natural history of child-hood cataracts. *Surv Ophthalmol* 2003; 48:125–144.

3. Pandey SK, Wilson ME. Chapter 2. Etiology and morphology of pediatric cataracts. In: Wilson ME, Trivedi RH, Pandey SK (eds). *Pediatric Cataract Surgery: Techniques, Complications, and Management*. Philadelphia: Lippincott, Williams & Wilkins; 2005. pp. 6–13.

4. Eckstein M, Vijayalakshmi P, Killedar M, *et al*. Aetiology of childhood cataract in south India. *Br J Ophthalmol* 1996; 80:628–632.

5. Wilson ME, Hennig A, Trivedi RH, *et al*. Clinical characteristics and early post-operative outcomes of pediatric cataract surgery with IOL implantation from Lahan, Nepal. *J Ped Ophth Strab* (submitted).

6. Wilson ME, Trivedi RH. Intraocular Lens Implantation in Pediatric Eyes with Posterior Lentiglobus. *T Am Ophthal Soc* 2006; 104:176–181.

7. Gilbert C, Foster A, Negrel AD, *et al*. Childhood blindness: a new form for recording causes of visual loss in children. *Bull World Health Organ* 1993; 71:485–489.

8. Foster A, Gilbert C, Rahi J. Epidemiology of cataract in childhood: a global perspective. *J Cataract Refr Surg* 1997; 23:601–604.

9. Kocur I, Resnikoff S. Visual impairment and blindness in Europe and their prevention. *Br J Ophthalmol* 2002; 86:716–722.

10. James LM. Maps of birth defects occurrence in the U.S., Birth Defects Monitoring Program (BDMP)/CPHA, 1970–1987. *Teratology* 1993; 48:551–646.

11. Edmonds LD, James LM. Temporal trends in the prevalence of congenital malformations at birth based on the birth defects monitoring program, United States, 1979–1987. *MMWR CDC Surveillance Summaries* 1990; 39:19–23.

12. Metropolitan Atlanta congenital defects program (MACDP) surveillance data, 1988–1991. *Teratology* 1993; 48:695–709.

13. Holmes JM, Leske DA, Burke JP, *et al*. Birth prevalence of visually significant infantile cataract in a defined U.S. population. *Ophthalmic Epidemiol* 2003; 10:67–74.

14. SanGiovanni JP, Chew EY, Reed GF, *et al*. Infantile cataract in the collaborative perinatal project: prevalence and risk factors. *Arch Ophthalmol* 2002; 120:1559–1565.

15. Hu DN. Prevalence and mode of inheritance of major genetic eye diseases in China. *J Med Genet* 1987; 24:584–588.

16. Stayte M, Reeves B, Wortham C. Ocular and vision defects in preschool children. *Br J Ophthalmol* 1993; 77:228–232.

17. Kohler L, Stigmar G. Vision screening of four-year-old children. *Acta Physiol Scand* 1973; 62:17–127.

18. Jensen H, Goldschmidt E. Visual acuity in Danish school children. *Acta Ophthalmol (Copenh)* 1986; 64:187–191.

19. Stoll C, Alembik Y, Dott B, *et al*. Epidemiology of congenital eye malformations in 131,760 consecutive births. *Ophthalmic Paed Gen* 1992; 13:179–186.

20. Hansen E, Flage T, Rosenberg T, *et al*. Visual impairment in Nordic children. III. Diagnoses. *Acta Ophthalmol (Copenh)* 1992; 70:597–604.

21. Wirth MG, Russell-Eggitt IM, Craig JE, *et al*. Aetiology of congenital and paediatric cataract in an Australian population. *Br J Ophthalmol* 2002; 86:782–786.

22. Rahi JS, Dezateux C, British Congenital Cataract Interest Group. Measuring and interpreting the incidence of congenital ocular anomalies: lessons from a national study of congenital cataract in the UK. *Invest Ophthalmol Vis Sci* 2001; 42:1444–1448.

23. Haargaard B, Wohlfahrt J, Fledelius HC, *et al.* Incidence and cumulative risk of childhood cataract in a cohort of 2.6 million Danish children. *Invest Ophthalmol Vis Sci* 2004; 45:1316–1320.

24. Mwende J, Bronsard A, Mosha M, *et al.* Delay in presentation to hospital for surgery for congenital and developmental cataract in Tanzania. *Br J Ophthalmol* 2005; 89:1478–1482.

25. Bronsard A, Geneau R, Shirima S, *et al.* Why are children brought late for cataract surgery? Qualitative findings from Tanzania. *Ophthalmic Epidemiol* 2008; 15:383–388.

26. Rahi JS, Dezateux C. Congenital and infantile cataract in the United Kingdom: underlying or associated factors. British Congenital Cataract Interest Group. *Invest Ophthalmol Vis Sci* 2000; 41: 2108–2114.

27. Haargaard B, Wohlfahrt J, Rosenberg T, *et al.* Risk factors for idiopathic congenital/infantile cataract. *Invest Ophthalmol Vis Sci* 2005; 46:3067–3073.

28. Johar SR, Savalia NK, Vasavada AR, *et al.* Epidemiology based etiological study of pediatric cataract in western India. *Indian J Med Sci* 2004; 58:115–121.

29. Reddy MA, Francis PJ, Berry V, *et al.* Molecular genetic basis of inherited cataract and associ-ated phenotypes. *Surv Ophthalmol* 2004; 49:300–315.

30. Hejtmancik JF. Congenital cataracts and their molecular genetics. *Semin Cell Dev Biol* 2008; 19:134–149.

31. Jin L, Thomas B. Application of molecular and sero-logical assays to case based investigations of rubella and congenital rubella syndrome. *J Med Virol* 2007; 79:1017–1024.

32. Robertson SE, Featherstone DA, Gacic-Dobo M, *et al.* Rubella and congenital rubella syndrome: global update. *Rev Panam Salud Pública* 2003; 14:306–315.

33. Moriarty BJ. Childhood blindness in Jamaica. *Br J Ophthalmol* 1988; 72:65–67.

34. Eckstein MB, Brown DWG, Foster A, *et al.* Congenital rubella in South India: diagnosis using saliva from infants with cataract. *Br Med J* 1996; 312:161.

35. Rahi J, Sripathi S, Gilbert CE, *et al.* Childhood blindness in India: causes in 1318 blind school stu-dents in 9 states. *Eye* 1995; 9:545–550.

36. Gutiérrez MN, Sáenz MC. Vaccination and postex-posure prophylaxis in health-care workers. *Rev Esp Quimioter* 2009; 22:190–200.

37. Robinson JL, Lee BE, Preiksaitis JK, *et al.* Prevention of congenital rubella syndrome — what makes sense in 2006? *Epidemiol Rev* 2006; 28:81–87. Epub 2006 Jun 14.

38. World Health Organization. Report of a meeting on preventing congenital rubella syndrome: immuniza-tion strategies, surveillance needs. WHO/V&B/00.10. Geneva: WHO; 2000.

39. American Academy of Pediatrics; Section on Ophthalmology; American Association for Pediatric Ophthalmology and Strabismus; American Aca-demy of Ophthalmology; American Association of Certified Orthoptists. Red reflex examination in neonates, infants, and children. *Pediatrics* 2008; 122:1401–1404.

40. Ledoux DM, Trivedi RH, Wilson ME Jr, *et al.* Pediatric cataract extraction with intraocular lens implantation: visual acuity outcome when measured at age four years and older. *J AAPOS* 2007; 11:218–224.

41. Gochnauer AC, Trivedi RH, Hill EG, *et al.* Interocular axial length difference as a predictor of postoperative visual acuity after unilateral pediatric cataract extraction with primary IOL implantation. *J AAPOS* 2010; 14:20–24.

42. Congdon NG, Ruiz S, Suzuki M, *et al.* Determinants of pediatric cataract program out-comes and follow-up in a large series in Mexico. *J Cataract Refr Surg* 2007; 33:1775–1780.

43. Chak M, Wade A, Rahi JS; British Congenital Cataract Interest Group. Long-term visual acuity and its predictors after surgery for congenital cataract: findings of the British congenital cataract study. *Invest Ophthalmol Vis Sci* 2006; 47:4262–4269.

44. Long V, Chen S, Hatt S. Surgical interventions for bilateral congenital cataract. *Cochrane Db Syst Rev* 2006; 3:CD003171. Review.

45. Birch EE, Swanson WH, Stager DR, *et al.* Outcome after very early treatment of dense congenital uni-lateral cataract. *Invest Ophthalmol Vis Sci* 1993; 34:3687–3699.

46. Lambert SR, Lynn MJ, Reeves R, *et al.* Is there a latent period for the surgical treatment of children with dense bilateral congenital cataracts? *J AAPOS* 2006; 10:30–36.

47. Infant Aphakia Treatment Study Group, Lambert SR, Buckley EG, *et al*. The infant aphakia treatment study: design and clinical measures at enrollment. *Arch Ophthalmol* 2010; 128:21–27.

48. Infant Aphakia Treatment Study Group, Lambert SR, Buckley EG, *et al*. A Randomized Clinical Trial Comparing Contact Lens to Intraocular Lens Correction of Monocular Aphakia During Infancy: Grating Acuity and Adverse Events at Age 1 Year. The Infant Aphakia Treatment Study (IATS) Study Report 1. *Arch Ophthalmol*; in press.

49. Wilson ME, Bartholomew LR, Trivedi RH. Pediatric cataract surgery and intraocular lens implantation: practice styles and preferences of the 2001 ASCRS and AAPOS memberships. *J Cataract Refr Surg* 2003; 29:1811–1820.

50. Wilson ME, Trivedi RH. Choice of intraocular lens for pediatric cataract surgery: survey of AAPOS members. *J Cataract Refr Surg* 2007; 33: 1666–1668.

51. Bayramlar H, Totan Y, Borazan M. Heparin in the intraocular irrigating solution in pediatric cataract surgery. *J Cataract Refr Surg* 2004; 30:2163–2169.

52. Rumelt S, Stolovich C, Segal ZI, *et al*. Intraoperative enoxaparin minimizes inflammatory reaction after pediatric cataract surgery. *Am J Ophthalmol* 2006; 141:433–437.

53. Wilson ME, Jr., Trivedi RH. Low molecular-weight heparin in the intraocular irrigating solution in pediatric cataract and intraocular lens surgery. *Am J Ophthalmol* 2006; 141:537–538.

54. Vasavada VA, Shah SK, Praveen MR, *et al*. Randomized Clinical Trial Evaluating Anti-inflammatory effect of Low Molecular-Weight Heparin in Pediatric Cataract and Intraocular Lens Surgery. Presented at the Annual Symposium of ASCRS, 2009, San Francisco, USA.

Glaucoma in children

MARIA PAPADOPOULOS AND PENG KHAW

14f.1	Introduction	341		14f.3	Treatment	345
14f.2	Classification, sub-types and incidence	342		14f.4	Implications for research	348
					References	349

14f.1   INTRODUCTION

Paediatric glaucoma encompasses a diverse group of conditions that have one thing in common — raised intraocular pressure (IOP) leading to optic-disc cupping as distinct from adult glaucoma, which may also occur in the presence of normal IOP.

It is a relatively rare condition. For example, it is estimated that a consultant ophthalmologist in a non-specialist centre in the Western world will expect to see a new case of **primary congenital glaucoma (PCG)** approximately every five years.[1] As a result of its rarity, paediatric glaucoma is sometimes misdiagnosed or suboptimally treated allowing irreversible corneal and optic nerve damage to occur. Consequently it accounts for a disproportionate percentage (up to 18%) of children in blind institutions around the world.[2,3] Overall, glaucoma is responsible for 5% of blindness in children worldwide.[4]

14f.1.1   Clinical features

The clinical manifestations of glaucoma in childhood are highly variable and largely determined by the magnitude of the elevated IOP and the age of onset. Very high IOP can present dramatically in a newborn with cloudy, enlarged corneas. However, a slower rise in IOP results in a less acute presentation of an infant with buphthalmos (prominent, enlarged eye) but no corneal clouding or photophobia (Plate 14f.1). Furthermore, the timing of the pressure rise influences the clinical features owing to the limited potential of the young eye to deform. The young eye is vulnerable to the effects of increased IOP, leading to buphthalmos in infancy owing to the immaturity of corneal and scleral collagen. The potential for corneal enlargement usually ceases by the age of three although the sclera remains deformable up until the age of ten.

Glaucoma from any cause in a neonate or infant is synonymous with the classic triad of lacrimation, blepharospasm and photophobia due to corneal oedema from elevated IOP. These signs are not entirely specific but are very suggestive of glaucoma, and may appear before the hazy cornea (most frequent physical sign) (Plate 14f.2) and characteristic buphthalmos become obvious. Beyond the age of three years, children are more likely to present with progressive myopia, strabismus or after having failed routine school vision testing. In late-onset presentations, the child may be asymptomatic until peripheral visual field defects cause them to bump into objects.

Glaucomatous changes of the optic nerve in children are similar to those occurring in adults, and are just as important in making a diagnosis and evaluating progression. Furthermore, in neonates, optic-disc cupping may be the only indicator of level of functional vision, with advanced disc-cupping suggestive of constricted visual fields. Glaucomatous optic-disc cupping in infants differs from adults in that it is often reversible if IOP reduction occurs before irreversible nerve atrophy.

Accurate measurement of IOP is very important but can be influenced by many factors. IOP measurement can be influenced by the type and depth of anaesthesia. The majority of anaesthetics lower IOP, exceptions being ketamine and chloral hydrate. Furthermore, the most accurate measurements are taken when a child is relaxed with the eyes in the primary position and motionless. There are other variables, including instrumentation; under anaesthesia the gold standard for tonometry in children is the Perkins hand-held tonometer used with a blue filter, and fluorescein instilled in the eye. Corneal oedema and scarring have long been known to influence IOP measurements, but more recently corneal thickness has been identified as an important variable. In the presence of a thin cornea, as is often the case in patients with PCG,[5] there is a tendency to under-read the IOP. Conversely an increase in corneal thickness, as is found in patients with aphakia[6] and aniridia,[7] may lead to an over-reading of IOP.

14f.2   CLASSIFICATION, SUB-TYPES AND INCIDENCE

Various classifications of paediatric glaucoma exist because of an incomplete understanding of the pathophysiology of many of the variants. However, it can be classified simply as (i) *primary*, where only a developmental abnormality of the anterior chamber angle exists, and (ii) *secondary*, where aqueous outflow is reduced owing to congenital or acquired ocular disease or systemic disorder (Table 14f.1). It is likely that the

classifications will change as we learn more about the genetics of each condition. Primary congenital glaucoma was found to account for 45% of newly diagnosed paediatric glaucoma in the UK prospectively over one year. This was followed by lens-related glaucoma (aphakia/pseudophakia) in 31% of children, the commonest secondary paediatric glaucoma.[8] The most commonly presenting glaucomas will be discussed.

14f.2.1   Primary glaucoma in children

Primary congenital glaucoma is characterized by a specific developmental abnormality of the anterior chamber angle (isolated trabeculodysgenesis) on which the diagnosis is largely based. It is typically bilateral (70–80%), asymmetrical, and usually manifests in the first year of life but can present at any age. In Europe and the USA, PCG occurs more frequently in males than females at a ratio of between 2–2.5:1 even though there does not seem to be a sex-linked inheritance pattern.[9,10] In Japan, the ratio was first thought to be reversed in a number of small studies,[11] but more recently has been shown to be similar to that found in other countries.[12] Familial cases both in the Middle East and the Slovak Gypsy population tend to have an equal sex distribution.[13–16] This is in contrast to secondary paediatric glaucoma, which tends not to have any sex predilection.

Incidence

Primary congenital glaucoma is the commonest glaucoma in infancy. It has an incidence of one in 10,000–20,000 live births in most Western countries.[8,17] The incidence rises in the Middle East to 1:8,200 live births in Palestinian Arabs[18] and 1:2,500 live births in Saudi Arabians.[19] The highest reported incidence in the literature is 1:1,250 in Slovakian Gypsies.[15] Parental consanguinity, especially cousin–cousin marriages, is thought to be responsible for the higher prevalence of PCG in certain ethnic and religious groups.[15,16,18]

Table 14f.1 *Classification of childhood glaucoma*

1. PRIMARY	2. SECONDARY cont.,
(a) Primary congenital glaucoma (isolated trabeculodysgenesis) **(b) Juvenile open-angle glaucoma**	**Inflammatory/infective disease** Juvenile chronic arthritis Idiopathic uveitis Congenital rubella Congenital syphyllis Cytomegalovirus Herpes simplex disease
2. SECONDARY **Anterior segment dysgenesis** Axenfeld–Rieger anomaly Peters anomaly Iris hypoplasia Congenital ectropion uveae Microcornea	**Ocular tumours** Benign — iris cysts, juvenile xanthogranuloma Malignant — retinoblastoma, leukaemia
Lens-related Congenital cataract surgery (i) aphakia (ii) pseudophakia Ectopia lentis Microspherophakia Lenticonus	**Metabolic disease** Oculo-cerebro-renal syndrome (Lowe Syndrome) Homocystinuria Mucopolysaccharidoses, e.g.Hurlers Cystinosis
Other ocular disease/treatment Aniridia Persistent hyperplastic primary vitreous Retinopathy of prematurity Microphthalmos Trauma-related — hyphema, angle recession Steroid-induced Post-retinal detachment surgery Oculodermal melanocytosis (nevus of ota) Sclerocornea	**Chromosomal disorders** Down's syndrome (trisomy 21) Patau's syndrome (trisomy 13–15) Turner's syndrome (XO) Prader–Willi syndrome
	Connective tissue abnormalities Marfan's syndrome Weil–Marchesani syndrome Homocystinuria Ehler–Danlos syndrome Sulphite oxidase deficiency Osteogenesis imperfecta
Phacomatoses Sturge–Weber syndrome Klippel–Trenaunay–Weber syndrome Neurofibromatosis (von Recklinghausen's disease) von-Hippel–Lindau syndrome	**Other systemic congenital disorders** Rubinstein–Taybi syndrome Pierre Robin syndrome Cutis marmorata telangiectasia congenita Stickler syndrome

Aetiology: genetics, pathogenesis and risk factors

Most cases of PCG are sporadic. A family history of glaucoma is reported in 10–40% of cases associated with autosomal recessive inheritance and variable penetrance ranging from 40–100%.[13] Insufficient data exists to confirm or reject multifactorial or dominant forms of the disease. Linkage studies suggest genetic heterogeneity and have mapped three loci at chromosome 2p21 (GCL3A), 1p36 (GLC3B) and 14q24 (GLC3C). Molecular genetic studies suggest the primary molecular defect underlying the majority of cases of PCG (87% of familial and 27% of sporadic cases) is related to mutations of the CYP1B1 gene associated with the GLC3A locus.[20] It encodes for enzyme cytochrome P4501B1, which is postulated to participate in the development and functioning of the eye. Genotype–phenotype correlation has been reported with specific CYP1B1 mutations possibly associated with moderate or severe angle abnormalities.[21]

The pathogenesis of PCG remains disputed. Pathology studies suggest that the appearance of an immature angle results from the developmental arrest of tissues derived from cranial neural crest cells in the third trimester of gestation. As regards the mechanism of glaucoma, obstruction to outflow was classically thought to be due to the presence an impermeable membrane (Barkan's membrane) related to mesoblastic remnants, but this has never been verified histopathologically or clinically. It is now thought to be due to thick, compacted trabecular sheets.[22] It seems likely that the way forward in understanding the pathogenesis of this condition will be to identify the responsible gene(s) and protein(s).

Juvenile open-angle glaucoma refers to a distinct group of children who have no anterior segment abnormalities, who present late in childhood with glaucoma. Often there is a strong family history of glaucoma. Several of these families have mutations of the *myocilin/TIGR (trabecular meshwork inducible glucocorticoid response) gene* at the GLC1A locus on chromosome 1q21–q31.[23] These patients typically have high pressures (40–50 mmHg), and do not respond well in the long-term to medical treatment, often requiring enhanced filtration surgery.

14f.2.2 Secondary glaucoma in children

Anterior segment dysgenesis

Anterior segment dysgenesis represents a spectrum of developmental diseases involving neural crest mesenchyme. Conditions include Axenfeld–Rieger anomaly and Peters anomaly. Axenfeld–Rieger anomaly is now thought to represent a spectrum of disease ranging from the presence of posterior embryotoxon (anteriorly displaced, prominent Schwalbe's line) with attached iris strands alone, or associated with iris changes such as corectopia (displacement of the pupil) or atrophy. In association with systemic anomalies, such as abnormal teeth and facial abnormalities, particularly hypertelorism, it is referred to as Axenfeld–Rieger syndrome. Families with Axenfeld–Rieger anomaly show an autosomal dominant pattern of inheritance. Two loci have been identified, namely RIEG1 at chromosome 4q25 associated with the RIEG/PITX2 gene[24] and RIEG2 at 13q14 with an unidentified gene. It is also associated with abnormalities in the FOXC1 gene and PAX6 gene. Genotype–phenotype correlations are known; for example, FOXC1 duplication is associated with an earlier onset and a higher incidence of glaucoma.[25]

Peters anomaly is characterized by a congenital central corneal opacity with underlying defects in stroma, Descemet's membrane and endothelium with iris strands, and sometimes lens attachment to the periphery of this opacity. It is typically bilateral (80%). Peters anomaly is usually sporadic and may result from abnormalities of the PAX6 gene on chromosome 11p13, RIEG/PITX2 and FOXC1 genes.

There is a sub-group of patients with a distinctive hypoplastic iris stroma who are probably part of the anterior segment dysgenesis spectrum. Iris hypoplasia is associated with a characteristic under-development of the anterior stromal layer of the iris and early onset glaucoma; it can have the same systemic features as Axenfeld–Rieger syndrome. Autosomal dominant iris hypoplasia is associated with RIEG/PITX2 gene mutations.

The risk of glaucoma with these anomalies is approximately 50–70%, hence lifelong surveillance is indicated. Glaucoma usually occurs in childhood or young adulthood, very rarely in infancy. The IOP is typically labile. The cause of outflow obstruction is believed to be due to the arrested maturation of angle structures.

Aniridia

Aniridia is characterized by bilateral variable absence of iris with findings such as photophobia, nystagmus, foveal hypoplasia, amblyopia and strabismus. Visual loss is further compounded by a high incidence of glaucoma, cataract, ectopia lentis and corneal surface abnormalities due to corneal epithelial stem cell failure. Aniridia results from abnormal neuroectodermal development secondary to PAX6 gene mutations at chromosome 11p13. Inheritance is usually autosomal dominant although recessive transmission is possible. Sporadic aniridia is associated with Wilm's tumour, genitourinary abnormalities and mental retardation (WARG) related to large deletions of 11p13, which encompasses PAX6 and the adjacent Wilm's tumour locus. Glaucoma associated with aniridia is usually due to progressive angle-closure from the iris stump, presenting often in pre-adolescence or early adulthood, with an incidence ranging from 6–75%.

Sturge–Weber syndrome

Sturge–Weber syndrome (encephalotrigeminal angiomatosis) is the commonest phakomatosis associated with glaucoma. It is a sporadic condition characterized by a facial cutaneous angioma (port wine stain) present at birth, which affects the regions innervated by the first and second divisions of the trigeminal nerve. Choroidal hemangiomas occur in 40% of patients, and of these 90% develop glaucoma.[26] Glaucoma can arise from elevated episcleral venous pressure secondary to abnormal episcleral vasculature and goniodysgenesis.

Other phakomatoses can be associated with glaucoma although with a lower incidence than Sturge–Weber syndrome. **Neurofibromatosis** is an autosomal dominant condition, which may first present with iris abnormalities, e.g. ectropion uveae and glaucoma before the systemic disease is apparent. Glaucoma occurs in 50% of patients with plexiform neuroma; these patients must be followed for life. It is typically unilateral and usually presents at or shortly after birth. Congenital ectropion uveae is a rare nonprogressive condition, which is strongly associated with glaucoma and may occur with neurofibromatosis.

Aphakic glaucoma

Aphakic glaucoma is one of the most serious causes of late visual loss following successful congenital cataract surgery (Plate 14f.1). Its pathogenesis is uncertain; chemical (inflammatory cells, lens remnants and vitreous-derived factors), mechanical (lack of ciliary body tension and trabecular meshwork collapse), and developmental theories (adverse influence of surgical insult on normal postnatal angle maturation) have been proposed. The incidence of glaucoma following childhood cataract surgery varies according to the definition of glaucoma and the duration of follow-up. It ranges from 5% with simple aspiration[27] to as high as 41% with

lensectomy and ocutome vitrectomy with at least five-year follow-up.[28] In the UK, the annual incidence of aphakic glaucoma is reported to be 5.25 per 100 childhood cataract operations.[29] Risk factors for aphakic glaucoma such as early surgery (especially at less than a month of age), microcornea, poor pupil dilation, the need for secondary surgery and nuclear cataract are well documented. Some authors suggest deferring surgery until four to five weeks of age in bilateral cases, especially with nuclear cataracts and microcornea, to reduce the risk of glaucoma.[30] The role of posterior capsule integrity and intraocular lens (IOL) implantation is less clear because of the confounding factor of age at the time of surgery. Certain studies have suggested that posterior capsulotomy and anterior vitrectomy may be risk factors for glaucoma,[31,32] whereas others have found no association once findings are adjusted for age at surgery.[33] Similarly, the suggested protective effect of an IOL[34] is lost once age of surgery is taken into account.[33,35] Poor vision in children with aphakia is multifactorial and includes: amblyopia (deprivation, strabismic, refractive), nystagmus, failure to maintain a clear visual axis, late glaucoma diagnosis and surgical complications. Children with aphakic glaucoma tend to have a worse visual prognosis when compared with other sub-types of paediatric glaucoma.[36,37]

Uveitic glaucoma

Uveitic glaucoma may arise following inflammation from any cause, but is most commonly seen in juvenile idiopathic arthritis (14–38%)[38,39] and congenital infective conditions. Glaucoma, which usually develops two to three years after diagnosis, is multifactorial due to chronic cellular trabecular obstruction, trabeculitis, peripheral anterior synechiae, pupil block, secondary to cataract removal, and following chronic topical steroid usage. Glaucoma is a major cause of blindness in these children, as high as 30%.[38]

14f.3 TREATMENT

Clinical research suggests that the prognosis of paediatric glaucoma is largely dependent on early, accurate diagnosis and successful treatment. This involves intraocular pressure control to a level where progression is unlikely to occur, along with the treatment of amblyopia.

The optimal care of children with glaucoma should be based on evidence from well-conducted randomized controlled trials which are adequately powered. But these are lacking because of the rarity and diversity of this condition, with children presenting at differing ages and stages of the disease. Furthermore, the initial shock of this potentially blinding diagnosis makes it difficult to convince parents to take part in a randomized, prospective study where there may be no perceivable immediate benefit of treatment owing to the long follow-up required in glaucoma. There are also a number of ethical issues facing paediatric researchers, leading to reluctance to participate in these studies. Consequently, most of the evidence is from uncontrolled, prospective case studies or, more commonly, retrospective studies with their associated biases. The two published randomized studies of the surgical treatment of congenital glaucoma to date are discussed below.[40,41] Three prospective observational studies are summarised.[42–44]

If left untreated or suboptimally treated, the prognosis of paediatric glaucoma is poor. The preservation of a lifetime of vision for children with glaucoma depends on early, accurate diagnosis followed by appropriate successful treatment, the objectives of which are, first, to control IOP to a level where progression is unlikely, and second, to prevent or minimize amblyopia.

Surgery is the definitive treatment for the control of IOP in paediatric glaucoma, although medical treatment is first line in secondary glaucoma because it is often successful in reducing the IOP short term. In a prospective, national population-based study of paediatric glaucoma in the United Kingdom (UK), after one year 94% (68/72 eyes) with PCG and 64% (44/69 eyes) with secondary paediatric glaucoma had surgery. The majority in both groups required a second operation within the first year to control IOP.[8] The available surgical procedures have varying indications with both advantages and disadvantages and potentially good success rates,

especially when performed at referral centres where there is sufficient volume to ensure both skilful surgery and safe anaesthesia. However, the approach to management and success varies around the world.

In the control of IOP, primary and secondary paediatric glaucomas differ in two major ways. In secondary glaucoma, the first-line treatment is usually medical followed promptly by surgery when ineffective. Angle surgery is usually associated with limited success. Although the approach to management varies throughout the world, the consensus is that the definitive treatment for IOP control is surgical. The different surgical procedures have varying indications and potentially good success rates, especially when performed at referral centres. The procedure of choice is largely determined by diagnosis, corneal clarity, the age of the patient and the surgeon's experience, but may further be influenced by the degree of optic nerve damage, race, history of previous surgery and the state of the fellow eye.

In PCG, as the IOP is raised owing to a developmental defect in the trabecular meshwork that reduces aqueous outflow, surgery has centred on incising the trabecular meshwork *ab interno*, goniotomy and *ab externo*, trabeculotomy (angle surgery). Providing an alternative drainage channel, trabeculectomy, has been the procedure of choice for most secondary paediatric glaucoma and in cases of PCG where angle surgery has failed. Drainage implant surgery is typically the treatment of choice for refractory paediatric glaucoma such as aphakic or uveitic glaucoma. The use of cyclodestruction is becoming less common due to its limited effectiveness in controlling IOP long-term in children.

14f.3.1   The evidence for angle surgery

There is no randomized, controlled study comparing goniotomy to trabulectomy. Observations from retrospective studies suggest that they share similar success rates because success is dictated more by the severity of the disease than the type of angle surgery procedure.[45] Angle surgery is the operation of choice for PCG rather than secondary paediatric glaucomas.[46,47]

Only two prospective studies regarding angle surgery exist. Senft and co-workers published a small randomized trial, comparing surgical goniotomy with Nd:YAG goniotomy in ten Saudi Arabian patients (20 eyes), less than one year old, with bilateral, symmetrical PCG and clear corneas.[40] The first eye of each patient was randomized in a double masked fashion to either surgical or Nd:YAG laser goniotomy. The fellow eye underwent the alternative treatment. The main outcomes were IOP and the percentage of IOP change (new IOP/initial IOP expressed as a percentage). Success was defined as IOP ≤22 mmHg with antiglaucoma medications or a reduction greater than 25%. Mean follow up was 9.5 months. There was a strong positive correlation ($r = 0.81$) of the percentage of IOP change between two treatments. However, only four eyes (40%) in each group met the criteria for success. The response to laser was generally found to mirror the surgical outcome of the contralateral eye.

This is a small study with very short follow-up. By allocating the alternative procedure to the fellow eye, the patients were thought to act as 'his/her own control', which may be problematic if the outcome in the two eyes is not completely independent. The overall success rate of 40% for either incisional or laser goniotomy is comparable with results of retrospective studies following one incisional goniotomy;[48,49] this usually increases to 70–90% when repeated.[45,50] That the outcome of either procedure was usually similar in the same patient supports observations from retrospective studies that success is influenced largely by the severity of the disease, that is, the degree of angle immaturity. Given the lack of long-term results for laser goniotomy, this evidence is insufficient to warrant a change from surgical goniotomy.

A prospective case series of trabeculotomies performed in 47 white and black American children (75 eyes) with congenital glaucoma has been reported.[43] Intraocular pressure was controlled in 85% of patients after the first trabeculotomy, increasing to 93.4% when repeated; this is similar to other studies of angle surgery. There was no relationship between successful outcome and

corneal diameter, age of onset, pre-operative IOP and race.

14f.3.2 Evidence for combined trabeculotomy–trabeculectomy: with or without antimetabolites

One advantage of trabeculotomy is that it can be combined with trabeculectomy, with some authors arguing that this is more effective than trabeculotomy alone. However, there is no randomized, controlled trial comparing trabeculotomy–trabeculectomy with other surgical techniques. A prospective case series evaluating trabeculotomy–trabeculectomy in nine Palestinian Arab children (16 eyes) less than one year old with congenital glaucoma has reported a cumulative probability of successful IOP control of 93.5% at 24 months,[42] similar to that reported for trabeculotomy alone.[43]

In a small prospective, randomized, double blind study, four minutes intraoperative application of 0.2 mg/ml **Mitomycin-C (MMC)** during trabeculotomy–trabeculectomy was compared with 0.4 mg/ml MMC.[41] It was performed in 16 Indian patients (30 eyes) less than or equal to seven years with congenital glaucoma. Success was defined as IOP control ≤20 mmHg at final follow-up, including antiglaucoma medications but without further surgery. After a follow-up of six months, the 0.4 mg/ml group had a 40% drop-out rate (three patients, six eyes). The decrease in IOP six months after surgery between the two groups was not statistically significant (Student's t test, $P = 0.64$). Surgical success without medications was achieved in 60% of patients who had received 0.2 mg/ml MMC, and 86.6% in those with 0.4 mg/ml at final follow-up of 18 months (chi-squared test, $P = 0.21$). With medications the success rate was 86.7% in both groups. Full details of randomization were not provided, beyond stating that patients were 'systematically randomized' and the two groups could only be accurately compared for six months, which is a short time. The success rates reported in both arms of the trial are comparable with those reported in previous observational studies.[51,52] However, there is no evidence that 0.4 mg/ml MMC is superior to 0.2 mg/ml MMC in trabeculotomy–trabeculectomy.

14f.3.3   Evidence for trabeculectomy with or without antimetabolites

One of the greatest obstacles to success in paediatric glaucoma surgery is the aggressive healing response in children. This is due to a thick Tenon's capsule with a large reservoir of fibroblasts. The availability of antimetabolites has had a significant positive impact on outcomes. In a small, prospective, randomized clinical trial, MMC trabeculectomy was compared with 5-fluorouracil (5FU) trabeculectomy, with both groups receiving postoperative 5FU injections over a follow-up period of 27 months.[53] Surgery was performed in 12 eyes of eight Israeli children with either primary or secondary glaucoma. Eight eyes underwent MMC trabeculectomy, and four eyes had 5FU trabeculectomy. Seven out of the eight eyes had controlled IOP without medications in the MMC group with two post-op 5FU injections, compared with none of the four eyes in the 5FU alone group, even with medications and six post-op 5FU injections.

This is a very small study and despite being randomized one group had double the numbers compared with the other group. The poor outcome with 5FU trabeculectomy has been reported by other workers.[54] Similar high success rates with MMC trabeculectomy have been reported;[55] however, the success rate decreases with age.[56]

14f.3.4   Evidence for drainage implants

There has been no randomized, controlled trial of drainage implants. In a prospective case series, the Ahmed valve implant was evaluated in 21 consecutive patients (24 eyes) of mixed ethnicity, aged less than 18 years (mean 4.8 years). Fifty-four percent were described as having 'congenital glaucoma' and all patients had either previously failed glaucoma surgery or else other surgery was considered inappropriate.[44] Cumulative probabilities of success were 78% at 12 months and 60.6% at 24 months. Race, sex, age, aphakia and number of previous surgeries were not associated with increased failure (**Cox regression**, P ≥0.15). These findings are similar to other observational studies of un-enhanced Baerveldt and Molteno implants without antifibrosis regimens in paediatric patients.[57,58]

14f.3.5 Prognosis

Visual loss in children with glaucoma occurs from a combination of intractable glaucoma and optic nerve damage, corneal pathology, uncorrected refractive errors and amblyopia. In a study looking at the visual prognosis of children with glaucoma, overall 29% had 6/12 or better vision. Children with PCG had the best prognosis and those with aphakia the worst. At 18 years of age 50% were legally blind.[36] Thus, although advances have been made over the years in the management of paediatric glaucoma, it is obvious that significant challenges remain. Furthermore, periodic examination must continue throughout life, not only because an increase in IOP can occur at any stage, but also because complications can occur many years after a seemingly successful operation.

14f.4   IMPLICATIONS FOR RESEARCH

Currently, clinical practice is based largely on observational data derived mainly from retrospective case series with varying diagnoses, ages, number of patients, criteria for success and follow-up. This makes comparisons difficult. The criteria for successful outcome often vary and include the level of IOP (measured with various anaesthetics and instruments) with or without medications, visual criteria or stability of signs.

The limited data available from prospective trials fail to address the major issues such as:

➢ What is the best primary procedure for IOP control in primary congenital glaucoma? A comparison of conventional 120° trabeculotomy to 360° suture trabeculotomy[59] would be useful.

> What is the procedure of choice to control IOP in primary congenital glaucoma refractory to angle surgery — enhanced trabeculectomy or drainage implants?

> *Trabeculotomy–trabeculectomy* in theory provides two major outflow pathways and so would be expected to be more successful than either procedure alone, but the clinical benefit over trabeculotomy or trabeculectomy alone is unclear from the available literature, and warrants further study.

> What is the role of angle surgery in certain secondary glaucomas? Some secondary glaucomas, such as those associated with infantile Sturge–Weber syndrome or uveitis,[60] may respond to angle surgery.

> Clinical data regarding concentration, duration of exposure and safety of antimetabolites in paediatric patients would also be worthwhile.

The answers to these questions will probably be found in multicentre studies, possibly performed in areas of high incidence of this condition, for example PCG in the Middle East.

REFERENCES

1. Walton DS. Primary congenital open-angle glaucoma. In: Chandler PA, Grant WM (eds). *Glaucoma*. Philadelphia: Lea & Febiger; 1979. pp. 329–343.

2. Tabbara KF, Badr IA. Changing patterns of childhood blindness in Saudi Arabia. *Br J Ophthalmol* 1985; 69:312–315.

3. Gilbert CE, Canovas R, Kocksch de Canovas R, *et al*. Causes of blindness and severe visual impairment in children in Chile. *Dev Med Child Neurol* 1994; 36:326–333.

4. Gilbert CE, Rahi JS, Quinn GE. Visual impairment and blindness in children. In: Johnson GJ, Minassian DC, Weale RA, West SK, (eds). *The Epidemiology of Eye Disease*. London: Edward Arnold Ltd; 2003. pp. 260–285.

5. Henriques MJ, Vessani RM, Reis FAC, *et al*. Corneal thickness in congenital glaucoma. *J Glaucoma* 2004; 13:185–188.

6. Muir KW, Duncan L, Enyedi LB, *et al*. Central corneal thickness: congenital cataracts and aphakia. *Am J Ophthalmol* 2007; 144:502–506.

7. Brandt JD, Casuso LA, Budenz DL. Markedly increased central corneal thickness: an unrecognised finding in congenital aniridia. *Am J Ophthalmol* 2004; 137:348–350.

8. Papadopoulos M, Cable N, Rahi J, *et al*. BIG Eye Investigators. The British Infantile and Childhood Glaucoma (BIG) Eye Study. *Invest Ophthalmol Vis Sci* 2007; 48:4100–4106.

9. McGinnity FG, Page AB, Bryars JH. Primary congenital glaucoma: twenty years' experience. *Irish J Med Sci* 1987; 156:364–365.

10. Jay MR, Rice NSC. Genetic implications of congenital glaucoma. *Metab Ophthalmol* 1978; 2: 257–258.

11. Waardenburg PJ, Franceschetti A, Klein D. *Genetics and Ophthalmology*. Oxford: Charles C. Thomas; 1961.

12. Nakajima A, Fujiki K, Tanabe U. Genetics of buphthalmos. *7th Congr Asia Pacific Acad Ophthalmology*, Karachi; 1979.

13. Sarfarazi M, Stoilov I. Molecular genetics of primary congenital glaucoma. *Eye* 2000; 14:422–428.

14. Debnath SC, Teichmann KD, Salamah K. Trabeculectomy versus trabeculotomy in congenital glaucoma. *Br J Ophthalmol* 1989; 73:608–611.

15. Gencik A. Epidemiology and genetics of primary congenital glaucoma in Slovakia. Description of a form of primary congenital glaucoma in gypsies with autosomal-recessive inheritance and complete penetrance. *Dev Ophthalmol* 1989; 16:76–115.

16. Turaçli ME, Aktan SG, Sayli BS, *et al*. Therapeutic and genetical aspects of congenital glaucomas. *Int Ophthalmol* 1992; 16:359–362.

17. François J. Congenital glaucoma and its inheritance. *Ophthalmologica* 1980; 181:61–73.

18. Elder MJ. Congenital glaucoma in the West Bank and Gaza Strip. *Br J Ophthalmol* 1993; 77: 413–416.

19. Jaafar MS. Care of the infantile glaucoma patient. In: Reinecke RD (ed). *Ophthalmology Annual*. New York: Raven Press; 1988. pp. 15–37.

20. Stoilov I, Akarsu AN, Sarfarazi M. Identification of three different truncating mutations in cytochrome P4501B1 (CYP1B1) as the principle cause of

primary congenital glaucoma (Buphthalmos) in families linked to the GLC3A locus on chromosome 2p21. *Hum Mol Genet* 1997; 6:641–647.

21. Hollander DA, Sarfarazi M, Stoilov I, *et al.* Genotype and phenotype correlations in congenital glaucoma: CYP1B1 mutations, goniodysgenesis and clinical characteristics. *Am J Ophthalmol* 2006; 142:993–1004.

22. Anderson DR. The development of the trabecular meshwork and its abnormality in primary congenital glaucoma. *T Am Ophthal Soc* 1981; 79:458–485.

23. Stone EM, Fingert JH, Alward WL, *et al.* Identification of a gene that causes primary open angle glaucoma. *Science* 1997; 275:668–670.

24. Semina EV, Reiter R, Leysens NJ, *et al.* Cloning and characterization of a novel bicoid-related homeobox transcription factor gene, RIEG, involved in Rieger syndrome. *Nat Genet* 1996; 14:392–399.

25. Strungaru MH, Dinu I, Walter MA. Genotype-- phenotype correlations in Axenfeld–Rieger malformation and glaucoma patients with FOC1 and PITX2 mutations. *Invest Ophthalmol Vis Sci* 2007; 48:228–237.

26. Fitzpatrick TB, Kitamura H, Kukita A, *et al.* Ocular and dermal melanocytosis. *Arch Ophthalmol* 1956; 56:830–832.

27. François J. Late results of congenital cataract surgery. *Ophthalmology* 1979; 86:1586–1598.

28. Simon JW, Mehta N, Simmons ST, *et al.* Glaucoma after pediatric lensectomy/vitrectomy. *Ophthalmology* 1991; 98:670–674.

29. Chak M, Rahi JS, British Congenital Cataract Interest Group. Incidence of and factors associated with glaucoma after surgery for congenital cataract: findings from the British Congenital Cataract Study. *Ophthalmology* 2008; 115:1013–1018.

30. Vishwanath M, Cheong-Leen R, Taylor D, *et al.* Is early surgery for congenital cataract a risk factor for glaucoma ? *Br J Ophthalmol* 2004; 88:905–910.

31. Michaelides M, Bunce C, Adams GG. Glaucoma following congenital cataract surgery-the role of early surgery and posterior capsulotomy. *BMC Ophthalmol* 2007; 7:13.

32. Rabiah PK. Frequency and predictors of glaucoma after pediatric cataract surgery. *Am J Ophthalmol* 2004; 137:30–37.

33. Haargaard B, Ritz C, Oudin A, *et al.* Risk of glaucoma after pediatric cataract surgery. *Invest Ophthalmol Vis Sci* 2008; 49:1791–1796.

34. Asrani S, Freedman S, Hasselblad V, *et al.* Does primary intraocular lens implantation prevent 'aphakic' glaucoma in children? *J AAPOS* 2000; 4:33–39.

35. Trivedi RH, Wilson ME Jr, Golub RL. Incidence and risk factors for glaucoma after pediatric cataract surgery with and without intraocular lens implantation. *J AAPOS* 2006; 10:117–123.

36. Biglan AW. Glaucoma in children: are we making progress? *J AAPOS* 2006; 10:7–21.

37. Chen TC, Walton DS, Bhatia LS. Aphakic glaucoma after congenital cataract surgery. *Arch Ophthalmol* 2004; 122:1819–1825.

38. Sijssens KM, Rothova A, Berendschott TT, *et al.* Ocular hypertension and secondary glaucoma in children with uveitis. *Ophthalmology* 2006; 113: 853–9.e2.

39. Kanski JJ. Uveitis in juvenile chronic arthritis: incidence, clinical features and prognosis. *Eye* 1988; 2:641–645.

40. Senft SH, Tomey KF, Traverso CE. Neodymium–YAG laser goniotomy vs surgical goniotomy. *Arch Ophthalmol* 1989; 107:1773–1776.

41. Agarwal HC, Sood NN, Sihota R, *et al.* Mitomycin-C in congenital glaucoma. *Ophthalmic Surg Las* 1997; 28:979–985.

42. Elder MJ. Combined trabeculotomy–trabeculectomy compared with primary trabeculectomy for congenital glaucoma. *Br J Ophthalmol* 1994; 78:745–748.

43. Luntz MH, Livingston DG. Trabeculotomy ab externo and trabeculectomy in congenital and adult-onset glaucoma. *Am J Ophthalmol* 1977; 83:174–179.

44. Coleman AL, Smyth RJ, Wilson MR, *et al.* Initial clinical experience with the Ahmed glaucoma valve implant in pediatric patients. *Arch Ophthalmol* 1997; 115:186–191.

45. Douglas DH. Reflections on buphthalmos and goniotomy. *T Ophthal Soc UK* 1970; 90: 931–937.

46. Rice NSC. The surgical management of congenital glaucoma. *Aust J Ophthalmol* 1977; 5:174–179.

47. Luntz MH. Congenital, infantile and juvenile glaucoma. *Ophthalmology* 1979; 86:793–802.

48. Shaffer RN. Prognosis of goniotomy in primary infantile glaucoma (trabeculodysgenesis). *T Am Ophthal Soc* 1982; 80:321–325.

49. Haas JS. Symposium: Congenital glaucoma. End results of treatment. *T Am Acad Ophthal Otolaryngol* 1955; 59:333–341.

50. Russell-Eggitt IM, Rice NSC, Jay B, *et al*. Relapse following goniotomy for congenital glaucoma due to trabecular dysgenesis. *Eye* 1992; 6: 197–200.

51. Mandal AK, Naduvilath TJ, Jayagandan A. Surgical results of combined trabeculotomy–trabeculectomy for developmental glaucoma. *Ophthalmology* 1998; 105:974–982.

52. Mullaney PB, Selleck C, Al-Awad A, *et al*. Combined trabeculotomy and trabeculectomy as an initial procedure in uncomplicated congenital glaucoma. *Arch Ophthalmol* 1999; 117:457–460.

53. Snir M, Lusky M, Shalev B, *et al*. Mitomycin C and 5-fluorouracil antimetabolite therapy for pediatric glaucoma filtration surgery. *Ophthalmic Surg Lasers* 2000; 31:31–37.

54. Marrakchi S, Nacef L, Kamoun N, *et al*. Results of trabeculectomy in congenital glaucoma. *J Fr Ophthalmol* 1992; 15:400–404.

55. Mandal AK, Walton DS, John T, *et al*. Mitomycin C — augmented trabeculectomy in refractory congenital glaucoma. *Ophthalmology* 1997; 104: 996–1003.

56. Al-Hazmi A, Zwaan J, Awad, A, *et al*. Effectiveness and complications of mitomycin C use during pediatric glaucoma surgery. *Ophthalmology* 1998; 105:1915–1920.

57. Muñoz M, Tomey KF, Traverso C, *et al*. Clinical experience with the Molteno implant in advanced infantile glaucoma. *J Pediat Ophth Strab* 1991; 28:68–72.

58. Fellenbaum PS, Sidoti PA, Heuer DK, *et al*. Experience with the Baerveldt implant in young patients with complicated glaucomas. *J Glaucoma* 1995; 4:91–97.

59. Beck AD, Lynch MG. 360° trabeculotomy for primary congenital glaucoma. *Arch Ophthalmol* 1995; 113:1200–1202.

60. Freedman SF, Rodriguez-Rosa RE, Rojas MC, *et al*. Goniotomy for glaucoma secondary to chronic childhood uveitis. *Am J Ophthalmol* 2002; 133: 617–621.

14g

Retinopathy of prematurity

SUBHADRA JALALI AND GRAHAM QUINN

14g.1	Introduction	353
14g.2	Historical perspective and regional variation	353
14g.3	Classification/grading systems	355
14g.4	Prevalence and incidence of ROP in preterm and low birth weight babies	356
14g.5	Risk factors for ROP	357
14g.6	Primary prevention of ROP	357
14g.7	Secondary prevention of ROP	359
14g.8	Tertiary prevention	360
14g.9	Programmes for detecting and treating ROP	360
14g.10	Conclusion	361
14g.11	Future areas of research	362
	Appendix to 14g	362
	References	363

14g.1 INTRODUCTION

Retinopathy of prematurity (ROP) is a potentially blinding vasoproliferative disorder of the retina that can affect the eyes of infants who are born prematurely. The condition occurs when the normal process of vasculogenesis is interrupted, leading to abnormal vessel development at the junction of vascular and avascular retina. Although spontaneous regression is common, progression to blinding retinal detachment can occur. The mainstay of control of visual loss from ROP lies in primary prevention of the condition through good neonatal care, and programmes of secondary prevention whereby babies at risk of ROP are examined to detect those needing treatment.

14g.2 HISTORICAL PERSPECTIVE AND REGIONAL VARIATION

Retinopathy of prematurity (ROP) emerged as a cause of blindness in children in industrialized countries during the late 1940s and 1950s, as a consequence of greater survival of preterm babies due to improvements in neonatal care including use of supplemental oxygen.[1-4] During the 1950s, ROP was the single most common cause of blindness in children in many industrialized countries (the 'first epidemic'). Hyperoxia was proposed as an important risk factor[5] that was largely supported by laboratory research and clinical and epidemiological studies.[6-7] The use of oxygen was restricted in the mid-1950s and was followed by a reduction in the incidence of blindness from ROP, but higher rates of infant mortality and cerebral palsy.[8] Oxygen was used more liberally in the 1960s, and blindness from ROP began to re-emerge.[6] The introduction of increasingly sophisticated technology, including accurate methods of monitoring oxygen, and better management of neonatal and perinatal complications in prematurely born infants in the 1970s, were probably the major factors responsible for the reduction of blinding ROP observed during this period.[9]

The risk of ROP is inversely related to **gestational age (GA)** and **birth weight (BW)**.[10] More **very low BW (VLBW**, <1,500 g) and **extremely low BW (ELBW**, <1,000 g) babies are surviving as neonatal services continue to improve.[11] The population of babies at risk is, therefore, increasing, and there is some evidence that blindness from ROP is increasing again in some industrialized countries (the 'second epidemic'). In industrialized countries, blindness from ROP is now largely restricted to infants in the ELBW group,[12–15] being different in this regard from the population at risk in the newly developing economies.[11]

ROP has been described with increasing frequency in regions with rapidly developing neonatal care. Data obtained from examining children in schools for the blind in different regions of the world suggest that ROP is an important cause of blindness, particularly in countries in Latin American and Eastern Europe, and in urban centres in Asia.[11,16–19] This has been termed the 'third epidemic' and, as suggested in Table 14g.1, the reasons for this epidemic are mixed: premature birth and low BW dominate in settings able to deliver high quality neonatal care, while exposure to other potentially modifiable risk factors, including oxygen, are important where resources are limited and optimum standards of care cannot be provided.[20] In many countries experiencing the third epidemic, screening and treatment programmes are also not consistently in place, and not all **new-born intensive care units (NICUs)** are included. Diverse approaches to control are, therefore, needed. Awareness needs to be increased among gynaecologists (as ROP is a potential complication of multiple births following assisted fertilization), neonatologists, ophthalmologists and neonatal nursing staff, as countries introduce increasingly sophisticated neonatal intensive care services.

The available evidence suggests that the risk of blindness from ROP is associated with **infant mortality rates (IMRs)**, which can be a useful proxy indicator[20] (Plate 14g.1). Countries with very high IMRs (>60/1,000 live births) tend not to have neonatal intensive care services and so preterm babies do not survive to develop ROP. On the other hand, countries with very low IMRs (<9/1,000 live births), have robust health systems, and ROP programmes are generally in place to detect and treat babies with severe stages of the condition. In these countries ROP does occur, but blindness is largely controlled.[18] Countries with IMRs in the range 9–60/1,000 live births are those at highest risk of blindness due to ROP because preterm babies survive, but

Table 14g.1 *Historical and current risk factors for ROP, and the population of babies at risk (adapted from Gilbert et al. 2008)*[20]

	Historical perspective of ROP		
	1940–1950s **1st epidemic**	**1960–1970s** **2nd epidemic**	**1980s–present**
Risk factors for ROP:			
— prematurity	+	++	++++
— low birth weight	+	++	++++
— high oxygen	++++	+++	+
— illness factors	+	+	+/−
< 1,000 g	High mortality No ROP	Mod mortality ROP +	Low mortality ROP +++
1,000–1,500 g	Improved survival ROP +++	Low mortality ROP ++	Very low mortality No ROP
Level of neonatal care provided	**Poor**	**Moderate**	**Excellent**

The current 'third epidemic' includes babies receiving all three levels of neo-natal care.

the health systems to detect and treat ROP are not widespread.[11]

14g.3 CLASSIFICATION/GRADING SYSTEMS

Prior to the early 1980s, there was no standard manner in which to report clinical findings in acute-phase ROP. Several different classifications were proposed[21–23] to replace a classification from the 1950s which predated the indirect ophthalmoscope.[24] In 1984 a group of experts developed and published the 'International Classification of Retinopathy of Prematurity' (ICROP),[25] which was elaborated on in 1987.[26] This classification was recently 'revisited'[27] and the following modifications were made: an intermediate form of the posterior pole vascular abnormalities seen in ROP was added as a particularly virulent form of ROP. As shown in Table 14g.2, the current classification of

ROP[25–27] takes into account four components of the ocular findings of acute phase retinopathy: severity (stage), anterior–posterior location of the retinopathy (zone), the extent of the disease along the circumference of the vascularized retina (expressed in terms of 30-degree sectors or clock hours), and the presence or absence of 'plus disease' defined as engorged and tortuous vessels of the posterior pole, indicating a more advanced and serious form of retinopathy. By convention, the ROP status of an eye is designated by the highest stage and the lowest zone observed, along with noting the presence or absence of plus disease.

Severity of the retinopathy is designated by indicating the abnormality at the junction of the vascular and avascular retina, with stages 1 and 2 usually indicating mild disease, stage 3 indicating more serious disease since there are vessels extending into the vitreous, and stages 4 and 5 indicating the presence of retinal detachment. In the 2005 ICROP-revisited, **aggressive posterior ROP**

Table 14g.2 *International classification of retinopathy of prematurity — revisited*[27]

Severity	Stage of ROP	Stage 1: demarcation line between vascularized central retina and peripheral avascular retina
		Stage 2: Ridge between vascularized and avascular retina
		Stage 3: Ridge with fibrovascular proliferation into vitreous cavity
		Stage 4: Subtotal retinal detachment
		4A: extrafoveal detachment
		4B: foveal detachment
		Stage 5: Total retinal detachment
	AP-ROP	Aggressive posterior ROP characterized by:
		1. severe dilation and tortuosity of posterior pole vessels
		2. difficult to distinguish ROP at junction between vascularized and avascular retina
		3. may occur in zone I or zone II
Anterior–posterior location		Zone I: the area of retina within a circle centred on the disc and which has a radius of twice the disc-foveal distance
		Zone II: a doughnut-shaped retinal region that extends from the edge of zone I to a circle which has a radius of the distance from the disc to the nasal ora serrata
		Zone III is the crescent-shaped retinal area peripheral to zone II
Extent		Number of 30-degree sectors or clock hours of retinopathy along the circumference of the vascularized retina
Posterior pole vascular abnormalities	Plus disease	Presence of dilated and tortuous vessels of the posterior pole, indicating more advanced and serious retinopathy*
	Preplus disease	Abnormal vascular dilation and tortuosity that is insufficient for diagnosis of plus disease*

* Vascular abnormality must be present in two or more quadrants

(**AP-ROP**) was included to indicate the most severe form of ROP which is usually seen in the smallest, most immature babies and is more difficult to recognize since the peripheral retinopathy is not as remarkable as the posterior pole vascular abnormalities of dilation and tortuosity.[27]

The antero-posterior location of the retinopathy has important prognostic significance[10–14] and is captured in ICROP by dividing the surface of the retina into three zones centred on the optic disc. The most severe retinopathy tends to occur in zone I, most ROP occurs in zone II, and ROP that occurs in the most peripheral zone (zone III) tends to be mild. The extent of disease is indicated by the number of clock hours or 30-degree sectors along the junction between the vascularized and avascular retina. Documenting the extent of disease in terms of sectors allows the examiner to indicate the presence of various stages of ROP along the junction.

Plus disease is characterized by tortuosity and/or dilation of the peripapillary arterioles and venules. The diagnosis is a clinical judgement based on the comparison of the vascular abnormalities with reference images used in clinical treatment trials in the USA,[12–14] and diagnosis requires that the arterioles and venules must be sufficiently abnormal in at least two quadrants. Recognizing that posterior pole vascular abnormalities in ROP represent a continuum from normal appearing vessels to plus disease, the 2005 ICROP classification[27] included 'pre-plus disease' to designate that the peripapillary vessels are not normal appearing, but they are not sufficiently abnormal to be designated as plus disease. The utility of including this diagnosis is not yet clear. Other signs of serious ROP activity include vitreous haze, iris vascular engorgement and pupillary rigidity (i.e. the pupil does not dilate well following instillation of mydriatics). Examples of these retinal appearances are shown in Plates 14g.4–9.

Several large natural history studies have shown that the earliest signs of ROP begin at about 31–32 weeks post-menstrual age (i.e. the number of weeks since the mother's last menstrual period) in the majority of cases.[10,14,28,29] The disease progresses over the next two–five weeks, with spontaneous regression commonly occurring in stages 1, 2 and

early stage 3 without plus.[10,30] Blindness or severe visual impairment can be a consequence of progression to retinal detachment or severe distortion of the posterior retina.[31–35] Disease in zone I carries a worse prognosis, starts early and progresses more rapidly than disease occurring in zone II, which has in turn a worse prognosis than disease occurring in zone III.[10] An important poor prognostic sign is the presence of 'plus disease' in eyes with either stage 2 or stage 3 in zone II or in association with any stage of ROP in zone I. Indeed, this constellation of signs are the current indications for treatment.[15]

14g.4   PREVALENCE AND INCIDENCE OF ROP IN PRETERM AND LOW BIRTH WEIGHT BABIES

The overall incidence of ROP in premature infants is reported to be between 19–65.8% in studies from the developed and developing countries.[10,28,36–39] Differences reported may reflect differences in referral patterns and case mix, survival rates, and the criteria used for examination as well as levels of maternal and neonatal care. Observer bias may also play a role. Comparison of data between units is, therefore, difficult.

All studies show that the incidence and severity of ROP increase with decreasing BW and GA at birth. The incidence of ROP in infants less than 1000 g has been reported to vary, being 96% in Brazil, 90% in India, 81.6% in the USA and 87.1% in units in the UK.[10,36–38] In the study by Gopal et al.[39] the incidence of ROP was 45.5% in babies with BWs less than 1500 g and 23.5% in those with BWs of more than 1500 g, while 42.9% in less than 32 weeks and 34.5% in more than 32 weeks GA. Hospital-based studies have shown that up to 60% of LBW babies develop ROP, which rises to 72% in ELBW babies. The proportion of VLBW babies which develop stage III 'plus disease' and subsequent blindness can be as high as 11% and 8% respectively.[10,14]

The prevalence of stages 1 and 2 without plus is generally much higher than stages 3 and beyond, or plus disease. In the majority of babies with stages 1 or 2 the condition regresses spontaneously and few progress to vision threatening levels or advanced

ROP related blindness.[10,14] Longitudinal studies undertaken in the same units show varying trends over time: in some units the incidence of severe ROP (i.e. stages 3 or more) was low at baseline, and did not change over time despite greater survival of the smallest infants (rate 3–3.2%).[40] In other units rates of severe ROP increased,[41] while in yet others the incidence of all stages of ROP remained stable but rates of disease needing treatment declined.[42] These findings are difficult to compare and interpret, but possibly indicate that better maternal, perinatal and neonatal management might have the ability to reduce the incidence and severity of ROP, particularly in larger babies.

14g.5   RISK FACTORS FOR ROP

Many case-control studies have been undertaken to elucidate risk factors for ROP. These studies are challenging to undertake as they require the collection of exposure data over the first four weeks of life, e.g. whether supplemental oxygen was administered and how this influences blood saturation levels, which fluctuate minute by minute; whether the infant was anaemic; and whether blood transfusions were given, and if so, how many and when. All studies identify low GA and low BW as major risk factors (Table 14g.3). The lower the GA the higher the risk of ROP, particularly ROP in posterior zones and AP-ROP.[10,14,36–39,43] Other risk factors for ROP include hyperoxia, hypoxia and fluctuating oxygen levels.[44,45] The following are also associated with ROP but are not necessarily causally associated as they are also markers of sickness, which are more likely in the more preterm baby: acidosis, intraventricular haemorrhage, exposure to light, vitamin E deficiency and septicaemia. Progression to advanced, potentially blinding disease seems to be determined by the immaturity of the retina and the degree of the early insult. The state of development of the retinal vasculature at birth may also be a risk factor for ROP.[46]

Other investigators are exploring whether weight gain and serum **insulin-like growth factor 1 (IGF-1)** levels, or weight gain alone, during the

Table 14g.3 *Risk factors for ROP*

Accepted as risk factors:
- Low gestational age
- Low birth weight
- Poor oxygen management (i.e. fluctuating hypoxia/hyperoxia; lack of monitoring)
- Lack of antenatal steroids

Associated with ROP but probably not causal:
- Poor post natal weight gain
- Respiratory distress syndrome
- Hyaline membrane disease
- Blood transfusions
- Sepsis
- Intraventricular haemorrhage
- Maternal anaemia/chronic *in utero* hypoxia
- Patent ductus arteriosus
- Vitamin E deficiency
- Low IGF-1 levels
- Genetic markers
- Light exposure

first four–six weeks of life can reliably predict ROP needing treatment. In European populations of preterm babies these measures of growth do hold some promise[47,48] but further larger studies are needed to confirm and refine these markers in a range of different settings.

Small studies of genetic markers for severe ROP or failure of treatment have implicated mutations and polymorphisms in the Norrie disease pseudoglioma (NDP) gene, endothelial nitric oxide synthetase (eNOS) gene and **vascular endothelial growth factor (VEGF)** gene. However, most studies failed to show a significant effect of the genetic abnormalities on ROP. Genetic influences on occurrence, course and severity of ROP need to be evaluated further and validated in varied patient populations and in larger cohorts.[49]

14g.6   PRIMARY PREVENTION OF ROP

Interventions which reduce the incidence of ROP require a multifaceted approach ranging from: increasing awareness of the disease; education of physicians and nurses caring for the premature babies; improving levels of neonatal care; and monitoring the oxygen levels and other factors that affect retinal vessel growth. Primary prevention of ROP requires meticulous neonatal care, and adequately equipped and staffed units. Clearly, the most effective intervention would be to decrease premature birth, but this remains a long-term goal.

The following interventions have been shown to reduce the incidence and severity of ROP:

1. Systemic parenteral steroids (dexamethasone or betamethasone) given to high-risk pregnant mothers during the second trimester of pregnancy, or even immediately prior to preterm birth, reduce the incidence of **respiratory distress syndrome (RDS)**, which in turn prevents the development and severity of ROP.[50] The mechanism is thought to be that steroids promote lung maturation. Treatment with natural or synthetic surfactant soon after birth to prevent or treat RDS does not influence the incidence of ROP among treated babies, but at a population level surfactant use has led to an increase in the number of babies affected on account of greater survival rates.[51]

2. A series of studies have suggested that lower target oxygen saturation levels, and closer attention to variations in the oxygen status of the baby, reduce the likelihood of serious ROP.[44,52,53] The practice of only giving supplemental oxygen when indicated should start in the delivery room, and protocols should be in place. Despite oxygen being such an important agent in neonatal care, appropriate oxygen saturation targets are still unclear and several large clinical trials are underway to address this issue.[40–42]

3. Anaemia of prematurity leads to reduction of the haematocrit in preterm babies, which may persist for up to a year. The low haemoglobin aggravates the hypoxic status in the eye. The effect of anaemia on ROP severity has been extensively examined and it appears that treatment with recombinant human erythropoietin lowers the risk of ROP.[54,55] Correction of anaemia in the presence of pre-threshold ROP has also led to rapid reduction of plus disease and better response to laser therapy.[55]

The following interventions are controversial or experimental:

1. Several randomized clinical trials have been undertaken to determine whether vitamin E supplementation prevents the development of ROP. Individually, these studies do not demonstrate a significant positive benefit, but a detailed meta-analysis of the randomized trials found that, not only did vitamin E supplementation reduce the risk of severe ROP and blindness, it also reduced the risk of intracranial haemorrhage. In addition it increased the risk of sepsis if administered in higher than physiologic doses early in life.[56,57] More investigations are warranted.[57]

2. In 2001, Hellstrom *et al.* showed in a cohort of babies in Sweden that IGF-1 is markedly deficient in premature infants after birth and found that those children in whom the recovery to normal IGF-1 serum levels is slow are likely to develop ROP.[58] In several follow-up studies, these and other investigators have demonstrated that monitoring rate of weight gain, essentially a non-invasive surrogate for growth hormone level, is effective in identifying those babies at high risk for developing ROP even before the retinopathy is manifest.[48,59,60] Such observations, along with extensive work in animal models of oxygen-induced retinopathy, open the way for the potential medical therapies that can be offered to high risk babies that may prevent ROP or at least modulate its severity.[54,61–64]

Challenges to implementing preventive measures

Barriers to monitoring and maintaining stable oxygen levels among all babies receiving supplemental oxygen include lack of awareness, high baby-to-nurse ratios, inadequate equipment for delivering oxygen (e.g. flow meters, humidifiers, pulse oximeters) and lack of consensus and strict comprehensive guidelines and protocols. Most nurseries follow an arbitrary cut-off of 90–94% SpO_2 levels of pulse oximeter when the infant is receiving oxygen. Controversies about optimal cut-offs at different postnatal ages need to be resolved.[65,66]

14g.7 SECONDARY PREVENTION OF ROP

14g.7.1 Surgical treatment

Interventions for secondary prevention currently rest on peripheral retinal ablation although medical therapies are being explored. Historically, the first large randomized clinical trial in ROP treatment was the **CRYO-ROP** study,[12,67] in which one eye each of preterm babies was randomized to retinal ablation with cryotherapy or no treatment. Babies randomized had advanced proliferative stages of ROP, termed threshold ROP (i.e. stage III, new vessels in five or more contiguous clock hours or eight or more non-contiguous disease with 'plus' disease of all four posterior pole vessels). The results of the study showed that treatment with cryotherapy almost halved the proportion of babies going on to develop blinding disease.[12,67,68] The treatment effect persisted until the children were ten years of age, both in terms of structure and function including distance and near visual acuity, visual field and contrast sensitivity.[69–71] However, although cryotherapy reduced rates of total retinal detachment and blindness, it did not preserve good vision. More than 44% of treated eyes had visual acuity worse than 20/200 at age ten years[71] and only 21.5% and 13.4% retained 20/60 or better and 20/40 or better visual acuity respectively. The need for strategies to improve visual outcomes was identified.

The **Early Treatment of ROP trial (ETROP)** was designed to address whether earlier treatment gave better structural and functional outcomes than treatment given at threshold disease. In this multicentre trial, one eye of each preterm baby was randomized once pre-threshold ROP had developed, where pre-threshold was defined as less severe disease but where the risk of progression was at least 15% using a diagnostic algorithm derived from CRYO-ROP data.[14,72] Randomized eyes were assigned to receive treatment either at this pre-threshold stage or only once the condition

Table 14g.4 *Indications for treatment according to ETROP (adapted from ETROP, 2003)*[15]

Zone I	No plus	Stage 1	Follow
		Stage 2	Follow
		Stage 3	**Treat**
Zone I	Plus	**Stage 1**	**Treat**
		Stage 2	**Treat**
		Stage 3	**Treat**
Zone II	No plus	Stage 1	Follow
		Stage 2	Follow
		Stage 3	Follow*
Zone II	Plus	Stage 1	Follow*
		Stage 2	**Treat**
		Stage 3	**Treat**

Note: Presence of plus and of new vessels are critically important for considering treatment.
*Rare presentations
Clinical judgement should be applied while using these guidelines.

had progressed to threshold. Results showed that the risk of blindness (VA <20/200 or worse) was reduced to less than 15.5% when eyes were treated at pre-threshold disease.[15] However, eyes treated at pre-threshold ROP were treated an average of one week earlier than eyes treated at threshold ROP. These babies had more apnoea and bradycardia, and were more likely to require incubation for an extended period, but no increased mortality or long-term morbidity was noted. More than 64% of early treated eyes retained normal grating visual acuity at nine months.[15] This study also brought to attention severe posterior disease that required early and aggressive treatment. Based on this study, new criteria for treatment were established (Table 14g.4). Further refinements in treatment criteria could achieve 20/40 or better vision in a higher proportion of eyes.[73] Another implication of earlier treatment is that the number of eyes/babies eligible for treatment has increased considerably.

A few small clinical trials have been undertaken, and a few case series have compared different treatment modalities (i.e. argon versus diode laser peripheral retinal ablation; confluent versus less confluent applications; cryo versus laser).[74] The results show that laser has several advantages over cryotherapy, i.e. less pain; less need for general anaesthesia; better direct visualization of delivery of treatment and less pigmentary reaction from the treatment.[74,75]

14g.7.2   Medical treatment

The Supplemental Treatment of Pre-threshold ROP study (STOP-ROP) was designed to address whether administration and maintenance of higher target levels of oxygen were efficacious in preventing progression of established moderately severe ROP (i.e. ROP with either plus disease or stage 3 disease). This large randomized trial not only showed no difference in progression to threshold ROP between the treatment arms but also showed that babies randomized to the higher target saturation levels had a higher incidence of pulmonary complications and longer hospital stays than those in the other arm of the trial.[76]

Recent approaches to ROP treatment have concentrated on non-destructive treatments using anti-vascular endothelial growth factors (anti-VEGF) injected intravitreally. To date more than 100 eyes have been reported where intravitreal Bevacizumab has been injected in varying doses.[77–83] No systemic side effects have been reported to date, but in most series the period of follow-up has been too short to allow assessment of neuro-developmental complications or long-term side effects. The drugs seem to cause regression of new blood vessels while allowing normal vascularisation to proceed, though at a slower pace than normal. Increased vitreoretinal traction after injection has been reported in some eyes with advanced disease.[81,82] Randomized controlled trials comparing safety and efficacy of Bevacizumab to standard laser treatment are under way. Because of the potential for systemic absorption, particularly in the preterm eye with plus disease where blood ocular barriers are, by definition, compromised, the use of anti-VEGF preparations should be subject to rigorous trials of safety as well as effectiveness before they can be recommended for widespread use.[84]

14g.8   TERTIARY PREVENTION

To date there have been no randomized clinical trials of surgical interventions for stages 4 or 5 ROP, and the reported case series need to be interpreted with caution as they are subject to observer bias and confounding. Surgery for stage 4a, especially in laser-failed cases, has been reported to give good to excellent anatomical and functional outcomes, particularly when lens-sparing vitrectomy techniques have been used.[85,86] Some stage 4b eyes can be salvaged by vitreoretinal surgery, giving fairly good ambulatory vision,[85] but surgery for stage 5 very rarely gives good functional outcomes even if the retina can be reattached.[85–89]

14g.9   PROGRAMMES FOR DETECTING AND TREATING ROP

14g.9.1   Examination and treatment by ophthalmologists

Current standard of care for ROP requires examination of babies at risk to identify the vision-threatening stages of the disease so that treatment can be given. Carefully timed retinal examination by trained ophthalmologists, using the binocular indirect ophthalmoscope, is recommended (Plate 14g.2). National guidelines for ROP screening have been developed or suggested in many countries (Appendix 14g.1). These guidelines are similar in many respects, with the major differences being the upper limits of BW and GA, beyond which routine screening is not necessary. These vary from 30–32 weeks and/or less than 1200–1700 g in developed countries and up to 34–35 weeks and/or less than 2000 g in emerging economies (Appendix 14g.1). Ideally, criteria and guidelines should be based on local evidence of the population of babies at risk of ROP, and these can be modified over time.[11]

Most guidelines recommend that the first retinal examination should occur between 31 and 33 weeks post-menstrual age, but usually not before age four weeks after birth. However, it is often difficult to ascertain an accurate post-menstrual age, and adopting a day-30 strategy (i.e. four weeks) as a deadline for the first eye examination, becomes an easy benchmark. However, smaller babies and those at risk of AP-ROP could need earlier examination, for which a day-20 strategy could be adopted.[73,90,91]

Ensuring that programmes for detecting and treating babies are effective and efficient requires constant surveillance to ensure that no eligible babies are missed.[20,91] Coordination between neonatologists, nurses and ophthalmologists is vital, particularly for arranging follow-up examinations for babies who have been discharged from the nursery.[92] In spite of national guidelines, audits have shown that compliance with and coverage of ROP programmes can often be improved.[93,94]

Many studies have addressed the barriers to effective ROP programmes in developing countries that would prevent ROP blindness.[11,17,18,20,95–97] The general theme of these reports is that, in resource-limited environments, awareness of the disease must be increased by education of caregivers, parents and governments, and that improving the quality of neonatal care and training, and equipping ophthalmologists to detect and treat ROP, will have a significant impact on ROP blindness. A major effort has been undertaken in developing countries to promote effective ROP programmes with neonatologists, NICU nurses and ophthalmologists, by conducting in-country workshops to raise awareness, determine the current status of ROP detection and treatment, as well as determining the BW, GA, and survival rates of babies currently developing serious ROP for that country.

14g.9.2 Digital imaging and ROP

Advances in digital imaging have provided the clinician with new opportunities and the ability to document the findings in acute-phase ROP, with minimal risk or discomfort to the baby; and digital images were integral to the development of ICROP-revisited.[27] Digital images are proving an important tool in ROP programmes as they allow change over time to be monitored. Images are also invaluable in the education of ophthalmologists,

for raising awareness and educating paediatricians, neonatologists, nurses, parents and administrators about a disease that was previously unseen. Further, computer-assisted digital analysis of vascular abnormalities (especially vessel dilation and tortuosity) may eventually allow development of quantitative scores that predict the likelihood of severe ROP, even before the severe disease is manifest.[98–106]

One of the commonly used cameras gives a wide, 130-degree field of view (Plate 14g.3). With this system, zone I is well visualized, as is much of zone II, allowing image capture in regions of the retina where serious disease is most likely to develop.[107–110] Other systems for digital imaging include narrow field cameras, which have been used to image the disc and surrounding retinal vessels,[111] and the video indirect ophthalmoscope.[112]

To date, there have been several, relatively small, studies that used different approaches, and examined different components of an overall system for ROP telemedicine. These reports give different, sometimes contradictory, results but have a common goal of developing and validating an effective system of telemedicine for ROP.[108,113] Should digital screening via telemedicine prove to have high levels of sensitivity, specificity and acceptability,[114] reliable services for treatment must be in place, and be able to be delivered within 48 hours, as in all screening programmes (see Chapter 8 for screening criteria).[114]

14g.10 CONCLUSION

Preventing blindness due to ROP is a race against time. Monitoring and maintaining stable oxygenation, haemoglobin and lung function is critical to reducing the incidence and severity of ROP. There is a small window of opportunity within one month of birth where the disease can be best treated if detected on time by careful retinal examination. A high level of awareness and coordination is required between neonatologists, neonatal intensive care nurses and ophthalmologists to achieve good anatomic and functional visual outcomes.

14g.11 FUTURE AREAS OF RESEARCH

Further epidemiological research is required:

To identify populations of babies at risk

1. To determine in which new industrializing counties ROP is becoming an important cause of blindness in children.

To explore factors that could lead to primary prevention

2. To identify risk factors in these settings (e.g. whether the incidence is influenced by ethnic origin).
3. To determine whether rate of growth in the first few weeks after birth predicts vision-threatening ROP in different settings.
4. To determine the best care practices for oxygen and blood transfusions in at risk babies.

To explore factors associated with secondary and tertiary prevention

5. To delineate the natural history of ROP in settings where bigger, more mature babies develop ROP, which might influence the timing of the first and subsequent examinations.
6. To develop appropriate guidelines for screening babies at risk. This is relevant as data from India and other developing countries suggest that babies with a BW of >1,500 g can develop threshold disease.[11] The recommendations for screening are likely to differ by country, depending on the neonatal care and survival of babies in that country or region.
7. To assess the validity, feasibility and cost-effectiveness of a telemedicine approach to screening babies for ROP.
8. To explore the role of fluorescein angiography and/or laser treatment posterior to the ridge in eyes which carry a poor prognosis, i.e. AP-ROP, or zone 1 disease.
9. To undertake clinical trials to compare the structural, functional and parent-related outcomes (i.e. economic and emotional cost) of surgery for stage 4b and stage 5 ROP.
10. To determine whether the outcome of laser treatment varies according to ethnic group, or whether the timing or nature of the treatment needs to be modified according to the geographical setting.
11. To investigate the efficacy, and short- and long-term safety, of anti-VEGF preparations in the treatment of ROP.

APPENDIX TO 14g

Reference list of National ROP screening guidelines/suggested guidelines in different countries.

Note: Screening guidelines have been constantly evolving and being updated and this is not a complete list. Arranged in descending order of year of publication.

1. Royal College of Ophthalmologists and Paediatric and Child Health. UK Retinopathy of Prematurity guideline May 2008. http://www.rcophth.ac.uk/docs/scientific/guideline_Retinopathy_of_Prematurity_2008.
2. Wilkinson AR, Haines L, Head K, et al. UK retinopathy of prematurity guideline. Eye 2008: Epub Oct 3.
3. Jandeck C, Kellner U, Lorenz B, et al. [Guidelines for ophthalmological screening of premature infants in Germany] [Article in German]. Klin Monatsbl Augenheilkd 2008; 225:123–130.
4. Misra A, Heckford E, Curley A, et al. Do current retinopathy of prematurity screening guidelines miss the early development of pre-threshold type 1 ROP in small for gestational age neonates? Eye 2008; 22:825–829. Epub 2007 Feb.
5. Grupo de Trabajo Colaborativo Multicéntrico para la Prevención de la Ceguera en la Infancia por Retinopatía del Prematuro. [Recommendations for Retinopathy of Prematurity screening in at-risk populations] [Article in Spanish]. Arch Argent Pediatr 2008; 106:71–76.

6. Binkhathian AA, Almahmoud LA, Saleh MJ, *et al.* Retinopathy of prematurity in Saudi Arabia: incidence, risk factors and the applicability of current screening criteria. *Br J Ophthalmol* 2008; 92:167–169.

7. Zin A, FlorÃªncio T, Fortes Filho JB, *et al.* Brazilian Society of Pediatrics, Brazilian Council of Ophthalmology and Brazilian Society of Pediatric Ophthalmology. [Brazilian guidelines proposal for screening and treatment of retinopathy of prematurity (ROP)] [Article in Portuguese]. *Arq Bras Oftalmol* 2007; 70:875–883.

8. Section on Ophthalmology American Academy of Pediatrics; American Academy of Ophthalmology; American Association for Pediatric Ophthalmology and Strabismus. Screening examination of premature infants for retinopathy of prematurity. *Pediatrics* 2006; 117:572–576. Erratum in: *Pediatrics* 2006; 118:1324.

9. Chen Y, Li X. Characteristics of severe Retinopathy of prematurity patients in China; a repeat of the first epidemic? *Br J Ophthalmol* 2006; 90:268–271.

10. Jalali S, Hussain A, Matalia J, *et al.* Modification of screening criteria for India and other middle-income group countries. *Am J Ophthalmol* 2006; 141:966–968.

11. Hautz W, Gra?ek M, Dobrza?ska A, *et al.* [Screening for retinopathy of prematurity — qualification criteria on the basis of our experience] [Article in Polish]. *Klin Oczna* 2006; 108:316–318.

12. Trinavarat A, Atchaneeyasakul LO, Udompunturak S. Applicability of American and British criteria for screening of the retinopathy of prematurity in Thailand. *Jpn J Ophthalmol* 2004; 48:50–53.

13. Chiang MC, Tang JR, Yau KI, *et al.* A proposal of screening guideline for retinopathy of prematurity in Taiwan. *Acta Paediatr Taiwan* 2002; 43:204–207.

14. Lee SK, Normand C, McMillan D, *et al.* Canadian Neonatal Network. Evidence for changing guidelines for routine screening for retinopathy of prematurity. *Arch Pediatr Adolesc Med* 2001; 155:387–395.

15. Goble RR, Jones HS, Fielder AR. Are we screening too many babies for retinopathy of prematurity? *Eye* 1997; 11:509–514.

REFERENCES

1. Flynn J. Retinopathy of prematurity. *Pediatr Clin N Am* 1987; 34:1487–1516.

2. Patz A, Hoeck L, De La Cruz E. Studies of the effect of high oxygen administration in retrolental fibroplasia: I. Norsery observations. *Am J Ophthalmol* 1952; 35:1248–1252.

3. Patz A. Clinical and experimental studies on role of oxygen in retrolental fibroplasia. *Trans Am Acad O&O* 1954; 58:45–50.

4. Patz A. The role of oxygen in retrolental fibroplasia. *Graef Arch Clin Exp Opthalmol* 1975; 195:77–85.

5. Campbell K. Intensive oxygen therapy as a possible cause of retrolental fibroplasia: a clinical approach. *Med J Aust* 1951; 2:48–50.

6. Flynn JT, Bancalari E, Snyder ES, *et al.* A cohort study of transcutaneous oxygen tension and the incidence and severity of retinopathy of prematurity. *N Engl J Med* 1992; 326:1050–1054.

7. Lanman J, Guy L. Retrolental fibroplasia and oxygen therapy. *JAMA* 1954; 155:223–226.

8. Cross CW. Cost of preventing retrolental fibroplasia. *Lancet* 1973; 2:954–956.

9. Gibson DL, Sheps SB, Schechter MT, *et al.* Retinopathy of prematurity: a new epidemic? *Pediatrics* 1989; 83:486–492.

10. Palmer EA, Flynn JT, Hardy RJ, *et al.* Incidence and early course of retinopathy of prematurity. The Cryotherapy for Retinopathy of Prematurity Cooperative Group. *Ophthalmology* 1991; 98:1628–1640.

11. Gilbert C, Fielder A, Gordillo L, *et al.* Characteristics of infants with severe retinopathy of prematurity in countries with low, moderate, and high levels of development: implications for screening programs. *Pediatrics* 2005; 115:518–525.

12. Cryotherapy for Retinopathy of Prematurity Cooperative Group, Multicenter Trial of Cryotherapy for Retinopathy of Prematurity: Preliminary Results. *Pediatrics* 1988; 81:697–706.

13. Cryotherapy for Retinopathy of Prematurity Cooperative Group, Incidence and Early Course of Retinopathy of Prematurity. *Ophthalmology* 1991; 98:1628–1640.

14. Good WV, Hardy RJ, Dobson V, *et al*. The incidence and course of retinopathy of prematurity: findings from the early treatment for retinopathy of prematurity study. *Pediatrics* 2005; 116:15–23.

15. Early Treatment For Retinopathy Of Prematurity Cooperative Group. Revised indications for the treatment of retinopathy of prematurity: results of the early treatment for retinopathy of prematurity randomized trial. *Arch Ophthalmol* 2003; 121:1684–1694.

16. Gilbert CE, Anderton L, Dandona L, *et al*. Prevalence of visual impairment in children: a review of available data. *Ophthal Epidemiol* 1999; 6:73–82.

17. Gilbert C, Foster A. Childhood blindness in the context of VISION 2020 — the right to sight. *Bull World Health Organ* 2001; 79:227–232.

18. Gilbert C, Rahi J, Eckstein M, *et al*. Retinopathy of prematurity in middle-income countries. *Lancet* 1997; 350:12–14.

19. Shah PK, Narendran V, Kalpana N, *et al*. Severe retinopathy of prematurity in big babies in India: history repeating itself? *Indian J Pediatr* 2009; 76:801–804.

20. Gilbert C. Retinopathy of prematurity: a global perspective of the epidemics, population of babies at risk and implications for control. *Early Hum Dev* 2008; 84:77–82.

21. Kingham J. Acute retroletnal fibroplasia. *Arch Ophthalmol* 1977; 95:39–47.

22. McCormick A. The retinopathy of prematurity in the newborn. *Curr Prob Pediatr* 1977; 7:28–42.

23. Quinn GE, Schaffer DB, Johnson L. A revised classification of retinopathy of prematurity. *Am J Ophthalmol* 1982; 94:744–749.

24. Reese A, King MJ, Owens WC. A classification of retrolental fibroplasia. *Am J Ophthalmol* 1953; 36:1333–1335.

25. The International Committee for the Classification of Retinopathy of Prematurity. An international classification of retinopathy of prematurity. *Arch Ophthalmol* 1984; 102:1129–1134.

26. The International Committee for the Classification of Retinopathy of Prematurity. An international classification of retinopathy of prematurity. *Arch Ophthalmol* 1987; 105:906–912.

27. International Committee for the Classification of ROP. The international classification of retinopathy of prematurity revisited. *Arch Ophthalmol* 2005; 123:991–999.

28. Reynolds JD, Dobson V, Quinn GE, *et al*. Evidence-based screening criteria for retinopathy of prematurity: natural history data from the CRYO-ROP and LIGHT-ROP studies. *Arch Ophthalmol* 2002; 120:1470–1476.

29. Fielder A, Shaw D, Robinson J. Natural history of retinopathy of prematurity: a prospective study. *Eye* 1992; 6:10.

30. Repka MX, Palmer EA, Tung B. Involution of retinopathy of prematurity. Cryotherapy for Retinopathy of Prematurity Cooperative Group. *Arch Ophthalmol* 2000; 118:645–649.

31. Dobson V, Quinn Ge, Tung B, *et al*. Comparison of recognition and grating acuities in very-low-birth-weight children with and without retinal residua of retinopathy of prematurity. Cryotherapy for Retinopathy of Prematurity Cooperative Group. *Invest Ophthalmol Vis Sci* 1995; 36:692–702.

32. Gilbert WS, Dobson V, Quinn GE, *et al*. The correlation of visual function with posterior retinal structure in severe retinopathy of prematurity. Cryotherapy for Retinopathy of Prematurity Cooperative Group. *Arch Ophthalmol* 1992; 110:625–631.

33. Vander Veen DK, Coats DK, Dobson V, *et al*. Prevalence and course of strabismus in the first year of life of infants with pre-threshold retinopathy of prematurity. Findings from the ETROP study. *Arch Ophthalmol* 2006; 124:766–773.

34. Gilbert WS, Quinn GE, Dobson V, *et al*. Partial retinal detachment at 3 months after threshold retinopathy of prematurity. Long-term structural and functional outcome. Multicenter Trial of Cryotherapy for Retinopathy of Prematurity Cooperative Group. *Arch Ophthalmol* 1996; 114:1085–1091.

35. Reynolds J, Dobson V, Quinn GE, *et al*. Prediction of visual function in eyes with mild to moderate posterior pole residua of retinopathy of prematurity. Cryotherapy for Retinopathy of Prematurity Cooperative Group. *Arch Ophthalmol* 1993; 111:1050–1056.

36. Charan R, Dogra MR, Gupta A, *et al.* The incidence of retinopathy of prematurity in a neonatal care unit. *Indian J Ophthalmol* 1995; 43:123–126.

37. Fielder AR, Shaw DE, Robinson J, *et al.* Natural history of retinopathy of prematurity: a prospective study. *Eye* 1992; 6:233–242.

38. Zin A. The increasing problem of retinopathy of prematurity. *Community Eye Health J* 2001; 14: 58–59.

39. Gopal L, Sharma T, Ramachandran S, *et al.* Retinopathy of prematurity: a study. *Indian J Ophthalmol* 1995; 43:59–61.

40. Lundqvist P, Kallen K, Hallstrom I, *et al.* Trends in outcomes for very preterm infants in the Southern region of Sweden over a 10-year period. *Acta Paediatr* 2009; 98:648–653.

41. Hameed B , Shyamanur K, Kotecha S, *et al.* Trends in the incidence of severe Retinopathy of Prematurity in a geographically defined population over a ten year period. *Paediatrics* 2004; 113:1653–1657.

42. Agarwal R, Deorari AK, Azad RV, *et al.* Changing profile of Retinopathy of Prematurity. *J Trop Pediatrics* 2002; 48:239–242.

43. Clemett R, Darlow B. Results of screening low-birth-weight infants for retinopathy of prematurity. *Curr Opin Ophthalmol* 1999; 10:155–163.

44. Silverman WA. A cautionary tale about supplemental oxygen: the albatross of neonatal medicine. *Pediatrics* 2004; 113:394–396.

45. Lucey J, Dangman B. A reexamination of the role of oxygen in retrolental fibroplasia. *Pediatrics* 1984; 73:82–96.

46. Jalali S, Madhavi C, Reddy GP, *et al.* Pilot study on *in vivo* evaluation of retinal vascular maturity in newborn infants in the context of retinopathy of prematurity. *Am J Ophthalmol* 2006; 142:181–183.

47. Fortes Filho JB, Bonomo PP, Maia M, *et al.* Weight gain measured at 6 weeks after birth as a predictor for severe retinopathy of prematurity: study with 317 very low birth weight preterm babies. *Graef Arch Clin Exp* 2009; 247: 831–836.

48. Lofqvist C, Andersson E, Sigurdsson J, *et al.* Longitudinal postnatal weight and insulin-like growth factor I measurements in the prediction of retinopathy of prematurity. *Arch Ophthalmol* 2006; 124:1711–1718.

49. Holmstorm G. Genetic suseptibility to ROP: the evidence from clinical and experimental studies. *Br J Ophthalmol* 2007; 91:1704–1708.

50. Higgins RD, Mendelsohn Al, DeFoe MJ, *et al.* Antenatal dexamethasone and decreased severity of retinopathy of prematurity. *Arch Ophthalmol* 1998; 116:601–605.

51. Soll R. Proplylactic natural surfactant extract for preventing morbidity and mortality in preterm infants. *Cochrane Db Syst Rev* 2000; 2: CD0000122.

52. Askie L. Appropriate levels of oxygen saturation for preterm infants. *Acta Paediatr Suppl* 2004; 93:26–28.

53. Tin W, Milligan D, Pennefather P, *et al.* Pulse oximetry, severe Retinopathy and outcomes at one year in babies less than 28 weeks gestation. *Archives Dis Child- Fetal* 2001; 84:PF106–F110.

54. Smith LE. Through the eyes of a child: understanding retinopathy through ROP the Friedenwald lecture. *Invest Ophthalmol Vis Sci* 2008; 49:5177–5182.

55. Chen J, Smith LE. A double-edged sword: erythropoietin eyed in retinopathy of prematurity. *J AAPOS* 2008; 12:221–222.

56. Brion LP, Bell EF, Raghuveer TS. Vitamin E supplementation for prevention of morbidity and mortality in preterm infants. *Cochrane Db Syst Rev* 2003; 4:CD003665.

57. Raju TN, Langenberg P, Bhutani V, *et al.* Vitamin E prophylaxis to reduce retinopathy of prematurity: a reappraisal of published trials. *J Pediatr* 1997; 131:844–850.

58. Hellstrom A, Perruzzi C, Ju M, *et al.* Low IGF-I suppresses VEGF-survival signaling in retinal endothelial cells: direct correlation with clinical retinopathy of prematurity. *Proc Natl Acad Sci USA* 2001; 98:5804–5808.

59. Hellstrom A, Engstrom E, Hard AL, *et al.* Postnatal serum insulin-like growth factor I deficiency is associated with retinopathy of prematurity and other complications of premature birth. *Pediatrics* 2003; 112:1016–1020.

60. Lofqvist C, Hansen-Pupp I, Andersson E, *et al.* Validation of a new retinopathy of prematurity screening method monitoring longitudinal postnatal weight and insulin-like growth factor I. *Arch Ophthalmol* 2009; 127:622–627.

61. Chen J, Smith LE. Retinopathy of prematurity. *Angiogenesis* 2007; 10:133–140.

62. Heidary G, Vanderveen D, Smith LE. Retinopathy of prematurity: current concepts in molecular pathogenesis. *Semin Ophthalmol* 2009; 24:77–81.

63. Lofqvist C, Niklasson A, Engstrom E, *et al.* A Pharmacokinetic and dosing study of intravenous insulin-like growth factor-I and IGF-binding protein-3 complex to preterm infants. *Pediatr Res* 2009; 65:574–579.

64. Mantagos IS, Vanderveen DK, Smith LE. Emerging treatments for retinopathy of prematurity. *Semin Ophthalmol* 2009; 24:82–86.

65. Gaynon MW. Rethinking STOP-ROP: is it worthwhile trying to modulate excessive VEGF levels in prethreshold ROP eyes by systemic intervention? A review of the role of oxygen, light adaptation state, and anemia in prethreshold ROP. *Retina* 2006; 26:S18–23.

66. York JR, Landers S, Kirby RS, *et al.* Arterial oxygen fluctuation and retinopathy of prematurity in very-low-birth-weight infants. *J Perinatol* 2004; 24:82–87.

67. Cryotherapy for Retinopathy of Prematurity Cooperative Group. Multicenter trial of cryotherapy for retinopathy of prematurity. One-year outcome — structure and function. Cryotherapy for Retinopathy of Prematurity Cooperative Group. *Arch Ophthalmol* 1990; 108:1408–1416.

68. Cryotherapy for Retinopathy of Prematurity Cooperative Group. Multicenter trial of cryotherapy for retinopathy of prematurity. Three-month outcome. Cryotherapy for Retinopathy of Prematurity Cooperative Group. *Arch Ophthalmol* 1990; 108:195–204.

69. Cryotherapy for Retinopathy of Prematurity Cooperative Group. Contrast sensitivity at age 10 years in children who had threshold retinopathy of prematurity. *Arch Ophthalmol* 2001; 119:1129–1133.

70. Cryotherapy for Retinopathy of Prematurity Cooperative Group. Effect of retinal ablative therapy for threshold retinopathy of prematurity: results of Goldmann perimetry at the age of 10 years. *Arch Ophthalmol* 2001; 119:1120–1125.

71. Cryotherapy for Retinopathy of Prematurity Cooperative Group. Multicenter trial of cryotherapy for retinopathy of prematurity: ophthalmological outcomes at 10 years. *Arch Ophthalmol* 2001; 119:1110–1118.

72. Hardy RJ, Palmer EA, Dobson V, *et al.* Risk analysis of prethreshold retinopathy of prematurity. *Arch Ophthalmol* 2003; 121:1697–1701.

73. Jalali S, Hussain A. We can aim at better results in coming years. *Arch Ophthalmol* 2006; 124:604–605; author reply 605–606.

74. Azad RV, Pasamula L, Kumar H, *et al.* Prospective randomized evaluation of diode-laser and cryotherapy in prethreshold retinopathy of prematurity. *Clin Exp Ophthalmol* 2004; 32:251–254.

75. White JE, Repka MX. Randomized comparison of diode laser photocoagulation versus cryotherapy for threshold retinopathy of prematurity: 3-year outcome. *J Pediat Ophth Strab* 1997; 34:83–87; quiz 121–122.

76. The STOP-ROP Multicenter Study Group. Supplemental therapeutic oxygen for prethreshold retinopathy of prematurity (STOP-ROP), a randomized, controlled trial. I: primary outcomes. *Pediatrics* 2000; 105:295–310.

77. Mintz-Hittner HA, Kuffel RR Jr. Intravitreal injection of bevacizumab (avastin) for treatment of stage 3 retinopathy of prematurity in zone I or posterior zone II. *Retina* 2008; 28:831–838.

78. Chung EJ, Kim JH, Ahn HS, *et al.* Combination of laser photocoagulation and intravitreal bevacizumab (Avastin) for aggressive zone I retinopathy of prematurity. *Graef Arch Clin Exp* 2007; 245:1727–1730.

79. Travassos A, Teixeira S, Ferreira P, *et al.* Intravitreal bevacizumab in aggressive posterior retinopathy of prematurity. *Ophthalmic Surg Las Im* 2007; 38:233–237.

80. Kong L, Mintz-Hittner HA, Penland RL, *et al.* Intravitreous bevacizumab as anti-vascular endothelial growth factor therapy for retinopathy of prematurity: a morphologic study. *Arch Ophthalmol* 2008; 126:1161–1163.

81. Kusaka S, Shima C, Wada K, *et al.* Efficacy of intravitreal injection of bevacizumab for severe retinopathy of prematurity: a pilot study. *Br J Ophthalmol* 2008; 92:1450–1455.

82. Lalwani GA, Berrocal AL, Murray TG, *et al.* Off-label use of intravitreal bevacizumab (Avastin) for

salvage treatment in progressive threshold retinopathy of prematurity. *Retina* 2008; 28:S13–18.

83. Quiroz-Mercado H, Martinez-Castellanos MA, Hernandez-Rojas ML, *et al.* Antiangiogenic therapy with intravitreal bevacizumab for retinopathy of prematurity. *Retina* 2008; 28:S19–25.

84. Darlow BA, Gilbert C, Quinn GE, *et al.* Promise and potential pitfalls of anti-VEGF drugs in retinopathy of prematurity. *Br J Ophthalmol* 2009; 93:986.

85. Bhende P, Gopal L, Sharma T, *et al.* Functional and anatomical outcomes after primary lens-sparing pars plana vitrectomy for Stage 4 retinopathy of prematurity. *Indian J Ophthalmol* 2009; 57:267–271.

86. El Rayes EN, Vinekar A, Capone A Jr. Three-year anatomic and visual outcomes after vitrectomy for stage 4B retinopathy of prematurity. *Retina* 2008. 28:568–572.

87. Quinn GE, Dobson V, Barr CC, *et al.* Visual acuity in infants after vitrectomy for severe retinopathy of prematurity. *Ophthalmology* 1991; 98:5–13.

88. Quinn GE, Dobson V, Barr CC, *et al.* Visual acuity of eyes after vitrectomy for retinopathy of prematurity: follow-up at 5 1/2 years. The Cryotherapy for Retinopathy of Prematurity Cooperative Group. *Ophthalmology* 1996; 103:595–600.

89. Trese MT, Droste PJ. Long-term postoperative results of a consecutive series of stages 4 and 5 retinopathy of prematurity. *Ophthalmology* 1998; 105:992–997.

90. Jalali S, Anand R, Kumar H, *et al.* Programme planning and screening strategy in retinopathy of prematurity. *Indian J Ophthalmol* 2003; 51: 89–99.

91. Misra A, Heckford E, Curley A, *et al.* Do current retinopathy of prematurity screening guidelines miss the early development of pre-threshold type 1 ROP in small for gestational age neonates? *Eye* 2008; 22:825–829.

92. Gold R, Sprague J, Jaafar M, *et al.* Retinopathy of prematurity: the relationship between the pediatric ophthalmologist and the hospital. *J Pediatr Ophth Strab* 2007; 44:145–149.

93. FIelder AR, Levene MI. Screening for retinopathy of prematurity. *Arch Dis Child* 1992; 67:860–867.

94. Ziakas NG, Cottrell DG, Milligan DW, *et al.* Regionalisation of retinopathy of prematurity (ROP) screening improves compliance with guidelines: an audit of ROP screening in the Northern Region of England. *Br J Ophthalmol* 2001; 85:807–810.

95. Chen Y, Li XX, Yin H, *et al.* Risk factors for retinopathy of prematurity in six neonatal intensive care units in Beijing, China. *Br J Ophthalmol* 2008; 92:326–330.

96. Fortes Filho JB, Barros CK, da Costa MC, *et al.* Results of a program for the prevention of blindness caused by retinopathy of prematurity in southern Brazil. *J Pediatr (Rio J)* 2007; 83:209–216.

97. Varughese S, Gilbert C, Pieper C, *et al.* Retinopathy of prematurity in South Africa: an assessment of needs, resources and requirements for screening programmes. *Br J Ophthalmol* 2008; 92:879–882.

98. Wilson CM, Cocker KD, Moseley MJ, *et al.* Computerized analysis of retinal vessel width and tortuosity in premature infants. *Invest Ophthalmol Vis Sci* 2008; 49:3577–3585.

99. Wallace DK, Freedman SF, Zhao Z, *et al.* Accuracy of ROPtool vs individual examiners in assessing retinal vascular tortuosity. *Arch Ophthalmol* 2007; 125:1523–1530.

100. Gelman R, Jiang L, Du YE, *et al.* Diagnosis of plus disease in ROP using retinal image multiscale analysis. *Invest Ophthalmol Vis Sci* 2005; 46: 4734–4738.

101. Shah DN, Karp KA, Ying GS, *et al.* Image analysis of posterior pole vessels identifies type 1 retinopathy of prematurity. *J AAPOS* 2009; 13:507–508.

102. Shah DN, Wilson CM, Ying GS, *et al.* Semiautomated digital image analysis of posterior pole vessels in retinopathy of prematurity. *J AAPOS* 2009; 13:504–506.

103. Grunwald L, Mills MD, Johnson KS, *et al.* The rate of retinal vessel dilation in severe retinopathy of prematurity requiring treatment. *Am J Ophthalmol* 2009; 147:1086–1091.

104. Mills MD. Evaluating the Cryotherapy for Retinopathy of Prematurity Study (CRYO-ROP). *Arch Ophthalmol* 2007; 125:1276–1281.

105. Johnson KS, Mills MD, Karp KA, *et al.* Quantitative analysis of retinal vessel diameter reduction after photocoagulation treatment for retinopathy of prematurity. *Am J Ophthalmol* 2007; 143:1030–1032.

106. Johnson KS, Mills MD, Karp KA, *et al.* Semiautomated analysis of retinal vessel diameter in retinopathy of prematurity patients with and

without plus disease. *Am J Ophthalmol* 2007;
143:723–725.

107. Ells AL, Holmes JM, Astle WF, *et al.* Telemedicine
approach to screening for severe retinopathy of
prematurity: a pilot study. *Ophthalmology* 2003;
110:2113–2117.

108. Schwartz SD, Harrison SA, Ferrone PJ, *et al.*
Telemedical evaluation and management of
retinopathy of prematurity using a fiberoptic
digital fundus camera. *Ophthalmology* 2000; 107:
25–28.

109. Yen KG, Hess D, Burke B, *et al.* Telephoto-
screening to detect retinopathy of prematurity:
preliminary study of the optimum time to employ
digital fundus camera imaging to detect ROP. *J
AAPOS* 2002; 6:64–70.

110. Chiang MF, Wang L, Busuioc M, *et al.*
Telemedical retinopathy of prematurity diagnosis:
accuracy, reliability, and image quality. *Arch
Ophthalmol* 2007; 125:1531–1538.

111. Skalet AH, Quinn GE, Ying GS, *et al.*
Telemedicine screening for retinopathy of prematurity in developing countries using digital retinal
images: a feasibility project. *J AAPOS*, 2008; 12:
252–258.

112. Wallace DK, Jomier J, Aylward SR, *et al.*
Computer automated quantification of in ROP.
JAAPOS 2003; 7:126–130.

113. Lorenz B, Bock M, Muller HM, *et al.*
Telemedicine based screening of infants at risk for
retinopathy of prematurity. *Stud Health Technol
Inform* 1999; 64:155–163.

114. Roth DB, Morales D, Feuer WJ, *et al.* Screening
for retinopathy of prematurity employing the
Retcam 120: sensitivity and specificity. *Arch
Ophthalmol* 2001; 119:268–272.

15

Dry eye disease

DEBRA SCHAUMBERG AND GIULIO FERRARI

15.1	Definition	369		15.7	Risk factors	379
15.2	Classification	369		15.8	Cost	384
15.3	Pathophysiology	371		15.9	Quality of life	384
15.4	Challenges for diagnosis in dry eye epidemiology	373		15.10	Therapy	384
15.5	Demographic distribution of dry eye disease	374		15.11	Summary	385
15.6	Incidence and natural history	378		15.12	Future research needs	385
					References	385

15.1 DEFINITION

Dry eye disease (DED) is one of the most frequently encountered ocular morbidities. Sjögren, a Swedish ophthalmologist, was the first to describe DED, using the term 'keratoconjuntivitis sicca'. In 1950 De Roetth introduced the term 'dry eye'.[1] For many years, DED was considered to be due solely to a reduction of the aqueous phase of the tear film. More recently, however, it became clear that DED is a complex, multifactorial disease of the ocular surface.

In 1995, expert members of a National Eye Institute/Industry Dry Eye Workshop[2] proposed the following definition of dry eye: 'Dry Eye is a disorder of the tear film due to tear deficiency or excessive evaporation, which causes damage to the interpalpebral ocular surface and is associated with symptoms of ocular discomfort.' The definition of DED was updated in the 2007 Report of the **International Dry Eye Workshop (DEWS)**,[3] based on a comprehensive review and

interpretation by an international group of recognized experts of the state of knowledge on dry eye. The updated definition takes into account the role of tear hyperosmolarity and ocular surface inflammation in dry eye, and its effects on visual function. The updated definition reads: 'Dry eye is a multifactorial disease of the tears and ocular surface that results in symptoms of discomfort, visual disturbance, and tear film instability with potential damage to the ocular surface. It is accompanied by increased osmolarity of the tear film and inflammation of the ocular surface.'

15.2 CLASSIFICATION

DED can be divided into two major subclasses: **aqueous tear deficient dry eye (ADDE)** and **evaporative dry eye (EDE)**, though these are recognized to be non-mutually exclusive (Fig. 15.1).

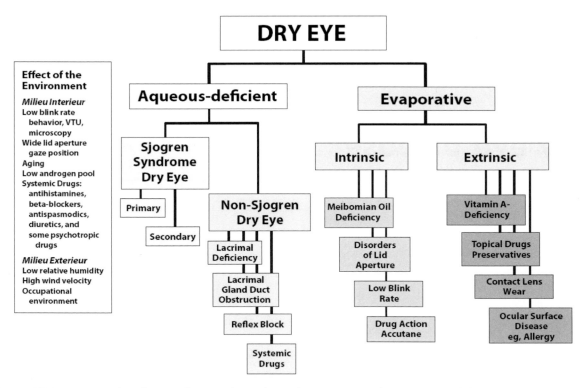

Figure 15.1 *Dry eye classification by aetiology (from the International Dry Eye Workshop, DEWS 2007; with permission)*

15.2.1   Aqueous tear deficient dry eye

ADDE is due to a failure of aqueous tear secretion, such as in lacrimal gland acinar destruction; this causes tear hyperosmolarity, which stimulates a cascade of inflammatory events such as release of inflammatory cytokines and matrix metalloproteinases.[4] It is not clear if tear evaporation is reduced or increased in ADDE.[5,6] It can be divided into two major subclasses: **Sjögren syndrome dry eye (SSDE)** and **non-Sjögren syndrome dry eye (NSSDE)**.

SSDE is an autoimmune disease in which the lacrimal and salivary glands are infiltrated by activated T-cells,[7] with consequent hyposecretion of tears and saliva. Sjögren's syndrome can occur as either a primary or secondary condition (the latter being associated with an overt autoimmune connective disorder, such as rheumatoid arthritis). The precise aetiology of SSDE is not known, but risk factors include genetic profile, low androgen pool, or environmental agents such as viral infections and polluted environments, as well as a

nutritional deficiency in omega-3 fatty acids and insufficient intake of vitamin C.[8]

NSSDE is due to lacrimal dysfunction that occurs in the absence of autoimmune features of SSDE. NSSDE can be found in association with a number of conditions, but it occurs most frequently as an age-related condition of unknown origin. Tear evaporation, volume, flow and osmolarity have been shown to change with age. In particular, tear evaporation, volume and flow were found reduced, while osmolarity increased with normal ageing in one study.[9] Other less frequent causes of NSSDE involving primary effects on the lacrimal gland are congenital alacrimia,[10] as in Allgrove syndrome, Addison's disease, autonomic dysautonomia, lacrimal gland infiltration (due to sarcoidosis,[11] lymphoma,[12,13] AIDS,[14] or graft versus host disease),[15] or lacrimal gland parasympathetic denervation.[16] NSSDE can also be induced by obstruction of the lacrimal gland ducts, which happens in cicatrizing conjunctivitis such as trachoma, pemphigoid, erythema multiforme, and chemical or thermal burns. Finally, NSSDE can be produced by nerve dysfunction affecting either the trigeminal (5th) cranial nerve or facial (7th) cranial nerve. The anterior segment of the eye is richly innervated by the trigeminal nerve, which continuously generates a sensory input responsible for tear secretion. Loss of trigeminal innervation reduces both tear secretion and blink rate. This condition is also named neurotrophic keratopathy, because pathologic findings such as punctate keratitis, oedema and sterile ulcers can develop in the cornea. Diabetes, contact lens wear, especially hard contact lenses, and refractive surgery such as LASIK[17,18] are responsible for alterations in trigeminal innervation and can contribute to development of DED symptoms in these patients.[19] Central damage to the facial nerve leads to dry eye owing to loss of lacrimal secretomotor function, which is aggravated by **lagophthalmos**.

15.2.2 Evaporative dry eye

Evaporative dry eye (EDE) is due to excessive water loss in the presence of a normal lacrimal secretory function. Causes of EDE can be divided into intrinsic (affecting the structure or function of the lids or Meibomian glands) and extrinsic. Intrinsic causes include Meibomian gland dysfunction,[20] disorders of lid aperture such as lagophthalmos, and a low blink rate[21] (such as happens when working at video terminals or in Parkinson's disease). Meibomian gland dysfunction is thought to be by far the most common underlying cause of EDE. Although its precise causes are unknown, and it is likely to be multifactorial in origin, some conditions have been hypothesized to contribute to Meibomian gland dysfunction. These include rosacea, seborrhoeic dermatitis, atopic dermatitis, and isotretinoin treatment (which leads to reversible Meibomian gland atrophy).

Extrinsic causes of EDE are thought to include vitamin A deficiency, which causes loss of goblet cells and lacrimal gland acinar damage; topical drugs and preservatives; contact lens wear; and allergic conjunctivitis. Many components of various therapeutic eye drop formulations can induce a toxic response from the ocular surface; among these, benzalkonium chloride — a preservative — is probably the most common culprit. Contact lens wearers were cited to number about 35 million in

the USA in the year 2000,[22] of whom about 50% report dry eye symptoms.[23]

15.3 PATHOPHYSIOLOGY

The ocular surface is part of a functional system termed the 'ocular surface system'.[24] This is defined as the wet-surfaced and glandular epithelia of the cornea, conjunctiva, and lacrimal gland, accessory lacrimal glands, nasolacrimal duct and Meibomian glands, and their apical and basal matrices, linked as a functional system by both continuity of epithelia, by innervation, and the endocrine and immune systems. The main purpose of the system is to maintain a smooth refractive surface for clear vision. At least in theory, an alteration in one or more its components can result in a change in the tear film composition (osmolarity, volume) and this can lead to desiccation and epithelial damage, which triggers a release of inflammatory mediators, leading to chronic damage of the ocular surface system as seen in DED. To further describe the pathophysiology of DED, the different components of the ocular surface system will be now considered.

15.3.1 Tears and tear film

The tear film is composed of three layers, namely an inner mucin layer (approximately 0.8 μ thick, composed of multiple mucins), an intermediate aqueous layer (8 μ), and an outer lipid layer (0.1 μm). Mucins are produced by the conjunctival goblet cells and by stratified squamous cells of the cornea and conjunctiva. The aqueous layer is produced by the main and accessory lacrimal glands, and contains water, electrolytes, antibacterial proteins and growth factors. The lipid layer is produced by the Meibomian tarsal glands, with a small contribution from the glands of Zeis. Functions of the tear film include lubrication of the ocular surface and eyelids; provision of a regular optical surface for the eye; removal of foreign material from the ocular surface; and the supply of nutrients to the ocular surface. It also provides antibacterial substances, and promotes tissue

(*Continued*)

(*Continued*)

maintenance and wound healing of the ocular surface. Alterations of tear composition in DED involve a reduction in the amount, increased osmolarity, reductions in specific protein content (e.g. lysozyme and lactoferrin), changes in matrix metallo proteinases and mucin concentration, and alterations in Meibomian lipid composition.[2]

15.3.2 *Surface of the eye*

The ocular surface is composed of the cornea and the conjunctiva. The corneal surface is covered by a multi-layered epithelium; the conjunctiva is a thin mucous membrane, consisting of an epithelial layer with goblet cells, which secrete mucins to comprise the innermost tear film layer. The normal wet-surfaced epithelium of the ocular surface forms a barrier to the outside environment. This function is lost in DED as is shown by an increased uptake of vital dyes owing to corneal and conjunctival epithelial cell damage. Moreover, anatomic changes such as reduction in mucin secreting cells in advanced DED,[25] and keratinization of conjunctival epithelial cells, have been documented. Corneal innervation and sensation are also altered in DED.[26,27] Conjunctival cells may actively sustain the pathologic process in DED by secreting pro-inflammatory mediators in response to various stimuli ranging from environmental to iatrogenic factors.

15.3.3. *Immune system*

Both T-cell populations and pro-inflammatory cytokines are increased in DED. A form of DED occurring in association with graft versus host disease is also associated with inflammation and immune cell infiltration of the lacrimal gland and the surface epithelia of the eye.[28] However, it is not clear whether immune activation is a cause or a consequence of the complex pathophysiology of DED. Schein *et al.* found no association of

(*Continued*)

(*Continued*)

DE symptoms with rheumatoid arthritis or the presence of auto-antibodies to the soluble nuclear antigens Ro/SS-A and La/SS-B. This was further supported by finding no association after restricting the DE group only to patients with both symptoms and abnormal tests (**Schirmer, Rose Bengal**).[29] Consequently, at least in the general elderly population, DE symptoms are unlikely to have an autoimmune basis. Nonetheless, such mechanisms have been shown to intervene once the degenerative process has started, and finally to contribute to perpetuating the vicious cycle of DED.

15.3.4 *Lacrimal glands*

The lacrimal glands are responsible for production of the aqueous tear component, and many but not all patients with DED show indications of insufficient aqueous tear secretion. Anatomical findings in the lacrimal gland in DE include a reduction in its innervations,[30] increased apoptosis[31] and fibrosis.[32] However, little is known about accessory lacrimal glands, which are embedded in the subconjunctival tissue at the ocular surface, and are considered to be important targets for topical therapeutic interventions. In DED associated with Sjögren's syndrome, infiltration of the lacrimal gland with lymphocytes has been demonstrated, together with Fas–Fas ligand expression.[31] The majority of these T-cells are autoreactive CD4+ that seem to surround B-cells.[33] DED has been also associated with HIV and hepatitis C (HCV) infection,[34] and postulated mechanisms include lacrimal gland infiltration by T-cells[35] in HIV, direct infection of the gland by HCV, and molecular mimicry between the gland and HCV leading to an immune reaction to lacrimal gland tissue. This immune reaction may be mediated by immune complex deposition and/or lymphocytic infiltration.[34] Finally, an auto-antibody against the M3 muscarinic acetylcholine receptor has been identified, and its increased serum

(*Continued*)

(Continued)

concentration is related to increased rose bengal staining scores.[36] It is possible that chronic interaction of these auto-antibodies would induce desensitization, internalization, and/or intracellular degradation finally contributing to the reduction of tear secretion in DED patients. It is not completely clear, however, how the main lacrimal gland, accessory lacrimal glands and the nasolacrimal duct interrelate in DED.

15.3.5 Meibomian glands

Meibomian glands are large modified sebaceous glands that produce the tear film lipid layer. It has been suggested that Meibomian gland dysfunction may be a contributing factor in over 60% of all DE patients.[37] More specifically, a reduction or alteration in the quality of Meibomian gland lipids,[38] together with a keratinization of ductal epithelium and orifice metaplasia, have been noticed. Of possible interest, nutrient intake (such as omega-3 fatty acids) has been associated with alterations in the polar lipid profiles of Meibomian gland secretions.[39]

15.4 CHALLENGES FOR DIAGNOSIS IN DRY EYE EPIDEMIOLOGY

The epidemiology of DE is still in its infancy, not having emerged before the mid-1990s, i.e. much later as compared with other ocular or systemic diseases (Fig.15.2).

Although a variety of diagnostic tests for DED are commonly used in clinical settings, and a number of questionnaire-based methods of assessment have been developed for use in both the clinic and in large-scale epidemiological studies, there is no single diagnostic test, or combination of tests, that can be performed in the field or in the clinic to distinguish reliably people with and without DED. Some of the difficulty relates to the relatively weak correlation between patients' irritative ocular symptoms and the results of selected clinical tests for dry eye. Other, and possibly related, difficulties include the lack of repeatability of many of the clinical tests, natural variability of the disease process, the subjective nature of symptoms, and presumed variability in pain thresholds and cognitive responses to questions about the physical sensations of the ocular surface. Some patients with DED may develop relative corneal anaesthesia with

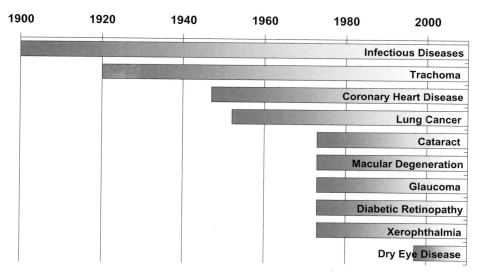

Figure 15.2 *Temporal development of modern epidemiology. Note that the epidemiology of dry eye has been studied only recently*

ageing, and with deteriorating disease this may affect their ability to sense dry eye symptoms.

In the light of these challenges, most researchers have recognized that, at its core, dry eye is a symptomatic disease, and that symptom questionnaires are among the most reliable and repeatable of the commonly used diagnostic tests. Symptomatic irritation is largely responsible for the public health burden of DED, and studies have also shown that symptom assessment is the single most important of all the available tests for dry eye in the clinic, and can provide an integrated view of the clinical condition over time. With these important issues in mind, individual research groups have formed, and used, a number of definitions of dry eye for purposes of their research, usually based on questionnaire assessment of symptoms and sometimes combined with additional clinical measures. When interpreting the epidemiological literature on DED and comparing study findings, it is consequently important to take these differences into account.

15.5 DEMOGRAPHIC DISTRIBUTION OF DRY EYE DISEASE

15.5.1 Prevalence

Comparison of age-specific data on the prevalence of dry eye from large epidemiological studies[40] reveals a range of about 5% to over 35% at various ages.[41] Such a large difference can be at least partly explained by the fact that different definitions of dry eye were used in these studies, but there may also be true differences in prevalence amongst various populations.

The largest epidemiological studies of dry eye to date come from the **Women's Health Study (WHS)**, and the **Physicians' Health Study (PHS)** cohorts. DED was defined by the presence of severe symptoms of DED (both dryness and irritation either constantly or often) or a clinical diagnosis of DED, based on a validated questionnaire-based assessment method.[42] Based on data from the 39,876 participants in the WHS and 25,444 participants in the PHS, it has been estimated that about 7.8% or 3.23 million women and

4.34% or 1.68 million men aged 50 years and older have dry eye in the USA. Millions more report less severe symptoms, and probably a more episodic manifestation of the disease, triggered by adverse contributing factor(s), such as wind, low humidity or contact lens wear.

USA

Other USA-based estimates come from the **Salisbury Eye Evaluation** (SEE) and the **Beaver Dam Eye Study** (BDES). In the former, the first large epidemiological study to undertake an assessment of DED, a dry eye questionnaire was administered to a population-based sample of 2,520 volunteers aged 65 to 84 years; approximately 15% of participants reported experiencing one or more of six DE symptoms often or all the time; 20% reported experiencing three or more symptoms sometimes, often or all the time. The frequencies of six symptoms were investigated: eyes feel dry, eyes feel gritty or sandy, eyes burn, eyes appear red, crust forms on lashes, and eyelids stick shut in the morning. Possible answers were: never, rarely, sometimes, often, or all the time. If a positive answer was taken to mean a symptom reported to 'occur often or all the time', then approximately 15% of the subjects reported DE symptoms. The study also evaluated clinical signs of DED, and 2.2% were both symptomatic and had a low Schirmer test (tear-flow) result, and 2% were symptomatic and had a high rose bengal test score. Furthermore, 3.5% were symptomatic and had either a low Schirmer score or a high rose bengal score, and 0.7% were symptomatic and had both a low Schirmer score and a high rose bengal score.

In the BDES, a population that was 48 to 91 years of age (n = 3,722) was asked a question regarding their experience of dry eye: 'For the past three months or longer, have you had dry eyes?' The prevalence of DE was found to be 14.4% and was significantly associated with age.[43]

Canada

In Canada the prevalence of DED was evaluated by **The Canada Dry Eye Epidemiology Study,**

(CANDEES). This clinic-based study evaluated, by means of a questionnaire, the prevalence of DE symptoms. The questionnaire return rate was 15.7%. Questionnaires were analyzed from 13,517 patients — of whom 60.7% were females aged from < 10 years to > 80 years. A total of 28.7% reported dry eye symptoms; severe symptoms were reported by 1 in 225 patients.[23] The data were collected from patients referred to optometric practices in Canada, which can explain why the DED prevalence was found higher than those studies addressing general population samples.

Australia

In Australia, two main studies of dry eye prevalence have been conducted within the **Blue Mountains Eye Study** (**BMES**),[44] and the **Melbourne Visual Impairment Project** (**VIP**)[40] study populations. The BMES examined 1,174 subjects 50 years or older, and found a prevalence of 16.6% of patients reporting at least one symptom of DED out of four symptoms asked (dry eye, grittiness, itchiness, discomfort), and 15.3% reporting three or more symptoms. Moderate to severe symptoms were more frequent in women, while no age-related trend or significant ocular association was observed. The VIP[40] examined 926 participants 40 years or older, and reported the prevalence of at least one of six severe symptoms not attributed by the subject to hay fever, and found a prevalence of 5.5%. The tested symptoms were discomfort, foreign body sensation, itching, tearing, dryness and photophobia. Examination of the eye was also performed. Overall, DE was diagnosed as follows: 10.8% by rose bengal, 16.3% by Schirmer's test, 8.6% by **tear film break-up time (BUT)**, 1.5% by **fluorescein staining**, 7.4% with two or more signs, and 5.5% with any severe symptom not attributed to hay fever. Age was found to be a significant risk factor for two or more clinical signs of DE. Moreover, women were significantly more likely to report severe symptoms of dry eye (OR = 1.85; 95% CL = 1.01, 3.41), but were not significantly more likely to have two or more signs of dry eye.

Asia

A population-based study conducted in Indonesia involving 1,058 subjects aged 21 years and older found a prevalence of DED of 27.5%.[45] DED was defined as a report of at least one of six symptoms of DED, often or all the time. The six symptoms assessed were dryness, grittiness or 'sandiness', burning, redness, crusting, and eyes stuck shut. A positive trend was found between age and prevalence of DED. The prevalence of DE was 1.4 times higher for men than for women and a protective effect of female sex (p < 0.001, OR 0.6; 95% CI 0.5–0.8) was found in relation to dry eye symptoms, but such a relation did not remain significant after multivariate adjustment. A study in Taiwan, using the same method of DED assessment, considered a population of 2,038 subjects aged 65 years and older, and found a prevalence of 33.7%. Women were more likely to report dry eye symptoms than men (OR 1.49; 95% CI 1.19–1.87); when the symptoms in the questionnaire were analyzed individually, only the symptoms of sticky and watery eyes were significantly related to gender (both p = 0.001). If these symptoms were omitted from the analysis, the gender difference for DE symptoms disappeared. This study did not find a significant association between DE symptoms and age, even if frequent dry eye symptoms were reported somewhat more often in the ≥ 80-year-old patients (37.5%) than in the 65–69 year old group (32.2%).[41] In Japan, a study was conducted on 2,500 subjects based on a 30-question self-administered questionnaire, and 33% of participants responded that they believed they had dry eye according to the self-diagnosis criteria, of which 25% used daily over-the-counter eye drops.[46] The prevalence of DED was also studied among Japanese high-school students[47] (age range 15–18 years). They consented to answer the three-question dry eye questionnaire used in the WHS and PHS[48] translated into Japanese and sent to them by mail. This consisted of the following question items: 1) Have you ever been diagnosed by a clinician as having dry eye syndrome? 2) How often do your eyes feel dry (not wet enough)? and 3) How often do your eyes feel irritated? DED was defined as the presence of either a previous clinical diagnosis of dry eye disease or severe symptoms (both dryness and irritation either constantly or often). Clinically diagnosed dry eye disease was present in 4.3% of the male and, significantly more, 8.0% of female subjects. Severe symptoms of dry eye disease were observed in 21.0% of boys and 24.4% of girls.

European studies

A recent study from Spain[49] addressed the prevalence of dry eye and its relationship with lifestyle and systemic factors in an adult population. Both signs and symptoms of DED were assessed. Symptoms were assessed using the questionnaire developed by Schein *et al.*[50] while clinical signs obtained included the Schirmer test, tear film break-up time, fluorescein and rose bengal stainings. Dry eye was defined as the simultaneous presence of symptoms and at least one sign. Subjects were considered symptomatic when at least one of the symptoms of the questionnaire was experienced often or all the time. Based on this definition, DE prevalence was found to be 11.0%. Dry eye was found to be more frequent in women (11.9%, 95% CI 8.8–15.1) than in men (9.0%, 95% CI 5.3–12.6) and was significantly associated with ageing ($p < 0.001$).

A summary of DE prevalence, as found from various studies is provided in Table 15.1.

Prevalence of DE clinical signs has been assessed in various studies, which used different cut-offs to define normal subjects. The results are summarized in Table 15.2.

Table 15.1 *Prevalence of dry eye disease in various populations, based on symptom assessment*

Study	Number	Age	Age association	Prevalence	More frequent in females	Female–male difference
US STUDIES						
Salisbury Eye Study	2,420	≥ 65 y	No	14.6%	Inconclusive	Females 5–8% express
Beaver Dam	3,722	≥ 48 y	Yes	14.4%	Yes	Females 17%, Males 11.1% (p < 0.001)
Women's Health Study*	36,995	≥ 49 y	Yes	7.8%	Study only included females	na
Physician's Health Study I and II*	25,655	≥ 50, 55 y	Yes	4.34%	Study only included males	na
EUROPEAN STUDIES						
Salnes Eye Study	654	40–96	Yes	11%	Yes	Females 11.9%, (95% CI 8.8–15.1) Males 9%, (95% CI 5.3–12.6)
AUSTRALIAN STUDIES						
Blue Mountains Eye Study	1,075	≥ 50 y	No	16.6% (1 symptom) 15.3% (≥ 3 symptoms)	Yes	OR 1.5, (95% CI 1.1–2.2)
Melbourne Visual Impairment Project	926	≥ 40 y	Yes	5.5%	Yes	OR 1.85; (95% CI 1.01,3.41)
ASIAN STUDIES						
Shihpai, Taiwan	2,038	≥ 65 y	No	33.7%	Yes	OR 1.49; (95% CI 1.19–1.87)
Sumatra, Indonesia	1,058	≥ 21 y	Yes	27.5%	No (protective effect of female versus DE symptoms)	OR 0.6; (95% CI 0.5–0.8)
Japan	2,500	Average	na	33%	Inconclusive	
Japan Ministry of Health	3,433	15–18 y	na	6.15%	Yes	Females 8% (95% CI 7.4%–8.4%) Males 4.3% (95% CI 3.9%–4.6%)

* These two studies of female health professionals and male physicians, respectively, were conducted using the same methodology and allowed for a direct comparison of the prevalence of dry eye in women versus men.

Table 15.2 *Dry eye disease clinical signs*

Study	Schirmer test		Tear break-up time		Rose bengal stain		Fluorescein stain	
	Prevalence	Cut-off	Prevalence	Cut-off*	Prevalence	Cut-off	Prevalence	Cut-off
Salisbury Eye Study	11.9%	≤ 5 mm	na	na	11.3%	≥ 5	na	na
Salnes Eye Study	37%	≤ 5 mm	15.6%	≤ 10 s	13%	≥ 3	7%	≥ 1
Melbourne Visual Impairment Project	16.3%	< 8 mm	8.6%	< 8 s	10.8%	> 3	1.5%	> 1/3
Shihpai Eye Study	21.1%	≤ 5 mm	26.6%	≤ 10 s	na	na	11.3%	≥ 1

* Seconds.

15.5.2   Differences by age and sex

Increasing age and female sex have been associated with a higher prevalence of DED in most studies (Table 15.1). Some have theorized that such differences can be explained by an increase in DED occurring after the menopause in women and a corresponding reduction of tear production around the sixth decade.[51] However, the weight of the evidence suggests that DED is more common among women than men at all ages, including among age groups in which the majority of women would be premenopausal. Moreover, in the WHS, menopause itself was not associated with the prevalence of DED.[52] There are inconclusive reports regarding possible effects of oral contraceptive use, pregnancy, hysterectomy and ovarian dysfunction on DED,[53, 54] and more research of these parameters is needed.

Ageing is thought to be associated with the development of Meibomian gland dysfunction, which promotes tear film instability and evaporative dry eye. Alterations in lacrimal secretion with age may also contribute to age-related differences in dry eye. There have been surprisingly few studies, however, of tear film characteristics and possible alterations in production of various tear components with normal ageing. In one small study, it was shown that there is a high correlation between ageing and tear volume (r = −0.64), Schirmer test (r = −0.63), and tear osmolarity (r = 0.59).[9] This study, however, did not separate subjects by gender, and contained more females than males. Craig *et al.*[55] found that age did not affect tear film osmolality (which is generally thought to be increased in DED) when all subjects were considered, but, when

separated by gender, a significant relationship was found to exist only for females. Moreover, no significant age effect was found for tear production in that study, suggesting that perhaps ageing alone does not result in alterations of tear production.

It has been hypothesized that alterations in androgen levels may contribute to a higher risk of dry eye among women, and, with ageing, in both sexes, thereby providing a unifying explanation for observations of a higher prevalence of DED in ageing, menopause, the complete androgen insufficiency syndrome, and Sjögren's syndrome.[56] In support of this view, some of the anatomical and physiological modifications of the Meibomian gland during ageing have been linked to androgen deficiency,[57] which tallies with what is known about androgenic control of sebaceous glands in the skin.[58] Androgen levels are lower in women than in men throughout life, and both sexes experience a decline in bioavailable androgen levels as they age.[59–62] The effects of this decline in androgen bioavailability with ageing are only beginning to be understood. In small clinic-based studies, chronic androgen deficiency, use of antiandrogen medications, and complete androgen insufficiency syndrome have been shown to be linked to Meibomian gland dysfunction and evaporative DED.[61–65]

15.5.3   Differences by race/ethnicity

The potential effect of race and ethnicity on dry eye is still little understood; however, data from the prevalence surveys conducted to date raise the possibility of a higher prevalence of DED among Asian populations as compared with the primarily white populations of the USA and Europe. Although differences in definition and methodology among these studies might account for some of the apparent differences, recent studies in the USA, Europe and Asia have used the same assessment methods and criteria for diagnosis of DED, and found a higher prevalence of DED in Asian populations. For example, a recent population-based study in Indonesia[45] has found that the age-adjusted prevalence of DE was 27.5%, and a similar study in Taiwan found a prevalence of 19.2%.[41] Both these estimates are substantially higher than the 14% prevalence found in the USA in the Salisbury study using the same assessment tool.[50] On the other hand, the prevalence of DED was found to be 11% in a Spanish population, with the same symptom questionnaire, similar to estimates derived from the Salisbury study in the USA.

Possible explanations for prevalence differences could include true differences due to anatomic differences in eye-lid structure or tear film components (though there is no evidence for the latter), possible bias in participation rates, population-based differences in the propensity to report symptoms, as well as possible differences in environmental conditions or other risk factors that might contribute to the development of DED. For example, it has been hypothesized that the higher levels of sunlight exposure and ambient temperature experienced by people in Indonesia may increase the frequency of DE symptoms, whereas high humidity in other environments could be protective. Interestingly, the Indonesian study found DE risk doubled in patients with pterygium, which affected 40% of the subjects. A case-control study[66] has found an association between pterygium and a shortened tear break-up time and Schirmer's test, and a decreased tear function index. Although these findings are supported by an earlier study,[67] conflicting results have also been obtained.[68] Pathological conjunctival, corneal or eyelid changes in pterygia could lead to a disturbed tear film function[69] or, conversely, an unstable tear film in dry eye could contribute to the initiation of pterygium. Pterygium may also well be a surrogate for the environmental factors associated with dry eye, as ultraviolet light, for example, has also been implicated in pterygium formation.[70]

It is to be noted that the Shiphai study found a higher prevalence of patients with low Schirmer test scores (21.1%) when compared with the Melbourne study (16.3%) and the Salisbury study (11.9%), but not with the Spanish population assessed in the Salnes study (37%). Low tear break-up time and high fluorescein staining were also found to be more frequently present in the Shihpai population in comparison with the Salnes and Melbourne study. However, such comparisons must be treated with care as the various studies used different cut-offs for the same tests, and the methodology of test performance was not standardized.

Finally, data from the WHS, in which a sizeable number of both white and minority US women were surveyed, also suggest the prevalence of dry eye symptoms may be greater in Asian as well as Hispanic women, as compared with non-Hispanic whites in the USA.[48] However, in the similarly conducted PHS, there was no significant difference in the prevalence of DED by race/ethnicity, though the proportion of minority participants in that study was small.

15.6 INCIDENCE AND NATURAL HISTORY

Data on the incidence and natural history of DED are scarce. At present, the incidence of dry eye in an adult population[71] (aged 43 to 84) has been reported only in the Beaver Dam Eye Study. The cumulative incidence of DED was based on participants' responses to the question: 'For the past three months or longer, have you had dry eyes?' The five-year cumulative incidence was found to be 13.3% (95% CI 12–14.7), whereas 21.6% (95% CI 19.9–23.3) had developed DED over ten years. The cumulative incidence of DED and was significantly higher with older age (Table 15.3), and was greater in women (ten-year cumulative incidence = 25.0%) than men (ten-year cumulative incidence = 17.2%, p < 0.001).[72]

In another USA study, Ellwein et al.[73] extracted data from fee-for-service physician claims from a 5% sample of Medicare beneficiaries 65 years and older. Use of eye care services and procedures, frequency of ocular diagnoses, and allowed charges were compared for each year from 1991 through 1998. Annual case incidence of DED ranged from 1.22 cases per 100 people in 1991 to 1.92 per 100 people in 1998 (57.4% increase). These data clearly underestimate the actual prevalence of DED as the study was based on Medicare diagnosis, and it is well known that not all cases of DED in a population are usually diagnosed. For example, in the Physician's Health Study[56] fewer than half (40.7%) of the men with severe DED symptoms (both dryness and irritation experienced at least often) reported being diagnosed with dry eye. Similar findings were also observed in the Women's Health Study.[48]

Table 15.3 *Odds for five- and ten-year incidence of dry eye for ten-year increase in baseline age in the Beaver Dam Eye Study*[71]

Characteristic	Incidence	P value	OR (95% CI)
Age, y	5 yrs cumulative incidence	0.04	1.14 (1.01–1.30)*
	10 yrs cumulative incidence	< 0.001	1.21 (1.09–1.34)*

* The data indicate, for example, that person who is 70 years old now would have a 14% higher chance of developing dry eye within five years, and a 21% higher chance of developing dry eye within ten years compared with a person who is 60 years old now.

The natural history of DED is still to be determined. Prognostic factors, rates of progression or remission of the disease, and treatment effects all remain to be fully elucidated.

15.7 RISK FACTORS

Epidemiological studies have only begun to address the evidence for potential lifestyle, dietary, behavioural and other risk factors for dry eye. Many studies to date have used a purely statistical non-hypothesis-driven approach to search for risk factors, and these findings must be viewed cautiously as spurious results are likely, and, at the same time, important associations could have easily been overlooked. It is also important to bear in mind that risk factors for aqueous deficient versus evaporative subtypes of dry eye might differ, which could invalidate associations in most studies where all forms of dry eye are combined.

15.7.1 Environmental influences

Relative humidity (RH), indoor environment and air pollution may play a role in the prevalence of DED. Relative humidity should be about 40%;[74] in an experiment involving contact lens wearers,[75] subjects in low humidity environments (less than 30%) showed significantly shorter break-up times (BUT) on the lens and more prominent lens deposits, than subjects in higher RH environments (RH of more than 40%). Of course, as many subjects living in lower humidity environments are completely asymptomatic, other parameters, such as room temperature, air velocity and indoor air pollution, may also be important. Complaints such as ocular burning, dryness, stinging and grittiness are often reported in epidemiologic studies of the health consequences of indoor air environments.[76] Extended visual tasks associated with computer or television use and prolonged reading, provoke symptoms of DED (as shown by Schindelar *et al.*, **ARVO** 2008, and Shimmura *et al.*[46]). Although the underlying cause of these symptoms remains unclear, it is plausible that low humidity, high room temperature and air velocity, decreased blink rate, or indoor pollution or air quality could lead to ocular dryness due to increased tear evaporation.[77,78] Other ultra-low humidity environments such as aircraft cabins have also been associated with dry eye symptoms.[79,80] Exposure to sun, dust and wind may exacerbate DED,[81] though epidemiological data on such factors are lacking.

15.7.2 Ocular factors

Contact lens wear

Long-term contact lens wear can precipitate and/or exacerbate DED, as it desensitizes the cornea over years of contact lens wear.[46,47,82] It has been suggested that potential mechanisms of contact lens-related dry eye include increased evaporation of the tear film,[2] reduced ability to produce adequate tears with concurrent increased osmolarity,[83] drying related to lack of biocompatibility of the lens surface,[84] or any combination of these. Yet the true aetiology of contact lens-related dry eye remains elusive.

As regards the relationship between DED and contact lens wear, it has been suspected for a long time that contact lens wear increases the occurrence of Meibomian gland dysfunction (the largest cause of EDE). However, the largest study comparing the prevalence of Meibomian gland dysfunction among contact lens wearers and non-wearers, showed only a small non-significant excess of Meibomian gland dysfunction in contact lens wearers (41%) versus non-wearers (38%), which is not likely to be clinically relevant.[85]

Nonetheless, symptoms of dry eye can reach estimates of 50–75% among contact lens wearers,[23,86–89] suggesting that as many as 17 million Americans may have at least transient DE when wearing contact lenses. One study of 415 contact lens wearers identified several factors that were more likely to be found among symptomatic wearers, including female sex, higher water content contact lenses, rapid prelens tear film thinning time, frequent usage of over-the-counter pain medication, limbal injection, and increased tear film osmolality.[90] Although such patients may not experience DED when not wearing contact lenses, their symptoms of dryness and discomfort are reported as the most frequent factor contributing to the abandonment of contact lens wear.[91] For example, in a study by Prichard and co-workers, 12% of contact lens patients discontinued lens wear within five years of starting owing to DE symptoms.[92]

Refractive surgery

Refractive surgery is associated with development of DE, as patients can experience significant DE for several months after corneal refractive surgery such as *laser in situ keratomileusis* (*LASIK*) or photorefractive keratectomy (PRK); this is probably due to the severing of corneal nerves during the operation.[93,94] Significant effort has been put into trying to determine whether measurable preoperative characteristics predispose patients to chronic dry eye after LASIK. One study by Konomi *et al.* has

shown that pre-operative tear volume may affect recovery of the ocular surface after LASIK, and may increase the risk for chronic dry eye.[95] In a second study, Albietz *et al.*[17] examined the relationship between chronic dry eye and refractive regression after LASIK for myopia; a retrospective analysis was done collecting data before and after LASIK. Regression after LASIK was related to chronic dry eye and it occurred in 12 (27%) of 45 patients with chronic dry eye and in 34 (7%) of 520 patients without (p < 0.0001). The risk for chronic DED was significantly associated with female sex, higher attempted refractive correction, greater ablation depth, and the following pre-LASIK variables: increased ocular surface staining; lower tear volume, tear stability, and corneal sensation; and dry-eye symptoms before LASIK. The rate of DED appears to be the highest immediately after surgery, and significantly associated with the extent of preoperative myopia and ablation depth.96 It has been estimated that the prevalence of DED in LASIK patient without a prior history of DED ranges from 0.25%[97] up to 48%.[98] However, some authors report a return of the Schirmer 1 test to baseline by one year postoperatively.[99] Wound healing may be compromised by DED, which has been associated with an increased risk of refractive regression.[17]

15.7.3 Social and dietary habits

Cigarette smoking and alcohol consumption

Social and dietary habits may also influence the development of DED. Cigarette smoking was identified as an independent risk factor for DED in one study,[45] and it seems reasonable to hypothesize that cigarette smoking could affect risk of DED through its effects on inflammatory mechanisms, nutrition, or possibly via direct toxicity to the ocular surface. A positive association between DED and smoking was also demonstrated by the Blue Mountains and Beaver Dam incidence studies. The Melbourne and Salisbury studies, however, failed to show such a correlation. Additional support for this hypothesis is currently lacking.

Regarding alcohol, the Melbourne and Salisbury studies failed to show a correlation with DED, but an association was found by the Blue Mountains study. Conflicting results have been shown by the Beaver Dam Eye Study, in which a protective effect of alcohol on the incidence of DED was observed, whereas the previous analysis from this group study found an association between heavy drink history and a higher prevalence of DED. It is thought that a strong biological rationale for alcohol consumption and DED is lacking, though indirect effects are possible.

Dietary factors

In a large study of USA women in the WHS, a greater dietary intake of omega-3 fatty acids was found to be associated with a lower prevalence of DED.[100] Each additional gram of omega-3 fatty acid consumption per day demonstrated a 30% reduction in risk of DED. Moreover, the ratio between ω-3 and ω-6 fatty acid appears to be important: the higher the ratio, the lower the risk of DED. Another study showed that women with Sjögren syndrome had a significantly lower intake of ω-3 fatty acids as compared with age-matched controls.[8] Intake of ω-3 fatty acids has also been correlated with alterations in the polar lipid pattern of Meibomian gland secretions in women with Sjögren's syndrome.[38]

In small clinical studies, supplementation of patients with DED using certain ω-6 fatty acids seems to improve symptoms and some signs of DED, even if the mechanism is still unclear. This could happen via the production of prostaglandin E1, an anti-inflammatory eicosanoid product of the ω-6 pathway.[101] Only one clinical trial so far has evaluated ω-3 supplementation effect in DED. In this study, approximately 3.3 g of α-linolenic acid were administered to the study group, obtaining significant DED sign and symptom improvement. Other studies evaluated the effect of supplementation with a combination of ω-6 and ω-3 fatty acids. Cruezot et al. found that docohexanoic acid, eicosapentaenoic acid (ω-3), α-linolenic and linoleic acid (ω-6) would improve signs,[102] even if not significantly. Finally, some trials have assessed ω-6 supplements. Specific ω-6 fatty acids have anti-inflammatory properties, as they lead to increased synthesis of 1-series prostaglandins that play a negative feedback role in chronic inflammation. Supplementation of certain ω-6 fatty acids (linoleic acid and α-linolenic acid) in one study improved the symptom of 'dryness' at three and six months ($p < 0.01$) among contact lens wearers, and also significantly improved overall lens comfort ($p < 0.01$) and tear meniscus height at six months ($p < 0.01$).[103] Another study of ω-6 supplementation obtained a statistically significant improvement in both signs (lissamine staining, ocular surface inflammation) and symptoms of DED. The supplement was in this case 28.5 mg of linoleic (LA) and 15 mg α-linolenic acid (GLA).[104] Finally, it is worth noting that the topical application of α-linolenic acid could reduce DE signs and inflammation in a mouse model of DE.[105]

15.7.4 Medications and medical interventions

Various medications, both topical and systemic, have been associated with the development of DED, and there is some emerging epidemiological information to support some relationships.

15.7.4.1 Topical medications

Topical beta blockers used in the treatment of glaucoma are known by clinicians and many patients to induce DED.[106] The use of preservative in topical ocular medication is also a well-known cause of DED. A clinical study evaluated two randomized groups of patients administered preservative-free or regular beta-blocker medications, and found dry eye symptoms to be significantly more pronounced in the preservative group (35% versus 16%).[107] Moreover, benzalkonium chloride, a widely used preservative, is able to induce DED in an animal model when applied topically.[108]

15.7.4.2 Systemic medications

Various studies have searched for relationships between a number of systemic medications and DED. This has been done for antihypertensives, antihistamines, antidepressants, hormones and antihormonal therapy. The evidence accumulated to date is summarized below.

Antihypertensive medication

A significant association between any use of antihypertensive medications and increased risk of DED was found in the PHS (OR 1.28; 95% CI 1.12–1.46). In contrast, the Beaver Dam study found a decreased incidence of DED in people using one specific class of antihypertensive drugs, angiotensin converting enzyme inhibitors, but a borderline increased incidence of DED with diuretic use; finally, incidence was not significantly associated with calcium channel blockers.[72]

Antihistamine medications

Two studies confirm an association between the use of antihistamine medication and DE (Salisbury and the Beaver Dam incidence studies). The use of antihistamine medications could suggest here a confounding factor, i.e. the presence of an allergy, which can induce ocular symptoms and signs similar to DE. Also, a potential confounding factor has to be taken into consideration as the studies do not specify whether the medications included topical antihistamine eye drops, and given the fact that preservative contained in eye drops can induce DED.

Antidepressants

Use of antidepressants has been associated with DED in the Blue Mountains, Beaver Dam incidence studies and the PHS, which found a twofold increase in DE prevalence in patients using these medications. Given the parallels between DED and other conditions associated with chronic pain, which can result in psychological sequelae including depression, the fact that such an association was found to be associated with incident DED supports these observations.

Antiandrogens

Indirect evidence to support this relationship can be derived from the PHS, in which the use of medications to treat benign prostatic hypertrophy (BPH) is associated with increased risk of DED. This could possibly relate to the use of antiandrogen therapy, as a prior clinical study showed that men receiving antiandrogen drugs developed significant pathologic changes of ocular surface.[61,62] Indeed, androgen deficiency could provide an explanation for observations of a higher prevalence of DED in ageing, menopause, complete androgen insufficiency syndrome, and Sjögren syndrome.[38,63–65] The lack of data specific to the use of antiandrogen medications in the PHS study is, however, a major limitation. Future study of the possible effects of these medications on the ocular surface is needed.

Oestrogens

In a study of over 25,000 women in the WHS, postmenopausal oestrogen therapy was associated with an increased prevalence of DED. The risk of DED was increased by about 30% among women who used oestrogen combined with progesterone/progestins, and by about 70% among women who used oestrogen alone.[52] A prospective analysis of data from this study showed that the initiation of oestrogen therapy preceded the diagnosis of DED. Moreover, duration of hormone use was significantly associated with risk of DED: for each additional three years of hormone use, the risk of dry eye was increased by 15%. Corroborating evidence was subsequently found in the Shihpai study,[41] and in the Blue Mountains Eye Study,[44] in which hormone therapy was associated with 28% and 70% increases in risk of dry eye, respectively, though the findings from the Shihpai study were not statistically significant.

15.7.5 Systemic diseases

Diabetes

Diabetes has been hypothesized to be an important risk factor for DED,[71] and was associated with DED in the Beaver Dam study[43] (OR 1.38; 95% CI 0.88–1.99). The Blue Mountains study failed to show an association with DED, but found one with individual DE symptoms. However, neither the

Salnes study nor the PHS found a significant association between diabetes and DED, with the PHS ruling out any strong association (OR 0.97; 95% CI 0.74–1.24). Reasons for these discrepant findings might relate to differences in study methodology, or positive findings might be explained by diagnostic bias, as people with diabetes tend to have more frequent eye exams and may consequently be more likely to be diagnosed with DED. Although results are thus far conflicting, there is a biological rationale to support the hypothesis that diabetes may increase the risk of DED. Diabetes can influence the health of the anterior segment of the eye, and might induce DE symptoms in various ways. There are some data to suggest that diabetic patients show tear secretion deficiency, peripheral neuropathy and hyperglycemia leading to corneal epitheliopathy with complications such as hyperosmolarity, punctate keratopathy, recurrent corneal erosions, persistent epithelial defects, and neurotrophic keratopathy,[109] which can all be related to DED. It is possible that the degree of glucose control might be relevant, so that DED might only develop in the setting of inadequate control. In this regard, it is interesting that in one study DED was seen more frequently in diabetic patients with diabetic retinopathy,[110] retinopathy being very strongly linked with inadequate glucose control.

Hypertension, serum cholesterol and cardiovascular disease

High blood pressure has been found to be associated with a higher risk of DED in the PHS (OR 1.28 95% CI 1.12–1.45);[56] however, this was likely to be due to the impact of antihypertensive medications. High blood pressure was not found to be associated with DED in either the Salnes or Beaver Dam studies. The Beaver Dam study found that an increased high density lipoprotein/total cholesterol ratio was significantly associated with DED, but did not observe any significant association with cardiovascular diseases.[43]

Allergic disease

A study conducted in Japan[46] and the Salnes study[49] each evaluated association of DED with allergic disease, but used different definitions of allergic disease. In the former study allergic conjunctivitis was found to be more prevalent among those with DED (p = 0.002), whereas in the latter study no significant association was found with systemic allergy. This could be at least partly explained with the use of antihistamine medications in this group. When asked what course of action they would take for relief, more than half reported that they buy over-the-counter eye drops. Interestingly, the Melbourne study of DED excluded subjects with hay fever allergy from the dry eye group, and it has been suggested this is one reason why they found a lower DED prevalence as compared with most other studies.

Arthritis

Arthritis has been found associated with DED in the Beaver Dam study (OR 1.91, 95% CI 1.56–2.33), in the Blue Mountains study (OR 1.8, 95% CI 1.3–2.5), and in the Melbourne study (OR 3.27, 95% CI 1.74–6.17). The PHS found a trend toward higher risk of DE among men with rheumatoid arthritis, but this was not significant, probably due to the small number of PHS participants with arthritis. When considering these data it is important to attend to the differences in the definition of arthritis used (e.g. the general term 'arthritis' in the Beaver Dam versus the more specific 'rheumatoid arthritis' in the PHS). Nonetheless, autoimmune conditions such as rheumatoid arthritis have long been thought by clinicians to be relevant to the development of DED, and these findings tend to be in accord with this clinical opinion.

Allogenic bone marrow transplantation

Allogenic bone marrow transplantation as a treatment for blood malignancies has expanded widely, and the survival rate is higher than ever before. Dry eye due to radiation therapy, systemic chemotherapy, or ocular graft versus host disease as a consequence of bone marrow transplantation can be seen in survivors,[111] especially in the paediatric population.[112] This is an increasingly recognized problem in these populations.

15.8 COST

Costs of dry eye can be divided into direct heath costs (health care system utilization, including office visits, surgery, medications and other non-pharmacological therapies) and indirect costs, which include lost work time and reduced productivity, mental health and quality of life.[113] However, no definite data exist on costs incurred by patients with DED, and new studies are expected to clear up this important epidemiological aspect. Direct resource utilization among dry eye sufferers includes healthcare professional visits, non-pharmacological therapies, pharmacological treatments, and surgical procedures, with the latter two categories being the major cost drivers. Regarding indirect costs, DED patients have been reported to lose two to five days of work per year, productivity was reduced as patients decreased their work time, and worked with symptoms for more than half the year; moreover, some patients changed their work because of this condition.[114]

15.9 QUALITY OF LIFE

The impact of DED on the quality of life (QoL) is mediated through a variety of mechanisms including pain, effect on general wellbeing, effect on visual function and impact on visual performance. Common activities such as driving, reading, working at the computer or watching television are affected, as well as social interactions, given the necessity of frequent lubricant instillation. A cross-sectional study conducted among 450 participants in the WHS and 240 participants in the PHS investigated such factors. After controlling for age, diabetes, hypertension and other factors, patients with DES were significantly two to three times more likely to report problems with reading, carrying out professional work, using a computer, TV watching, and driving during the day and at night.

Another study[115] evaluated the relation between dry eye severity and quality of life measured with the OSDI (Ocular Surface Disease Index) and VFQ-25 (Visual Function Questionnaire-25) questionnaires. Scores on both questionnaires indicated that patients suffering DED have greater problems

with visual functioning compared with normal subjects. Another study based on utility assessment, which allows one to compare how different diseases affect QoL, showed that DED ranked about the same as moderate angina in terms of its impact on patients' QoL.[116] Such data show that DED is associated with a measurable adverse impact on several common tasks of daily living; hence it must be considered an important public health problem deserving increased attention and resources.[117]

Visual symptoms are a common complaint of DED patients, though the effect of DED on visual function has not been widely studied. Both punctual occlusion and application of lubricants in DED patients have been shown to improve visual acuity, contrast sensitivity, and corneal epithelium.[118] Epithelial desiccation, tear film instability, and evaporation are common in DED and can all induce visual symptoms. Measuring visual function in DED patients is problematic, and high-contrast visual acuity, which is tested routinely at a practitioner's office, does not always capture the real impact of DED on patients' vision. To address this issue, a quick way of measuring visual function has been proposed which aims to measure the monocular recognition acuity during a 30-second blink-free period.[119] Other methods have been suggested using corneal topography examination methods to detect subtle changes induced by DED on the ocular surface. The Tear Stability Analysis System (TSAS)[120] uses ten consecutive corneal topograms, one per second for ten seconds, to detect small changes with time in the tear film; it derives data from the distortion of the mire rings.

15.10 THERAPY

Therapy for DED[121] is based on environmental strategies (humidified environment), tear supplementation (artificial tears and gels), tear retention (occlusion of the lacrimal puncta, moisture spectacles, contact lenses), anti-inflammatory therapy (topical cyclosporine, corticosteroids and tetracyclines), and ω-3 fatty acid supplementation. It is worth noting that topical Cyclosporine (Restasis®) is the only prescription drug in the USA for the treatment of DED, and there are anecdotal reports of only variable effectiveness of this drug in the dry eye population. Ongoing trials are targeting other inflammatory molecules such as interleukin-1 receptor, and these are thought to show promise for the development of more effective dry eye therapies. Effective therapies are sorely needed, as many patients with DED find little relief from available ones.

15.11 SUMMARY

Since being initiated in earnest in the mid-1990s, the study of the epidemiology of DED has made great strides toward improving our understanding of this common and bothersome eye disease. Several well-conducted prevalence studies have provided useful information on the extent of the problem across the globe, showing DED to be a condition affecting a high percentage of the adult population. The weight of the evidence shows an increase in DED with ageing and among females. There is also evidence that Asian populations may be particularly susceptible. The study of risk factors for dry eye has suggested that a number of factors may contribute to its development, including dietary factors such as an inadequate intake of omega-3 fatty acids, wearing of contact lenses, having refractive surgery, and the use of a number of medications including antihistamines, antidepressants, certain antihypertensives, antiandrogen drugs, and oestrogens. Though it rarely leads to blindness or permanent visual impairment using the standard definition, studies have indicated that DED has an adverse effect on a person's quality of life, both in quality of vision and in terms of overall wellbeing. Further research to describe the epidemiology and public health consequences of dry eye should be encouraged.

15.12 FUTURE RESEARCH NEEDS

➤ More studies would be desirable to understand better the global distribution and public health consequences of DED.
➤ Although some risk factors for DED have been identified, additional ones are likely to be involved.
➤ More thorough studies of risk factors are still needed, however, and there is a strong need for prospective studies of this disease.
➤ It would be useful to add DED to the repertoire of possible adverse outcomes in studies of novel pharmaceuticals.
➤ The relationship between corneal nerves and DED needs more attention, in particular the origin of pain symptoms.
➤ The development of biomarkers for diagnosis of DED might be useful to assist in standardization of operational definitions of DED, such as the measurement of tear film osmolarity, which may gain widespread use due to the development of practical, user-friendly osmometers.
➤ Interesting new therapeutic options that could become available soon involve purinergic receptors and novel inflammatory mediators.

REFERENCES

1. Murube J. Andrew de Roetth (1893–1981): dacryologist who introduced the term dry eye. *Ocul Surf* 2004; 2:225–227.
2. Lemp MA. Report of the national eye institute/industry workshop on clinical trials in dry eyes. *CLAO J* 1995; 21:221–232.
3. Herrero-Vanrell R, Peral A. International Dry Eye Workshop (DEWS). Update of the disease [Article in Spanish]. *Arch Soc Esp Oftalmol* 2007; 82:733–734.
4. De Paiva CS, Corrales RM, Villarreal AL, et al. Corticosteroid and doxycycline suppress MMP-9 and inflammatory cytokine expression, MAPK activation in the corneal epithelium in experimental dry eye. *Exp Eye Res* 2006; 83:526–535.
5. Tsubota K, Yamada M. Tear evaporation from the ocular surface. *Invest Ophthalmol Vis Sci* 1992; 33:2942–2950.
6. Mathers WD, Daley TE. Tear flow and evaporation in patients with and without dry eye. *Ophthalmology* 1996; 103:664–669.
7. Hayashi Y, Arakaki R, Ishimaru N. The role of caspase cascade on the development of primary Sjögren's syndrome. *J Med Invest* 2003; 50:32–38.

8. Cermak JM, Papas AS, Sullivan RM, *et al.* Nutrient intake in women with primary and secondary Sjögren's syndrome. *Eur J Clin Nutr* 2003; 57:328–334.

9. Mathers WD, Lane JA, Zimmerman MB. Tear film changes associated with normal ageing. *Cornea* 1996; 15:229–234.

10. Davidoff E, Friedman AH. Congenital alacrima. *Surv Ophthalmol* 1977; 22:113–119.

11. James DG, Anderson R, Langley D, *et al.* Ocular sarcoidosis. *Br J Ophthalmol* 1964; 48:461–470.

12. Heath P. Ocular lymphomas. *Trans Am Ophthalmol Soc* 1948; 46:385–398.

13. Heath P. Ocular lymphomas. *Am J Ophthalmol* 1949; 32:1213–1223.

14. Itescu S, Brancato LJ, Winchester R. A sicca syndrome in HIV infection: association with HLA-DR5 and CD8 lymphocytosis. *Lancet* 1989; 2:466–468.

15. Ogawa Y, Okamoto S, Wakui M, *et al.* Dry eye after haematopoietic stem cell transplantation. *Br J Ophthalmol* 1999; 83:1125–1130.

16. Maitchouk DY, Beuerman RW, Ohta T, *et al.* Tear production after unilateral removal of the main lacrimal gland in squirrel monkeys. *Arch Ophthalmol* 2000; 118:246–252.

17. Albietz JM, Lenton LM, McLennan SG. Chronic dry eye and regression after laser *in situ* keratomileusis for myopia. *J Cataract Refract Surg* 2004; 30:675–684.

18. Albietz J, Lenton L, McLennan S. The effect of tear film and ocular surface management on myopic LASIK outcomes. *Adv Exp Med Biol* 2002; 506:711–717.

19. Seifart U, Strempel I. The dry eye and diabetes mellitus [Article in German]. *Ophthalmologe* 1994; 91:235–239.

20. Bron AJ, Tiffany JM. The contribution of meibomian disease to dry eye. *Ocul Surf* 2004; 2:149–165.

21. Abelson MB, Ousler GW 3rd, Nally LA, *et al.* Alternative reference values for tear film break-up time in normal and dry eye populations. *Adv Exp Med Biol* 2002; 506:1121–1125.

22. McMahon TT, Zadnik K. Twenty-five years of contact lenses: the impact on the cornea and ophthalmic practice. *Cornea* 2000; 19:730–740.

23. Doughty MJ, Fonn D, Richter D, *et al.* A patient questionnaire approach to estimating the prevalence of dry eye symptoms in patients presenting to optometric practices across Canada. *Optom Vis Sci* 1997; 74:624–631.

24. Gipson IK. The ocular surface: the challenge to enable and protect vision: the Friedenwald lecture. *Invest Ophthalmol Vis Sci* 2007; 48:4390; 4391–4398.

25. Lievens CW, Connor CG, Murphy H. Comparing goblet cell densities in patients wearing disposable hydrogel contact lenses versus silicone hydrogel contact lenses in an extended-wear modality. *Eye Contact Lens* 2003; 29:241–244.

26. Dastjerdi MH, Dana R. Corneal nerve alterations in dry eye-associated ocular surface disease. *Int Ophthalmol Clin* 2009; 49:11–20.

27. Bourcier T, Acosta MC, Borderie V, *et al.* Decreased corneal sensitivity in patients with dry eye. *Invest Ophthalmol Vis Sci* 2005; 46:2341–2345.

28. Rojas B, Cuhna R, Zafirakis P, *et al.* Cell populations and adhesion molecules expression in conjunctiva before and after bone marrow transplantation. *Exp Eye Res* 2005; 81: 313–325.

29. Schein OD, Hochberg MC, Munoz B, *et al.* Dry eye and dry mouth in the elderly: a population-based assessment. *Arch Intern Med* 1999; 159:1359–1363.

30. Rivas L, Murube J, Toledano A. Innervation of the lachrymal gland in patients with primary Sjogren's syndrome. An immunohistopathological study [Article in Spanish]. *Arch Soc Esp Oftalmol* 2002; 77:623–629.

31. Tsubota K, Fujita H, Tsuzaka K, *et al.* Quantitative analysis of lacrimal gland function, apoptotic figures, Fas and Fas ligand expression of lacrimal glands in dry eye patients. *Exp Eye Res* 2003; 76:233–240.

32. Obata H, Yamamoto S, Horiuchi H, *et al.* Histopathologic study of human lacrimal gland. Statistical analysis with special reference to ageing. *Ophthalmology* 1995; 102: 678–686.

33. Fox RI, Kang HI. Pathogenesis of Sjogren's syndrome. *Rheum Dis Clin North Am* 1992; 18:517–538.

34. Zegans ME, Anninger W, Chapman C, *et al.* Ocular manifestations of hepatitis C virus infection. *Curr Opin Ophthalmol* 2002; 13:423–427.

35. Research in dry eye. Report of the Research Subcommittee of the International Dry Eye WorkShop (2007). *Ocul Surf* 2007; 5:179–193.

36. Bacman S, Perez Leiros C, Sterin-Borda L, *et al.* Autoantibodies against lacrimal gland M3 muscarinic acetylcholine receptors in patients with primary Sjogren's syndrome. *Invest Ophthalmol Vis Sci* 1998; 39:151–156.

37. Shimazaki J, Sakata M, Tsubota K. Ocular surface changes and discomfort in patients with meibomian gland dysfunction. *Arch Ophthalmol* 1995; 113:1266–1270.

38. Sullivan DA, Yamagami H, Liu M, *et al.* Sex steroids, the meibomian gland and evaporative dry eye. *Adv Exp Med Biol* 2002; 506:389–399.

39. Sullivan RM, Cermak JM, Papas AS, *et al.* Economic and quality of life impact of dry eye symptoms in women with Sjogren's syndrome. *Adv Exp Med Biol* 2002; 506:1183–1188.

40. McCarty CA, Bansal AK, Livingston PM, *et al.* The epidemiology of dry eye in Melbourne, Australia. *Ophthalmology* 1998; 105:1114–1119.

41. Lin PY, Tsai SY, Cheng CY, *et al.* Prevalence of dry eye among an elderly Chinese population in Taiwan: the Shihpai Eye Study. *Ophthalmology* 2003; 110:1096–1101.

42. Gulati A, Sullivan R, Buring JE, *et al.* Validation and repeatability of a short questionnaire for dry eye syndrome. *Am J Ophthalmol* 2006; 142:125–131.

43. Moss SE, Klein R, Klein BE. Prevalence of and risk factors for dry eye syndrome. *Arch Ophthalmol* 2000; 118:1264–1268.

44. Chia EM, Mitchell P, Rochtchina E, *et al.* Prevalence and associations of dry eye syndrome in an older population: the Blue Mountains Eye Study. *Clin Exp Ophthalmol* 2003; 31:229–232.

45. Lee AJ, Lee J, Saw SM, *et al.* Prevalence and risk factors associated with dry eye symptoms: a population based study in Indonesia. *Br J Ophthalmol* 2002; 86:1347–1351.

46. Shimmura S, Shimazaki J, Tsubota K. Results of a population-based questionnaire on the symptoms and lifestyles associated with dry eye. *Cornea* 1999; 18:408–411.

47. Uchino M, Dogru M, Uchino Y, *et al.* Japan Ministry of Health study on prevalence of dry eye disease among Japanese high school students. *Am J Ophthalmol* 2008; 146:925–929, e922.

48. Schaumberg DA, Sullivan DA, Buring JE, *et al.* Prevalence of dry eye syndrome among US women. *Am J Ophthalmol* 2003; 136:318–326.

49. Viso E, Rodriguez-Ares MT, Gude F. Prevalence of and associated factors for dry eye in a Spanish adult population (the Salnes Eye Study). *Ophthalmic Epidemiol* 2009; 16:15–21.

50. Schein OD, Munoz B, Tielsch JM, *et al.* Prevalence of dry eye among the elderly. *Am J Ophthalmol* 1997; 124:723–728.

51. Lamberts DW, Foster CS, Perry HD. Schirmer test after topical anesthesia and the tear meniscus height in normal eyes. *Arch Ophthalmol* 1979; 97:1082–1085.

52. Schaumberg DA, Buring JE, Sullivan DA, *et al.* Hormone replacement therapy and dry eye syndrome. *JAMA* 2001; 286:2114–2119.

53. Connor CG, Flockencier LL, Hall CW. The influence of gender on the ocular surface. *J Am Optom Assoc* 1999; 70:182–186.

54. Schechter JE, Pidgeon M, Chang D, *et al.* Potential role of disrupted lacrimal acinar cells in dry eye during pregnancy. *Adv Exp Med Biol* 2002; 506:153–157.

55. Craig JP, Tomlinson A. Age and gender effects on the normal tear film. *Adv Exp Med Biol* 1998; 438:411–415.

56. Schaumberg DA, Dana R, Buring JE, *et al.* Prevalence of dry eye disease among US men: estimates from the Physicians' Health Studies. *Arch Ophthalmol* 2009; 127:763–768.

57. Belanger A, Candas B, Dupont A, *et al.* Changes in serum concentrations of conjugated and unconjugated steroids in 40- to 80-year-old men. *J Clin Endocrinol Metab* 1994; 79:1086–1090.

58. Labrie F, Belanger A, Cusan L, *et al.* Marked decline in serum concentrations of adrenal C19 sex steroid precursors and conjugated androgen metabolites during ageing. *J Clin Endocrinol Metab* 1997; 82:2396–2402.

59. Labrie F, Luu-The V, Belanger A, *et al.* Is dehydroepiandrosterone a hormone? *J Endocrinol* 2005; 187:169–196.

60. Liu PY, Beilin J, Meier C, *et al.* Age-related changes in serum testosterone and sex hormone binding globulin in Australian men: longitudinal analyses of two geographically separate regional cohorts. *J Clin Endocrinol Metab* 2007; 92:3599–3603.

61. Krenzer KL, Dana MR, Ullman MD, *et al.* Effect of androgen deficiency on the human meibomian gland and ocular surface. *J Clin Endocrinol Metab* 2000; 85:4874–4882.

62. Sullivan BD, Evans JE, Krenzer KL, *et al.* Impact of antiandrogen treatment on the fatty acid profile of neutral lipids in human meibomian gland secretions. *J Clin Endocrinol Metab* 2000; 85:4866–4873.

63. Sullivan DA, Sullivan BD, Evans JE, *et al.* Androgen deficiency, Meibomian gland dysfunction, and evaporative dry eye. *Ann N Y Acad Sci* 2002; 966:211–222.

64. Cermak JM, Krenzer KL, Sullivan RM, *et al.* Is complete androgen insensitivity syndrome associated with alterations in the meibomian gland and ocular surface? *Cornea* 2003; 22:516–521.

65. Sullivan BD, Evans JE, Cermak JM, *et al.* Complete androgen insensitivity syndrome: effect on human meibomian gland secretions. *Arch Ophthalmol* 2002; 120:1689–1699.

66. Ishioka M, Shimmura S, Yagi Y, *et al.* Pterygium and dry eye. *Ophthalmologica* 2001; 215:209–211.

67. Taylor HR. Studies on the tear film in climatic droplet keratopathy and pterygium. *Arch Ophthalmol* 1980; 98:86–88.

68. Ergin A, Bozdogan O. Study on tear function abnormality in pterygium. *Ophthalmologica* 2001; 215:204–208.

69. Brewitt H, Sistani F. Dry eye disease: the scale of the problem. *Surv Ophthalmol* 2001; 45:S199–202.

70. Khoo J, Saw SM, Banerjee K, *et al.* Outdoor work and the risk of pterygia: a case-control study. *Int Ophthalmol* 1998; 22:293–298.

71. Moss SE, Klein R, Klein BE. Incidence of dry eye in an older population. *Arch Ophthalmol* 2004; 122:369–373.

72. Moss SE, Klein R, Klein BE. Long-term incidence of dry eye in an older population. *Optom Vis Sci* 2008; 85:668–674.

73. Ellwein LB, Urato CJ. Use of eye care and associated charges among the Medicare population: 1991–1998. *Arch Ophthalmol* 2002; 120:804–811.

74. Wolkoff P, Kjaergaard SK. The dichotomy of relative humidity on indoor air quality. *Environ Int* 2007; 33:850–857.

75. Nilsson SE, Andersson L. Contact lens wear in dry environments. *Acta Ophthalmol (Copenh)* 1986; 64:221–225.

76. Skyberg K, Skulberg KR, Eduard W, *et al.* Symptoms prevalence among office employees and associations to building characteristics. *Indoor Air* 2003; 13:246–252.

77. Wolkoff P, Nojgaard JK, Troiano P, *et al.* Eye complaints in the office environment: precorneal tear film integrity influenced by eye blinking efficiency. *Occup Environ Med* 2005; 62:4–12.

78. McCulley JP, Aronowicz JD, Uchiyama E, *et al.* Correlations in a change in aqueous tear evaporation with a change in relative humidity and the impact. *Am J Ophthalmol* 2006; 141:758–760.

79. Lindgren T, Andersson K, Dammstrom BG, *et al.* Ocular, nasal, dermal and general symptoms among commercial airline crews. *Int Arch Occup Environ Health* 2002; 75:475–483.

80. Sato M, Fukayo S, Yano E. Adverse environmental health effects of ultra-low relative humidity indoor air. *J Occup Health* 2003; 45:133–136.

81. Khurana AK, Choudhary R, Ahluwalia BK, *et al.* Hospital epidemiology of dry eye. *Indian J Ophthalmol* 1991; 39:55–58.

82. Farris RL. The dry eye: its mechanisms and therapy, with evidence that contact lens is a cause. *CLAO J* 1986; 12:234–246.

83. Gilbard JP, Gray KL, Rossi SR. A proposed mechanism for increased tear-film osmolarity in contact lens wearers. *Am J Ophthalmol* 1986; 102:505–507.

84. Thai LC, Tomlinson A, Simmons PA. In vitro and in vivo effects of a lubricant in a contact lens solution. *Ophthalmic Physiol Opt* 2002; 22:319–329.

85. Hom MM, Martinson JR, Knapp LL, *et al.* Prevalence of Meibomian gland dysfunction. *Optom Vis Sci* 1990; 67:710–712.

86. Brennan NA, Efron N. Symptomatology of HEMA contact lens wear. *Optom Vis Sci* 1989; 66:834–838.

87. Vajdic C, Holden BA, Sweeney DF, *et al.* The frequency of ocular symptoms during spectacle and daily soft and rigid contact lens wear. *Optom Vis Sci* 1999; 76:705–711.

88. Begley CG, Caffery B, Nichols KK, *et al.* Responses of contact lens wearers to a dry eye survey. *Optom Vis Sci* 2000; 77:40–46.

89. Nichols JJ, Ziegler C, Mitchell GL, *et al.* Self-reported dry eye disease across refractive modalities. *Invest Ophthalmol Vis Sci* 2005; 46:1911–1914.

90. Nichols JJ, Sinnott LT. Tear film, contact lens, and patient-related factors associated with contact lens-related dry eye. *Invest Ophthalmol Vis Sci* 2006; 47:1319–1328.

91. Richdale K, Sinnott LT, Skadahl E, *et al.* Frequency of and factors associated with contact lens dissatisfaction and discontinuation. *Cornea* 2007; 26:168–174.

92. Pritchard N, Fonn D, Brazeau D. Discontinuation of contact lens wear: a survey. *Int Contact Lens Clin* 1999; 26:157–162.

93. Ang RT, Dartt DA, Tsubota K. Dry eye after refractive surgery. *Curr Opin Ophthalmol* 2001; 12:318–322.

94. Donnenfeld ED, Solomon K, Perry HD, *et al.* The effect of hinge position on corneal sensation and dry eye after LASIK. *Ophthalmology* 2003; 110:1023–1029; discussion 1029–1030.

95. Konomi K, Chen LL, Tarko RS, *et al.* Preoperative characteristics and a potential mechanism of chronic dry eye after LASIK. *Invest Ophthalmol Vis Sci* 2008; 49:168–174.

96. De Paiva CS, Chen Z, Koch DD, *et al.* The incidence and risk factors for developing dry eye after myopic LASIK. *Am J Ophthalmol* 2006; 141:438–445.

97. Hammond MD, Madigan WP Jr, Bower KS. Refractive surgery in the United States Army, 2000–2003. *Ophthalmology* 2005; 112:184–190.

98. Hovanesian JA, Shah SS, Maloney RK. Symptoms of dry eye and recurrent erosion syndrome after refractive surgery. *J Cataract Refract Surg* 2001; 27:577–584.

99. Battat L, Macri A, Dursun D, *et al.* Effects of laser in situ keratomileusis on tear production, clearance, and the ocular surface. *Ophthalmology* 2001; 108:1230–1235.

100. Miljanovic B, Trivedi KA, Dana MR, *et al.* Relation between dietary n-3 and n-6 fatty acids and clinically diagnosed dry eye syndrome in women. *Am J Clin Nutr* 2005; 82:887–893.

101. Aragona P, Bucolo C, Spinella R, *et al.* Systemic omega-6 essential fatty acid treatment and pge1 tear content in Sjögren's syndrome patients. *Invest Ophthalmol Vis Sci* 2005; 46:4474–4479.

102. Creuzot C, Passemard M, Viau S, *et al.* Improvement of dry eye symptoms with polyunsaturated fatty acids [Article in French]. *J Fr Ophtalmol* 2006; 29:868–873.

103. Kokke KH, Morris JA, Lawrenson JG. Oral omega-6 essential fatty acid treatment in contact lens associated dry eye. *Cont Lens Anterior Eye* 2008; 31:141–146; quiz 170.

104. Barabino S, Rolando M, Camicione P, *et al.* Systemic linoleic and gamma-linolenic acid therapy in dry eye syndrome with an inflammatory component. *Cornea* 2003; 22:97–101.

105. Rashid S, Jin Y, Ecoiffier T, *et al.* Topical omega-3 and omega-6 fatty acids for treatment of dry eye. *Arch Ophthalmol* 2008; 126:219–225.

106. Ohtsuki M, Yokoi N, Mori K, *et al.* Adverse effects of beta-blocker eye drops on the ocular surface [Article in Japanese]. *Nippon Ganka Gakkai Zasshi* 2001; 105:149–154.

107. Jaenen N, Baudouin C, Pouliquen P, *et al.* Ocular symptoms and signs with preserved and preservative-free glaucoma medications. *Eur J Ophthalmol* 2007; 17:341–349.

108. Xiong C, Chen D, Liu J, *et al.* A rabbit dry eye model induced by topical medication of a preservative benzalkonium chloride. *Invest Ophthalmol Vis Sci* 2008; 49:1850–1856.

109. Alves Mde C, Carvalheira JB, Modulo CM, *et al.* Tear film and ocular surface changes in diabetes mellitus. *Arq Bras Oftalmol* 2008; 71:96–103.

110. Manaviat MR, Rashidi M, Afkhami-Ardekani M, *et al.* Prevalence of dry eye syndrome and diabetic retinopathy in type 2 diabetic patients. *BMC Ophthalmol* 2008; 8:10.

111. Bray LC, Carey PJ, Proctor SJ, *et al.* Ocular complications of bone marrow transplantation. *Br J Ophthalmol* 1991; 75:611–614.

112. Suh DW, Ruttum MS, Stuckenschneider BJ, *et al.* Ocular findings after bone marrow transplantation

in a pediatric population. *Ophthalmology* 1999; 106:1564–1570.

113. Reddy P, Grad O, Rajagopalan K. The economic burden of dry eye: a conceptual framework and preliminary assessment. *Cornea* 2004; 23:751–761.

114. Nelson JD, Helms H, Fiscella R, *et al*. A new look at dry eye disease and its treatment. *Adv Ther* 2000; 17:84–93.

115. Garcia-Catalan MR, Jerez-Olivera E, Benitez-Del-Castillo-Sanchez JM. Dry eye and quality of life [Article in Spanish]. *Arch Soc Esp Oftalmol* 2009; 84:451–458.

116. Schiffman RM, Walt JG, Jacobsen G, *et al*. Utility assessment among patients with dry eye disease. *Ophthalmology* 2003; 110:1412–1419.

117. Miljanovic B, Dana R, Sullivan DA, *et al*. Impact of dry eye syndrome on vision-related quality of life. *Am J Ophthalmol* 2007; 143:409–415.

118. Goto E, Yagi Y, Matsumoto Y, *et al*. Impaired functional visual acuity of dry eye patients. *Am J Ophthalmol* 2002; 133:181–186.

119. Ishida R, Kojima T, Dogru M, *et al*. The application of a new continuous functional visual acuity measurement system in dry eye syndromes. *Am J Ophthalmol* 2005; 139:253–258.

120. Kojima T, Ishida R, Dogru M, *et al*. A new non-invasive tear stability analysis system for the assessment of dry eyes. *Invest Ophthalmol Vis Sci* 2004; 45:1369–1374.

121. O'Brien PD, Collum LM. Dry eye: diagnosis and current treatment strategies. *Curr Allergy Asthma Rep* 2004; 4:314–319.

122. Methodologies to diagnose and monitor dry eye disease. Report of the Diagnostic Methodology Subcommittee of the International Dry Eye WorkShop (2007). *Ocul Surf* 2007; 5:108–152.

16

Corneal and external diseases

16a	Microbial keratitis	393
16b	Viral Infectious keratoconjunctivitis	403
16c	Acanthamoeba keratitis	409
16d	Ocular manifestations of leprosy	419

16e	Vernal keratoconjunctivitis	429
16f	Mooren's ulcer	435
16g	Climatic droplet keratopathy	439
16h	Pterygium	447

16   EDITORS' NOTE

The following sections are all sub-chapters of chapter 16. They represent a collection of different conditions with varied causations. They are arranged beginning with infectious causes. These sub-chapters have been contributed by authors with a particular interest in the entities concerned.

Microbial keratitis

JOHN WHITCHER, MATHUA SRINIVASAN AND MADAN UPADHYAY

16a.1	Definition	393	16a.5	Risk factors	397
16a.2	Clinical features and classification	393	16a.6	Prevention	398
16a.3	Prevalence	395	16a.7	Management	399
16a.4	Incidence and geographical distribution	396	16a.8	Epidemiological research priorities	400
				References	401

16a.1 DEFINITION

Microbial keratitis, also referred to as infective keratitis, suppurative keratitis, or central corneal ulceration, is by definition a suppurative infection of the corneal stroma with an associated overlying epithelial defect and signs of inflammation. The pathogens that are usually responsible for the infection are bacterial or fungal, but, in the strict definition of the term, other organisms can also produce a central corneal ulcer. Free living pathogens such as Acanthamoeba are a cause of central corneal ulceration, and viruses including *Herpes simplex* (**HSV**) and *Herpes zoster* (**HZV**) can produce large central geographic ulcers with underlying stromal infiltrates that mimic bacterial or fungal infections. However, for reasons of classification and clinical description these organisms are usually excluded as specific causes of microbial keratitis. For purposes of the present discussion, the terms microbial keratitis and central corneal ulceration will be used exclusively to describe suppurative corneal infections caused by bacterial and fungal pathogens. Viral and parasitic corneal infections will be discussed in Sections 16b and 16c.

16a.2 CLINICAL FEATURES AND CLASSIFICATION

Patients who develop a corneal ulcer usually cite a history of redness, pain and sensitivity to light with an associated decrease in vision. The distinction between central and peripheral corneal ulcers is sometimes arbitrary, and a large suppurative area of infection does not have to occupy the visual axis to be included in the central corneal ulceration category. Microbial keratitis is characterized by the presence of a white or yellowish stromal infiltrate with an associated epithelial defect. The eye exhibits signs of inflammation: conjunctival and scleral injection, purulent discharge, an anterior chamber reaction, and possibly a **hypopyon**. Because of increasingly severe pain in the eye and marked photophobia, the patient usually presents as an acute emergency. Both bacterial and fungal ulcers may present with a large area of central necrosis and a significant hypopyon. If there is a delay in receiving treatment, as happened frequently in a study in Nepal where patients had to walk for weeks to reach the hospital,[1] there may be total necrosis of the stroma on presentation, with corneal perforation and endophthalmitis. Because of the delay in diagnosis and treatment, microbial keratitis in developing countries is often much more severe on initial presentation than it is in countries where health facilities are readily accessible.

Although attempts at an aetiological diagnosis from clinical signs and symptoms are potentially fraught with disaster, there are several clinical findings and historical clues that may aid in differentiating between a corneal ulcer caused by a bacterium from one caused by a fungus.

16a.2.1   Bacterial keratitis

Patients with bacterial corneal infections frequently associate the beginning of their symptoms with a specific traumatic event that occurred only a few days previously. A corneal abrasion, over-wear of a contact lens, or a minor traumatic abrasion usually predates a rapidly evolving course, with the ulcer developing over a few hours to several days. Pathogenic organisms such as *Pseudomonas sp.*, *Streptococcus pneumoniae* and *Moraxella sp.* produce rapid and extensive destruction of the corneal stroma.

Characteristically, *Pseudomonas sp.* produces a large, dense, yellowish infiltrate with a copious yellowish-green purulent discharge. The entire corneal stroma is hazy, there is frequently an associated immune ring around the infiltrate, and a hypopyon is present. Corneal perforation can occur quickly (Plate 16a.1). *Streptococcus pneumoniae* usually starts more peripherally and has a serpiginous appearance. The ulcer progresses towards the centre of the cornea leaving the surrounding corneal stroma relatively clear. Perforation is less common but does occur (Plate 16a.2). *Moraxella sp.*, in spite of its rather indolent biochemical properties, can produce severe stromal necrosis with an associated hypopyon that may contain a layered **hyphaema**. Moraxella ulcers progress slowly and inexorably with a prolonged healing time even with appropriate therapy (Plate 16a.3). Other common causes of bacterial keratitis include *Staphylococcus aureus* and *Staph. epidermidis*, *Serratia sp.* and *Streptococcus viridans*. Even though these bacterial pathogens are common causes of central corneal ulceration, almost all bacterial species are capable of producing a corneal infection under the appropriate conditions.

16a.2.2   Fungal keratitis

In contrast to patients with bacterial corneal infections, patients with fungal keratitis typically cite a history of corneal trauma, sometimes almost insignificant, a few weeks to several months before developing symptoms. Although severe symptoms can develop quickly after trauma, in general the clinical course of a fungal ulcer is much more indolent than a bacterial infection. The traumatic agent may be organic in nature, but this is not essential. In developing countries, where most corneal trauma is caused by vegetable or animal material, no definite association is found to exist between injury with organic matter and the development of a fungal ulcer.[2] However, in South Florida the opposite is the case. Fungal keratitis was found to occur predominantly in young males who had a previous history of ocular trauma that occurred outdoors or in association with agricultural occupations.[3]

Unlike bacterial ulcers, fungal ulcers usually pursue an indolent course in the early stages. A persistent fungal stromal infiltrate is frequently inadvertently treated with antibiotic-steroid drops because of its recalcitrant nature, and the initial effect is beneficial, only to enhance later necrosis and inflammation when the drops are discontinued. At this point the fungal stromal infiltrate becomes diffuse and feathery in appearance, and satellite lesions may develop around the original infiltrate. The corneal epithelium often heals over the central ulcer and a waxing and waning hypopyon is observed. As the stromal infiltrate enlarges, a fibrin plaque often forms on the endothelium immediately posterior to the lesion (Plate 16a.4).[4] If an aetiological diagnosis is not made and appropriate therapy is not started, the ulcer can eventually involve the entire cornea, progressing to perforation, endophthalmitis and loss of the eye.

Even though hundreds of fungal species have been reported as causes of fungal keratitis, three organisms account for the majority of infections: *Fusarium sp.*, *Aspergillus sp.* and *Candida sp.*

16a.3 PREVALENCE

The prevalence of bacterial pathogens causing microbial keratitis has changed dramatically in industrialized countries during the past 50 years. Prior to the antibiotic era, *Strep. pneumoniae* was considered to be the only true corneal pathogen, and was the most common cause of corneal ulceration.[5] By the 1980s, with increasing numbers of people wearing contact lenses, especially extended-wear soft contact lenses, the most common cause of bacterial keratitis in the USA was *Pseudomonas aeruginosa*. This trend toward an increase in 'opportunistic' bacterial pathogens has continued so that *Strep. pneumoniae* is now responsible for less than 10% of all cases of bacterial keratitis. *Moraxella sp.*, *Staphylococcus sp.* and various species of streptococci have also increased in importance as the prevalence of the pneumococcus has declined. In contrast, several studies in developing countries[1,2,6] have demonstrated that *Strep. pneumoniae* is frequently the most common cause of bacterial corneal ulceration in populations where contact lens wear is rare (Table 16a.1).[7] These findings are not consistently observed in all developing countries. *Staphylococcus sp.* has been found to be the most common cause of bacterial keratitis in two African populations,[8,9] and *Pseudomonas sp.* is the most common corneal bacterial pathogen in Bangladesh (Table 16a.1).[10]

The prevalence of fungal pathogens causing corneal ulceration is more difficult to determine. In the past the number of reported cases has been relatively small, but a few epidemiological associations are apparent. Areas where the climate is warm and humid, especially near the equator, appear to have proportionately more cases of fungal keratitis: South Florida,[3] Bangladesh,[10] Ghana[9] and South India.[2] In fact, in Ghana and South India fungal ulcers were found to occur more frequently than bacterial ulcers (Table 16a.1).[2,8] In Burma fungi are reported to be the infectious organism in one third of corneal ulcers, mixed fungal and bacterial pathogens in one third, and pure bacteria in a third. However, these observations have not been well substantiated.[11] Interestingly, in Bhutan, fungal ulcers are seen only rarely.[12] In most areas where fungi are an important cause of microbial keratitis, *Fusarium sp.* is the dominant fungal corneal pathogen. In more temperate areas, such as Nepal,[1] *Aspergillus sp.* predominates. *Candida sp.*, which is rarely seen in warm humid climates or in a developing country setting, seems preferentially to infect compromised corneas in industrialized countries with temperate climates. While not based on any firm evidence, the obvious conclusion from the anecdotal observations appears to be that the prevalence of fungal corneal infections in a community is somehow influenced by altitude, temperature, or humidity

Table 16a.1 *Central corneal ulcers in the developing world (geographical comparison)*[7]

	South Africa[6]	South Africa[6]	Nepal[1]	Bangladesh[10]	West Africa[9]	South India[2]
Date of study	1985	1987	1991	1994	1995	1997
Number of ulcers	91	131	405	142	199	434
Culture positive (%)	68	65	80	82	57	68
Bacteria (%)	90	96	79	59	49	47
Most frequent pathogens*						
Streptococcus pneumoniae (%)	40	16	31	32	13	44
Staphylococcus species (%)	13	61	22	3	29	16
Pseudomonas species (%)	17	6	11	48	25	14
Other bacteria (%)	30	17	36	17	33	26
Fungi (%)	10	4	21	41	51	53

*Each species as a percentage of the total number of bacteria cultured.

with high, dry, cool climates being protective against developing fungal keratitis. Some investigators feel that the incidence of fungal keratitis has dramatically increased worldwide in the last several decades because many more cases have been reported in the literature, especially since the advent of corticosteroid therapy.[4] Even though this observation is not supported by population-based data, there is no doubt that many large eye centres around the world are reporting an increase in cases of fungal keratitis.[13] A case in point is the recent worldwide epidemic of fungal keratitis associated with the use of particular brands of contact lens cleaning solutions.[14] In most of these cases *Fusarium sp.* have been the offending organisms.

The prevalence of blindness worldwide secondary to microbial keratitis is currently unknown. Corneal ulceration is rarely a bilateral condition.[15] Most individuals who have microbial keratitis, especially in the developing world, become monocularly blind but continue to work as before, at increased risk of bodily injury and disability. Of the 30 to 40 thousand individuals who develop suppurative keratitis every year in the USA, many are eventually fitted with hard contact lenses to compensate for scarring of the cornea, or, in severe cases, undergo corneal surgery in an attempt to achieve useful vision. This is not the case for an estimated several million individuals in Asia and Africa who become monocularly blind every year as a result of microbial keratitis.[15] These individuals, whose corneas are permanently scarred, are predominantly from the ranks of the working poor, and their blindness is frequently under-reported, and often neglected. Population-based surveys in developing countries hint at the magnitude of the problem. In the Nepal Blindness Survey in 1980[16] it was found that the second leading cause of blindness in Nepal after cataract was corneal scarring, accounting for 37,216 (7.9%) of all blind eyes examined. In Uganda[17] corneal ulceration was found to be second only to cataract as the main cause of blindness in children. Of 1,135 children with subnormal vision, 30.7% had visual impairment secondary to cataracts or poor surgical outcome, and 22.0% had visual loss as a result of corneal ulceration. It is likely that similar prevalence rates of blindness exist in many countries of the developing world. As monocular corneal blindness becomes recognized as the final common pathway for many ocular diseases (trachoma, vitamin A deficiency, neonatal ophthalmia and ocular injuries, to name a few) microbial keratitis also will be recognized as the unfortunate event that is ultimately responsible.[18]

16a.4 INCIDENCE AND GEOGRAPHICAL DISTRIBUTION

Microbial keratitis from either bacterial or fungal infection exists in all parts of the world. All populations are at risk of developing corneal infections, but some are at greater risk than others. It is known from the Olmsted County Study[19] conducted from 1950 to 1988 that the incidence of corneal ulceration in that particular defined population in Minnesota in the last decade of the study, was 11 per 100,000. All subsequent estimates of the incidence of microbial keratitis in the USA have been based on that study, including the national estimate of 35,000 to 40,000 cases of microbial keratitis annually. In 1996 Gonzales *et al.* found in a retrospective study of corneal ulceration in South India[20] that the annual incidence of microbial keratitis in Madurai District was 113 per 100,000 population, or ten times the incidence in the USA. Generalizing these findings to all of India, it was estimated that 840,000 people a year in that country develop a bacterial or fungal corneal ulcer every year. In rural Bhutan the annual incidence of ulceration was reported by Getshen *et al.* to be 306 per 100,000.[12] And in a two-year prospective study in Bhaktapur, Nepal, an even higher incidence was reported by Upadhyay *et al.*; they found an incidence of 799 per 100,000 in this defined rural population in Kathmandu Valley.[21] All things being equal, this is seven times the incidence in South India and seventy times the incidence in Olmsted County, Minnesota. Corneal ulcer incidence studies are presently being conducted by the World Health Organization in other countries in Asia to define the magnitude of this potentially serious public health problem. In African countries, because of the absence of population-based studies, the incidence of microbial keratitis is unknown, but it is reasonable to assume that it is probably as high as it is in South East Asia, if not higher.

16a.5 RISK FACTORS

A number of risk factors may render an individual susceptible to developing microbial keratitis. In industrialized countries, pre-existing corneal diseases such as healed HSV and HZV infections, dry eyes, neurotrophic keratitis and exposure keratitis, are all risk factors for corneal ulceration, but the major risk factor appears to be contact lens wear, especially extended-wear soft contact lenses. In the Olmsted County Study[19] the incidence of microbial keratitis increased 435% over a 38-year period, and this increase was paralleled by a similar increase in contact lens wear. Schein *et al.*[22] reported that not only do contact lens wearers have a higher incidence of microbial keratitis than non-contact lens wearers, but users of disposable soft contact lenses have a 13.33-fold excess risk of developing ulcerative keratitis compared with daily-wear soft contact lens wearers, with overnight wear being the main risk factor for the development of corneal ulceration. Undoubtedly contact lens wear, especially soft contact lens wear, has also led to an increased risk for pseudomonas corneal infections. *Pseudomonas sp.* are ubiquitous in the environment and a common contaminant of contact lens cases. Also, the slimy biofilm that commonly develops on the posterior surface of soft contact lenses provides a perfect environment for growth of the organism. This propensity of *Pseudomonas sp.* to grow on the surface of soft contact lenses, combined with the microcystic oedema and microscopic corneal abrasions that are invariably produced by extended-wear soft contact lenses, especially when they are worn overnight, has created all the elements of an epidemiological disaster. There is no doubt that the widespread use of contact lenses in industrialized countries has led to an increase in the incidence of microbial keratitis as well as to an increase in the prevalence of *Pseudomonas* and other virulent opportunistic organisms.

Although trauma is still the main risk factor for the development of fungal keratitis in industrialized countries, contact lens wear has become increasingly important as a risk factor in these patients as well.[23] The recent multi-country outbreak of fungal keratitis associated with ReNu contact lens solution is a case in point.[24] A dramatic increase in the number of cases of fungal keratitis caused by *Fusarium spp.* was observed in Hong Kong, Singapore and the USA from 2004–2006. This 'epidemic' was eventually found to be caused by the temperature instability of ReNu with MoistureLoc.[25] When the product was exposed to prolonged temperature elevation it was found to lose its *in vitro* fungistatic activity. And this loss of fungal inhibition occurred to a much greater extent in ReNu than it did in other comparable contact lens solutions when subjected to similar temperature elevation.

In countries of the developing world, as in industrialized nations, a number of risk factors may lead to corneal ulceration. In South India[2] many patients with keratitis were found to have chronic dacryocystitis, leprosy, exposure keratitis, and corneal anaesthesia following HSV or HZV infections; but the overwhelming risk factor for corneal ulceration was the history of a recent injury to the cornea (65.4%). In Nepal[1] the most common risk factor was also recent trauma to the cornea (52.8%). There was no reported contact lens wearer in either of these two populations. Corneal trauma in developing countries is frequent and often trivial. The usual agents are vegetable or animal in origin and, as the majority of work is agricultural, the injuries occur in the course of normal daily activity.[1,2] The use of traditional eye medicines, often plant-based and usually non-sterile, increase the likelihood of introducing pathogens to eyes with corneal abrasions.

However, the precise risk of corneal ulceration after corneal trauma is not known. Even though many researchers feel that there is a definite increase in risk for fungal ulceration following trauma with an organic agent,[3,4,26] this association has also not been confirmed in countries where fungal keratitis was responsible for more than 50% of all cases (Table 16a.1).[2,9] As previously mentioned, it is also noteworthy that the risk of fungal keratitis increases with proximity to the equator and that the most likely fungal pathogen to be isolated in warm humid climates is *Fusarium sp.*[2,9]

16a.6   PREVENTION

Prevention of microbial keratitis in industrialized countries is complicated by the diversity of ocular diseases that place the individual at risk for developing a corneal ulcer. The issue of contact lens wear, however, as the overwhelming risk factor for suppurative keratitis, should be addressed at a national level. Cosmetic extended-wear soft contact lenses should never be worn overnight; a warning to this effect should be posted prominently on all contact lens packaging. Physicians, contact lens manufacturers, allied healthcare providers and public health workers should jointly develop a plan for risk reduction among contact lens wearers.

Prevention of corneal ulceration in developing countries is a much greater problem because of the sheer numbers of individuals who are at risk of infection. With an incidence of ulceration 10–70 times higher than the incidence in the USA, countries of the developing world face an enormous public health problem. Fortunately, at present, contact lens wear is uncommon there, and the expected increases in more virulent corneal pathogens such as *Pseudomonas sp.* have not yet occurred. Because 52.8–65.4% of all patients with microbial keratitis report corneal trauma just prior to onset of the infection, public health efforts at risk reduction should be focused in this area. Upadhyay and co-workers reported the results of such a study in Nepal,[21] in which they demonstrated that the application of Chloramphenicol ointment three times a day for three days to the eyes of 442 patients who had suffered corneal abrasions dramatically reduced the rate of corneal infection to only 4%. Moreover, none of the 284 patients who presented for treatment within the first 18 hours after injury developed an ulcer, but as the time interval increased more cases of ulceration occurred.

Even though ethical considerations prevented the use of a control group, the large number of patients surveyed over the two-year period of this prospective population-based study provided compelling evidence that antibiotic prophylaxis may be effective in preventing corneal ulceration after abrasion. This outcome was achieved in 96% of patients if the treatment was administered, within the first 48 hours after trauma. It is of interest in this study that screening of the population of 34,902 individuals over the two-year period was carried out by 81 primary eye care workers, who referred all cases of ocular trauma and infection to local secondary eye centres for examination, treatment and follow-up. It is essential that the recognition and triage of corneal trauma and infection in developing countries is handled at the grass roots level. As was implied by the Nepal study, these same eye care workers could also be trained to treat corneal abrasions prophylactically with antibiotic ointment, and thereby prevent the development of most of the corneal ulcers that occur after trauma.

Similar corneal ulcer prevention studies have been successfully carried out in Bhutan,[12] Burma,[11] and South India,[27] demonstrating that following corneal epithelial abrasions both bacterial and fungal ulcers can be prevented by simple prophylaxis. In Bhutan[12] all individuals in the study area with a confirmed corneal abrasion were treated with Chloramphenicol ointment three times a day for three days: none of them developed a corneal ulcer. The occurrence of fungal keratitis is extremely rare in Bhutan, even less than in Nepal, so using concomitant antifungal prophylaxis was not considered necessary. In Burma,[11] where a third of all corneal ulcers are caused by fungal pathogens, and another third are mixed bacterial and fungal, 1% Chloramphenicol ointment plus an antifungal, 1% Clotrimazole ointment, were both applied three times a day for three days to all eyes with a confirmed corneal abrasion. No case of microbial keratitis occurred in the study area.

In South India,[27] where half of all cases of microbial keratitis are fungal and half are bacterial,[2] there were 50,000 individuals in the study area, and everyone who presented with a confirmed corneal abrasion was randomized into one of two groups. One group was treated with Chloramphenicol and Clotrimazole ointment and the other group with Chloramphenicol and a placebo ointment three times a day for three days. Surprisingly, no corneal ulcers, either bacterial or fungal, occurred in either of the two groups. There may be several explanations for this unexpected outcome. Application of any ointment, even a placebo, to a corneal abrasion may speed up epithelialization.

Ointment may also prevent pathogens on the lids from gaining access to the corneal stroma. However, it has been reported that some antibiotics, including Chloramphenicol, have a modest anti-fungal effect *in vitro* against *Fusarium* and *Aspergillus*.[28,29] This may explain reports that describe a positive therapeutic effect of antibiotics in patients with proven fungal keratitis,[13,30] and it may also explain why, in the South Indian study, Chloramphenicol prevented the occurrence of both bacterial and fungal keratitis after epithelial corneal abrasion.

16a.7 MANAGEMENT

Even though bacterial and fungal corneal ulcers often display different clinical characteristics, a specific aetiological diagnosis cannot be made without laboratory confirmation.[26] Scrapings of the leading edge of the ulcer should be performed with a platinum Kimura spatula (in the absence of a spatula, with a large gauge needle) and smeared on several glass slides to be examined with Giemsa stain for morphology of both bacteria and fungi, Gram stain for identification of bacteria, and lactophenol cotton blue, **Gomori's methenamine silver (GMS)** or other specific fungal stains for identifying fungi. A **potassium hydroxide (KOH)** wet mount is often useful for identifying fungi in large ulcers where many organisms are present. A culture should then be prepared using the heat-sterilized platinum spatula or a cotton-tipped applicator moistened with sterile broth. The scraping should be inoculated directly onto blood agar and chocolate agar and into thioglycolate broth if bacterial pathogens are suspected, and onto Sabouraud's dextrose agar or to potato dextrose agar if fungal organisms are suspected. In practice, both bacterial and fungal media are inoculated in all cases of microbial keratitis. Special media may also be inoculated if unusual pathogens such as *Mycobacterium sp.* (Lowenstein–Jensen medium) or nutritionally deficient *Streptococcus* (Brucella agar) are suspected. Growth of an organism on two solid media at the site of inoculation is confirmatory. Corneal smears help guide antibiotic or antifungal therapy until cultures are available. Antibiotic sensitivity testing is performed on all isolated bacterial pathogens. As a guide to treatment, antifungal sensitivities are, however, generally less reliable than antibiotic sensitivities.

If a bacterial keratitis is suspected clinically and corneal scrapings reveal bacterial organisms, the patient should be started on broad spectrum antibiotic such as a fourth generation fluoroquinolone until an etiologic diagnosis is confirmed by culture. Moxifloxacin or gatifloxacin are good first choices. In developing countries these antibiotics may not be available.[31] Because Gram-positive pathogens, specifically streptococcal species, require different conventional antibiotics for treatment than do Gram-negative organisms, dual therapy is then required. In general, topical cefazolin (50 mg/ml) and tobramycin or ciprofloxacin every hour should be started immediately. Therapy should be modified once smears and cultures are available and the response to treatment has been reviewed. In severe cases, subconjunctival antibiotics (cefazolin and tobramycin) can also be given at the initial examination.[32]

If a fungal keratitis is suspected on clinical examination and corneal scrapings examined with Giemsa, GMS or a KOH wet mount are confirmatory, the patient should be started on topical 5% Natamycin (pimaricin) drops and 0.15% Amphotericin B drops every hour. In general, pimaricin is more effective against filamentous fungi and Amphotericin B is more effective against yeasts, but the sensitivities vary, and the two drugs are usually used together until drug toxicity begins to become a problem. Recently 1% voriconazole eye drops were used successfully in the treatment of a number of cases of fungal keratitis caused by both yeasts and filamentous fungi.[33] Even though voriconazole is fungistatic, not fungicidal, it penetrates the corneal stroma easily and can be detected in therapeutic concentrations in the aqueous.[34] It also crosses the blood–brain barrier and can be given in high doses systemically. This property may lead to its usefulness as an adjunct to topical treatment in severe cases of fungal keratitis where perforation is likely.[35,36]

Unlike antibiotic sensitivities, antifungal sensitivities are not often helpful and treatment success is judged by clinical response. When the ulcer is refractory to treatment, other antifungal topical medications should be tried, such as Miconazole (10 mg/ml) or 1% Clotrimazole (or possibly myconazole 10 mg/ml if nothing else available). For severe keratitis invading the anterior chamber or sclera, systemic antifungal is given. Voriconazole is now the treatment of choice (expensive); itraconazole is probably second choice. If necessary, voriconazole can be injected into the eye (50 μg in 0.1 ml) or directly into the corneal stroma. Amphotericin is very toxic, but if nothing else was available, might be given subconjunctivally (50 μg per ml as 0.1 ml injection) after an injection of local anaesthetic.

In treating both bacterial and fungal keratitis, adjunctive therapeutic modalities should be employed. The pupil should be sufficiently dilated on a daily basis to prevent the formation of posterior synechiae. Topical corticosteroids may be used in the treatment of bacterial keratitis after sufficient time has elapsed for sterilization of the ulcer to occur. The possible, but unproven, exception to this rule is in the treatment of ulcers caused by *Pseudomonas sp*. It has been postulated anecdotally that corticosteroids will enhance the production of collagenase in pseudomonas ulcers, leading to corneal perforation in the ulcer bed. These effects may be counteracted by oral doxycycline (100 mg orally twice daily) and by large doses of vitamin C (500 mg orally four times a day). Fungal keratitis, however, should never be treated with corticosteroids except in rare cases where it is proven that the ulcer no longer has viable organisms. The growth of filamentous fungi and yeasts is enhanced by corticosteroids, and even with antifungal coverage the outcome may be disastrous.

16a.8 EPIDEMIOLOGICAL RESEARCH PRIORITIES

The global impact of microbial keratitis from the standpoint of blindness, visual disability, social and economic implications, and of cost to the healthcare infrastructure has not been adequately assessed in any meaningful way. In industrialized countries, the visual loss secondary to corneal scarring is not tolerated, and invariably an inordinate amount of healthcare resources is spent on corneal transplants and other sophisticated surgical procedures to restore vision. In the developing world, microbial keratitis affects predominantly the poorest of the poor, who cannot afford medical treatment for a corneal ulcer, much less the cost for a corneal transplant. These individuals, even by conservative estimates, number several million every year. A problem of this size deserves further research and the development of effective programmes of prevention.

Epidemiological research should address several areas:

➢ First, the true magnitude of the problem of microbial keratitis must be assessed. The incidence of corneal ulceration in the developing world has to date been investigated in only two areas using population-based data: South India[20] (113 cases per 100,000) and Nepal[21] (799 cases per 100,000). Reliable incidence studies are needed in other countries to determine whether these figures are too high, or whether the problem of microbial keratitis is, indeed, much greater than we have previously thought.

➢ Second, we need to understand the epidemiology of microbial keratitis in all of its nuances in different geographical areas. What are the risk factors specific to each region? What are prevalences of bacterial and fungal pathogens? Why does climate seem to have such a pronounced effect on the ratio of bacterial to fungal ulcers?

➢ Third, there is a need for much larger, better funded, and better regulated studies of the prevention of microbial keratitis. Studies like the Bhaktapur Eye Study[21] need to be performed in different countries where there are different risk factors, where prevalence of pathogens differs, and where there are different ratios of bacterial to fungal keratitis. For instance, we know that in Nepal 52.8% of corneal ulcer patients suffer corneal trauma before developing keratitis[1] and that in South India the figure is 65.4%,[2] but why do the other 47.2% and 34.6%, respectively, of patients develop corneal ulcers? Are there other risk factors that are amenable to prevention?

Finally, there is a need for research and development of new antibiotic and antifungal agents. If prophylactic treatment indeed prevents 96 to 100% of patients who have suffered a corneal abrasion from developing a corneal ulcer, as was shown in the Bhaktapur Study,[21] will a similar regimen be effective in an area where half of the ulcers are caused by fungi?[2,11] This question appears to have now been initially answered by the study in South India.[27] The results, however, need to be confirmed by similar studies in other countries to prove that antibiotic prophylaxis after corneal abrasion is an acceptable public health intervention for preventing both bacterial and fungal ulcers on a global scale.[37] As was shown by village health workers in Nepal,[21] a model exists to identify and triage patients with corneal abrasions at the grass roots level.

As the epidemiology of microbial keratitis in the developing world becomes better understood, evidence-based prevention and treatment programmes can be implemented. Hopefully, at the same time less costly and more effective antibiotic and antifungal agents will also become available to treat those ulcers that have so far eluded prevention.

REFERENCES

1. Upadhyay M, Purna C, Karmacharya M, *et al.* Epidemiologic characteristics, predisposing factors, and etiologic diagnosis of corneal ulceration in Nepal. *Am J Ophthalmol* 1991; 111:92–99.
2. Srinivasan M, Gonzales C, George C, *et al.* Epidemiology and aetiological diagnosis of corneal ulceration in Madurai, South India. *Br J Ophthalmol* 1997; 81:965–971.
3. Liesegang TJ, Forster RK. Spectrum of microbial keratitis in South Florida. *Am J Ophthalmol* 1980; 90:38–47.
4. Thygeson P. Keratomycosis. *Trans Pac Coast Oto-Ophthalmol Soc* 1976; 57:351–356.
5. Ostler HB, Okumoto M, Wilkey C. The changing pattern of the etiology of central bacterial corneal (hypopyon) ulcer. *Trans Pac Coast Oto-Ophthalmol Soc* 1976; 57:235–246.
6. Carmichael TR, Wolpert M, Koornhof HJ. Corneal ulceration at an urban African hospital. *Br J Ophthalmol* 1985; 69:920–926.
7. Whitcher JP, Srinivasan M, Upadhyay M. Prevention of corneal ulceration in the developing world. *Int Ophthalmol Clin* 2002; 42:71–77.
8. Ormerod DL. Causation and management of microbial keratitis in subtropical Africa. *Ophthalmology* 1987; 94:1662–1668.
9. Hagan M, Wright E, Newman M, *et al.* Causes of suppurative keratitis in Ghana. *Br J Ophthalmol* 1995; 79:1024–1028.
10. Dunlop AAS, Wright ED, Howlader SA, *et al.* Suppurative corneal ulceration in Bangladesh: A study of 142 cases examining the microbiological diagnosis, clinical and epidemiological features of bacterial and fungal keratitis. *Aust NZ J Ophthalmol* 1994; 22:105–110.
11. Maung N, Thant CC, Srinivasan M, *et al.* Corneal ulceration in South East Asia II: A strategy for the prevention of fungal keratitis at the village level in Burma. *Br J Ophthalmol* 2006; 90:968–970.
12. Getshen K, Srinivasan M, Upadhyay MP, *et al.* Corneal ulceration in South East Asia. I: A model for the prevention of bacterial ulcers at the village level in rural Bhutan. *Br J Ophthalmol* 2006; 90:276–278.
13. Khor W, Aung T, Saw S, *et al.* An outbreak of Fusarium keratitis associated with contact lens wear in Singapore. *JAMA* 2006; 295:2867–2873.
14. Margolis TP, Whitcher JP. Fusarium — A new culprit in the contact lens case. *JAMA* 2006; 296:985–987.
15. Whitcher JP, Srinivasan M. Corneal ulceration in the developing world — a silent epidemic. *Br J Ophthalmol* 1997; 81:622–623.
16. Brilliant LB, Pokhrel RP, Grasset NC, *et al.* Epidemiology of blindness in Nepal. *Bull World Health Organ* 1985; 63:375–386.
17. Waddell K. Childhood blindness and low vision in Uganda. *Eye* 1998; 12:184–192.
18. Whitcher JP, Srinivasan M, Upadhyay MP. Corneal blindness: a global perspective. *Bull World Health Organ* 2001; 79:214–221.
19. Erie JC, Nevitt MP, Hodge DO, *et al.* Incidence of ulcerative keratitis in a defined population from 1950 through 1988. *Arch Ophthalmol-chic* 1993; 111:1665–1671.
20. Gonzales C, Srinivasan M, Whitcher JP, *et al.* Incidence of corneal ulceration in Madurai

District, South India. *Ophthalmic Epidemiol* 1996; 3:159–166.

21. Upadhyay M, Karmacharya S, Koirala S, *et al.* The Bhaktapur eye study: ocular trauma and antibiotic prophylaxis for the prevention of corneal ulceration in Nepal. *Br J Ophthalmol* 2001; 85:388–392.

22. Schein OD, Buehler PO, Stamler JP, *et al.* The impact of overnight wear on the risk of contact lens-associated ulcerative keratitis. *Arch Ophthalmol-chic* 1994; 112:186–190.

23. Rosa RH, Miller D, Alfonso EC. The changing spectrum of fungal keratitis in South Florida. *Ophthalmology* 1994; 101:1005–1013.

24. Ma S, SO K, Chung P, *et al.* A multi-country outbreak of fungal keratitis associated with a brand of contact lens solution: the Hong Kong experience. *Int J Infect Dis* 2009; 13:443–448.

25. Bullock J, Warwar R, Elder B, *et al.* Temperature instability of ReNu with MoistureLoc: a new theory to explain the worldwide Fusarium keratitis epidemic of 2004–2006. *Arch Ophthalmol-chic* 2008; 126:11493–11498.

26. Ostler HB. *Diseases of the External Eye and Adnexa.* Baltimore: Williams & Wilkins; 1993. pp. 173–191.

27. Srinivasan M, Upadhyay MP, Priyadarsini B, *et al.* Corneal ulceration in South East Asia III: prevention of fungal keratitis at the village level in South India using topical antibiotics. *Br J Ophthalmol* 2006; 90:1472–1475.

28. Mehta A, Chopra S, Mehta P. Antibiotic inhibition of pectolytic and cellulolytic enzyme activity in two *Fusarium* species. *Mycopathologia* 1993; 124:185–188.

29. Day S, Lalitha P, Haug S, *et al.* Activity of antibiotics against *Fusarium* and *Aspergillus*. *Br J Ophthalmol* 2009; 93:116–119.

30. Chodosh J, Miller, Tu E, *et al.* Tobramycin-responsive *Fusarium oxysporum* keratitis. *Can J Ophthalmology* 2000; 35:29–30.

31. Guidelines for the Management of Corneal Ulcer at Primary, Secondary, and Tertiary Care health facilities in the South-East Asia Region. SEA/Opthal/126. World Health Organization Regional Office for South-East Asia; 2004:1–36.

32. Srinivasan M. Guidelines for management of corneal ulcer at the primary, secondary and tertiary levels. *J Aravind Eye Care System* 2009; 9:1–15.

33. Lor A, Hong K, Lee S, *et al.* Practice patterns in the management of fungal keratitis. *Cornea* 2009; 28:856–859.

34. Vorwerk C, Streit F, Binder L, *et al.* Aqueous humor concentration of voriconazole after topical administration in rabbits. *Graef Arch Clin Exp* 2008; 246:1179–1183.

35. Bunya V, Hammersmith K, Rapuano C, *et al.* Topical and oral voriconazole in the treatment of fungal keratitis. *Am J Ophthalmol* 2007; 143:151–153.

36. Lee S, Lee J, Kim S. Topical and oral voriconazole in the treatment of fungal keratitis. *Korean J Ophthalmol* 2009; 23:46–48.

37. Upadhyay M, Srinivasan M, Whitcher JP. Microbial keratitis in the developing world: does prevention work? *Int Ophthalmol Clin* 2007; 47:17–25.

16b

Viral infectious keratoconjunctivitis

STEPHEN TUFT AND BITA MANZOURI

16b.1	Definition	403
16b.2	Clinical picture	403
16b.3	Prevalence and incidence	404
16b.4	Geographical distribution	405

16b.5	Risk factors	405
16b.6	Summary of management	405
16b.7	Epidemiological research priorities	407
	References	407

16b.1   DEFINITION

Viral keratoconjunctivitis is an important cause of ocular morbidity and visual loss, producing characteristic ocular changes that can be amplified by co-existent local or systemic disease. The most frequent infections are by members of the herpes virus group (*Herpes simplex* **virus** (**HSV**), *Varicella zoster* **virus** (**VZV**), adenovirus and enterovirus.

16b.2   CLINICAL PICTURE

Primary infection with HSV may be subclinical and remote from the site of recurrent disease. Primary ocular HSV is characterized by blepharoconjunctivitis, vesicles on the lids, subconjunctival haemorrhages, follicles, punctate keratitis and microdendrites; 60% of ocular cases involve the cornea. Keratitis resulting from recurrent HSV can cause infectious epithelial lesions (dendritic ulcer, geographic ulcer), neurotrophic keratitis, stromal disease (necrotizing keratitis, immune keratitis) and endothelialitis (disciform keratitis).[1]

After primary infection at a site that can be remote from the eye, the virus is carried to the sensory ganglion where a latent infection is established. Up to 10% of seropositive patients, especially children and the immune-compromised, periodically shed HSV and are contagious. Stimuli such as fever, hormonal change, ultraviolet radiation, trauma and trigeminal injury may then reactivate HSV, which is transported in axons to the periphery to cause recurrent disease. It is also possible that viruses may maintain latency within the cornea, and HSV can be spread by corneal transplantation.[2] Following a first episode of keratitis the rate for recurrence of ocular HSV is estimated to increase from 20% at two years post-infection, to 40% by five years and 70% by seven years. The pattern of disease changes and stromal disease accounts for only 2–6% of initial infection but 20–48% of recurrent disease. Visual complications are therefore associated with recurrent HSV. Bilateral disease occurs in 11.9% of patients, especially in atopes and the immunosuppressed. After the first episode of corneal involvement 32–40% of the patients experience a recurrent herpetic ulcer, 25% experience disciform or irregular stromal keratouveitis, 5% experience ocular hypertension, and 6% develop scarring sufficient to decrease visual acuity.[3]

The clinical picture may vary over time and multiple features may be present in the same cornea. The strain HSV1 is usually responsible for ocular or labial disease, whereas HSV2 causes urogenital infection and is the strain associated with herpetic ophthalmia neonatorum. HSV1 and HSV2 reside equally in almost all ganglia, and local factors favour HSV1 reactivation from the trigeminal ganglion.[4] VZV can similarly become latent in sensory ganglia in up to 100% of primary infections. The diagnosis of primary VZV infection and reactivation is usually clinical, although polymerase chain reaction (PCR) testing can be used for confirmatory of primary infection.

Epithelial keratitis, the result of virus replication, is the most common presentation of recurrent ocular HSV. Viral antigen is detectable in stromal disease but replication is not thought to be an important component of the disease. Lymphocytes (Th1) are essential for stromal inflammation, Langerhans antigen-presenting cells participate in the immune response, and polymorphonuclear neutrophils are critical for viral clearance but also mediate tissue destruction.

In many parts of the world adenoviral keratoconjunctivitis is the most common viral infection of the ocular surface, typically causing community or medical facility-based epidemics. The clinical signs of the ocular pathogenic strains (serotypes 8, 19 and 37) are indistinguishable, but viral serotyping permits epidemiological tracing of outbreaks. The signs are acute lid swelling, follicular conjunctivitis and pseudomembrane formation. Immune-mediated subepithelial infiltrates are common but rarely cause permanent visual loss. The fact that there may be four to ten days of virus shedding before clinical disease is apparent, and the ability of adenovirus to survive on dry surfaces, both facilitate the spread of infection. Diagnosis can be confirmed by PCR testing.[5]

Acute haemorrhagic conjunctivitis is caused by enterovirus 70 or coxsackie virus A24.[6] It has a rapid onset and resolution with characteristic petechial subconjunctival haemorrhages, but without permanent corneal change. The infection is spread by direct inoculation and the use of traditional eye medicines, rather than the usual faecal–oral route. Confirmation of infection is by PCR.[7]

16b.3   PREVALENCE AND INCIDENCE

Herpes simplex virus is the most common infectious cause of corneal blindness in developed countries. Because primary HSV infections may be asymptomatic in two thirds of cases, clinical surveys underestimate the incidence and prevalence.[8] Serology is used to define the prevalence of prior infection, and this reflects latency. Age, geographical location and socio-economic status are known to affect the prevalence. Using PCR the detection of HSV in the trigeminal ganglion increases from 18.2% at 20 years of age to almost 100% in people over 60 years of age. However, in the lowest socio-economic groups 70–80% have HSV1 antibodies by adolescence. In their study in Minnesota, Liesegang et al.[9] found an incidence of 8.4 new cases of ocular HSV per 100,000 person-years, increasing to 20.7 per 100,000 including recurrences, with a prevalence of a history of ocular HSV infection of 149 per 100,000 people. Therefore, as many as ten million people worldwide may have herpetic eye disease; 90–94% of patients maintain vision of >6/12 but 3% have 6/36 or worse.[3] The prevalence of HSV in developing countries is unknown, although 60% of corneal ulcers in Tanzania were thought to be attributable to infection with HSV.[4] Less than 1% of corneal disease is caused by HSV2. HSV is a rare cause of follicular conjunctivitis accounting for < 5% of cases in one large study from Japan.[10]

In developed countries, VZV affects about 1% of the population per year, but antibodies to VZV are found in 90% of the population by the age of 60 years. Herpes zoster has an incidence of 130 per 100,000 patient-years. One series reported that 9–16% of patients had trigeminal involvement, of whom 50–72% had ocular involvement, and 20% had corneal involvement. The peak is in the fourth to seventh decades.[11,12]

Adenovirus is a common cause of infectious conjunctivitis. A British study, in primary care, of children with acute infective conjunctivitis found that 8% of cases were due to adenovirus infection.[8] An American study of adults and children, in an ophthalmic emergency room, found that 62% of acute infective conjunctivitis cases had an adenoviral cause.[13]

16b.4 GEOGRAPHICAL DISTRIBUTION

There is no evidence for differences in racial or sexual susceptibility to HSV infection, but recurrence may be more common in men. The rate of infection does not vary with the season. Crowding may increase the risk of early exposure, and in Africa 70–80% of the population have antibodies by the age of adolescence.

Large outbreaks of acute haemorrhagic conjunctivitis caused by enterovirus 70 or coxsackie virus A24 occurred in central Africa and Asia in the 1980s.

16b.4.1 Changes in prevalence and geographical distribution with time

In the USA the age-related prevalence of HSV1 antibodies has dropped over the past 40 years, indicating later exposure, whereas the prevalence of HSV2-positive serology has increased to 22–30% over the past 20 years. There is increasing genital infection with HSV1, but it is not known if there is increasing ocular HSV2 infection. Corneal disease associated with HSV infection accounts for 3–10% of penetrating keratoplasties (PK) performed in the UK and the USA. However, recent data published by Branco *et al.* indicate that HSV-associated keratitis has declined significantly as an indication for PK during the period 1972–2001, and most dramatically in the 1980s.[14] This decline may reflect better medical management options and a reluctance to perform surgery for recurrent HSV keratitis, rather than a reduction in the incidence of HSV keratitis. A marked increase in the incidence and prevalence of shingles and **Herpes Zoster Ophthalmicus (HZO)** is attributed to diminishing cell-mediated immunity in an ageing population, the increase in cases of acquired immune deficiency syndrome, and an increase in cancer and associated immunosuppression.

16b.5 RISK FACTORS

Patients with atopy are at risk of severe herpes simplex keratitis, and 40% develop bilateral disease. Disease associated with HSV is more severe in children and in patients with acquired immune deficiency syndrome, in whom viral shedding and recurrences are more common. Transmission of HSV is facilitated in conditions of crowding and poor hygiene. Malnutrition, measles and malaria may suppress cell-mediated immunity and, in an observational case series, they were associated with severe unilateral and bilateral HSV infection (see Section 14d).[15] Maternal genital HSV is a risk for transmitting herpetic ophthalmia neonatorum (see Section 14c). Application of topical steroid is associated with the development of geographical HSV infection, and there is a six-fold increase risk in epithelial herpes disease after PK for non-herpetic disease.

16b.6 SUMMARY OF MANAGEMENT

Epithelial HSV disease is the result of viral replication, and is therefore treated with an antiviral agent. Stromal disease is treated with steroid to reduce destructive inflammation but covered with an antiviral agent to prevent enhanced viral replication. Latent virus cannot be eliminated, but viral resistance is not usually a problem except in the immunosuppressed, because each reactivation occurs with naive virus.

Treatments for HSV disease use purine or pyrimidine analogues that are incorporated to form abnormal viral DNA. Idoxuridine and adenine arabinoside (Ara-A, vidarabine) are poorly soluble and relatively toxic, but are still used where cost containment is critical. Trifluorothymidine (F_3T, trifluridine) and acycloguanosine (aciclovir) have low toxicity and achieve virucidal concentrations in the stroma and anterior chamber, and effectively cover adjunctive steroid treatment; aciclovir has the advantage that it can be used systemically. Both F_3T and aciclovir are active against HSV1 and HSV2. A **meta-analysis** of clinical studies[16] indicates that topical F_3T, aciclovir and vidarabine are similar in relative effectiveness in treating dendritic and geographical epithelial keratitis, but more effective than idoxuridine. Other topical agents, such as ganciclovir and foscarnet, were equivalent to F_3T or aciclovir. Topical interferon may have a small additional effect when used in conjunction with a topical antiviral. Oral aciclovir did not hasten healing when used in combination with topical treatment. Debriding infected corneal epithelium is effective, but adjunctive virucidal agents are needed to avert a recrudescence of epithelial keratitis.[16] Signs of treatment toxicity include superficial punctate erosions, follicular conjunctivitis and punctal occlusion.

The Herpes Eye Disease Study Group conducted a series of randomized controlled studies, which provide important management guidelines. They found that for stromal disease, topical steroid (1% prednisolone phosphate four times daily) in conjunction with antiviral cover, reduced recovery time by 68%, with no increased risk of recurrence at six months.[17] They found no additional effect of oral aciclovir (400 mg five times a day for ten weeks) over topical steroid and F_3T when treating stromal keratitis.[18] After epithelial HSV, a three-week course of oral aciclovir (400 mg five times a day) did not prevent stromal disease in the subsequent year.[19] Prophylactic treatment with aciclovir (400 mg twice a day) reduces epithelial and stromal recurrences by about 50% over 12 months, with no evidence of rebound or sustained benefit. However, stromal recurrences were only reduced in patients with prior stromal disease, with the greatest effect in patients with multiple recurrences.[20] Oral aciclovir (400 mg twice a day for six months) also reduces the risk of HSV recurrence after PK.[21] Stromal inflammation can be controlled with a topical non-steroidal anti-inflammatory agent or topical ciclosporin, combined with a topical antiviral agent, as alternatives to steroid.

A successful vaccine against HSV has yet to be developed. Vaccines against HSV surface glycoprotein have the potential to prevent primary infection, latency and reactivation, while a replication-impaired mutant HSV1 strain could occupy the neuronal site of latency and prevent colonization with wild-type HSV. Fundamental to a successful vaccine is its ability to prevent person-to-person transmission.[22]

Oral antivirals reduce the severity of acute HZO, but have no proven effect on reducing late complications such as neurotrophic keratitis.[23,24] For non-ocular disease valaciclovir (1 g three times a day), famciclovir (500 mg three times a day) to brivudin (BVDU) are more effective than aciclovir (800 mg five times a day for three days given within 72 hours of onset) in resolving acute pain of herpes zoster and have more convenient dosing regimens.[25,26] Live attenuated vaccine is widely used in the USA with up to 97% protection, but it is unknown whether a vaccination programme reduces the shingles and postherpetic neuralgia.[27,28]

There is no controlled trial that shows a benefit of topical steroid or antiviral therapy for adenoviral keratoconjunctivitis or enterovirus, and treatment is based on symptomatic relief.[29] Topical steroid may be used if there is visual reduction secondary to keratitis,[30] if there is a membranous conjunctivitis, or uveitis, although steroid and ciclosporin may increase the period of virus shedding. However, conjunctival scarring is not progressive, and is rarely a clinically significant problem. Topical steroid is also unlikely to precipitate corneal epithelial disease even if there is HSV conjunctivitis.[10] Topical cidofovir 1% may be effective in reducing the severity and duration of adenoviral keratoconjunctivitis, although its usefulness is limited by local toxicity.[31] In general, topical non-steroidal agents,[32] interferon and antivirals (aciclovir, trifluorothymidine) have no convincing effect. Specific adenovirus serotype vaccines are available. The lack of an effective treatment has led to the development of strict protocols to limit nosocomial (originating in a hospital or clinic) virus spread in the clinical setting.[33]

Limitation of acute haemorrhagic conjunctivitis relies on education and infection control. The outcome is usually benign, although a polio-like paralysis (radiculomyelitis) develops in approximately one in 10,000 patients infected with enterovirus 70. It is not possible to predict at present which patients it will affect.[34]

16b.7 EPIDEMIOLOGICAL RESEARCH PRIORITIES

➤ The impact of factors such as malnutrition, malaria, measles and xerophthalmia on the severity of HSV keratitis needs to be evaluated further. Cheap and potent antiviral agents are required that need less frequent dosing schedules. Studies are required on ways to suppress HSV recurrences, which are the primary cause of visual loss, and to identify the optimum target group for prophylaxis.

➤ Studies are required to document the increasing prevalence of HSV2 and to determine whether it is related to an increase in ocular disease.

➤ An answer is needed to whether the introduction of vaccination for VZV will eventually reduce the incidence and severity of HZO.

➤ Research is needed to identify the best way to limit the spread of adenoviral keratoconjunctivitis. A cheap, rapid, clinic-based technique is required to identify early cases.

➤ It is desirable to develop a vaccine to protect against the type of enterovirus infection causing acute haemorrhagic conjunctivitis.

REFERENCES

1. Holland EJ, Schwartz GS. Classification of herpes simplex virus keratitis. *Cornea* 1999; 18:144–154.

2. Remeijer L, Maertzdorf J, Doornenbal P, *et al.* Herpes simplex virus 1 transmission through corneal transplantation. *Lancet* 2001; 357:442.

3. Liesegang TJ. Herpes simplex virus epidemiology and ocular importance. *Cornea* 2001; 20:1–13.

4. Kaye S, Choudhary A. Herpes simplex keratitis. *Prog Retin Eye Res* 2006; 25:355–380.

5. Heim A, Ebnet C, Harste G, *et al.* Rapid and quantitative detection of human adenovirus DNA by real-time PCR. *J Med Virol* 2003; 70:228–239.

6. Palacios G, Oberste MS. Enteroviruses as agents of emerging infectious diseases. *J Neurovirol* 2005; 11:424–433.

7. Xiao XL, Wu H, Li YJ, *et al.* Simultaneous detection of enterovirus 70 and coxsackievirus A24 variant by multiplex real-time RT-PCR using an internal control. *J Virol Methods* 2009; 159:23–28.

8. Rose PW, Harnden A, Brueggemann AB, *et al.* Chloramphenicol treatment for acute infective conjunctivitis in children in primary care: a randomised double-blind placebo-controlled trial. *Lancet* 2005; 366:37–43.

9. Liesegang TJ, Melton LJ 3rd, Daly PJ, *et al.* Epidemiology of ocular herpes simplex. Incidence in Rochester, Minn, 1950 through 1982. *Arch Ophthalmol* 1989; 107:1155–1159.

10. Uchio E, Takeuchi S, Itoh N, *et al.* Clinical and epidemiological features of acute follicular conjunctivitis with special reference to that caused by herpes simplex virus type 1. *Br J Ophthalmol* 2000; 84:968–972.

11. Womack LW, Liesegang TJ. Complications of herpes zoster ophthalmicus. *Arch Ophthalmol* 1983; 101:42–45.

12. Liesegang TJ. Herpes zoster ophthalmicus natural history, risk factors, clinical presentation, and morbidity. *Ophthalmology* 2008; 115:S3–12.

13. Sambursky RP, Fram N, Cohen EJ. The prevalence of adenoviral conjunctivitis at the Wills Eye Hospital Emergency Room. *Optometry* 2007; 78:236–239.

14. Branco BC, Gaudio PA, Margolis TP. Epidemiology and molecular analysis of herpes simplex keratitis requiring primary penetrating keratoplasty. *Br J Ophthalmol* 2004; 88:1285–1288.

15. Foster A, Sommer A. Corneal ulceration, measles, and childhood blindness in Tanzania. *Br J Ophthalmol* 1987; 71:331–343.

16. Wilhelmus KR. Therapeutic interventions for herpes simplex virus epithelial keratitis. *Cochrane Db Syst Rev* 2008:CD002898.

17. Wilhelmus KR, Gee L, Hauck WW, *et al.* Herpetic Eye Disease Study. A controlled trial of topical corticosteroids for herpes simplex stromal keratitis. *Ophthalmology* 1994; 101:1883–1895.

18. Barron BA, Gee L, Hauck WW, *et al.* Herpetic Eye Disease Study. A controlled trial of oral acyclovir for herpes simplex stromal keratitis. *Ophthalmology* 1994; 101:1871–1882.

19. The Herpetic Eye Disease Study Group. A controlled trial of oral acyclovir for the prevention of stromal keratitis or iritis in patients with herpes simplex virus epithelial keratitis. The Epithelial Keratitis Trial. *Arch Ophthalmol* 1997; 115:703–712.

20. The Herpetic Eye Disease Study Group. Oral acyclovir for herpes simplex virus eye disease: effect on prevention of epithelial keratitis and stromal keratitis. *Arch Ophthalmol* 2000; 118:1030–1036.

21. van Rooij J, Rijneveld WJ, Remeijer L, *et al.* Effect of oral acyclovir after penetrating keratoplasty for herpetic keratitis: a placebo-controlled multicenter trial. *Ophthalmology* 2003; 110:1916–1919; discussion 9.

22. Whitley RJ, Roizman B. Herpes simplex viruses: is a vaccine tenable? *J Clin Invest* 2002; 110:145–151.

23. Colin J, Prisant O, Cochener B, *et al.* Comparison of the efficacy and safety of valaciclovir and acyclovir for the treatment of herpes zoster ophthalmicus. *Ophthalmology* 2000; 107:1507–1511.

24. Tyring S, Engst R, Corriveau C, *et al.* Famciclovir for ophthalmic zoster: a randomised aciclovir controlled study. *Br J Ophthalmol* 2001; 85:576–581.

25. Dworkin RH, Johnson RW, Breuer J, *et al.* Recommendations for the management of herpes zoster. *Clin Infect Dis* 2007; 44:S1–S26.

26. Gross G, Schofer H, Wassilew S, *et al.* Herpes zoster guideline of the German Dermatology Society (DDG). *J Clin Virol* 2003; 26:277–289.

27. Reynolds MA, Chaves SS, Harpaz R, *et al.* The impact of the varicella vaccination program on herpes zoster epidemiology in the United States: a review. *J Infect Dis* 2008; 197:S224–227.

28. Liesegang TJ. Varicella zoster virus vaccines: effective, but concerns linger. *Can J Ophthalmol* 2009; 44:379–384.

29. Ward JB, Siojo LG, Waller SG. A prospective, masked clinical trial of trifluridine, dexamethasone, and artificial tears in the treatment of epidemic keratoconjunctivitis. *Cornea* 1993; 12:216–221.

30. Laibson PR, Dhiri S, Oconer J, *et al.* Corneal infiltrates in epidemic keratoconjunctivitis. Response to double-blind corticosteroid therapy. *Arch Ophthalmol* 1970; 84:36–40.

31. Hillenkamp J, Reinhard T, Ross RS, *et al.* The effects of cidofovir 1% with and without cyclosporin a 1% as a topical treatment of acute adenoviral keratoconjunctivitis: a controlled clinical pilot study. *Ophthalmology* 2002; 109:845–850.

32. Shiuey Y, Ambati BK, Adamis AP. A randomized, double-masked trial of topical ketorolac versus artificial tears for treatment of viral conjunctivitis. *Ophthalmology* 2000; 107:1512–1517.

33. Dart JK, El-Amir AN, Maddison T, *et al.* Identification and control of nosocomial adenovirus keratoconjunctivitis in an ophthalmic department. *Br J Ophthalmol* 2009; 93:18–20.

34. Wright PW, Strauss GH, Langford MP. Acute haemorrhagic conjunctivitis. *Am Fam Physician* 1992; 45:173–178.

16c

Acanthamoeba keratitis

STEPHANIE WATSON AND JOHN DART

16c.1	Definition	409		16c.5	Risk factors	412
16c.2	Classification	410		16c.6	Management	413
16c.3	Prevalence of blindness from acanthamoeba keratitis	410		16c.7	Epidemiological research priorities	415
16c.4	Geographical distribution and incidence	410			References	416

16c.1 DEFINITION

Acanthamoeba spp. are cyst-forming, free-living amoeboid protozoans. They are ubiquitous in air, soil, dust and water[1-3] and are commonly found in the upper respiratory tracts of humans.[4,5] *Acanthamoeba spp.* may occasionally cause a meningoencephalitis, as well as granulomatous infections in a variety of other non-ocular tissues that typically occur in the immune-compromised. Acanthamoeba keratitis differs from these non-ocular infections in that it affects healthy individuals predisposed to keratitis by **contact lens (CL)** wear or corneal trauma, and has become increasingly common.[3,6,7] Other amoebae, such as *Hartmanella spp.*, *Naeglaeria spp.*, and *Vahlkampfia spp.* have been isolated from cases of keratitis.

Acanthamoebae exist either as actively metabolizing motile trophozoites or, under adverse conditions, dormant cysts that are able to survive desiccation, temperature extremes and noxious chemicals.[8] *Acanthamoeba* cysts are therefore difficult to treat and eradicate (Plate 16c.1 and 16c.2).[8-10]

16c.1.1 Acanthamoeba keratitis

Acanthamoeba keratitis (AK) is often painful and disabling,[11] and may also result in scleritis[9,12,13] and chorioretinitis.[14] The pain on presentation is typically severe and out of proportion to the clinical signs, although absence of pain does not preclude the diagnosis.[3,9,11,15-17] Radial keratoneuritis is said to be pathognomonic for Acanthamoeba keratitis (Plate 16c.3),[18] but is neither invariably present[3,15,17] nor specific, having also been reported in Pseudomonas keratitis.[19] In early disease, punctate keratopathy, pseudodendrites, epithelial infiltrates and diffuse or focal subepithelial infiltrates are common (Plate 16c.4).[11,20] Recognition of these early signs is important in order to avoid the common pitfall of misdiagnosis as herpes simplex or fungal keratitis.[1,9,10,15,17] Ring infiltrates and indolent or relapsing corneal ulceration are usually signs of late disease, although they can be seen in the first month (Plate 16c.5).[20] Limbitis is common in all disease phases.[21]

A good prognosis is associated with early diagnosis and the use of effective medical therapy.[3,8-11,18] Advanced disease has a poorer prognosis and is often complicated by factors such as persistent epithelial defect, bacterial super-infection, chronic or recurrent corneal or scleral inflammation, severe pain and glaucoma.[3,9–11,15]

Despite the large number of corneal cases now recorded, spread of *Acanthamoeba* from the cornea into other ocular and non-ocular tissues has been reported only very rarely.[12,14,21]

16c.2   CLASSIFICATION

Acanthamoeba spp. have been classified subjectively, based on their cyst morphology or, more recently, using isoenzyme or **mitochondrial deoxyribonucleic acid (mtDNA)**. Over 30 species of *Acanthamoebae* have now been identified.[3] At least eight species have been reported to cause keratitis: *A. castellani, A. polyphagia, A. hatchetii, A. culbertsoni, A. rhysodes, A. lugdenesis, A. quina* and *A. griffini.*

16c.3   PREVALENCE OF BLINDNESS FROM ACANTHAMOEBA KERATITIS

Earlier diagnosis and better anti-amoebic therapy have improved the prognosis of Acanthamoeba keratitis, so that loss of the eye is now uncommon.[3,8,10,22] A poorer prognosis is associated with a delay in the start of effective therapy of more than three weeks from the onset of symptoms.[18,22] Two large national surveys in the United Kingdom reported a final visual acuity of 6/6 or better in 65.5% and of 6/9 to 6/12 in 30.5%.[11] The main reason for poor visual outcome (< 6/12) is corneal scarring.[10,18,22] Eyes lost because of infection with *Acanthamoeba* are the result of pain or scleritis. Factors associated with a poor outcome include delayed diagnosis or misdiagnosis, inappropriate antimicrobial treatment, resistant organisms, severe scleritis, deep stromal involvement and a ring infiltrate.[10,12,17,18,22,23]

The need for penetrating keratoplasty in Acanthamoeba keratitis has been greatly reduced by the improved outcomes of medical therapy.[10] At one centre in 1984–1992, 30% of Acanthamoeba keratitis cases required penetrating keratoplasty,[17] compared with 9% of cases in 1992–1995.[10] Recently, in the UK, corneal grafting was required in 11% of cases.[11] Multiple corneal grafts with a poor visual outcome

may be required to treat Acanthamoeba keratitis that is unresponsive to medical therapy.[24] The outcome of penetrating keratoplasty in Acanthamoeba keratitis is good in uninflamed eyes but poor if inflammation or uncontrolled infection is present, when graft failure and/or recurrence are common.[21,22,24]

16c.4   GEOGRAPHICAL DISTRIBUTION AND INCIDENCE

Acanthamoeba keratitis is an uncommon acute disease, rarely persisting for years. Consequently, population-based cross-sectional studies of prevalence would be impractical, as these would require huge sample sizes of more than a million individuals. Incidence figures, however, are available, derived from surveillance data (disease notification data) in large general populations and in contact lens wearers. Wide geographical variations in incidence have been reported.[7,15,25–29] These have been related to differences in the prevalence of wear and care of contact lenses, environmental factors, and variations in the use of diagnostic techniques for Acanthamoeba keratitis.[30]

Population-based estimates for the annual incidence of Acanthamoeba keratitis in the whole population vary from as low as 0.15–0.18 per million in the USA to as high as 1.4 per million in the UK and 1.35 per million in Sweden, with other countries for which figures are available, such as Australia and New Zealand, having intermediate incidences.[31] These differences have been shown, at least in large part, to relate to the prevalence of contact lens (CL) use, the contamination of domestic water and swimming pools by *Acanthamoeba*, the amoebicidal efficacy of CL care systems, regional variations in the availability of different CL care systems, the use of reusable soft contact lenses, and the frequency of the use of diagnostic techniques for Acanthamoeba keratitis. These risks are described in more detail below.

Acanthamoeba keratitis in non-lens users

In non-contact lens wearers, Acanthamoeba keratitis is often overlooked, leading to its late diagnosis. Of all Acanthamoeba keratitis cases, 3–15% occur in non-contact lens wearers.[27,32] In India, where

CL use is much less widespread, it has been reported in 1% of culture positive cases of microbial keratitis,[31,33,34] compared with 4–8% for countries where CL use is common.[25,35]

Acanthamoeba keratitis in contact lens users

AK is responsible for less than 5% of CL related microbial keratitis cases[25,31,35] and is typically unilateral, though in a UK survey 8/106 (7.5%) cases were reported as bilateral.[32] Male and female CL wearers are affected equally.[15,27] National incidence estimates for CL users vary widely from 1.65–2.01 per million in the USA to 17.53–19.50 per million in the UK.[32] These incidence data are summarized in Table 16c.1.

16c.4.1 Changes in incidence and geographical distribution with time

An increased incidence of Acanthamoeba keratitis during the summer/early autumn has been reported and is probably related to the increased presence of Acanthamoeba in the environment during warmer weather.[2,25,28,30,32,36] However, there have been longer-term and more substantial temporal and regional changes in the incidence of Acanthamoeba keratitis[3] as a result of changing trends in the care and use of contact lenses[3,26,27] and of other environmental factors.

Table 16c.1 *Summary of the incidence of AK (population data from internet)*

Location	Annual incidence of AK per million population	Annual incidence of AK per million CLW[A]	Year
UK[8,32]	1.4	19.5	1992–1996
	1.26	21.14	1997–1998
	1.13	17.53	1998–1999
USA[39]	0.15–0.18	1.65–2.01	1985–1987
West Scotland[65]		149	1999
Canada[6]			
Netherlands[26,42]		2.9	1996
Sweden[66,67]	1.35		1991–1993
Sweden[66]		12.91	1989–1991
New Zealand[46]	0.28	25	1998
Australia[46,68]	0.56		1984–1997
Hong Kong[25]	3	5 cases in CLW	1997–1998

[A] CLW = contact lens wearer

Acanthamoeba keratitis was first reported in 1974 in the USA, and by 1984 only 11 further cases had been recorded; most of these were associated with minor ocular trauma.[27] The first case in a CL user, as a result of exposure to contaminated water from a hot tub, was reported in 1984, and by 1985 the association with CL wear was established.[37] Subsequently, similar cases were reported in the UK, and then in many other countries.[3,28] An epidemic was recognized in the USA in the 1980s,[27] and an association with CL wear became apparent, and was probably linked to an increase in the number of CL users, the use of homemade saline for lens care, swimming in lenses and poor lens hygiene.[9,27,38] The estimated incidence in the USA from 1985 to 1987 was between 1.65 and 2.01 per million contact lens wearers.[27,39]

In the UK the main increase in cases occurred during the 1990s.[17] This was accounted for by an increased prevalence of contact lens wear and a deterioration of contact lens hygiene practice. This was associated with the introduction of frequently replaced (one to four weeks) soft lenses, together with the greater use of chlorine-based contact lens cleaning systems.[3,28,40] Chlorine disinfection is relatively ineffective against Acanthamoeba spp. and accounted both for the increased incidence of Acanthamoeba keratitis during the 1990s in the UK and for the association with swimming and CL wear.[41]

The occurrence of Acanthamoeba keratitis in CL wearers, the role of chlorine-based cleaning systems and poor CL hygiene in promoting the disease, attracted intense media attention in the UK. Widespread discussion and increased education of CL wearers followed, and the incidence fell dramatically in 1996.[42] Currently there has been a reported increase in cases of Acanthamoeba keratitis in the USA, similar to the outbreak in the UK. On this occasion the association has been with the use of a multipurpose contact lens solution (AMO Complete MoisturePlus), probably compounded by poor use of the hygiene systems.[43] Previous studies have also identified one-step hydrogen peroxide systems as a probable risk factor for Acanthamoeba keratitis.[25,28] Table 16c.2 summarizes factors that have so far been iden-tified in the intra-regional incidence of Acanthamoeba keratitis with time.

Table 16c.2 *Risk factors for Acanthamoeba keratitis*

Risk factors for Acanthamoeba keratitis
CL-related
Swimming in CL[28,38,46,65]
Irregular disinfection[28,32,38,65]
Chlorine disinfection[32,40,65]
Non-sterile water[65]
Homemade saline[9,28,38,46]
One-step hydrogen peroxide systems[32]
Poor CL case hygiene,[32,65] e.g. not leaving case to dry[65]
Orthokeratology lenses[47]
Non-CL-related
Trauma in an agricultural or outdoor setting[15,27,28,32,69]
Exposure to unclean water, e.g. lake, sea or spring water[70,71]
Flooding[44]
Tank-fed water in the home[2,9,42]
Warmer weather[2,28,44]
Poor socio-economic conditions[15,44]

Environmental factors, such as flooding or the emergence of more virulent strains, may have contributed to the increased incidence in some regions of the USA.[44] This may also be an unrecognized factor elsewhere. Regional flooding has been identified as a potential cause of a localized increase in incidence in a part of the USA, although the diagnostic criteria were weak and the disease atypical, raising the possibility that these cases were due to a different pathogen.[45]

Changes in the reported incidence are likely to continue with the following developments:

➢ An increase due to the more widespread inclusion of screening tests for *Acanthamoeba* in diagnostic protocols for keratitis. Currently there is limited availability of the specialist tissue stains, culture techniques, **polymerase chain reaction (PCR)** for *Acanthamoeba* DNA, and confocal microscopy, which can all contribute to, or confirm, the diagnosis.

➢ Changes in the prevalence of CL wear, which is likely to increase the incidence. However, the potential increase in incidence among CL wearers could be offset by improved CL hygiene and the efficacy of contact lens care systems against *Acanthamoeba*.

16c.5   RISK FACTORS

16c.5.1   Contact lenses and lens types

Contact lens wear is the most widely recognized risk factor for occurrence of Acanthamoeba keratitis.[9,10,27,28,38,46] However, epidemiological studies of Acanthamoeba keratitis have neither been designed nor powered appropriately to measure the risks associated with different CL types. Daily-wear rigid lenses probably have a lower risk than soft lenses.[6,28] Planned-replacement soft lenses, which need to be cleaned daily and stored overnight, probably have a higher risk than daily disposable lenses, possibly due to hygiene issues.[32] Cases of Acanthamoeba keratitis have been associated with orthokeratology lenses, which are rigid and worn overnight to flatten the cornea and improve the unaided vision during the day,[47] as well as with cosmetic contact lenses that are used to change the eye colour.[48] The development of Acanthamoeba keratitis in CL users is much more strongly related to poor lens hygiene and water contamination than is bacterial keratitis, for which wearing lenses overnight remains the main factor. The preferential adhesion of *Acanthamoeba* to some contact lens materials may also have a role in CL-associated Acanthamoeba keratitis.[3,51] Additional factors probably include tear film stagnation, ocular surface compartmentalization behind the lens, a reduction in corneal epithelial cell turnover and alterations in corneal epithelial cell mannose expression, amongst other factors.[49,50]

16c.5.2   Contaminated water and contact lens use

Contaminated water is important to the pathogenesis of AK both in CL and in non-lens users. For CL users the same risk factors have been demonstrated in a number of epidemiological studies carried out in different countries; all have shown the importance of exposure to contaminated water in swimming pools and to tap water in the home, failures of various CL hygiene systems, and poor CL hygiene practices.[6,25,27,28,32,40,43,52] Up to 90% of cases can be attributed to avoidable risk factors.[28] The relatively low incidence of Acanthamoeba keratitis in New Zealand (Table 16c.1) has been ascribed to the lack of availability of chlorine-release disinfection,[46] as well as the small total number (30,000–50,000) of soft CL wearers.

In the UK *Acanthamoeba* has been found in limescale in domestic water taps. This could result from the favourable environment provided by the limescale, coupled with contamination by *Acanthamoeba* of tank-stored domestic water.[2,42] An epidemiological study found a three-fold increase in the risk of Acanthamoeba keratitis in hard water areas.[32] This circumstantial evidence for the importance of domestic water contamination in the UK has been shown for AK cases where identical organisms, demonstrated by gene sequencing, have been recovered from the eye and domestic water supply of 6/27 AK cases. This study demonstrated free living amoebae in 24/27 domestic supplies of which 8/27 grew *Acanthamoeba*.[53] In Korea, similar methodology was used to demonstrate that 4/5 CL cases were contaminated by the same organism as found in the domestic supply.[54] An increase in the incidence of AK cases in Chicago in 2003–2005 has been circumstantially related to alterations in disinfection policy affecting the contamination of local water supplies.[52] Tap water has also been implicated in Hong Kong, where the organism is found in the domestic water of 8% of homes, perhaps because of the warm weather.[25] Swimming in CLs has been identified as a risk factor since the first epidemic of AK was investigated in the 1980s.[27]

16c.5.3 Contact lens solution and lens hygiene practice

A case-controlled study established that lens solutions and lens hygiene were major risk factors for Acanthamoeba keratitis in CL users in the epidemiological investigation of the outbreak in the USA in the 1980s. This was linked to an increase in the number of CL users, the use of homemade saline lens care solution, swimming with lenses and poor lens hygiene.[27] An epidemic of AK occurred in the early 1990s in the UK but with causes different from the epidemic in the USA. A case-control study demonstrated that the risk of developing Acanthamoeba keratitis was largely confined to users of the recently introduced planned replacement (one to four week) soft CLs. This was due both to absent or poor contact lens hygiene in users of these lenses (increasing the risk up to 50x), and because of the use, in addition to the poor implementation, of a chlorine-based CL disinfection system that was marketed with this lens type (increasing the risk 14 to 40 times). The increasing prevalence of CL wear was also implicated.[41] The intense media attention in the UK that followed this publication led to widespread awareness of the disease, increased education of CL users and a dramatic fall in incidence.[42]

The recent increase in cases of AK in the USA, similar to the outbreak described a decade earlier in the UK, has been associated with the use of a multipurpose contact lens solution (AMO Complete MoisturePlus), probably compounded by poor use of the hygiene systems.[43] Previous studies have also identified one-step hydrogen peroxide systems as a probable risk factor for Acanthamoeba keratitis.[25,28] No other CL hygiene solution has yet been implicated.

16c.5.4 Non contact lens users

In non-wearers of contact lenses, AK has been attributed to environmental factors. Exposure to contaminated water or soil, often with agricultural trauma, is the main risk factor in this group.[15,29,33,38] The occurrence of AK has been linked to flooding,[44] tank-fed water in the home,[2,9,42] warmer weather,[2,28,44] and poor socio-economic conditions.[15,44] Acanthamoeba keratitis has also been reported after penetrating keratoplasty and radial keratotomy.[3] Table 16c.2 summarizes risk factors for AK.

16c.6 MANAGEMENT

16c.6.1 Diagnosis

The diagnosis of AK is based on the clinical picture and laboratory investigations, including the culture and histology of corneal scrapes and/or biopsies.[9,55] Corneal scrapes are taken from the corneal stroma for culture on non-nutrient agar overlaid with *Escherichia coli*, and if available smears are sent for PCR and/or stained with calcafluor white and immunostains. Sensitivity testing of isolates *in vitro* is possible in some centres but only the biguanides have been shown to be consistently cysticidal.[56] Confocal microscopy allows rapid confirmation of AK and is the preferred diagnostic test in some centres.[57–59] The sensitivity and specificity of confocal microscopy for AK have been reported to exceed 90% for individual unmasked observers. The efficacy of confocal microscopy has, however, not been confirmed in well-designed masked studies nor compared with culture- or histology-positive cases. PCR has been shown in one study to have a sensitivity of over 80% and specificity of 100% for the diagnosis of AK.[60] In another study only 24 of 31 cases of AK diagnosed by confocal microscopy were confirmed by PCR.[45] The high sensitivity and specificity reported for confocal microscopy in AK may be centre-related and therefore not representative of what may be expected elsewhere. Reliance on confocal microscopy alone may lead either to misdiagnosis or a missed diagnosis of AK. Until further confirmatory data are available on confocal microscopy, it should be used in the initial evaluation of cases, but not for making a definitive diagnosis in cases with a negative tissue diagnosis (culture, histology of biopsies/smears, or PCR) and a poor response to therapy.[11]

Contact lenses and lens cases should also be tested and routine bacterial and fungal investigations performed, including microscopy of contact lens case fluid.[3] However *Acanthamoeba* is a common contaminant of CL cases (up to 6% of asymptomatic users in some series,[61] and its presence in the case does not indicate that a keratitis is due to *Acanthamoeba*. Conversely, Acanthamoeba keratitis is uncommon in patients from whose lens cases it cannot be cultured or identified by microscopy.

Biopsy is undertaken if initial investigations are negative in progressive cases, or before graft surgery to determine whether there is active infection. A 3 mm skin trephine is used to mark an area off the visual axis, and a lamellar button is removed with a lamellar corneal dissection knife (e.g. a Paufique or scleral pocket knife); in cases with large necrotic abscesses, the necrotic material is removed with a lamellar dissection together with some relatively unaffected tissue peripheral to the ulcer. The specimen is divided for histology, and for culture after homogenization. The success rate of microscopy investigations is 48% for epithelial biopsies/scrapes, 65% for formal corneal biopsies (Plate 16c.2) and 66% for whole corneal buttons.[17]

16c.6.2 Medical therapy

Topical treatment usually results in a medical cure, especially if it is commenced in the early stages of infection.[10,56]

Drug susceptibility and availability

The only consistently cysticidal agents are the biguanides, chlorhexidine and **polyhexamethyl biguanide (PHMB)**. Chlorhexidine is usually used as a 0.02% (200 μg/ml) solution, and occasionally as a 0.2% (2000 μg/ml) solution in cases that have been resistant to therapy. PHMB is also used as a 0.02% and, in cases that are resistant to therapy, as a 0.06% (600 μg/ml) solution.[8] These drugs are available from Moorfields Pharmaceuticals, London, UK and manufacturing pharmacies elsewhere. The diamidines, propamidine isethionate 0.1% (Brolene, May and Baker, Dagenham, UK) or hexamidine 0.1% (Desomedine, Chauvin, Montpellier, France) have also been widely used; but some organisms are fully resistant to these *in vitro*, and this has been associated with poor clinical outcomes.[10,11,56] Resistance may develop during therapy and is difficult to manage. Alexidine and the amidoamine myristamidopropyl dimethylamine are biguanides with good *in vitro* anti-acanthamoebal efficacy, but are not in clinical use.[62,63]

Drug administration

After tissue is taken for diagnosis, therapy with a biguanide and a diamidine is commenced. This treatment is empiric as there is no clinical evidence to suggest that dual therapy is more effective than monotherapy with a biguanide alone. Topical therapy is administered, according to the authors' protocol, hourly for 48 hours and then hourly during daytime only for three days. Intensive therapy is given initially as cysts are more susceptible before they may have fully matured. Toxicity is common if the dosage is maintained at this frequency, thus therapy is then reduced to two-hourly by day for three to four weeks.[1,10,11] If toxicity is suspected, Brolene (or hexamidine) is reduced or stopped as PHMB less often causes a toxic response.[10] After the clinical signs have fully resolved, therapy is then continued four times daily for a further month to prevent the recrudescence of active infection from viable cysts (Plate 16c.1); this may take several weeks.

The management of advanced disease is often complicated by persistent epithelial defects, with or without bacterial superinfection, keratitis and scleritis, severe pain and/or glaucoma. Keratitis may persist in the absence of any viable organisms. Scleritis, although occurring in up to 10% in some series, has only once been associated with scleral invasion by *Acanthamoeba*. The clinical problem of establishing whether persistent keratitis is due to viable organisms or not, leads to substantial difficulty in management. Oral non-steroidal anti-inflammatory agents are useful for pain management and for control of less severe scleritis and limbitis. Topical and/or systemic immunosuppressive therapy may be needed, in addition to antimicrobial therapy, to control the severe inflammatory complications.[13] The use of topical steroids is controversial. If topical steroids are needed for severe persistent inflammation, we do not use them until completion of two weeks of biguanide therapy to ensure, as far as possible, that viable organisms have been eliminated. Topical biguanide therapy is always used during topical steroid use, and continued for four weeks after the steroid treatment has ceased. In advanced disease, prolonged periods of anti-amoebic therapy are required and treatment may be needed for 12 months or more.

16c.6.3   Surgical therapy

Extensive debridment of the epithelium can be used to obtain specimens for diagnosis, to treat intraepithelial disease and to improve drug penetration.[11,64]

In inflamed eyes, corneal graft surgery is reserved for the management of corneal perforation, intumescent cataract or severe unremitting keratitis that has failed medical therapy.[11,17,24] Anti-amoebic therapy is continued after keratoplasty, at least until either culture results from the host corneal button have been shown to be negative or there have been no signs of a relapse of infection within four weeks of the transplant. Recurrence is usually dramatic and widespread and typically occurs within three to 21 days postoperatively,[55] although recurrence several months after keratoplasty has been seen by the authors. Topical, and sometimes systemic immunosuppressive agents, may be needed to control severe post keratoplasty ocular inflammation. Graft surgery in the presence of active disease carries a poor prognosis[24] and we avoid this if at all possible.

Double freeze–thaw cryotherapy of the cornea may be used when medical therapy has failed, as it is thought to potentiate drug penetration into cysts.[11]

16c.7   EPIDEMIOLOGICAL RESEARCH PRIORITIES

➢ Epidemiological studies have provided a good understanding of the etiological factors, distribution and features of AK, especially in CL wearers.[17,27,28,32,38,61] Further studies are needed to define the risk factors, epidemiology and clinical features of AK in non-wearers of contact lenses, as this group still faces considerable delays in diagnosis and treatment, with a poorer prognosis in consequence.[10,11,15,28]

➢ The potential of prophylaxis for AK after ocular injuries in agricultural communities, by the provision of clean water for irrigation and the topical application of inexpensive broadspectrum disinfectants, such as propamidine, has not been evaluated. Interventional trials could be used to evaluate their use in prophylaxis for all types of keratitis, including AK (see Section 16a).

➢ For CL wearers, ongoing surveillance studies are needed to determine the current incidence of AK, as it varies with the ever-changing trends in CL use.[28,32] Trends in CL materials, wearing patterns (daily disposable, frequent- and infrequent-replacement daily wear, and overnight wear) and care systems (chlorine, one-step peroxide, and some multipurpose solutions),[3,26,32] have affected the incidence of AK in the past and may do so in the future.

> *Acanthamoeba* levels in domestic water, resistance patterns to anti-amoebic treatments, and the colonization of CL cases and solutions should be evaluated to identify areas for intervention. There is a requirement to educate CL wearers and CL practitioners about the risks of poor hygiene and the use of ineffective hygiene systems.[28,55] Epidemiological studies have shown that most AK in contact lens wearers is associated with avoidable risk factors, rendering this condition potentially more susceptible to preventive measures than any other cause of keratitis in CL users.[32]

> Acanthamoeba keratitis has been found to be more common than expected in many countries once laboratory tests for its identification have been included in the routine investigation of keratitis cases. These tests should be included in any keratitis surveillance studies in order to identify the early changes in the incidence of AK that are needed to develop effective prevention and treatment strategies.[33]

REFERENCES

1. Mathers WD, Sutphin JE, Folberg R, *et al*. Outbreak of keratitis presumed to be caused by Acanthamoeba. *Am J Ophthalmol* 1996; 121:129–142.

2. Seal D, Stapleton F, Dart J. Possible environmental sources of *Acanthamoeba spp.* in contact lens wearers. *Br J Ophthalmol* 1992; 76:424–427.

3. Illingworth CD, Cook SD. Acanthamoeba keratitis. *Surv Ophthalmol* 1998; 42:493–508.

4. Wang SS, Feldman HA. Isolation of hartmannella species from human throats. *N Engl J Med* 1967; 277:1174–1179.

5. Cerva L, Serbus C, Skocil V. Isolation of limax amoebae from the nasal mucosa of man. *Folia Parasitol (Praha)* 1973; 20:97–103.

6. McAllum P, Bahar I, Kaiserman I, *et al*. Temporal and seasonal trends in Acanthamoeba keratitis. *Cornea* 2009; 28:7–10.

7. Carvalho FR, Foronda AS, Mannis MJ, *et al*. Twenty years of Acanthamoeba keratitis. *Cornea* 2009; 28:516–519.

8. O'Day DM, Head WS. Advances in the management of keratomycosis and Acanthamoeba keratitis. *Cornea* 2000; 19:681–687.

9. Moore MB, McCulley JP, Luckenbach M, *et al*. Acanthamoeba keratitis associated with soft contact lenses. *Am J Ophthalmol* 1985; 100:396–403.

10. Duguid IGM, Dart JK, Morlet N, *et al*. Outcome of Acanthamoeba keratitis treated with polyhexamethyl biguanide and propamidine. *Ophthalmology* 1997; 104:1587–1592.

11. Dart JK, Saw VP, Kilvington S. Acanthamoeba keratitis: diagnosis and treatment update 2009. *Am J Ophthalmol* 2009; 148:487–499.

12. Mannis MJ, Tamaru R, Roth AM, *et al*. Acanthamoeba sclerokeratitis. Determining diagnostic criteria. *Arch Ophthalmol* 1986; 104:1313–1317.

13. Lee GA, Gray TB, Dart JK, *et al*. Acanthamoeba sclerokeratitis: treatment with systemic immunosuppression. *Ophthalmology* 2002; 109:1178–1182.

14. Johns KJ, O'Day DM, Feman SS. Chorioretinitis in the contralateral eye of a patient with *Acanthamoeba* keratitis. *Ophthalmology* 1988; 95:635–639.

15. Sharma S, Garg P, Rao GN. Patient characteristics, diagnosis, and treatment of non-contact lens related Acanthamoeba keratitis. *Br J Ophthalmol* 2000; 84:1103–1108.

16. Tabin G, Taylor H, Snibson G, *et al*. Atypical presentation of Acanthamoeba keratitis. *Cornea* 2001; 20:757–759.

17. Bacon AS, Frazer DG, Dart JKG, *et al*. A review of 72 consecutive cases of Acanthamoeba keratitis. *Eye* 1993; 7:719–725.

18. Bacon AS, Dart JK, Ficker LA, *et al*. Acanthamoeba keratitis. The value of early diagnosis. *Ophthalmology* 1993; 100:1238–1243.

19. Feist RM, Sugar J, Tessler H. Radial keratoneuritis in Pseudomonas keratitis. *Arch Ophthalmol* 1991; 109:774–775.

20. Patel DV, McGhee CN. Acanthamoeba keratitis: a comprehensive photographic reference of common and uncommon signs. *Clin Exp Ophthalmol* 2009; 37:232–238.

21. Perez-Santonja JJ, Lee GA, Fulcher T, *et al.* Acanthamoeba keratitis. *Comprehensive Ophthalmology Update* 2001; 2:93–104.

22. Claerhout I, Goegebuer A, Van Den Broecke C, *et al.* Delay in diagnosis and outcome of Acanthamoeba keratitis. *Graefes Arch Clin Exp Ophthalmol* 2004; 242:648–653.

23. Tu EY, Joslin CE, Sugar J, *et al.* Prognostic factors affecting visual outcome in Acanthamoeba keratitis. *Ophthalmology* 2008; 115:1998–2003.

24. Kitzmann AS, Goins KM, Sutphin JE, *et al.* Keratoplasty for treatment of Acanthamoeba keratitis. *Ophthalmology* 2009; 116:864–869.

25. Houang E, Lam D, Fan D, *et al.* Microbial keratitis in Hong Kong: relationship to climate, environment and contact-lens disinfection. *Trans R Soc Trop Med Hyg* 2001; 95:361–367.

26. Cheng KH, Kijlstra A. Contact-lens-associated microbial keratitis in The Netherlands and Scotland. *Lancet* 2000; 355:144.

27. Stehr-Green JK, Bailey TM, Visvesvara GS. The epidemiology of Acanthamoeba keratitis in the United States. *Am J Ophthalmol* 1989; 107:331–336.

28. Radford CF, Lehmann OJ, Dart JKG. National Acanthamoeba Study Group. Acanthamoeba keratitis: multicentre survey in England 1992–1996. *Br J Ophthalmol* 1998; 82:1387–1392.

29. Kunimoto DY, Sharma S, Garg P, *et al.* Corneal ulceration in the elderly in Hyderabad, south India. *Br J Ophthalmol* 2000; 84:54–59.

30. Ibrahim YW, Boase DL, Cree IA. Factors affecting the epidemiology of Acanthamoeba keratitis. *Ophthalmic Epidemiol* 2007; 14:53–60.

31. Acharya NR, Lietman TM, Margolis TP. Parasites on the rise: a new epidemic of Acanthamoeba keratitis. *Am J Ophthalmol* 2007; 144:292–293.

32. Radford CF, Minassian D, Dart JK. Acanthamoeba keratitis in England and Wales: incidence, outcome, and risk factors. *Br J Ophthalmol* 2002; 86: 536–542.

33. Srinivasan M, Gonzales CA, George C, *et al.* Epidemiology and aetiological diagnosis of corneal ulceration in Madurai, South India. *Br J Ophthalmol* 1997; 81:965–971.

34. Bharathi MJ, Ramakrishnan R, Meenakshi R, *et al.* Microbial keratitis in South India: influence of risk factors, climate, and geographical variation. *Ophthalmic Epidemiol* 2007; 14:61–69.

35. Butler TK, Males JJ, Robinson LP, *et al.* Six-year review of Acanthamoeba keratitis in New South Wales, Australia: 1997–2002. *Clin Exp Ophthalmol* 2005; 33:41–46.

36. Ibrahim YW, Boase DL, Cree IA. Factors affecting the epidemiology of Acanthamoeba keratitis. *Ophthalmic Epidemiol* 2007; 14:53–60.

37. Moore MB, McCulley JP, Luckenbach M, *et al.* Acanthamoeba keratitis associated with soft contact lenses1. *Am J Ophthalmol* 1985; 100:396–403.

38. Stehr-Green JK, Bailey TM, Brandt FH, *et al.* Acanthamoeba keratitis in soft contact lens wearers. A case-control study. *JAMA* 1987; 258:57–60.

39. Schaumberg DA, Snow KK, Dana MR. The epidemic of Acanthamoeba keratitis: where do we stand? *Cornea* 1998; 17:3–10.

40. Radford CF, Dart JK, Minassian DC. Risk factors for acanthamoeba keratitis. *Br Med J* 1996; 312:183.

41. Radford CF, Bacon AS, Dart JK, *et al.* Risk factors for acanthamoeba keratitis in contact lens users: a case-control study. *Br Med J* 1995; 310:1567–1570.

42. Morlet N, Duguid G, Radford C, *et al.* Incidence of acanthamoeba keratitis associated with contact lens wear. *Lancet* 1997; 350:414.

43. Joslin CE, Tu EY, Shoff ME, *et al.* The association of contact lens solution use and Acanthamoeba keratitis. *Am J Ophthalmol* 2007; 144:169–180.

44. Mathers WD, Sutphin JE, Lane JA, *et al.* Correlation between surface water contamination with amoeba and the onset of symptoms and diagnosis of amoeba-like keratitis. *Br J Ophthalmol* 1998; 82:1143–1146.

45. Mathers WD, Nelson SE, Lane JL, *et al.* Confirmation of confocal microscopy diagnosis of Acanthamoeba keratitis using polymerase chain reaction analysis. *Arch Ophthalmol* 2000; 118: 178–183.

46. Murdoch D, Gray TB, Cursons R, *et al.* Acanthamoeba keratitis in New Zealand, including two cases with *in vivo* resistance to polyhexamethylene biguanide. *Aust NZ J Ophthalmol* 1998; 26:231–236.

47. Watt KG, Swarbrick HA. Trends in microbial keratitis associated with orthokeratology. *Eye Contact Lens* 2007; 33:373–377.

48. McKelvie J, Patel D, McGhee C. Cosmetic contact lens-related Acanthamoeba keratitis. *Clin Exp Ophthalmol* 2009; 37:419–420.

49. Dart JK, Radford CF, Minassian D, *et al.* Risk factors for microbial keratitis with contemporary contact lenses: a case-control study 3. *Ophthalmology* 2008; 115:1647–1654.

50. Stapleton F, Keay L, Edwards K, *et al.* The incidence of contact lens-related microbial keratitis in Australia. *Ophthalmology* 2008; 115:1655–1662.

51. Gorlin AI, Gabriel MM, Wilson LA, *et al.* Effect of adhered bacteria on the binding of Acanthamoeba to hydrogel lenses. *Arch Ophthalmol* 1996; 114: 576–580.

52. Joslin CE, Tu EY, McMahon TT, *et al.* Epidemiological characteristics of a Chicago-area Acanthamoeba keratitis outbreak. *Am J Ophthalmol* 2006; 142:212–217.

53. Kilvington S, Gray T, Dart J, *et al.* Acanthamoeba keratitis: the role of domestic tap water contamination in the United Kingdom. *Invest Ophthalmol Vis Sci* 2004; 45:165–169.

54. Jeong HJ, Lee SJ, Kim JH, *et al.* Acanthamoeba: keratopathogenicity of isolates from domestic tap water in Korea. *Exp Parasitol* 2007; 117:357–367.

55. Meisler D. Acanthamoeba keratitis. In: Tabbara KHR, (ed). *Infections of the Eye.* Boston: Little, Brown and Company; 1995. pp. 685–695.

56. Larkin DFP, Kilvington S, Dart JKG. Treatment of Acanthamoeba keratitis with topical polyhexamethylene biguanide. *Ophthalmology* 1992; 99:185–191.

57. Mathers WD. Acanthamoeba: a difficult pathogen to evaluate and treat. *Cornea* 2004; 23:325.

58. Tu EY, Joslin CE, Sugar J, *et al.* The relative value of confocal microscopy and superficial corneal scrapings in the diagnosis of Acanthamoeba keratitis. *Cornea* 2008; 27:764–772.

59. Parmar DN, Awwad ST, Petroll WM, *et al.* Tandem scanning confocal corneal microscopy in the diagnosis of suspected acanthamoeba keratitis. *Ophthalmology* 2006; 113:538–547.

61. Larkin DF, Kilvington S, Easty DL. Contamination of contact lens storage cases by Acanthamoeba and bacteria. *Br J Ophthalmol* 1990; 74:133–135.

62. Seal DV. Acanthamoeba keratitis update — incidence, molecular epidemiology and new drugs for treatment. *Eye* 2003; 17:893–905.

63. Kilvington S, Hughes R, Byas J, *et al.* Activities of therapeutic agents and myristamidopropyl dimethylamine against Acanthamoeba isolates. *Antimicrob Agents Chemother* 2002; 46: 2007–2009.

64. Sun X, Zhang Y, Li R, *et al.* Acanthamoeba keratitis: clinical characteristics and management. *Ophthalmology* 2006; 113:412–416.

65. Seal DV, Kirkness CM, Bennett HG, *et al.* Population-based cohort study of microbial keratitis in Scotland: incidence and features. *Cont Lens Anterior Eye* 1999; 22:49–57.

66. Nilsson SE, Montan PG. The annualized incidence of contact lens induced keratitis in Sweden and its relation to lens type and wear schedule: results of a 3-month prospective study. *CLAO J* 1994; 20:225–230.

67. Skarin A, Floren I, Kiss K, *et al.* Acanthamoeba keratitis in the south of Sweden. *Acta Ophthalmol Scand* 1996; 74:593–597.

68. Jackson TN, Heinze JB, Tuxen J, *et al.* Successful medical treatment of a corneal ulcer due to Acanthamoeba polyphaga. *Aust NZ J Ophthalmol* 1986; 14:139–142.

69. Whitcher JP, Srinivasan M. Corneal ulceration in the developing world — a silent epidemic. *Br J Ophthalmol* 1997; 81:622–623.

70. Chang PC, Soong HK. Acanthamoeba keratitis in non-contact lens wearers. *Arch Ophthalmol* 1991; 109:463–464.

71. Sharma S, Srinivasan M, George C. Acanthamoeba keratitis in non-contact lens wearers. *Arch Ophthalmol* 1990; 108:676–678.

16d

Ocular manifestations of leprosy

PAUL COURTRIGHT AND SUSAN LEWALLEN

16d.1 Introduction   419
16d.2 Eye disease in leprosy   421
16d.3 The magnitude of blindness   425
       in leprosy
16d.4 Prevention and control   425
16d.5 Epidemiological research needs   427
       References   427

16d.1 INTRODUCTION

Leprosy is a chronic inflammatory disease caused by *Mycobacterium leprae*, an acid-fast bacillus related to *Mycobacterium tuberculosis*. It is an obligate human parasite, not yet cultivated *in vitro*. The organism is slowly growing, having a doubling time of 12 days, the longest of any known bacterium.

Infection by *M. leprae* results in a complex humoral and cellular immune response. The disease displays a wide clinical spectrum related to the host ability to develop a specific cell-mediated response. The organism infects most people exposed to it, but most do not develop recognizable clinical disease because they mount an adequate immune response that limits bacterial multiplication. The determinants of an individual's immune response to *M. leprae*, including the possible role of infective dose and route of infection, are still not completely understood.

16d.1.1 The systemic disease

Leprosy consists of a spectrum of disease, determined by an individual's immunologic response to the infection (Fig. 16d.1). At one end there are **paucibacillary (PB)**, previously known as tuberculoid type patients, with localized lesions restricted to skin and peripheral nerves. They have relatively intact cellular immune function. Acid-fast bacilli are scanty in the skin tissue, hence the term 'paucibacillary'. At the other end of the spectrum there are **multibacillary (MB)**, previously known as lepromatous patients, with markedly impaired cellular immunity and very high bacillary loads throughout the body, including the skin, upper respiratory tract and eyes. The relationship between number of bacilli harboured, the patient's cell-mediated immunity status, and the resulting disease type are shown in Fig 16d.1. Many patients, known as *borderline*, lie between the two extremes and have variable degrees of cellular immunity towards *M. leprae*. The immune response against *M. leprae* in a borderline patient is unstable and may shift in either direction. These shifts may occur quietly or be clinically manifest during so called leprosy '*reactions*', which are immunologically-mediated inflammatory episodes. The cause of these reactions is not known, but they are responsible for a great deal of the nerve and skin damage that characterize leprosy. Reactions are characterized as two

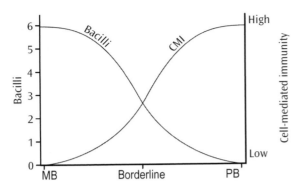

Figure 16d.1 *The clinical spectrum of leprosy. MB = Multibacillary disease; PB = Paucibacillary disease; CMI = cell-mediated immunity*

types: **Type I reactions** are due to increasing cell-mediated hypersensitivity, while **Type II reactions** (erythema nodosum leprosum, or ENL) are due to immune complex disease.[1] Type II reactions occur only in MB patients, and it is during these reactions that acute iridocyclitis and scleritis are most likely to occur.

Skin smear or biopsy is generally used in determining leprosy type although it is not always a clear determination. Nonetheless the type is used to determine duration of treatment as described below.

M. leprae grows best at temperatures of less than 37°C; hence it infects cooler regions of the body including the skin, nasal mucosa, certain cranial and peripheral nerves, and the anterior segment of the eye. Damage to these structures can result from massive infiltration by the bacilli (in MB types) and from inflammation. Nerve damage, probably the most important consequence of leprosy, occurs as a result of acute and chronic inflammation in the Schwann cells of infected nerves; it is responsible for many of the deformities that stigmatize leprosy, including **lagophthalmos**. Motor nerve damage results in clawing of hands and feet; loss of sensation renders digits highly susceptible to recurrent minor traumas, which eventually destroy the tissues.

16d.1.2   Effect of treatment

The use of leprosy chemotherapy determines much of the 'epidemiology' of the disease.

Dapsone, the first effective drug used, was administered daily for a minimum of five years to PB patients and for life to MB patients. Because it was slow acting and weakly bactericidal, little clinical improvement was apparent, poor patient compliance was common, and dapsone-resistant strains of *M. leprae* emerged. In 1982 the World Health Organization (WHO) recommended **multidrug therapy (MDT)**, comprising dapsone, rifampicin and clofazimine.[2] The aim of MDT is two-fold — to cure individual patients and to interrupt further transmission of the disease. Most significantly, the WHO declared that after six months of treatment for PB disease and one year for MB disease, patients would be regarded as 'cured' and released from treatment. This resulted in a dramatic decrease in the official prevalence of the disease. However, an unknown number of patients have already sustained irreversible nerve and other tissue damage at the time of leprosy diagnosis, and will progress after 'cure' to develop disabilities (including eye disease) secondary to their pre-existing nerve damage. Such patients still require healthcare and rehabilitation, but are likely to be ignored by the healthcare system when defined as 'cured'.[3] These people are referred to as 'released from treatment' (RFT). With these definitions in mind, during the last ten years approximately five million people have been newly diagnosed with leprosy. For the five years from 2004 to 2008 the number of new cases of leprosy has ranged between 250,000–400,000 per year.[4] However, many leprologists believe that the true global burden could be much higher.[3]

The introduction and expansion of MDT has changed the leprosy profile in all endemic countries and reduced complications due to the disease. Compared with dapsone alone, MDT is better accepted by patients and prevents development both of drug resistance and disabilities. The prevention of disabilities has been attributed to MDT's effectiveness in reducing bacterial loads and, indirectly, to improvements in case detection and management secondary to improved patient compliance. In spite of all the important benefits of MDT, however, there is little evidence that it has changed the epidemiology of leprosy and the actual incidence of the disease may have remained static.[5]

16d.1.3   Prevalence and incidence

In the past leprosy occurred in almost all tropical and temperate countries. It is generally recognized that the distribution of leprosy is linked to socio-economic status. In Norway and elsewhere in Europe, where the disease was once endemic, the reduction in incidence preceded the introduction of effective anti-leprosy chemotherapy. The worldwide prevalence has continued to decline, so that registered leprosy cases at the beginning of 2009 were 213,036. The geographical distribution in 1997 is shown in Fig. 16d.2.

The number of new cases reported by 121 countries in 2008 was 249,007. Data from 2004–2008 suggest that the majority of new cases came from India (about 55%), Brazil (about 16%) and Indonesia (about 7%).[5] The top ten countries in terms of numbers of new cases also include Bangladesh, Democratic Republic of the Congo, Nigeria, Nepal, Ethiopia, Myanmar and Tanzania. For many years these countries have consistently had the highest number of newly registered cases. In leprosy-endemic areas, the peak age of incidence for MB leprosy is said to be 20–35 years, while PB is detected somewhat younger. In most races the incidence is higher in men than women.

16d.2   EYE DISEASE IN LEPROSY

Obtaining accurate information about the prevalence and incidence of ocular manifestations of leprosy has been hindered by several factors. Varying case definitions of leprosy have been used, sometimes also including only patients under treatment and sometimes patients who have been released from treatment, but may still have or develop ocular disease. Another problem has been the definition of 'eye disease'; for example, some studies have reported manifestations of leprosy, which include non-visually significant changes such as loss of eyebrows and lashes. At a meeting of experts in 2001 it was suggested that only visually threatening lesions should be considered in reporting.[20]

The **Longitudinal Study of Ocular Leprosy (LOSOL)** was a multicentre study of MB patients that ran for ten years starting in 1988. This provided important information on prevalence of ocular pathology at diagnosis and incidence throughout treatment and beyond. Findings are noted below, we will in appropriate sections.

The three major causes of visual disability and blindness in leprosy patients are corneal disease (primarily a result of exposure secondary to lagophthalmos), uveal disease (in particular, chronic uveitis) and cataract (both complicated and age-related). The distribution of these across populations with leprosy depends on three interrelated factors: the distribution of leprosy type (PB or MB), the age of the population, and the penetration of MDT in the population. We will discuss what is known about each of the clinical aspects in relation to these factors.

16d.2.1   The effect of leprosy type

In general, the ocular manifestations of leprosy vary depending on whether the patient is PB or MB type; however, as noted, these are not always clear distinctions. With declining prevalence of new cases, there has been a predominance of MB disease globally; whether this is due to changing epidemiology or better detection of MB disease compared with PB disease remains unclear. Globally, it is likely that over 65% of new leprosy patients are MB. The proportion of new cases with advanced deformities, an indication of the length of time the disease has gone untreated, can be as high as 25%, indicating that there is a significant delay in leprosy diagnosis.[5]

16d.2.2   Lagophthalmos

Lagopthalmos (literally 'hare eye'), the primary factor associated with corneal disease in leprosy patients, is a result of damage in the zygomatic branch

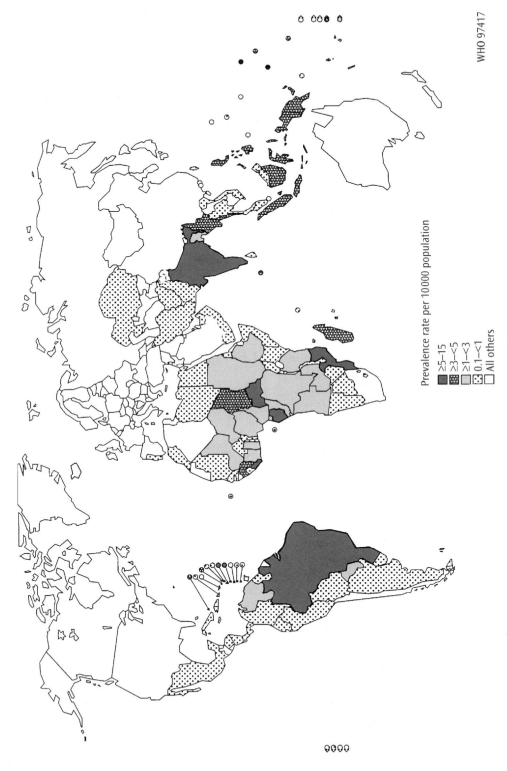

WHO 97417

Prevalence rate per 10000 population

≥5–15
≥3–<5
≥1–<3
0.1–<1
All others

Figure 16d.2 *The prevalence of registered leprosy cases in the world as of 1997 (reproduced by kind permission of the World Health Organization)*

or the temporal branch of the eighth nerve. Together with corneal anaesthesia due to inflammation of the fifth nerve, lagophthalmos causes corneal damage from exposure keratitis, trichiasis, trauma and infection (Plate 16d.1). Among Chinese patients, the risk of corneal disease was 67 times (95% CI 26–175) higher in the presence of lagohthalmos than in its absence.[6]

Lagophthalmos occurs in both PB and MB patients but the aetiologies are different. Among PB patients, lagophthalmos is primarily associated with the presence of facial patches, areas where skin is infiltrated with bacilli over the malar region or around the eye (Plate 16d.2).[7] Damage to the facial nerve, where it traverses the facial patch, presumably occurs from increased inflammation during a reaction. In this Indian study,[7] 85% of PB patients with recent lagophthalmos had both a facial patch involving the lid and a history of Type I reaction.

Among MB patients, lagophthalmos may be related to nerve damage secondary to proliferation of bacilli in the nerve tissue. In the MB patients in the LOSOL Study lagophthalmos prevalence was 3.3% at the time of diagnosis.[8] This is consistent with findings among newly diagnosed Chinese MB patients where lagophthalmos was present in 3.8% of cases.[6] Older age and a reaction involving the face were associated with lagophthalmos in the LOSOL patients. The incidence of lagophthalmos during MDT was low, being only 1.2% (95% CI 0.5–2.8) of patients per year over two years of anti-leprosy treatment.[9] Incident lagophthalmos during MDT was associated with grade 2 deformity in all limbs. After completion of MDT the annual incidence of lagopthalmos declined further, and was estimated to be 0.24% (95% CI 0.10–0.37) per patient year.[10] Available information on lagophthalmos is summarized in Table 16d.1.

Table 16d.1 *Summary of prevalence and incidence estimates for lagophthalmos and chronic uveitis in leprosy*

Lagophthalmos	Prevalence (*)	Incidence (*)
At leprosy diagnosis	PB: 2%[6] MB: 3%[8]	
During MDT (2 yrs for MB)		PB: no data MB: 1.2%/year[9]
After MDT		PB: no data MB: 0.2%/year[10]
Population-based surveys	PB: 2%[11] MB: 5%[12]	

Chronic uveitis([†])	Prevalence (*)	Incidence (*)
At leprosy diagnosis	4%[8]	
During MDT (2 yrs)		5.1%/year[9]
After MDT		3.8%/year[10]
Population-based surveys	6–20%[7,9,17,18]	

* Primary references for estimates.
† Defined as posterior synechiae or constricted pupil (by slit lamp examination) and reported for MB patients only.
PB = paucibacillary leprosy.
MB = multibacillary leprosy.
MDT = multidrug therapy.

Further evidence for different aetiologies of lagophthalmos in PB and MB patients is provided by the finding that lagophthalmos in PB disease is primarily unilateral and develops early, while in MB patients it is primarily bilateral, sometimes developing many years after diagnosis.

An estimate of the magnitude of lagophthalmos worldwide (Table 16d.2) is based on the expected lagophthalmos prevalence rates in MB and PB patients and an assumption that the ratio of MB to PB patients worldwide is 65:35. With this assumption, among the five million newly diagnosed patients in the past ten years, there are approximately 198,000 leprosy patients with lagophthalmos, about 100,000 fewer than

Table 16d.2 *Estimate of the global distribution of leprosy and lagophthalmos*

	SE Asia	Africa	Americas	Other*	Total
Leprosy patients (million)	3.75	0.55	0.60	0.10	5.0
Estimated lagophthalmos cases	148,000	22,000	24,000	4,000	198,000

Assumptions: At a minimum, lagophthalmos will be found among 2% of PB (paucibacillary) patients and 5% of MB (multibacillary) patients.

previous estimates.[11] This reduction is most likely due to (non-specific) mortality in leprosy patients diagnosed before the implementation of MDT.

16d.2.3   Chronic uveitis

So-called chronic uveitis occurs primarily among MB patients, although it has been recognized among PB patients in Nepal and Uganda.[12,13] PB patients with uveitis were older and had a longer duration of disease than those without. The process is insidious and may be the result of nerve damage as well as low-grade inflammation and results in a small pupil (Plate 16d.3).

Among newly diagnosed MB patients in Nepal and Sichuan, China, chronic uveitis was detected in 2% and 4.3% of patients respectively.[12,14] In newly diagnosed MB patients in the LOSOL study, chronic uveitis was recognized in 4.1% at the time of leprosy registration; older age was the only factor associated with its prevalence.[8] During two years of MDT in an Indian population, it was noted that the annual incidence was 5.1% (95% CI 3.3–7.8), with grade 2 deformity in all limbs and older age being the only predictors.[9] In the same group of patients, after the completion of MDT, the annual incidence remained high at 3.78% per patient year (95% CI 2.96–4.83).[10] Incident uveal involvement was associated with increasing age, grade 2 deformity and smear positivity at baseline. Thus, it appears that the more severely infected MB patients and those with serious deformity before treatment may be at a higher risk of continuing immunologically mediated disease.

16d.2.4   Cataracts

Chronic uveitis predisposes patients to complicated cataracts. Data from a cross-sectional study in Uganda showed that leprosy patients with evidence of chronic uveitis have a three-fold risk (95% CI 1.6, 5.5) of cataract, compared with leprosy patients without uveitis, independent of age.[13]

Another cross-sectional study found that, among males, cataract occurred at a significantly younger age in multibacillary patients compared to paucibacillary, but whether this was related with more uveitis in the MB group was not clear.[15]

16d.2.5   Other ocular manifestations

The incidence of acute uveitis in leprosy patients is not known. An increased risk is recognized in MB patients during a Type II reaction but its magnitude is unknown.

In addition to the potentially blinding complications mentioned above, there are a number of other manifestations of leprosy in the eye and ocular adnexa. Some of them are unique to leprosy but tend to be either rare or visually insignificant, and include such entities as avascular keratitis, beading of corneal nerves, formation of iris pearls, scleral nodules and madarosis (loss of eyebrows). They generally occur in MB patients and reflect the high bacillary load. In addition to acute iridocyclitis, scleritis may occur in patients undergoing Type II reactions.

Ocular disease is often present at the time of leprosy diagnosis. In Nepal 5% of newly diagnosed leprosy patients (both MB and PB) already had leprosy-related sight threatening pathology (defined as lagophthalmos, corneal hypoaesthesia or iris involvement) and 18% had lens changes.[12] Evidence from China suggests that about 10% of patients will have pre-existing ocular pathology at the time of disease diagnosis.[6] Eleven percent of MB patients in the LOSOL study had potentially blinding leprosy pathology (lagophthalmos, trichiasis, chronic uveitis) at the time of their leprosy registration.[8] MDT cannot reverse this pathology.

16d.2.6   The effect of age of the population

Ocular pathology and blindness in leprosy develop as a result of chronic factors, and most ocular morbidity and blindness in leprosy occur in adulthood. Older populations everywhere in developing countries are expected to have more blindness due to age-related cataract; this occurs in leprosy populations at least as commonly as in non-leprosy populations. Cataract is the major cause of blindness and visual impairment in leprosy patients. It is likely that they often have less access to whatever services exist than do the elderly without leprosy, since those with physical deformities may have to overcome the barriers related to the stigma of leprosy.[16]

16d.2.7 The effect of MDT

The LOSOL study demonstrated that MDT does not eliminate incident leprosy-related ocular disease. During the two years of follow-up, the annual incidence of leprosy-related ocular pathology (defined as muscle weakness, lagophthalmos, ectropion, entropion, trichiasis, episceritis, scleritis, corneal nerve beading, punctate keratis and uveal involvement) was 9.9% (95% CI 7.2–13.7).[9] If only lagophthalmos and uveal involvement were included as potentially blinding leprosy-related pathology, the annual incidence was 5.8% (95% CI 3.9–8.8%). The LOSOL cohort also showed that after completion of MDT (at which time patients were generally removed from control efforts) incident leprosy-related ocular pathology ranged from 5.65% (95% CI 4.51–7.09) per patient year for overall pathology to 3.86% (95% CI 3.00–4.95) per patient year for potentially blinding leprosy-related ocular pathology.[10] These findings are consistent with an earlier report from Korea which found that 14.7% developed one or more sight threatening lesions (lagophthalmos, keratitis or posterior synechiae) over an 11-year period.[17] This is likely due to the many years of undertreated leprosy.

Thus, to summarize, populations with more MB disease, those with more elderly people and those with the greatest lag time between infection and treatment will have the greatest prevalence of ocular disease.

16d.3 THE MAGNITUDE OF BLINDNESS IN LEPROSY

In 1988 it was estimated that there were approximately 250,000 blind among the (then) 12 million total leprosy patients,[12] a prevalence rate of 2.1%. No estimate has been made since then. It is worth noting that, at diagnosis, 2.8%, (age-adjusted) of the 691 LOSOL MB patients were blind (defined as best-eye vision of <6/60) and 29 (5.2%) were visually impaired (6/24–6/60).[8] Most of this blindness, however, was unrelated to leprosy. Current data suggest that approximately 0.5–1% of leprosy patients would be blind owing to the disease, and an additional 2–3% owing to causes other than leprosy (age-related cataract, in particular). Based upon these assumptions, among the total five million recognized leprosy patients 100,000 to 200,000 are likely to be blind. Evidence from population based surveys[13,16] and LOSOL[8] suggests that cataract is the leading cause of blindness in leprosy patients. The transition from corneal blindness, the major cause in the pre-MDT era, is likely due to the success of MDT in reducing the incidence of lagophthalmos.

16d.4 PREVENTION AND CONTROL

Generally, the best strategy for prevention of the ocular manifestations of leprosy is early case detection and prompt treatment of patients with MDT. However, even in the best programmes there will be patients who have ocular problems at the time of diagnosis and also some who will develop problems during and after treatment. The evidence for interventions for specific problems derives primarily from assessment in limited groups of patients.

Preventing corneal disease should focus on educating patients about the hazards of anaesthetic corneas and foreign bodies, preventing lagophthalmos, and providing surgical intervention when it has occurred. Lagophthalmos that has been present for less than six months may be reversed by giving oral steroids.[19] Once lagophthalmos is established, however, eyelid surgery is required to prevent corneal damage. A large number of different surgical procedures are used worldwide, but there are no valid clinical trials to compare procedures in leprosy patients.

Prevention of chronic uveitis and complicated cataract is impeded by our poor understanding of the pathophysiology of this condition and our inability to recognize it in its early stage. Long-term use of dilating agents, commonly suggested, has not been studied in a trial. The persistent finding of incident chronic uveitis, even after release from treatment, suggests that some patients, particularly those with high bacterial loads or grade 2 disability at time of diagnosis require long-term follow up.

For leprosy patients with cataract, whether complicated or age-related, surgery is recommended and modern techniques with intraocular lenses have been shown to give good results in studies from India,[20] Brazil[21] and Korea.[16] Leprosy patients face all the barriers experienced by any elderly poor rural people in getting good quality cataract surgery, but an additional challenge is sometimes found in getting the eye services to accept leprosy patients.

Recommendations for prioritization of leprosy patients for screening and follow-up for eye care have been published.[22–23]

16d.4.1   Future needs and trends

Leprosy remains a disease associated with poverty and marginalized populations; providing eye care in these environments will remain a challenge. Case detection for leprosy is passive in most settings, and health workers are expected to report cases to national health authorities when they present. Rarely, active case-finding campaigns may take place but these have decreased dramatically in the past decade. Current guidelines recommend that all patients be screened for eye disease at the time of their leprosy diagnosis and at discharge from the anti-leprosy treatment programme.[20] Any patients with visual impairment or blindness, lagophthalmos, a facial patch or a persistent red eye should have routine follow-up. The political will, resources and management necessary to implement these guidelines remain elusive.

MDT should theoretically reduce the general incidence of leprosy by continuing to reduce the mycobacterial load in the community. However, there is little documented evidence of reductions in incidence.[3] Reducing mycobacterial load in the individual should reduce the propensity for ocular damage. It is important to keep in mind, however,

a number of factors that will limit the impact of MDT on the incidence and severity of ocular pathology.

First, coverage of MDT is not 100% in every programme. Researchers and policy makers have expressed concern regarding the reduction of active case-finding programmes (leading to under-diagnosis) and the late presentation among new cases identified (leading to high prevalence of disabilities).[4]

Second, even with the expansion of MDT, a significant proportion of leprosy patients alive today and cured microbiologically years ago have a history of dapsone mono-therapy. The prevalence of ocular complications is high in this group. Evidence from Korea suggests that pre-existing pathology (in particular chronic uveitis) may be progressive in nature, or may only become clinically apparent after the completion of MDT. An interesting note from the histological work in Nepal was that among 29 cured MB patients acid-fast bacilli were found in the iris specimens of five cases.[15] Although it is important from a societal standpoint that patients released from treatment no longer be considered leprosy patients, from the perspective of eye care and blindness prevention, many of these people should continue to be routinely monitored.

The general worldwide increase in life expectancy in developing countries is having an impact on the epidemiology of the ocular complications of leprosy. Although life expectancy is generally increasing, the pre-MDT cohort is dying. Over the next 20 years the number of patients in this group (among whom ocular complications and blindness are greatest) will decrease. Conversely, many leprosy patients, especially in newly industrialized countries, have increased visual needs and demands, which some programmes are starting to address.

Third, the consistent finding that both an older age and a longer duration between disease onset and leprosy diagnosis are independently associated with an increased risk of ocular pathology suggests that expansion of MDT coverage alone is inadequate. Even where MDT coverage is excellent, 5–10% of leprosy patients will have potentially blinding ocular pathology present at the time of leprosy diagnosis. Although two-year MDT reduces the incidence of ocular pathology, the LOSOL findings show that it does not eliminate *M. leprae* related ocular pathology. Furthermore, there is no information on the impact of the adoption of the more recent short-course (one-year) MDT on incident ocular pathology.

16d.5 EPIDEMIOLOGICAL RESEARCH NEEDS

➢ The completion of the LOSOL study of MB patients provided much needed epidemiological and clinical information. Following this cohort for additional years would further our understanding of the incidence of eye disease in MB leprosy. The anticipated low incidence of eye disease in PB patients (and the declining proportion of PB patients) would make it difficult to justify a longitudinal study among these individuals.

➢ Existing recommended practical guidelines for eye care in leprosy[20,21] need to be implemented. Operational research on the ability of the programme to recognize, refer and manage eye disease in leprosy patients would help to refine strategies to meet these guidelines.

➢ Cataract extraction will be the primary ocular surgery required by leprosy patients in the coming decades, and recent reports suggest that good outcomes can be achieved. Operational research is needed to determine the best approaches for increasing uptake of cataract surgery.

➢ Research is required into appropriate community educational activities to ensure that once patients are mycobacteriologically cured they are no longer considered leprosy patients. This will assist in improving the community and patient acceptance of leprosy as a curable disease. At the same time, there is the need to identify cured leprosy patients who can be included in eye care without having attention drawn to them as having once had leprosy. Research is needed to determine how this can be done practically, particularly given the fact that grade 2 disability (clinically obvious deformity) at the time of disease diagnosis is a major risk factor for leprosy-related eye disease.

➢ Finally, addressing social and economic factors will become increasingly important as life expectancy continues to climb and leprosy patients must face additional years with eye disease or vision loss. Leprosy may have been eliminated globally as a 'public health problem', but the challenges of reducing the impact of eye disease in leprosy patients remains.

REFERENCES

1. Saunderson P. The epidemiology of reactions and nerve damage. *Leprosy Review* 2000; 71(supplement): S106–110.

2. World Health Organization Study Group. Chemotherapy of leprosy for control programmes. WHO Technical Report Series No. 675. Geneva: WHO, 1982.

3. Burki T. Old problems still mar fight against ancient disease. *Lancet* 2009; 373:287–288.

4. World Health Organization. Global leprosy situation 2009. *WHO Wkly Epidemiol Rec* 2009; 84:333–340.

5. Saunderson PR. Leprosy elimination: not as straightforward as it seemed. *Public Health Reports* 2008; 123:213–216.

6. Courtright P, Hu LF, Li HY, *et al.* Multidrug therapy and eye disease in leprosy: a cross-sectional study in the People's Republic of China. *Int J Epidemiol* 1994; 23:835–842.

7. Hogeweg, M, Kiran KU, Suneetha S. The significance of facial patches and Type I reaction for the development of facial nerve damage in leprosy. A retrospective study among 1226 paucibacillary leprosy patients. *Lepr Rev* 1991; 62: 143–149.

8. Courtright P, Daniel E, Rao S, *et al.* Eye disease in multibacillary leprosy patients at the time of their leprosy diagnosis: findings from the Longitudinal Study of Ocular Leprosy (LOSOL) in India, the Philippines and Ethiopia. *Lepr Rev* 2002; 73: 225–238.

9. Daniel E, ffytche TJ, Sundar Rao PSS, *et al.* Incidence of ocular morbidity among multibacillary leprosy patients during a 2-year course of multidrug therapy. *Br J Ophthalmol* 2006; 90:568–573.

10. Courtright P, Daniel E, Ffytche TJ, *et al.* Incidence of ocular complications in patients with multibacillary leprosy after completion of a 2-year course of multidrug therapy. *Br J Ophthalmol* 2006; 90: 949–954.

11. Courtright P, Lewallen S. Current concepts in the surgical management of lagophthalmos in leprosy. *Lepr Rev* 1995; 66:220–223.

12. Lubbers WJ, Schipper A, Hogeweg M, *et al.* Eye disease in newly diagnosed leprosy patients in eastern Nepal. *Lepr Rev* 1994; 65:231–238.

13. Waddell KM, Saunderson PR. Is leprosy blindness avoidable? The effect of disease type, duration, and treatment on eye damage from leprosy in Uganda. *Br J Ophthalmol* 1995; 79:250–256.

14. Courtright P, Lewallen S, Li HY, *et al.* Lagophthalmos in a multibacillary population under multidrug therapy in the People's Republic of China. *Lepr Rev* 1995; 66:214–219.

15. Brandt F, Kampik A, Malla OK, *et al.* Blindness from cataract formation in leprosy. *Dev Ophthal* 1983; 7:1–12.

16. Courtright P, Lewallen S, Tungpakorn N, *et al.* Cataract in leprosy patients: cataract surgical coverage, barriers to acceptance of surgery, and outcome of surgery in a population-based survey in Korea. *Br J Ophthalmol* 2001; 85:643–647.

17. Lewallen S, Tungpakorn NC, Kim SH, *et al.* Progression of eye disease in 'cured' leprosy patients: implications for understanding the pathophysiology of ocular disease and for addressing eye care needs. *Br J Ophthalmol* 2000; 84:817–821.

18. Courtright P, Johnson GJ. *Prevention of Blindness in Leprosy*, 1st Edition. London: International Centre for Eye Health; 1998.

19. Kiran KU, Hogeweg M, Suneetha S. Treatment of recent facial nerve damage with lagophthalmos, using a semistandard steroid regimen. *Lepr Rev* 1991; 62:150–154.

20. Courtright P, Tamplin M. Guidelines for the management of eye care in leprosy: recommendations from ILEP supported meeting. *IAPB News* 2001; 32:8–9.

21. Courtright P, Lewallen S. *Prevention of Blindness in Leprosy*, 2nd Edition. Greenville, SC: American Leprosy Missions; 2006.

22. Anand S, Neethiodiss P, Xavier JW. Intra- and postoperative complications and visual outcomes following cataract surgery in leprosy patients. *Lepr Rev* 2009; 80:177–186.

23. Dias RJN, Maakaroun MJ, deCastro AV. Phacoemuslification with intraocular lens implantation in leprosy patients: case control study. *Arq Bras Oftalmol* 2006; 69:345–348.

16e

Vernal keratoconjunctivitis

STEPHEN TUFT AND BITA MANZOURI

16e.1	Definition	429	16e.5	Risk factors	431
16e.2	Clinical features	429	16e.6	Management	432
16e.3	Classification	430	16e.7	Epidemiological research priorities	432
16e.4	Prevalence and geographical distribution	431		References	433

16e.1   DEFINITION

Atopy is a predisposition to mount an allergic response to environmental allergens. The mild ocular allergic diseases are seasonal and perennial allergic conjunctivitis. The severe variants are **vernal keratoconjunctivitis (VKC)**, which has an early onset with a high expectation for eventual resolution, and atopic keratoconjunctivitis, which is unremitting and typically develops in older patients with severe pre-existing eczema.

16e.2   CLINICAL FEATURES

VKC usually develops in the first decade of life (82% by age ten years with a mean age of seven years), and in 95% of cases there is remission by the late teens.[1,2] New cases are rare in adults.[2] Symptoms consist of itch, blepharospasm, photophobia, foreign body sensation, blurred vision and mucous discharge. The clinical signs are often asymmetric. The skin of the lids may be eczematous and fissured at the canthi with secondary ptosis. There is diffuse papillary hypertrophy over the upper tarsal plate with cellular infiltration that obscures the underlying vessels (Plate 16e.1). Giant papillae (>1 mm) have a cobblestone appearance and, in active disease, mucus accumulates between the papillae. When papillae form at the limbus they appear as gelatinous and vascular mounds. White Horner–Trantas dots (aggregates of degenerated eosinophils and epithelial cells) can form on the apices of limbal papillae. Eventually, reticular scarring develops over the upper tarsal plate, although this is rarely of clinical significance.[3]

Punctate epithelial erosions on the superior and central cornea may be the only corneal change in mild disease. If there is active palpebral disease, mucus is deposited on the superior corneal epithelium, which may stimulate the formation of new superficial corneal vessels. Severe upper lid disease may result in corneal epithelial necrosis (macroerosion) caused by toxic agents (e.g. eosinophilic major basic protein) released from the epithelium of the upper tarsal conjunctiva.[4] An epithelial erosion may heal completely with appropriate treatment, but mucus and calcium deposition on Bowman's layer can prevent re-epithelialization. The resulting vernal plaque (shield ulcer; Plate 16e.2) rarely vascularizes, but there is a risk of secondary infection, and, after control of inflammation, a superficial keratectomy may be required before re-epithelialization will occur. In recurrent limbal disease an arcuate infiltrate can develop adjacent to areas of papillae (pseudogerontoxon), and there may be cystic degeneration of the conjunctiva in previously affected areas. Limbal VKC can be severe in tropical regions, where it can be an important cause of visual loss. Patients with chronic allergic eye disease are more susceptible to severe attacks of herpes simplex keratitis, and in Turkey, keratoconus has been reported in up to 26% of patients with VKC. A characteristic anterior capsular cataract has been described in up to 8% of atopic patients in the past.[5]

Giant papillae, whether tarsal or limbal, consist of a central vascular core of mononuclear cells surrounded by oedematous connective tissue infiltrated with granulocytes, plasma cells, mast cells, activated eosinophils and lymphocytes.[6] There is squamous metaplasia of the overlying epithelium that may contain mast cells but a reduced number of goblet cells. Scar tissue (collagen type III) is formed in the fibrovascular core of the papillae. The conjunctival cellular infiltrate is rich in **T-lymphocytes** with clusters of **B-lymphocytes** beneath the epithelium. A subpopulation of T-lymphocytes (Th2) is abnormally expanded, and these drive the disease process via the type I **(immunoglobulin E (IgE)**-mediated) immediate hypersensitivity response. The Th2 cells generate cytokines and interleukins (IL-3, IL-4 and IL-13) promoting B-cell synthesis of IgE.[7,8] When an allergen comes into contact with conjunctival mast cells coated with IgE antibodies specific to that allergen, the mast cells degranulate and release histamine and other cytokines that recruit other inflammatory cells, such as eosinophils, which in turn attract more inflammatory cells.[9] Several inflammatory mediators are then released into the tissue and tears.[10]

A diagnosis of VKC is normally based on the characteristic clinical signs. Investigations to support the diagnosis are not widely available. Examination of tears shows elevated histamine, tryptase and IgE. In patients with VKC who have associated eczema, the total serum IgE and tear IgE are almost always elevated, and measurement of this is therefore not always helpful in confirming an allergic basis of eye symptoms. In contrast, measurement by radio-allergosorbent test (RAST) of local IgE production by the conjunctiva, as opposed to passive leakage of IgE into the tear film, supports the presence of allergic conjunctivitis.[2,11] Cytology, taken by swabbing the conjunctiva, will contain eosinophils and MC_T mast cells (tryptase positive, chymase negative) if there is severe allergic eye disease.[12] Testing for immediate hypersensitivity by skin prick challenge to environmental allergens (pollens, house dust mite etc.) can support an atopic basis for the disease. However, the results may not help guide treatment, as patients may react to several allergens. In temperate regions, epidermal or conjunctival challenge testing shows that at least 50% of patients are sensitive to house dust mite allergen, pollens and animal dander.[2,11] Allergen-specific conjunctival provocation may reveal sensitivity to allergens that do not provoke a response by skin testing; in the same individual the allergens provoking asthma and allergic conjunctivitis may be different.

16e.3 CLASSIFICATION

VKC is classified as palpebral, limbal or combined disease according to the distribution of the giant papillae. An observational study performed in London showed that corneal ulceration, the primary cause of visual reduction, is almost exclusively associated with palpebral disease. Palpebral or combined limbal and palpebral diseases behave similarly, whereas isolated limbal disease is a more benign variant of VKC in temperate regions.[13] Disease activity is best reflected by the presence of mucous between the papillae over the upper tarsal plate, with mucous adherent to the corneal epithelium, as well as corneal epithelial breakdown and ulceration. A grading system for severity of disease based on the size of superior tarsal papillae and associated scarring, the presence of limbal papillae, the extent of encroachment of the papillae onto the peripheral cornea, and secondary corneal changes, has been proposed as a basis for initiating treatment and as a suitable template for assessing the outcome of clinical trials.[14] Incorporating an assessment of quality of life changes into clinical trials would help quantify any subjective response to treatment.[15]

16e.4 PREVALENCE AND GEOGRAPHICAL DISTRIBUTION

There is very little information from population-based studies on the prevalence of VKC. The available information comes either from surveys of clinic attendances or surveys of school children. This information suggests that the prevalence of VKC varies greatly. Sixty years ago in Africa, India and the Middle East it constituted a substantial public health problem, accounting for 3% of new ophthalmic disease presenting to clinics.[5] More recently it was responsible for 9.8% of outpatient attendances.[16] Surveys of schools report that it affects 3–10% of children in Africa and the Middle East.[17] In tropical areas it can account for up to 6% of all ophthalmic referrals and up to 90% of new ophthalmic referrals in children.[18] In contrast, by extrapolation from outpatient attendances, the prevalence in the UK has been estimated to be 0.02%,[19] and 0.03% in Western Europe as a whole.[2,17]

VKC is more common in males (male:female ratio of up to 6:1),[2] although the gender difference is less marked in the tropics.[20] The reason for the increased incidence of atopic disease in males is unknown. In temperate regions, 45% to 75% of patients have a personal history of asthma or eczema,[2,21] while in tropical regions this is lower (0–40%), although the histological features are still suggestive of an allergic basis for the disease.[18] The risk of visual loss is generally greatest in tropical regions, and varies between 0% and 10%. Reports of up to 20% of patients becoming legally blind include complications of unsupervised steroid treatment.[22] The higher rate of visual loss in tropical areas may be related to poor access to treatment, reporting bias towards severe disease, or the presence of coexistent disease, such as trachoma and bacterial conjunctivitis, which might aggravate VKC in these regions. Corneal complications from scar, vascularization and irregular astigmatism (including keratoconus) can affect vision, and in developed countries minor visual loss from corneal scar occurs in about 6% of patients.[23] It has been estimated that about 25% of patients with VKC in Western Europe (0.8/10,000 inhabitants) have corneal complications.[17]

16e.4.1 Changes in prevalence and geographical distribution with time

Hospital-based epidemiological studies, principally in Scotland, Switzerland and Japan, suggest that in developed countries there has been approximately a four-fold increase in the prevalence of seasonal allergic rhinoconjunctivitis and other allergic conditions between the 1950s and the 1990s, and increased IgE levels in some communities. This is thought to be the result of changes in environmental factors, because allergen exposure has actually reduced in some areas that have experienced an increase in atopic diseases. Although it is likely, there is no evidence for an increase in the prevalence of VKC. In some developing countries, the severity of disease may be decreasing as access to treatment improves and as co-morbidity factors such as superinfection with microbial conjunctivitis reduces.

16e.5 RISK FACTORS

The pattern of exposure to allergens influences expression of disease, which may be perennial in tropical climates, or related to dry and wet seasons rather than temperature. The specific plant and animal allergens causing disease may vary according to geographical location; for example, Japanese cedar pollen is a common allergen in Japan, while olive pollen is a common allergen in Spain. There are few data on allergens responsible for VKC in tropical countries. Mechanical irritation can precipitate a clinical picture similar to VKC, and the role of secondary irritation (diesel particles, infection or smoke) has not been fully explored. It is not known why VKC is more severe in tropical regions. Although it is possible that conjunctivitis or trachoma may increase the severity of VKC, severe VKC also occurs in areas of sub-Saharan Africa where trachoma is not endemic. The role of vitamin A deficiency is unclear, and in tropical regions intestinal parasitic roundworm infection is more common in patients with VKC.[20]

16e.5.1   Genetics

The inheritance of atopy is polygenic, with the several components of the disease (e.g. IgE secretion, mast cell degranulation) each determined by different loci. No genetic marker or HLA type has yet been associated with VKC. There is a family history of atopy in 50% of patients, although the expression (eczema, asthma, allergic rhinitis etc.) may vary in different family members.[1] Limbal VKC is more frequently found in patients of African or Asian descent; this racial predisposition persists after migration to temperate regions.[24]

16e.6   MANAGEMENT

There is the potential to retain good vision in the majority of cases of VKC, and iatrogenic disease must be avoided. Investigation for potential allergens is not indicated for the majority of patients, but advice should be sought from a specialist allergist if the disease is refractory. Allergens are often locally distributed, but geographical treatment by relocation, although effective, is not always practical.

Apart from topical corticosteroid, a variety of topical medications have been shown to be more effective than placebo for the treatment of allergic conjunctivitis, but there is a lack of evidence to support the use of any one agent.[25] Medical management is based on an incremental treatment proportional to symptoms and signs, with topical steroid reserved for crises.[14] For mild disease topical histamine (H_1) antagonists (levocobastine 0.05%, emedastine 0.05%) produce rapid symptomatic relief, while oral antihistamines help sleep and reduce nocturnal eye rubbing. Topical cromones (sodium cromoglycate 2–4%, nedocromil sodium 2%) and other mast cell stabilizers (lodoxamide 0.1%) prevent mast cell degranulation. Dual action agents active against H1 receptors and mast cell degranulation (e.g. olopatadine 0.1%) have also been introduced. All these agents are safe for long-term

maintenance therapy, and can reduce the number and severity of exacerbations and the need for supplementary steroid. Topical acetylcysteine 10% reduces mucus adherence to the cornea during exacerbations. The role of topical non-steroidal agents (diclofenac 0.1%, ketorolac 0.5%), potentially safe options, needs to be fully evaluated.

For more severe disease topical steroid is very effective; but patients should be carefully monitored for side effects (glaucoma, cataract, potentiation of ocular herpetic infection).[22] Synthetic steroids (fluorometholone, loteprednol, rimexolone) may reduce the risk of glaucoma and cataract. Steroid injected into the supratarsal space after lid eversion (0.5–1.0 ml of either dexamethasone (4 mg/ml) or triamcinolone (40 mg/ml) is reserved for cases that are non-compliant with topical treatment, or given during surgery for excision of plaque. Ciclosporin A (0.05% to 2%) is an alternative to topical steroid, but less effective and more expensive.[26] The potential use and safety of antimetabolites such as mitomycin 0.01% needs to be evaluated.[27]

Systemic immunosuppression with corticosteroids, ciclosporin A, tacrolimus, or azathioprine is reserved for severe unremitting disease. Leukotriene receptor antagonists (e.g. montelukast) and molecular antagonists of IgE (e.g. omalizumab) are very expensive and have not yet been fully evaluated for allergic eye disease.[28] Surgical excision or cryotherapy of papillae produce only temporary remission, but application of mitomycin 0.02% after excision may reduce the rate of recurrence.[29]

16e.7   EPIDEMIOLOGICAL RESEARCH PRIORITIES

➢ Better population-based information is needed on the geographical distribution of VKC, the local severity of the disease and the prevalence of sight-threatening complications.
➢ More information is needed on the risk factors and co-morbidities that affect the severity of disease.
➢ Adoption of an agreed system for grading the severity of disease and assessment of quality of life would improve the conduct and interpretation of clinical trials.

> As new, effective, safe and cheap topical treatments, based on research into the mechanisms of VKC, become available, they require evaluating in developing countries.

REFERENCES

1. Bonini S, Lambiase A, Marchi S, *et al*. Vernal keratoconjunctivitis revisited: a case series of 195 patients with long-term followup. *Ophthalmology* 2000; 107:1157–1163.

2. Leonardi A, Busca F, Motterle L, *et al*. Case series of 406 vernal keratoconjunctivitis patients: a demographic and epidemiological study. *Acta Ophthalmol Scand* 2006; 84:406–410.

3. Kumar S. Vernal keratoconjunctivitis: a major review. *Acta Ophthalmol* 2009; 87:133–147.

4. Trocme SD, Hallberg CK, Gill KS, *et al*. Effects of eosinophil granule proteins on human corneal epithelial cell viability and morphology. *Invest Ophthalmol Vis Sci* 1997; 38:593–599.

5. Beigelman MN. *Vernal Conjunctivitis*. Los Angeles: University of Southern California Press; 1950.

6. Kato N, Fukagawa K, Dogru M, *et al*. Mechanisms of giant papillary formation in vernal keratoconjunctivitis. *Cornea* 2006; 25:S47–52.

7. Maggi E, Biswas P, Del Prete G, *et al*. Accumulation of Th-2-like helper T cells in the conjunctiva of patients with vernal conjunctivitis. *J Immunol* 1991; 146:1169–1174.

8. Kumagai N, Fukuda K, Fujitsu Y, *et al*. Role of structural cells of the cornea and conjunctiva in the pathogenesis of vernal keratoconjunctivitis. *Prog Retin Eye Res* 2006; 25:165–187.

9. Abu El-Asrar AM, Struyf S, Al-Kharashi SA, *et al*. The T-lymphocyte chemoattractant Mig is highly expressed in vernal keratoconjunctivitis. *Am J Ophthalmol* 2003; 136:853–860.

10. Leonardi A, Sathe S, Bortolotti M, *et al*. Cytokines, matrix metalloproteases, angiogenic and growth factors in tears of normal subjects and vernal keratoconjunctivitis patients. *Allergy* 2009; 64: 710–717.

11. Lambiase A, Minchiotti S, Leonardi A, *et al*. Prospective, multicenter demographic and epidemiological study on vernal keratoconjunctivitis: a glimpse of ocular surface in Italian population. *Ophthalmic Epidemiol* 2009; 16:38–41.

12. Irani AM, Butrus SI, Tabbara KF, *et al*. Human conjunctival mast cells: distribution of MCT and MCTC in vernal conjunctivitis and giant papillary conjunctivitis. *J Allergy Clin Immunol* 1990; 86: 34–40.

13. Tuft SJ, Dart JK, Kemeny M. Limbal vernal keratoconjunctivitis: clinical characteristics and immunoglobulin E expression compared with palpebral vernal. *Eye* 1989; 3:420–427.

14. Bonini S, Sacchetti M, Mantelli F, *et al*. Clinical grading of vernal keratoconjunctivitis. *Curr Opin Allergy Clin Immunol* 2007; 7:436–441.

15. Sacchetti M, Baiardini I, Lambiase A, *et al*. Development and testing of the quality of life in children with vernal keratoconjunctivitis questionnaire. *Am J Ophthalmol* 2007; 144:557–563.

16. O'Shea JG. A survey of vernal keratoconjunctivitis and other eosinophil-mediated external eye diseases amongst Palestinians. *Ophthalmic Epidemiol* 2000; 7:149–157.

17. Bremond-Gignac D, Donadieu J, Leonardi A, *et al*. Prevalence of vernal keratoconjunctivitis: a rare disease? *Br J Ophthalmol* 2008; 92: 1097–1102.

18. Tuft SJ, Cree IA, Woods M, *et al*. Limbal vernal keratoconjunctivitis in the tropics. *Ophthalmology* 1998; 105:1489–1493.

19. Jones BR, Andrews BE, Henderson WG, *et al*. The pattern of conjunctivitis at Moorfields during 1956. *Trans Opthal Soc UK* 1957; 77:291–302.

20. Ajaiyeoba A. Vernal keratoconjunctivitis and intestinal parasitic infestations in black children. *J Natl Med Assoc* 2005; 97:1529–1532.

21. Buckley RJ. Long term experience with sodium cromoglycate in the management of vernal keratoconjunctivitis. In: Pepys J, Edwards, AM (eds). *The Mast Cell: Its Role in Health and Disease*. London: Pitman Medical; 1979.

22. Khan MD, Kundi N, Saeed N, *et al*. A study of 530 cases of vernal conjunctivitis from the North West Frontier Province of Pakistan. *Pakistan J Ophthalmol* 1986; 2:111–114.

23. Bonini S, Lambiase A, Sgrulletta R. Allergic chronic inflammation of the ocular surface in vernal keratoconjunctivitis. *Curr Opin Allergy Clin Immunol* 2003; 3:381–387.

24. Montan PG, Ekstrom K, Hedlin G, *et al.* Vernal keratoconjunctivitis in a Stockholm ophthalmic centre — epidemiological, functional, and immunologic investigations. *Acta Ophthalmol Scand* 1999; 77:559–563.

25. Mantelli F, Santos MS, Petitti T, *et al.* Systematic review and meta-analysis of randomised clinical trials on topical treatments for vernal kerato-conjunctivitis. *Br J Ophthalmol* 2007; 91:1656–1661.

26. Pucci N, Novembre E, Cianferoni A, *et al.* Efficacy and safety of cyclosporine eyedrops in vernal keratoconjunctivitis. *Ann Allergy Asthma Immunol* 2002; 89:298–303.

27. Jain AK, Sukhija J. Low dose mitomycin-C in severe vernal keratoconjunctivitis: a randomized prospective double blind study. *Indian J Ophthalmol* 2006; 54:111–116.

28. Lambiase A, Bonini S, Rasi G, *et al.* Montelukast, a leukotriene receptor antagonist, in vernal keratoconjunctivitis associated with asthma. *Arch Ophthalmol* 2003; 121:615–620.

29. Tanaka M, Takano Y, Dogru M, *et al.* A comparative evaluation of the efficacy of intra-operative mitomycin C use after the excision of cobblestone-like papillae in severe atopic and vernal keratoconjunctivitis. *Cornea* 2004; 23:326–329.

Mooren's ulcer

STEPHEN TUFT AND BITA MANZOURI

16f.1	Definition	435	16f.5	Risk factors	436
16f.2	Clinical description	435	16f.6	Mechanisms	436
16f.3	Classification	435	16f.7	Management	437
16f.4	Prevalence and geographical distribution	436	16f.8	Epidemiological research priorities	437
				References	438

16f.1 DEFINITION

Mooren's ulcer is an idiopathic peripheral corneal ulceration that is bilateral in approximately one half of patients. The diagnosis depends upon identification of the clinical features and exclusion of other pathologies that may cause **peripheral ulcerative keratitis (PUK)**.

16f.2 CLINICAL DESCRIPTION

The disease typically starts as discrete peripheral stromal infiltrates, often in the interpalpebral zone or at the site of previous surgery. Severe pain is common and the eye may be intensely inflamed and photophobic. If left untreated, stromal thinning progresses inexorably circumferentially and centrally with a leading edge that is undermined and infiltrated (Plate 16f.1). Thinning also spreads peripherally to involve the limbus, but there is no scleral melt. Although the disease principally involves the stroma there is often a linear epithelial defect at the central margin. There may be a mild anterior uveitis but the endothelium is not involved.[1,2]

In established disease, new vessels grow to the leading edge of the ulceration, but not beyond. Secondary bacterial infection, glaucoma and cataract can develop. Corneal thinning can lead to astigmatism and ectasia; perforation occurs in between 11% and 36% of eyes, sometimes following minor trauma. Even with treatment it has been reported that vision is reduced to light perception in 17–19% of eyes, whereas, if untreated, the disease eventually results, within 6–18 months, in blindness due to a thinned and vascularized cornea.[1-3]

16f.3 CLASSIFICATION

Wood and Kaufman[4] suggested that Mooren's ulcer could be grouped as either a unilateral disease that occurred in older patients with an equal sex distribution, was slowly progressive, and responded well to treatment; or as a second group that had bilateral disease, which was rapidly progressive and poorly responsive to treatment. This latter group was reported to be more common in West Africa in otherwise healthy young males.

Lewallen and Courtright[5] pointed out that this classification was not supported by a review of the published cases. The classification of Wood and Kaufman[4] has now generally been abandoned. It is now accepted that bilateral disease, irrespective of age or race, is the aggressive form of the disease.[3] A further classification based on angiographic evidence of capillary closure or leakage has been proposed.[6]

16f.4   PREVALENCE AND GEOGRAPHICAL DISTRIBUTION

The prevalence of Mooren's ulcer, and blindness caused by it, is unknown. The disease is rare in the northern hemisphere but more common in southern and central Africa, China and the Indian subcontinent. It is more common in males than females (between 1.3:1 and 4.7:1) and very rare in children. The incidence varies from approximately one case per year attending specialist corneal clinics in Europe and North America, to between 1 in 350 and 1 in 2,200 clinic visits in India and Nigeria.[1] However, there are no comparative data on the case mix of the respective clinics, the catchment population or the referral base. There have been large case series from China (715 eyes treated over 36 years) and southern India (242 eyes treated over ten years), and in China the incidence was estimated to be 0.03% of the population.[3,7] There is no evidence that the prevalence or geographical distribution is changing.

16f.5   RISK FACTORS

Recent studies suggest that there may be an auto-immune process directed against a specific target antigen in the corneal stroma, possibly triggered by trauma in genetically susceptible individuals. The reported rate of previous trauma, surgery or infection in eyes with Mooren's ulcer varies between 11% and 68%.[1,2] A recent study of a large cohort of patients with Mooren's ulcer in southern India (242 eyes of 166 patients) identified predisposing risk factors as being prior corneal surgery (22%), corneal

trauma (17%) and corneal infection (2%).[7] Two cases have been described from the USA of bilateral Mooren's ulcer associated with a chronic hepatitis C infection.[8] However, no increase in the rate of hepatitis C infection has been found in patients with Mooren's ulcer[9] from India or China.

An increased risk of Mooren's ulcer may persist in second-generation immigrants.[10] As any potential environmental risk factors would probably have changed, this observation suggests a genetic as well as an environmental basis for the disease. Case-control studies of Asian and black African patients show that there is an increased prevalence of human leukocyte antigens HLA-DR17(3) and/or HLA-DQ2 in patients with Mooren's ulcer, which supports an immune pathogenesis for the disease as it may confer susceptibility.[10,11] In a case-control study in southern India an association with helminthiasis was noted in older males, but Mooren's ulcer can develop in its absence, and, even where helminthiasis is endemic, Mooren's ulcer is still rare.[12]

16f.6   MECHANISMS

The aetiology of Mooren's ulcer is uncertain. Corneal tissue from affected patients contains polymorphonuclear leukocytes, lymphocytes, plasma cells, mast cells and eosinophils, and the keratocytes have an increased expression of major histocompatibility class II antigen. There is a significant reduction in the number of CD8 (clonal deletion or T-suppressor) cells in the blood, and an imbalance between the ratio of CD4 and CD8 cells could lead to overproduction of antibody and immune complex deposition in the peripheral cornea. The conjunctiva adjacent to active lesions contains increased immunoglobulin A and a B-cell infiltrate, and immunoglobulins and complement are fixed both to the conjunctiva and the peripheral cornea.[2,13]

When compared with unaffected controls, the serum of patients with Mooren's ulcer contains increased levels of an antibody against a cornea-associated stromal antigen (calgranulin C). It has been proposed that trauma or inflammation may induce autoimmunity to this previously hidden antigen.[14] The resulting inflammation then releases tissue matrix metalloproteinases from the conjunctiva or cornea, which cause corneal ulceration. Interestingly, the same antigen is also found on the surface of some filarial nematodes, and molecular mimicry could increase the risk of autoimmunity to corneal stromal antigen. An alternative explanation for these observations is that the presence of corneal autoantibodies is the result rather than the cause of corneal destruction.

The major differential diagnosis of Mooren's ulcer is PUK resulting from vasculitis (rheumatoid arthritis, Wegener's granulomatisis, polyarteritis nososa, systemic lupus erythematosis) or microbial keratitis. Although previously undiagnosed vasculitis is uncommon in patients with peripheral ulcerative keratitis, an assessment by a physician is recommended. Initial screening for vasculitis should include antinuclear antibodies, rheumatoid factor, antineutrophil cytoplasmic antibodies (ANCA), herpes simplex virus type 1, hepatitis C virus antibodies and a chest X-ray.[2]

16f.7 MANAGEMENT

There is no single effective treatment for Mooren's ulcer. The primary goal is control of inflammation and prevention of corneal perforation. A wide range of therapies has been described in case reports or case series. The outcome of management is therefore difficult to determine because of the different treatments and poor case definition. There are no randomized studies comparing management strategies. Several authors have recommended a graded therapeutic strategy, according to the severity of the disease and the response to initial treatments.[1,13] Such a strategy would include initial treatment with topical steroid, tacrolimus 0.1% or ciclosporin 1.0%, followed by conjunctival resection, systemic immunosuppression and, finally, corneal surgery. Systemic immunosuppression should be considered earlier for bilateral disease, or if, at first examination, the disease were advanced with extensive corneal thinning.[15] Other topical treatments reported to be effective, are artificial tears or a therapeutic contact lens to prevent drying, collagenase inhibitors (acetylcysteine 10%,

L-cysteine 0.2 mol/L), and topical interferon alpha 2a.[16] The use of autologous serum drops has also been recommended as supplementary treatment.[17] Systemic immunosuppression has traditionally been with high dose oral steroid initially with cyclophosphamide, but more recently, ciclosporin A (5 mg/kg) has been shown to be effective. In recalcitrant cases molecular therapies such as infliximab or adalimumab (anti-tumour necrosis factors) or anti-lymphocyte therapy (alemtuzumab) may be effective, but they are very expensive and require close supervision.[18–20]

Surgical options include conjunctival resection or cryotherapy, with or without excision of necrotic tissue, which should extend 4 mm back from the limbus and 2 mm beyond the margins of the lesion. This, however, is not effective as sole therapy for severe (bilateral) disease. Conjunctival excision may be combined with keratoepithelioplasty to produce a physical barrier against conjunctival regrowth and further melting;[21] amniotic membrane transplantation may have a similar short-term effect.[22,23] In cases of advanced disease, excision of the residual central corneal island by lamellar dissection may remove the stimulus for further inflammation. Corneal perforation is initially managed with cyanoacrylate glue and immunosuppression to prevent further tissue destruction. Reconstruction, if required, should be with lamellar surgery if possible, and surgery should be covered by immunosuppression to reduce the risk of recurrence. Without systemic immunosuppression, the recurrence rate after surgery is about 25%. Finally, although initial corneal surgery is usually contraindicated, some authors have reported good results with a primary lamellar keratoplasty combined with topical ciclosporin A. Using this regimen, Chen et al. achieved a cure of 74% at the first procedure and a final cure rate of 95%.[3]

16f.8 EPIDEMIOLOGICAL RESEARCH PRIORITIES

➤ There is a need to reach a consensus on case definition of Mooren's ulcer, and some older studies may not have had access to facilities to exclude all underlying pathologies.

➤ The development of a specific marker for disease, rather than a diagnosis of exclusion, would be helpful.

➤ In future studies there must be stratification of results according to whether the cases are unilateral or bilateral, and uniform documentation of outcome to permit a comparison of results.

➤ The rarity of the disease has made it difficult to conduct masked clinical trials, which may only be possible from single centres in countries such as India or China, where large case series have been reported. Multicentre enrolment would be an alternative approach.

REFERENCES

1. Zegans ME, Srinivasan M. Mooren's ulcer. *Int Ophthalmol Clin* 1998; 38:81–88.

2. Sangwan VS, Zafirakis P, Foster CS. Mooren's ulcer: current concepts in management. *Indian J Ophthalmol* 1997; 45:7–17.

3. Chen J, Xie H, Wang Z, *et al.* Mooren's ulcer in China: a study of clinical characteristics and treatment. *Br J Ophthalmol* 2000; 84:1244–1249.

4. Wood TO, Kaufman HE. Mooren's ulcer. *Am J Ophthalmol* 1971; 1:417–422.

5. Lewallen S, Courtright P. Problems with current concepts of the epidemiology of Mooren's corneal ulcer. *Ann Ophthalmol* 1990; 22:52–55.

6. Watson PG. Management of Mooren's ulceration. *Eye* 1997; 11:349–356.

7. Srinivasan M, Zegans ME, Zelefsky JR, *et al.* Clinical characteristics of Mooren's ulcer in South India. *Br J Ophthalmol* 2007; 91:570–575.

8. Moazami G, Auran JD, Florakis GJ, *et al.* Interferon treatment of Mooren's ulcers associated with hepatitis C. *Am J Ophthalmol* 1995; 119:365–366.

9. Wang QS, Yuan J, Zhou SY, *et al.* Chronic hepatitis C virus infection is not associated with Mooren's ulcer. *Eye* 2008; 22:697–700.

10. Taylor CJ, Smith SI, Morgan CH, *et al.* HLA and Mooren's ulceration. *Br J Ophthalmol* 2000; 84:72–75.

11. Zelefsky JR, Taylor CJ, Srinivasan M, *et al.* HLA-DR17 and Mooren's ulcer in South India. *Br J Ophthalmol* 2008; 92:179–181.

12. Zelefsky JR, Srinivasan M, Kundu A, *et al.* Hookworm infestation as a risk factor for Mooren's ulcer in South India. *Ophthalmology* 2007; 114:450–453.

13. Chow CY, Foster CS. Mooren's ulcer. *Int Ophthalmol Clin* 1996; 36:1–13.

14. Gottsch JD, Liu SH, Minkovitz JB, *et al.* Autoimmunity to a cornea-associated stromal antigen in patients with Mooren's ulcer. *Invest Ophthalmol Vis Sci* 1995; 36:1541–1547.

15. Foster CS. Systemic immunosuppressive therapy for progressive bilateral Mooren's ulcer. *Ophthalmology* 1985; 92:1436–1439.

16. Erdem U, Kerimoglu H, Gundogan FC, *et al.* Treatment of Mooren's ulcer with topical administration of interferon alfa-2a. *Ophthalmology* 2007; 114:446–449.

17. Mavrakanas NA, Kiel R, Dosso AA. Autologous serum application in the treatment of Mooren's ulcer. *Klin Monbl Augenheilkd* 2007; 224:300–302.

18. Fontana L, Parente G, Neri P, *et al.* Favourable response to infliximab in a case of bilateral refractory Mooren's ulcer. *Clin Exp Ophthalmol* 2007; 35:871–873.

19. Cordero-Coma M, Benito MF, Fuertes CL, *et al.* Adalimumab for Mooren's ulcer. *Ophthalmology* 2009; 116:1589.

20. van der Hoek J, Azuara-Blanco A, Greiner K, *et al.* Mooren's ulcer resolved with campath-1H. *Br J Ophthalmol* 2003; 87:924–925.

21. Kinoshita S, Ohashi Y, Ohji M, *et al.* Long-term results of keratoepithelioplasty in Mooren's ulcer. *Ophthalmology* 1991; 98:438–445.

22. Chen KH, Hsu WM, Liang CK. Relapsing Mooren's ulcer after amniotic membrane transplantation combined with conjunctival autografting. *Ophthalmology* 2004; 111:792–795.

23. Lambiase A, Sacchetti M, Sgrulletta R, *et al.* Amniotic membrane transplantation associated with conjunctival peritomy in the management of Mooren's ulcer: a case report. *Eur J Ophthalmol* 2005; 15:274–276.

16g

Climatic droplet keratopathy

GORDON JOHNSON

16g.1	Definition and classification	439
16g.2	Pathology of abnormal material	440
16g.3	Prevalence and geographical distribution	441
16g.4	Incidence	442
16g.5	Time trends	442

16g.6	Genetic predisposition	442
16g.7	Aetiological risk factors	442
16g.8	Control and management	444
16g.9	Future research priorities	444
	References	445

16g.1 DEFINITION AND CLASSIFICATION

Climatic droplet keratopathy (CDK) is a degenerative condition of the cornea. It is characterized by the accumulation of translucent protein material looking like small 'droplets' in the superficial corneal stroma. It is confined to the exposed, interpalpebral strip of each cornea, beginning in the nasal and temporal periphery of both eyes (Fig. 16g.1), and extending centrally (Fig. 16g.2). Progressive accumulation of the abnormal material later in life can involve the entire area of the cornea exposed between the eyelids and can lead to visual impairment (Fig. 16g.3 and Plate 16g.1). People leading an outdoor life are those at risk. The subject was comprehensively reviewed in 1992.[1] Additions to the literature since then have been few because, although CDK remains an important cause of visual impairment in areas of climatic extremes, these are not places where ophthalmologists interested in investigation are often visiting.

16g.1.1 Nomenclature

A profusion of names has been applied to what is likely to be a single pathological response in the cornea. These names have been based on race (Eskimo keratopathy), geography (Labrador keratopathy), occupation (fisherman's keratitis), clinical appearance (nodular band-shaped hyaline keratopathy), presumed nature of the deposits (keratinoid corneal degeneration; corneal elastosis) or the author's name (Bietti's nodular dystrophy).

The term climatic droplet keratopathy has found broad acceptance. It recognizes the occurrence in geographical regions with extreme climatic conditions, and 'droplet' is descriptive of the appearance under the slit-lamp, although it is understood that fluid-filled spaces will not be found.

16g.1.2 Classification

Fraunfelder and Hanna distinguished three clinical and pathological categories,[2] not only primary and secondary corneal forms, but also a conjunctival

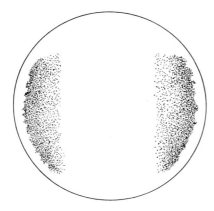

Figure 16g.1 *Drawing of Grade 1 climatic droplet ker-atopathy, as seen with the slit-lamp. The clear zones, free of droplets, are seen between the limbus and the irregular outer peripheral edges of the involved zones*

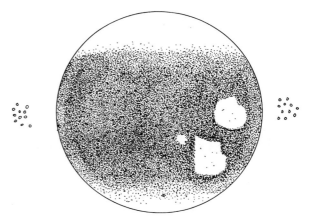

Figure 16g.3 *Drawing of Grade 3 climatic droplet ker-atopathy. The irregular clear 'windows' represent areas where the degenerated superficial cornea appears to have flaked off*

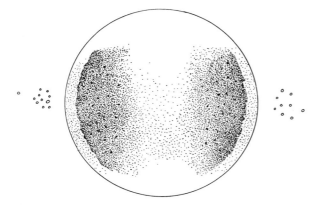

Figure 16g.2 *Drawing of Grade 2 climatic droplet ker-atopathy, showing extension of droplets to the optic axis, and larger droplets in the adjacent conjunctiva*

Table 16g.1 *Grading of climatic droplet keratopathy*

Grade	Description
1	Involvement of nasal and temporal interpalpebral strips, usually bilaterally, with sparing of central cornea
2	Central cornea affected, but not densely enough to affect vision or obscure the details of the pupil margins
3	Central cornea affected, vision reduced, and details of pupil margin partially obscured
4	Elevated nodules present in addition to findings of Grade 3

16g.1.3   Grading

A practical grading scheme (Table 16g.1) has evolved from the original observations and grading suggested by Freedman.[3] The typical appearance of Grade 4 as seen in the Red Sea area is shown in Rodger's illustrations from the Dahlak Islands[4] and in Plate 16g.2.

16g.2   PATHOLOGY OF ABNORMAL MATERIAL

Light microscopy shows homogenous, globular deposits of various sizes in Bowman's layer and the superficial stroma[5] (Plate 16g.3). These deposits stain positive for many different proteins, such as fibrin, fibrinoid and elastosis, but are not fully

form. In people exposed to severe environmental conditions throughout life, the primary corneal type of CDK involves both corneas, without evidence of pre-existing ocular disease. The corneal deposits in the secondary type are histologically identical with the primary forms, but are associated with pre-existing, often unilateral, ocular pathology. The deposits tend to be larger than those in the cornea and golden-yellow in colour. Other subjects may have more pronounced deposits in the conjunctiva than in the cornea, often in association with pinguecula.

The remainder of this section will be devoted to the primary corneal form.

characteristic of any one protein. They are sharply demarcated from the surrounding collagen and have a different amino acid composition. Electron microscopy shows the bodies to be round, with smooth margins and very electron-dense. The 'droplets' are always extracellular, with no evidence of secretory activity from epithelial or stromal cells.

Immunoperoxidase and immunofluorescent techniques show the deposits to be surrounded by a mixture of plasma proteins, which are known to be normally diffusing from the limbal vessels through the superficial stroma towards the centre. They are thought to be acted upon by an environmental influence to become denatured and deposited within the superficial cornea.

16g.3 PREVALENCE AND GEOGRAPHICAL DISTRIBUTION

Climatic droplet keratopathy occurs throughout the world. It is rare in temperate climates and mid-latitudes, although Grade 1 is occasionally seen in clinics in England among people who have spent all their lives working outdoors as farmers or gardeners.

Those geographical areas where CDK is both severe and has high prevalence are those where snowfall persists late into the summer in the northern hemisphere (Labrador, Greenland, Siberia, Mongolia). At lower latitudes CDK occurs in dry, sandy or desert areas, as in the Arabian Peninsula, Iran and Australia. It is particularly common on sea coasts where there is white coral sand or the sand is impregnated with salt (Red Sea coasts, Somalia, Dahlak Islands), or where people are working in salt pans (southern India or the soda lakes in the Rift Valley of East Africa).

Examples of prevalence studies are given in Table 16g.2; these percentages include all grades.

16g.3.1 Prevalence of blindness

There is limited information on the proportion of blindness caused by CDK in the populations listed in Table 16g.2. In a total population of all ages in Labrador it was 25% of the small number with bilateral blindness and accounted for 19% of all blind eyes.[8] In Mongolia, corneal disease was the third cause of blindness, 7.2% of the total after glaucoma and cataract.[14] CDK was also the third cause of blindness in clinics in Somalia. Rodger found that 57% of all cases of blindness in the Dahlak Islands in the Red Sea were caused by CDK.[4]

Table 16g.2 *Prevalence of climatic droplet keratopathy, arranged by date of publication*

Date of publication	Location	Age	Males	Females	Overall	Reference
1973	Dahlak Islands	All ages	45.7	42.0		4
1976	N Cameroon	10+	21.7	12.6	17.2	6
		40–49	44.1	36.4	40.3	
		50+	65.2	52.0	60.6	
1980	Australia, Aborigines	All ages			0.7	7
		>45	41.0	8.0		
1981	Labrador	All ages			18.9	8
1985	South Africa, semi-arid	All ages	14.0	10.4	11.7	9
1988	Chad, subdesert	40+			15	10
	Sahel	40+			7.0	
	tropical	40+			1.7	
1989	South Africa, rural Transkei	All ages	14.0	10.4	11.7	11
1989	Chesapeake Bay, male watermen	30+	19.3		19.0	12
1991	Djibouti, rural	All ages			2.8	13
	urban	All ages			0.5	
1994	Mongolia	40+	32.2	24.1	28.0	14

16g.4   INCIDENCE

There has been no longitudinal study of populations or individuals from the areas with high frequency and severity. There have been a few reports where the number of 'microspheric granules' in the corneas of individual subjects had increased significantly in number over two to three years.

16g.5   TIME TRENDS

Similarly, the trend in prevalence has not been studied over time in the same population. As the way of life changes from outdoors to indoor occupations in some areas, and with greater availability and use of protective sunglasses, the overall prevalence may be expected to decrease with time.

16g.6   GENETIC PREDISPOSITION

There is no evidence for a racial or familial predisposition to developing CDK. In Labrador, three groups of people live side by side, either in the same village or in adjacent villages at the same latitude — Inuit (Eskimos), North American Indians and white settlers. The degree of CDK in these three groups is the same when they are living the same traditional outdoor life of hunting and fishing throughout the year.[15]

Several members of a family may be affected, but the severity is in direct proportion to the time spent outdoors. Thus, for example, two brothers who have spent all their lives outdoors have Grade 3 or 4 CDK; a third brother has hunted only part-time and is found to have Grade 2; while a fourth brother, who has no CDK, turns out to be a light-house keeper and has not participated in the traditional way of life.

16g.7   AETIOLOGICAL RISK FACTORS

16g.7.1   Evidence for an environmental factor

The restriction of the corneal lesions to the exposed inter-palpebral band of cornea argues strongly in favour of an external environmental factor acting directly on the cornea. In Labrador the condition was invariably bilateral and usually symmetrical unless associated with marked strabismus, ptosis or voluntary closing of one eye because bright light reflected from snow was present. No epidemiological study has found evidence that malnutrition is a risk factor.

16g.7.2   Age and gender

The distributions of different grades of CDK in the total populations aged 25 years and over in two small villages at different locations are given in Figs. 16g.4–7. With the exception of the man aged 79 years with no CDK at latitude 50°23′, who was a teacher and then a store keeper, all the males lived the traditional life of hunting and cutting wood in the snow in the forests in the winter, hunting seals on the ice in the spring, and fishing in the summer. The graphs show the greater prevalence and severity with age at the more northern latitude. The females in these villages had a similar pattern of prevalence, but the severity was not greater than Grade 1.

In those areas of the world where women are affected as severely as men, it is found that they

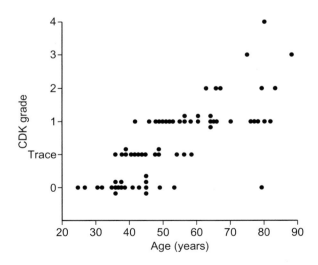

Figure 16g.4 *Distribution of different grades of climatic droplet keratopathy by age in all males 25 years and older in a community on the Northern Peninsula of Newfoundland, at latitude 50° 23′N*

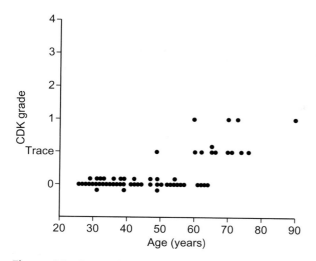

Figure 16g.5 *Distribution of different grades of climatic droplet keratopathy by age in total female population 25 years and older in a community on the Northern Peninsula of New Foundland at latitude 50° 23′N*

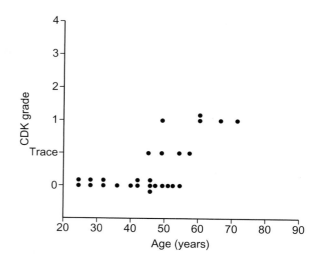

Figure 16g.7 *Distribution of different grades of climatic droplet keratopathy in total population of Caucasian females aged 25 years and over in Makkovik at latitude 55° 05′N*

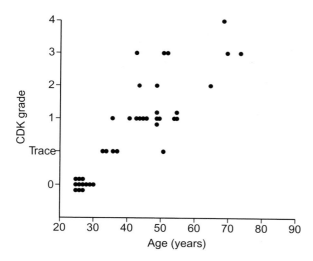

Figure 16g.6 *Distribution of different grades of climatic droplet keratopathy in total population of Caucasian males aged 25 years and over in Makkovik, latitude 55° 05′N on the Labrador coast*

spend an equal amount of time out of doors exposed to the elements, as in the Dahlak Islands.

16g.7.3　Ultraviolet radiation

A number of authors have pointed to the opportunities for exposure to excessive **ultraviolet**

radiation (UVR) that exist in all areas where a high prevalence of CDK has been reported. In a cross-sectional study of Australian aborigines, Taylor found that CDK was strongly related to occupation as a stockman (workman engaged in care of farm livestock, especially cattle), male sex and age, but did not find a significant correlation with levels of UVR.[16]

The major evidence from an ecological study was carried out along the eastern Canadian coast.[15] A series of total population surveys at different latitudes, and also data recorded with the same criteria from clinics at each latitude, established that the peak prevalence and severity of CDK was at latitude 55°–57°N. The prevalence and severity declined progressively going north towards the high Arctic, or going south in the island of Newfoundland. The total ambient UV flux received at different latitudes was then calculated, and combined with ground records and satellite maps of the duration of snow and ice cover, to give an annual total of UV at different wavelengths, which could be reflected back towards the eyes of people travelling or hunting outdoors.

The index thus derived was strongly associated with the geographical distribution of CDK (Fig. 16g.8). The peak of exposure was explained

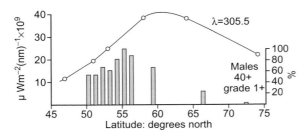

Figure 16g.8 *Geographical distribution of climatic droplet keratopathy in males in the clinic population compared with the total annual ultraviolet (UV) flux, at wavelength 305.5 nm, which could be reflected upwards from snow and ice at six latitudes*

by the fact that further north the increasing obliqueness of the sun's rays caused more short-wave UV to be filtered out by the ozone layer of the atmosphere, despite almost permanent snow cover. Further south in Newfoundland, although the sun was higher, the snow and ice melted much earlier in the spring, and therefore there was less opportunity for UV light to be reflected. The fact that the peak of distribution and peak of reflected UVR exposure are not in an identical position is probably because of the assumptions that had to be made to calculate the UVR.

Other suggested environmental factors, such as low humidity, low temperature or high wind-chill factor, showed an inverse relationship. The only other suggested factor, which showed a weak association, was wind velocity. It is possible to speculate that microtrauma from wind-blown ice crystals, or sand particles in desert areas, might increase hyperaemia at the limbus and the leakage of plasma proteins into the cornea, thereby contributing to the development of CDK under the influence of UVR.

The evidence based on estimation of individual long-term exposure to UVR comes from a cross-sectional study in watermen in Chesapeake Bay, Maryland, USA.[12] Taylor and associates combined field and laboratory-derived data for UV exposure of the face with published ambient **UVB** measurements and personal exposure histories to show a significant association between CDK and UVB. The odds ratio for those in the highest quarter of exposure compared with those in the lowest quarter was 6.4 (95% CI 3.5–11.7). Further analysis

showed the increased risk of CDK was also present with **UVA** exposure.

16g.7.4   Conclusions on aetiology

The circumstantial evidence for UVR as the major aetiological factor is strong. This appears to be a purely environmentally determined condition, without interaction with genetic factors. What is so striking, in those geographical areas with a high prevalence, is that it is possible from an estimation of the age of a person walking into a clinic, and his or her general appearance, to predict the grade of CDK that will be found on slit-lamp examination of the corneas. Although the exact chemical nature of the proteinaceous corneal deposits remain uncertain, it is likely that they represent a mixture of photochemically degraded plasma proteins.

16g.8   CONTROL AND MANAGEMENT

Spectacles that filter out UV wavelengths, particularly if they wrap around the face or have side pieces, are likely to prevent the condition. Their long-term efficacy has not yet been subjected to a clinical trial. The traditional Inuit goggles made from caribou bone or antler, with a narrow slit, protect against snow blindness, and no doubt also against CDK. Many surgical approaches to treatment have been tried, including scraping off dense superficial deposits, superficial keratectomy, lamellar keratoplasty and penetrating keratoplasty. The condition appears to be a good candidate for application of excimer laser phototherapeutic keratectomy.[17]

16g.9   FUTURE RESEARCH PRIORITIES

➢ Future epidemiological studies of aetiological risk factors should measure individual exposure to UVR and estimate individual cumulative long-term exposure. If a UV causation can be firmly established, CDK can be used as a biological marker of cumulative UV exposure in further studies of conditions which may be associated with UV, including pinguecula, pterygium and, particularly, cortical cataract.

- Further histological and biochemical studies of the exact nature and origin of the protein deposits.
- A long-term randomized trial or community trial of the efficacy of protective UV-filtering glasses in prevention.

REFERENCES

1. Gray RH, Johnson GJ, Freedman A. Climatic droplet keratopathy. *Surv Ophthalmol* 1992; 36:241–253.

2. Fraunfelder FT, Hanna C. Spheroid degeneration of the cornea and conjunctiva. 1: Clinical course and characteristics. *Am J Ophthalmol* 1972; 74:821–828.

3. Freedman A. Climatic droplet keratopathy. 1: Clinical aspects. *Arch Ophthalmol* 1973; 89:193–197.

4. Rodger FC. Clinical findings, course and progress of Bietti's corneal degeneration in the Dahlak Islands. *Br J Ophthalmol* 1973; 57:657–664.

5. Johnson GJ, Overall M. Histology of spheroidal degeneration of the cornea in Labrador. *Br J Ophthalmol* 1978; 62:53–61.

6. Anderson J, Fuglsang H. Droplet degeneration of the cornea in North Cameroon. Prevalence and clinical appearances. *Br J Ophthalmol* 1976; 60:256–262.

7. The National Trachoma and Eye Health Program. Sydney: The Royal Australian College of Ophthalmologists; 1980.

8. Johnson GJ, Paterson GD, Green JS, *et al.* Ocular conditions in a Labrador community. In: Harvald B, Hart-Hansen J (eds). *Proceedings of the 5th International Symposium on Circumpolar Health, Copenhagen, Report 33.* Copenhagen: Nordic Council for Arctic Medical Research; 1981. pp. 352–359.

9. Hill JC. The prevalence of corneal disease in the coloured community of a Karoo town. *S Afr Med J* 1985; 67:723–727.

10. Resnikoff S. Epidemiology of Bietti's keratophathy. Study of risk factors in central Africa (Tchad) [Article in French]. *J Fr Ophtalmol* 1988; 11:733–740.

11. Hill JC, Maske R, van de Walt S, *et al.* Corneal disease in rural Transkei. *S Afr Med J* 1989; 75:469–472.

12. Taylor HR, West SK, Rosenthal FS, *et al.* Corneal changes associated with chronic UV radiation. *Arch Ophthalmol* 1989; 107:1481–1484.

13. Resnikoff S, Filliard G, Dell'Aquila B. Climatic droplet keratopathy, exfoliation syndrome and cataract. *Br J Ophthalmol* 1991; 75:737–736.

14. Baasanhu J, Johnson GJ, Burendei G, *et al.* Prevalence and causes of blindness and visual impairment in Mongolia: a survey of populations aged 40 years and older. *Bull World Health Organ* 1994; 72:771–776.

15. Johnson GJ. Aetiology of spheroidal degeneration of the cornea in Labrador. *Br J Ophthalmol* 1981; 65:270–283.

16. Taylor HR. Aetiology of climatic droplet keratopathy and pterygium. *Br J Ophthalmol* 1980; 64:154–163.

17. Badr IA, Al-Rajhi A, Wagoner MD, *et al.* Phototherapeutic keratectomy for climatic droplet keratopathy. *J Refract Surg* 1996; 12:114–122.

Pterygium

GORDON JOHNSON

16h.1	Definition	447		16h.7	Pathogenesis	451
16h.2	Grading	447		16h.8	Management	451
16h.3	Prevalence and incidence	447		16h.9	Future research priorities	451
16h.4	Geographical distribution	449			References	452
16h.5	Heredity	449				
16h.6	Aetiological risk factors	449				

16h.1   DEFINITION

A pterygium (plural 'pterygia') is a radially-arranged, triangular or 'wing'-shaped fibrovascular growth extending over the corneal limbus onto the cornea. It usually starts from the nasal limbus, within the area exposed between the eyelids. In advanced cases, pterygia may be bilateral and affect both temporal and nasal aspects of each cornea. It is uncommon for an isolated temporal pterygium to occur. Pterygia may be irritating, are frequently unsightly, and the higher grades cause astigmatism. Advanced cases cause visual impairment and sometimes blindness.

In the past it has been classified as a 'degenerative' disease. As will become apparent from the evidence presented, it can now be regarded more as a proliferative condition, a dysplasia, or even a benign neoplasm.

16h.2   GRADING

Early clinic or population-based studies used a simple grading system based on the extent in millimetres to which the apex of a pterygium extended from the limbus towards the centre of the cornea.

In a population-based survey in Indonesia, Gazzard and co-workers applied a grading system described by Tan, which takes into account the thickness of the invading pterygium, and is based on the visibility of the underlying episcleral blood vessels as an indicator of severity.[1] T1 ('atrophic') was defined as episcleral vessels clearly visible; T2 ('intermediate') as vessels partially visible; and T3 ('fleshy, opaque') as vessels wholly obscured. In addition, size was measured with callipers as both the chord length of the corneal limbus involved and the greatest distance from the limbus to the apex of the lesion.

16h.3   PREVALENCE AND INCIDENCE

No incidence studies of pterygium have been reported. Much of the early information was taken from clinic reports and based on the frequency with which pterygia were seen in private practice. The condition is a particular problem in Australia and the Pacific Islands. The very high rate amongst

Table 16h.1 *Prevalence rates of pterygium, arranged by latitude*

Latitudes (degrees)	Location	Ethnic group	Setting and occupation	Ages	n	Prevalence (%)			Ref.
						Overall	Men	Women	
57 N	Labrador	Mainly Inuit	Hunting, fishing	All	646	2.6			6
39 N	Chesapeake Bay MD, USA	White	Fishermen	30+		16.6			7
34.5 N	Qinghai-Tibetan plateau, China	Mongolian	Altitude 3450 m Yearly mean temp −3C	40+	2,112	17.9	17.2	18.7	8
31.5–32 N	Arizona USA	Mexican American (Latinos)		40+	4,767	16.2	23.7	11.5	9
21 N	Meiktila, Myanmar	Burman		40+	2,076	19.6	19.3	19.7	10
13 N	Barbados	Black		40–84	2,617	23.4	24.0	23.1	11
		Mixed		40–84	97	23.7			
		White		40–84	59	10.2			
1.5 N	Singapore	Chinese		40–79	1,232	9.7	16.4	4.3	12
1 N	Sumatra, Indonesia	Indonesian/Malay		21+	1,210	10.0			1
				41+	403	16.8	16.1	17.6	
0.5 N	Riau Archipelago	Indonesian	Fishing community		477	17.0	22.7	12.4	13
Equator	Amazonas State, Brazil	American Indian							14
		Arawak + Tukano	Riverside, fishing	Adult	265	36.6			
		Yanomani + Maku	Forest, hunting	Adult	359	5.0			
31.5 S	Transkei, SA	Bantu	Rural			0.46	nil	0.75	15
32.5 S	Karoo, SA		Semi-arid	All		5.7	5.0	6.2	16
34 S	Blue Mountains, Australia						11.0	4.5	17
37–38 S	Victoria, Australia	White	Urban + rural	40+		2.83			18
			Urban	40+	3239	1.2	1.76	0.71	
			Rural	40+	1473	6.7	9.78	3.83	

Australian Aborigines was documented in the Australian National Trachoma and Eye Health Program (age 60+ years 14.0%; all ages 3.2%).[2] Data from clinic studies, operation rates and surveys were compiled in a global 'pterygium map' by Cameron.[3] Information on frequency and prevalence available up to 2000 was summarized in a monograph.[4]

Recent population-based sample surveys (Table 16h.1), show a spread from approximately 2.5% to 24%, in general populations, according to latitude and exposure to risk factors.

The condition has not often featured in published surveys of causes of blindness. Reports from South East Asia, particularly Thailand, specific areas of South America, and among Europeans in tropical Queensland, demonstrate that bilateral pterygia can cause blindness. In Elliott's report from Western Samoa in 1960, pterygium was the sole cause of blindness in 15 out of 136 blind people.[5] In a recent survey of pterygium in central Myanmar, two of the 84 people blinded in both eyes were bilaterally blind from pterygium.[10]

16h.4   GEOGRAPHICAL DISTRIBUTION

Although pterygia occur in all countries of the world, there is an uneven distribution. Cameron drew attention to the fact that they are most common in populations within 40° latitude north or south of the equator,[3] with a general trend of higher rates with decreasing latitude (Table 16h.1).

Pterygia are observed uncommonly in Europe, North America and Asia north of 40° latitude, except in specific areas of the sub-Arctic and Arctic, where people lead a largely outdoor way of life and the terrain is covered by snow and ice for much of the year (for example, prevalence of 2.6% in all age groups in a total population in Labrador at 57°N).[6] Norn supplemented this information from studies in clinics in Aqaba (Jordan), Greenland and Copenhagen, where pterygia occurred in 12%, 9% and 1% of patients respectively.[19]

16h.5   HEREDITY

A genetic predisposition to pterygium has been recognized for some time. Examples of pedigrees were reviewed by Duke-Elder, indicating dominant inheritance with reduced penetrance.[20] Hilgers found a high prevalence in the non-negroid population of the island of Aruba, and recorded two families with distribution of pterygium over four generations.[21] These authors thought it was not the actual lesion that was inherited, but rather the tendency of the eye to react in a particular way to environmental stimuli.

Genetic alterations, such as loss of heterozygosity, have been found in pterygium.[22] The involvement of tumour suppressor genes in the pathogenesis has been suggested.[23]

16h.6   AETIOLOGICAL RISK FACTORS

16h.6.1   Personal factors

The prevalence increases with age. Pterygium typically first occurs between the ages of 20 and 30, and then the prevalence usually has an approximately linear increase with age, sometimes reaching a plateau in the age group 50 years and over.[1] There have been, however, some situations such as the Blue Mountains Study, where this association with age was weak, and not statistically significant.[17]

Males are affected more often than females, from a ratio of 2:1 in the Australian National Trachoma and Eye Health Program,[2] to 4:1 for unilateral pterygia and 10:1 for bilateral pterygia in Singapore,[12] presumably linked to outdoor occupation. Pterygium is usually associated with occupations such as farming, fishing or construction. However, when localities are surveyed where the exposure of the two sexes to outdoor environmental factors is the same, the prevalence in the two genders is similar.

In Singapore, after controlling for age and sex, an association with occupation persisted not only with labouring and agricultural occupation (odds ratio, OR 3.3, 95% CI 1.6, 7.0) but also for indoor factory workers, production workers and machine operators (OR 3.1, 95% CI 1.5, 6.3) compared with professionals and office workers.[12] The study in Victoria showed an association with rural residence compared with that for urban Melbourne.[18]

16h.6.2   Sunlight and ultraviolet light

The occurrence of pterygia in hot, dry and dusty countries, and in males in outdoor occupations, led the early workers to attribute them to the effects of microtrauma and drying of the cornea. The same geographical variation, however, led Cameron and others to suggest that the distribution is better explained by ocular exposure to solar **ultraviolet radiation (UVR)**.[39] This was supported by ecological studies from Australia.[24] In studying the fishermen of Chesapeake Bay, Maryland, USA, a method was evolved for estimating lifetime exposure to **UVB** and other wavelengths of sunlight, using direct measurement of ambient radiation and a detailed UVR questionnaire.[7] UVR was the main risk factor for pterygium in these 'watermen'. The same approach was applied in the Victoria survey, where lifetime ocular sun exposure was an independent risk factor for pterygium (OR 1.63, 95% CI, 1.18–2.25).[18] The result was the same when ocular UVB exposure was substituted in the model for broadband sun exposure. The **attributable risk** of sunlight and pterygium in this population was 44%.

A case-control study in Perth, Western Australia, found that pterygium was strongly related to ocular sun exposure, with a dose–response relationship, the curve flattening with higher levels of exposure.[25] A case-control study in Brisbane showed that the risk of pterygium was increased among patients who, in their third decade of life, worked outdoors in an environment with high surface reflectance of ultraviolet radiation compared with those who worked indoors. The level of risk was raised several hundred-fold among those subjects who worked mainly on sand compared with those who worked indoors.[26]

There has been no agreement as to the most important period of life at which exposure occurs. In Brisbane, for example, there was significant risk in living close to the equator (less than 30 degrees) and spending more than 50% of the time outdoors during the first 5 years of life.[25] However, in Victoria, residence during the first years of life was not related to the development of pterygium.[18]

Coroneo has proposed an explanation for the characteristic location of a pterygium at the nasal limbus.[27] The anterior part of the eye is regarded as acting as a lens, with light incident on the temporal cornea being focused by off-axis refraction across the anterior chamber onto the nasal limbus. Using computer-assisted optical ray tracing techniques, the peak light power density at the nasal limbus was calculated to be potentially 20 times the power density of the incident light. This applies to both visible light and wavelengths in the UV band. Thus the limbal stem cells are at risk of intense exposure to UVR from behind.

Sliney investigated the geometry of exposure of the eye to solar UVR.[28] Assumptions based on the behaviour of the visible wavelengths are misleading in connection with UV. Because of the position of the eyebrow ridge and the upper eyelid, as well as the wearing of hats, the cornea is seldom exposed to direct rays from the overhead sun. Ultraviolet-B can be reflected off clouds or buildings, and hazy skies cause scattering of UVB so that more comes horizontally. One of the most important factors in determining ocular exposure to UVB is the ground-surface reflection for these wavelengths. Measures to protect the eyes fully from UV exposure must take into account all the different directions from which radiation may reach the cornea and conjunctiva.

16h.6.3   Other risk factors

Desiccation and microtrauma have been considered as aetiological factors in hot, dry and dusty countries. Examinations of the tear film in eyes with pterygia have proved normal. Evidence for particulate injury comes from studies of sawmill workers,[29] as is also suggested by the high odds ratio for factories in the Singapore survey.[12] Other suggestions, for which there may be anecdotal evidence, include irritation by smoke (as with indoor cooking fires) and chemicals. The evidence for chronic inflammation and infection is not epidemiological but histological.

Four studies, in four different ethnic groups, have now demonstrated a protective effect of cigarette smoking. Amongst Latinos in Arizona, current smoking was protective compared with 'never having smoked' (OR 0.75, 95% CI 0.59–0.94).[9] In Indonesia 'ever smoked' was protective for pterygium compared with 'never smoked' (OR 0.46, 95% CI 0.27–0.78).[1] Amongst African-Caribbeans in Barbados cigarette smoking had a protective OR of 0.59 (95% CI 0.39–0.90),[11] while in the Caucasian population of Melbourne the apparent protective effect of smoking was seen in univariate, but not multivariate, analysis of the Visual Impairment Project.[18] The mechanism or explanation of this apparently protective effect is unknown.

Herpes simplex virus and human papilloma virus have been demonstrated in the tissue of pterygia in some series,[30,31] but not others. Both viruses possess oncogenic potential. Herpes simplex virus is involved in a multi-stage process of tumour transformation. The postoperative recurrences were more common in patients with simultaneous detection of herpes simplex virus and human papilloma virus.

16h.6.4 Conclusions on aetiology

Unlike climatic droplet keratopathy (discussed previously in Chapter 16g), where UVR is the essential cause of the disease, and the severity appears to be directly proportional to the cumulative UV dose reaching the cornea, pterygium occurs less predictably in a particular location or individual subject. Although UV is likely to be the most important environmental risk factor, genetic predisposition is sometimes evident and other risk factors have been associated with the presence of pterygium, so that the causation is multifactorial. In these respects it is behaving more like a tumour or, at least, a proliferative disorder, rather than being directly proportional to one environmental exposure. Indeed, it may now be considered to be a low-grade neoplastic condition. Further evidence for this view comes from examination of excised tissue, when squamous carcinoma cells have sometimes been found.

16h.7 PATHOGENESIS

It has been proposed that the initial event in pterygium formation is an alteration, due to chronic UV exposure, of limbal stem cells. These normally form a junctional barrier between the conjunctival and corneal epithelial cells.

The tumour suppressor gene p53 has been detected in pterygia specimens, suggesting they have undergone mutation, and indicating aberrant regulation of apoptosis in the limbal basal epithelial cells.[32] Tumour-like development in these cells is consistent with UVR damage. Mutation of other genes could progressively occur. Dushku and Reid found that in primary and recurrent pterygia the cornea was invaded by vimentin-expressing altered limbal epithelial basal cells.[23] They proposed a model for the pathophysiology, in which the pterygium cells are tumour-like altered epithelial basal cells, which invade into normal corneal basement membrane, drawing conjunctival epithelial cells with them. The altered basal cells are positive for proteases, including matrix metalloproteinases, which can promote the invasion of the cornea and the dissolution of Bowman's membrane.[33] Kowk and Corones developed a computational algorithm of the movement of stimulated and unstimulated epithelial cells.[34] They assumed that the peak UV stimulation was at the mid-point of the nasal limbus (three o'clock position in the right eye), the intensity decreasing to zero 1.6 mm circumferentially above and below its peak. The final shape computed if epithelial cells migrated in centripetal streams into the cornea was a wing-shaped mass, with a curved leading edge, closely resembling a clinical pterygium.

16h.8 MANAGEMENT

Although no clinical trial has yet been carried out of the effect of long-term protection of the eyes from reflected UVR or total solar radiation, wearing sunglasses has been protective in a case-control analysis.[26]

The surgical management of pterygium has traditionally relied on excision, leaving a bare sclera, often with supplementary β-irradiation or antimetabolites such as mitomycin intraoperatively or thiotepa, applied postoperatively as drops. A valuable advance has been the introduction of free autografts of superior bulbar conjunctiva to cover the bare sclera; the graft is taken from the same or the opposite eye.

16h.9 FUTURE RESEARCH PRIORITIES

➤ Improved methods of assessment of all aspects of UVR exposure at the eye level , in particular how to assess lifetime exposure in an individual.

➤ If the position of pterygia at the nasal limbus is a result of the same UVR wavelengths to which are also attributed early infero-nasal cortical cataracts (see Chapter 10), why are they not in the same position? The relationship of these two conditions requires further consideration.

➤ The apparent protective effect of cigarette smoking in four recent studies requires further exploration.

➤ Long-term clinical trials of protection of the eyes from UV, including protective side pieces to dark glasses.

REFERENCES

1. Gazzard G, Saw S-M, Farook M, *et al*. Pterygium in Indonesia: prevalence, severity and risk factors. *Br J Ophthalmol* 2009; 86:1341–1346.

2. The Royal Australian College of Ophthalmologists. The National Trachoma and Eye Health Program. Sydney: The Royal Australian College of Ophthalmologists; 1980.

3. Cameron ME. Pterygium throughout the world. Springfield, IL: Charles C Thomas; 1965.

4. Taylor HR (ed). *Pterygium*. The Hague: Kugler; 2000.

5. Elliott, R. Ophthalmic disease in Western Samoa. *Trans Ophthal Soc New Zeal* 1960; 12:87–97.

6. Johnson GJ, Paterson GD, Green JS, *et al*. Ocular conditions in a Labrador community. In: Harvald B, Hart-Hansen J (eds). *Proceedings of the 5th International Symposium on Circumpolar Health, Copenhagen, Report 33*. Copenhagen: Nordic Council for Arctic Medical Research; 1981. pp. 352–359.

7. Taylor HR, West SK, Rosenthal FS, *et al*. Corneal changes associated with chronic UV irradiation. *Arch Ophthalmol* 1989; 107:1481–1484.

8. Lu J, Wang Z, Lu P, *et al*. Pterygium in an aged Mongolian population: a population-based study in China. *Eye* 2009; 23: 421–427.

9. West S, Munoz B. Prevalence of pterygium in Latinos: Proyecto VER. *Br J Ophthalmol* 2009; 93: 1287–1290.

10. Durkin SR, Abhary S, Newland HS, *et al*. The prevalence, severity and risk factors for pterygium in central Myanmar: the Meiktila Eye Study. *Br J Ophthalmol* 2008; 92:25–29.

11. Luthra R, Nemesure BB, Wu SY, *et al*. Frequency and risk factors for pterygium in the Barbados Eye Study. *Arch Ophthalmol* 2001; 119:1827–1832.

12. Wong TY, Foster PJ, Johnson GJ, *et al*. The prevalence and risk factors for pterygium in an adult Chinese population in Singapore: the Tanjong Pagar Survey. *Am J Ophthalmol* 2001; 131:126–131.

13. Tan CSH, Lim TH, Koh WP, *et al*. Epidemiology of pterygium on a tropical island in the Riau Archipelago. *Eye* 2006; 20: 908–912.

14. Paul JS, Thorn F, Cruz AAV. Prevalence of pterygium and cataract in indigenous populations of the Brazilian Amazon rain forest. *Eye* 2006; 20:533–536.

15. Hill JC, Maske R, Van Der Walt S, Coetzer P. Corneal disease in rural Transkei. *S Afr Med J* 1989; 75:469–472.

16. Hill JC. The prevalence of corneal disease in the coloured community of a Karoo town. *S Afr Med J* 1983; 67:723–727.

17. Panchapakesan J, Hourihan F, Mitchell P. Prevalence of pterygium and pinguecula: the Blue Mountains Eye Study. *Aust NZ J Ophthalmol* 1998; 26:52–55.

18. McCarty CA, Fu CL, Taylor HR. Epidemiology of pterygium in Victoria, Australia. *Br J Ophthalmol* 2000; 84:289–292.

19. Norn MS. Spheroid degeneration, piguecula, and pterygium among Arabs in the Red Sea Territory, Jordan. *Acta Ophthalmol* 1982; 60:949–954.

20. Duke-Elder S. *System of Ophthalmology, Volume VIII. Diseases of the Outer Eye*. London: Henry Kimpton; 1965. pp. 574–575.

21. Hilgers JHC. Pterygium: its incidence, heredity, and etiology. *Am J Ophthalmol* 1960; 50: 635.

22. Spandidos DA, Sourvinos G, Kiaris H, *et al*. Micro satellite instability and loss of heterozygosity in human pterygia. *Br J Ophthalmol* 1997; 81:493–496.

23. Dushku N, Reid TW. P53 expression in altered limbal basal cells of pingueculae, pterygia, and limbal tumours. *Curr Eye Res* 1997; 16:1179–1192.

24. Taylor HR. Aetiology of climatic droplet keratopathy and pterygium. *Br J Ophthalmol* 1980; 84:154–163.

25. Threlfall TJ, English DR. Sun exposure and pterygium of the eye: a dose–response curve. *Am J Ophthalmol* 1999; 128:280–287.

26. Mackenzie FD, Hirst LW, Battistutta D, *et al*. Risk analysis in the development of pterygia. *Ophthalmology* 1992; 99:1056–1061.

27. Coroneo MT. Pterygium as an early indicator of ultraviolet insolation: a hypothesis. *Br J Ophthalmol* 1993; 77:734–739.

28. Sliney DH. The focusing of ultraviolet radiation in the eye and ocular exposure. In: Taylor HR (ed). *Pterygium*. The Hague: Kugler; 2000. pp. 29–40.

29. Detels R, Dhir SP. Pterygium: a geographical study. *Arch Ophthalmol* 1967; 78:485–491.

30. Gallagher MJ, Giannoudis A, Herrington CS, Hiscott P. Human papilloma-virus in pterygium. *Br J Ophthalmol* 2001; 85:782–784.

31. Detorakis ET, Sourvinos G, Spandidos DA. Detection of herpes simplex virus and human papilloma virus in ophthalmic pterygium. *Cornea* 2001; 20:164–167.

32. Tan DTH, Tang WY, Liu YP, *et al.* Apoptosis and apoptosis-related gene expression in normal conjunctiva and pterygium. *Br J Ophthalmol* 2000; 84:212–216.

33. Di Givolamo N, Wakefield D, Coroneo MT. Differential expression of matrix metalloproteinases and their tissue inhibitors and the advancing pterygium head. *Invest Ophthalmol Vis Sci* 2000; 41:4142–4149.

34. Kwok LS, Coroneo MT. A model for pterygium formation. *Cornea* 1994; 13:219–224.

Epidemiology of trachoma

SHEILA WEST AND ROBIN BAILEY

17.1	Introduction	455
17.2	Chlamydia: The pathogen	456
17.3	Trachoma: The clinical signs	459
17.4	Epidemiology of trachoma	464

17.5	Control strategy: SAFE	473
17.6	Future research	478
	References	479

17.1 INTRODUCTION

The leading infectious cause of blindness world-wide, trachoma is caused by an ocular infection with *Chlamydia trachomatis*. Once endemic in most countries, trachoma has largely disappeared from Europe and the Americas, the disappearance predating the advent of antibiotics. Famous hospitals established to treat trachoma, Massachusetts Eye and Ear Infirmary and Moorfield's Hospital in London, saw little trachoma by the 1930s. In the USA, infection with *C. trachomatis* became better known as a sexually transmitted disease than as an ocular infection. Because of its absence in developed countries, trachoma was largely forgotten as a public health issue until a renewed focus by the World Health Organization, resulting in a resolution by the World Health Assembly, rekindled interest in eradicating blinding trachoma by 2020.[1]

Trachoma continues to be endemic in many of the poorest and most remote areas of Africa, Asia, Australia and the Middle East. Communities with trachoma are often those with the fewest resources to take on health issues, and trachoma strikes the most vulnerable members of those communities, women and children. There are over 1.3 million

blind and 8 million with trichiasis, which makes them at risk for subsequent blindness.[1,2] The total productivity loss from trachoma is estimated at $5.3 billion (2003, US dollars) and health economists suggest an even greater burden when factoring in disability due to trichiasis prior to visual impairment, which would increase the figure by 50%.[3]

In this chapter, we will summarize the characteristics of chlamydial infection, the detection of agent and the clinical presentation of trachoma, the epidemiology and important risk factors for trachoma that have led to the multifaceted control strategy currently being implemented in several countries.

17.1.1 Historical perspective

Trachoma is an ancient disease, with evidence of its existence in China as early as the 27th century BC.[4] In Egypt, the features of trachoma were described in the Ebers Papyrus, a collection of writings by ancient Egyptians physicians found by Ebers in 1889 (cited by Duke-Elder[5]), and epilation devices used for removing in-turning eyelashes, a consequence of trachoma, were present in Egyptian tombs as early as the 19th century BC.[6] Ancient Greek physicians, including Hippocrates, wrote descriptions of treating trachoma and the chronic sequelae of infection.[6–7] In fact, trachoma is derived from the Greek words for 'rough', and 'swelling'.[5]

Trachoma spread to Europe in the early 1800s following the battles between England, France and Turkey for control of Egypt. Much of the blindness was probably gonococcal conjunctivitis, but simultaneous infection with trachoma was likely.[6] By 1897, the supervising Surgeon General rendered the opinion that trachoma in immigrants to the United States was grounds for immediate denial of entry and return to the port of origin.[8] The United States Public Health Service spent more than 80% of its resources between 1897 and 1925 on medical inspections at seaports and borders, primarily for trachoma.[9] Despite American public opinion that trachoma was a disease of poor immigrants, trachoma was a common cause of blindness in Native Americans and in endemic populations of Appalachia. The history of this ancient organism is covered more fully in Taylor's book.[10]

Descriptions of the disease that appeared in the early 1900s included possible preventive or public health strategies to control transmission.[6,8,11] In 1920, Elliot recommended practicing fly control and avoiding hand/eye contact as mechanisms to decrease the spread of infection.[11] A public health approach to trachoma as a disease of the entire community is the most effective way to control trachoma in endemic areas.

17.2   CHLAMYDIA: THE PATHOGEN

Chlamydia trachomatis, the causative agent of trachoma, is an obligate intracellular organism with no known animal reservoir. Chlamydiae are eubacteria, and are given a place in their own order, Chlamydiales. Within *C. trachomatis*, the primary **serovars** responsible for trachoma are A, B, Ba, and C, while the serovars D to K are associated with genital infections. L1 to L3 are the lymphogranuloma venereum serovars. The genome of *C. trachomatis* (serovar D) has been sequenced and contains a 1,042,519 base-pair chromosome with 894 likely protein-coding genes, and a 7,493 base-pair plasmid.[12] The sequencing project has

provided considerable insight into the biology of the organism.

Chlamydiae have a unique developmental cycle distinguished by two specialized forms (Fig. 17.1). The **elementary body (EB)** is the metabolically inert, infectious particle which, through endocytosis, infects susceptible host cells. Through invagination of the host cell membrane, the EBs are encased in a vesicle that matures into the **inclusion body**. The chlamydial inclusion inhibits phagolysosome fusion, allowing the organisms to avoid host cell lysosomal killing. Within two hours of infection in an *in vitro* tissue culture system, transformation of the EB into a **reticulate body (RB)** occurs. The RB, although non-infectious, is metabolically active and multiplies rapidly over the next 15 to 30 hours. Approximately 18–30 hours after infection, the RBs begin transformation into EBs. The RBs and EBs remain enclosed in the inclusion, which can occupy up to 90% of the cell cytoplasm. At 40–48 hours post infection, the cell will lyse, releasing EBs into the extracellular space to infect other cells. In the last several years, exciting research on the active interaction of Chlamydia with the host cell has emerged, including data that Chlamydia modulate apoptosis in infected cells.[13] The trachoma serovars target columnar and squamocolumnar epithelial cells, and are thus infections of the conjunctiva, genital, respiratory and intestinal tissues. How the developmental cycle described above might be modified or delayed *in vivo* is still under active research, although such modifications may explain some features of infection. *In vitro*, in response to nutrient deprivation or exogenous immune factors such as gamma interferon (IFNγ), reticulate bodies may experience a prolonged life cycle resulting in persistent intracellular infection, but the significance of this type of persistence in human infections of ocular serovars is unclear.

The outer membrane of *C. trachomatis* contains many principal antigens from an immunologic perspective, and mediates adhesion between the Chlamydia and the host cell. The **major outer membrane protein (MOMP**, also called *omp1*) is immunodominant in the humoral immune response, accounting for 60% of the outer membrane proteins. The antigenic heterogeneity as a

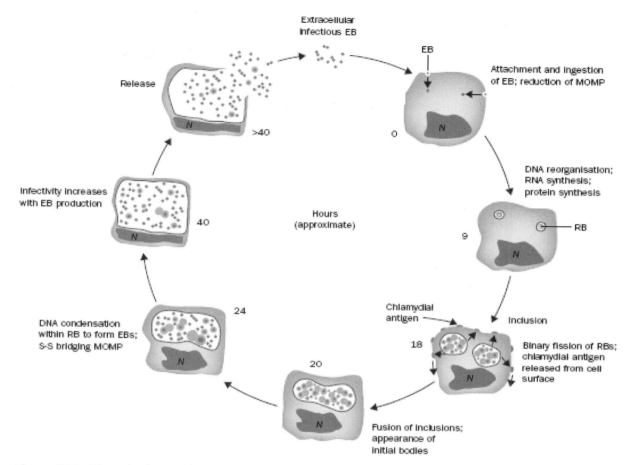

Figure 17.1 *Life cycle of C. trachomatis*

result of diversity in the four variable domains of MOMP is the basis for the distinction of *C. trachomatis* into different serovars. Genotyping studies, typically of the *ompA* gene, which codes for *omp1*, done in trachoma endemic areas, suggest that a number of **genovars** may be present within a given serovar, implying more variants than previously known on the basis of serovar studies; however, most of the polymorphisms are based on point mutations. Research suggests this genetic diversity may be associated with high prevalence of trachoma in a community, but more work is needed.[14]

The inclusion membrane (Inc) proteins and polymorphic proteins (Pmp) occupy 12–19% of the genomic sequence. Sequence variation within pmpH distinguishes ocular and genital serovars, and work is ongoing in using these protein antigens, particularly PmpD, as vaccine candidates.

17.2.1 Detection of chlamydial infection

The detection of infection with *C. trachomatis* in the laboratory can be done using cytological examination of stained slides of conjunctival swabs, growing the organism in tissue cultured cells, or by detection of antigen or nucleic acids. Serologic tests or tear tests for antibody are not helpful for determining current infections.

Determining the sensitivity and specificity of laboratory tests for *C. trachomatis* is tricky, as clearly the **nucleic acid amplification tests (NAATS)** are the most sensitive and specific, compared with older methods. Comparison against the clinical signs of disease is not optimal because many cases of follicular trachoma no longer have agent; the follicular reaction takes time to resolve once the infection is gone. Moreover, subclinical or pre-clinical infections are well-recognized entities, and a laboratory test may well be positive in the absence of clinical signs. The sensitivity and specificity of the tests are affected greatly by the collection, handling, and storage of the samples in the field and in the laboratory. For example, poor handling of specimens for tissue culture can change the sensitivity by as much as 50%. Many of the studies have used Chlamydia culture as the gold standard, although the newer techniques are clearly more sensitive.

The major advantage of tissue culture is the nearly 100% specificity. Ideally, the sensitivity of tissue culture should be 90% or better, but sensitivity is highly dependent on the degree to which strict requirements for transport and storage are maintained. Moreover, negative cultures in clearly symptomatic individuals positive for Chlamydia using other techniques have been reported.[15–16]

Direct antigen detection tests for diagnosing chlamydial infections, such as enzyme immunoassays or direct immunofluorescence assays, were popular in the past. However, nucleic acid amplification tests are currently in wide use. These tests are highly sensitive and specific for *C. trachomatis*. A number of commercial kits, and a number of in-house **polymerase chain reaction (PCR)** tests, use different **DNA** or **RNA** regions as targets for amplification. A major target sequence is the cryptic plasmid, which is present at seven to ten copies per EB. Thus, these tests theoretically can detect less than one EB in a sample. The recent emergence of a rare, plasmid-free variant in sexually transmitted Chlamydia would not be detected by these methods, but plasmid-free ocular strains have not been reported.[17] Commercial tests currently in use for sexually transmitted Chlamydia include strand displacement amplification (SDA) technology, a real time PCR method (Cobas TaqMan CT), and a transcription-mediated amplification (TMA) to detect a specific 23S ribosomal RNA target, which is present in hundreds of copies in each organism. These tests have been used for ocular specimens to detect the presence of *C. trachomatis* for research purposes, and in one study, it appeared that the **rRNA (ribosomal RNA)**-based test was more sensitive than the DNA-based test for plasmid, as expected,[18] but the significance of finding rRNA in the absence of chlamydial DNA is unclear.

Nucleic acid amplification techniques require meticulous attention to the handling of specimens in order to avoid contamination, as false positivity can easily result. For low to medium areas of endemicity (less than 40% prevalence), pooling multiple specimens into a single test may be a feasible approach for prevalence studies, although there is an increased risk of contamination, and the possibility of false negativity if diluted specimens are not mixed thoroughly.[19]

Concerns for the use of these tests for trachoma have been raised, especially in terms of 'false positivity' as evidence of contamination when trachoma is absent clinically. In all population-based studies, a certain percentage of those 'without trachoma' are PCR positive, the percentage depending somewhat on the degree of endemicity. PCR positivity has shown good correlation with severity of disease. In hyper-endemic communities in Tanzania, 70% of PCR positive cases without trachoma were mild, having 1–4 follicles and thus falling below the level defined as trachoma (see next section).[20] In the Gambia, the clinically negative subjects who were PCR positive were more likely to develop signs of trachoma one to six months later.[21] These findings suggest that some of the PCR-positive–clinically-negative cases are either incubating the disease or are such mild cases that they do not meet the WHO definitions of trachoma. However, contamination, if field techniques are not scrupulous, is always an issue.

These tests are not realistic options for monitoring infection in trachoma endemic countries because of the expense and lack of facilities for processing specimens. As more formerly trachoma-endemic countries move towards low prevalence of disease, the ability to test communities for remaining infection or re-emergent infection is a high priority. The development of a simple, inexpensive, rapid, point-of-care test for Chlamydia that is robust under field conditions is a high priority. One such test was initially somewhat encouraging, but was not robust, with too many false positives in dusty, hot conditions.[22] There is avid competition for the development of such a test for use in sexually transmitted *C. trachomatis*, and it is hoped such tests would be useful for trachoma as well.

17.3 TRACHOMA: THE CLINICAL SIGNS

The clinical signs of infection by *C. trachomatis* are the result of immunopathology, and the host response to infection, discussed in the next section, is key to understanding the manifestations of trachoma including the sequelae induced by repeated, or persistent, episodes of infection. A single episode of acute chlamydial conjunctivitis, as seen in newborns in Europe and North America, is not considered trachoma because there is virtually no risk of prolonged inflammation or the blinding complications that characterize eyes exposed to multiple or prolonged bouts of infection in trachoma endemic areas.[23–24] In a monkey model of trachoma, naive animals receiving weekly inoculations of *C. trachomatis* showed a waning of the inflammatory response after two months, but maintained a follicular response as long as the reinoculation of the ocular challenge was maintained.[24]

In trachoma endemic communities, trachoma is a chronic disease. The community pool of active inflammatory disease resides in the children who may have persistent signs of active trachoma as a result of repeated or persistent infections. Children with active trachoma present with follicles and papillae, the markers for the intensity of the inflammation (Plates 17.1 and 17.2). Follicles are yellow or white 'spots' in the tarsal conjunctiva, and consist of lymphoid tissue containing **B-lymphocytes**. Severe, inflammatory trachoma presents as thickening of the conjunctiva with inflammation obscuring the deep tarsal vessels. The presence of pus with severe inflammation usually indicates a bacterial infection, which may co-exist with trachoma. Corneal changes may occur during active inflammation, but these signs are not a sensitive indicator of trachoma. Limbal follicles may appear, and new vessels develop, producing corneal pannus. Once the limbal follicles resolve, depressions remain on the cornea, resulting in the pathognomic sign of trachoma, 'Herbert's pits'.

Multiple infections and/or prolonged, severe infection are followed by evidence of scarring of the conjunctiva (Plate 17.3). Even in late childhood and early adulthood, the scarring may be prominent and obscure evidence of active disease, although in some cases of scarring without evidence of active disease there is laboratory evidence of *C. trachomatis* infection.[25] The scarring can be significant enough to cause entropion and trichiasis, or in-turned eyelashes (Plate 17.4). Entropion/trichiasis eventually requires lid surgery to correct the eyelashes rubbing on the globe and prevent visual loss from corneal opacification.

Corneal damage from trachoma, which leads to the visual consequences with this disease, is felt to be the result of multiple processes. Scarring may affect the Meibomian orifices and result in atrophy of the glands and development of features of dry eye. Similarly, the lacrimal ducts may be affected resulting in aqueous deficiency. In-turned eyelashes abrade the corneal surface, which may be drier than normal, and allow secondary infections. Ultimately, the cornea develops opacities that are irreversible (Plate 17.5).

In 1987, the World Health Organization published a simple classification scheme for assessing trachoma based on clinical signs (Table 17.1).[26] Each of the signs has relevance for understanding the epidemiology of trachoma in a population. The prevalence of active disease is represented by the proportion of the population with **follicular trachoma (TF)** and/or **trachoma-intense (TI)**; those with TI are most infectious and need prompt treatment; the prevalence of **trachomatous trichiasis (TT)** provides an indication of need for surgical services; and the prevalence of **corneal opacity (CO)** is an indication of the magnitude of impact of trachoma on the blindness rates in the community. The WHO trachoma grading scheme is reliable, easy to teach to eye nurses and other eye health workers, and has been used in a number of surveys.

For research purposes, there are complicated grading systems available which have more detailed levels of severity for each sign.[27] Early complex systems had poor reliability, but newer expanded grading schemes for active trachoma, scarring and trichiasis have reported good reproducibility.[28–30]

Several cross-sectional population studies have reported the absence of infection in anywhere from

Table 17.1 *World Health Organization. Simplified trachoma grading classification system*

Sign	Description
TF	Follicular trachoma: the presence of five or more follicles in the upper tarsal conjunctiva of at least 5 mm.
TI	Inflammatory trachoma: pronounced inflammatory thickening of the upper tarsal conjunctiva that obscures more than half of the normal deep tarsal vessels (not to be confused with scarring, which may also obscure the tarsal vessels). TI may be severe enough to obscure follicles.
TS	Trachomatous scarring: the presence of easily visible scarring in the tarsal conjunctiva.
TT	Trichiasis: evidence of at least one eyelash touching the globe. Evidence of recent removal of in-turned eyelashes is also graded as TT.
CO	Corneal opacity: the presence of easily visible corneal opacity, which obscures at least part of the pupillary margin.

50% to 70% of cases of TF and 10% to 50% of cases of TI. Using these signs to predict evidence of infection is not recommended, as predictive probability of a positive or negative sign at the community level is poor.[a] The lack of high correlation is understandable, as infection disappears and clinical signs wane more slowly over time. It was never intended that clinical signs be used to predict infection with *C. trachomatis*, and this lack of concordance is only an issue in the context of community treatment with antibiotics. As discussed below, mass treatment with antibiotics is recommended for trachoma-endemic communities when the prevalence rate of TF in children is above 10%. However, in these communities TF alone is relatively poor as a surrogate for the presence of infection, which is the real target for the antibiotic. As communities approach 10% prevalence of TF, infection may in fact be absent,[31] or conversely, at rates of TF less than 10%, infection may still be present that would warrant treatment.[a]

17.3.1 Trachoma: an immunopathological disease

Understanding trachoma as a clinical disease in its various manifestations, and key to any attempt at vaccine development, requires understanding the host immunological response to infection. Chlamydial infection elicits both an innate and an adaptive immunological response from the host. The innate response has not been well characterized. The antibody response does not appear to be protective for subsequent infections, and clearing of infection likely depends on the cellular immune response. The cellular immune response is also likely to lead to the immunopathological consequences of repeated infection, and the degree to which there is dysregulation of the immune response may explain those at increased risk of severe inflammatory trachoma, scarring and trichiasis. We provide a further overview of immunological responses to infections, and to chlamydial infection in particular in the box below.

Immunology of Trachoma

Various kinds of human immune response have been established as playing a role in host defences against intracellular infections like trachoma. These include the development of 'neutralizing' antibodies, which recognize the chlamydial surface and are capable of blocking chlamydial attachment to, or infection of, host cells; and cellular responses in which **T-lymphocytes** (thymus-derived lymphocytes) recognize Chlamydiae or chlamydial-infected

(Continued)

[a] Stare D, Munoz B, Mkocha H *et al.* Use of clinical signs of trachoma to guide mass treatment. *PLoS NTD*, submitted 2010.

(Continued)

cells using **HLA (human leukocyte antigens)** antigens and other surface receptors. These T-cells then influence the outcome of infection by secreting proteins (cytokines) such as gamma interferon or directly attacking the infected cell themselves. There are two kinds of T-lymphocytes involved, which are distinguished by the presence of **cellular differentiation (CD)** markers **CD4** or **CD8** on their surface. HLA antigens have now been recognized to have a key role in the recognition of infecting microorganisms and infected cells by T-lymphocytes.

CD4[+] lymphocytes recognize antigen using class II HLA molecules and are important in defence against microorganisms. Following recognition of antigen, they produce cytokines, proteins with diverse actions on the host. An increasing number of 'patterns' of cytokine secretion by CD4[+] cells have been described, with two of the best characterized being **Th1 phenotype**, characterized mainly by gamma interferon production and **Th2** phenotype, in which **interleukin-4 (IL-4)** and **interleukin-10 (IL-10)** predominate. The balance between Th1 and Th2 responses appears to be important in determining the outcome of some intracellular infections, like trachoma. CD8[+] or cytotoxic T-cells (CTL) recognize microbial antigens presented by HLA class I molecules at the surface of infected host cells, and try to kill these cells either by producing cytokines or by direct attack.

These cellular immune responses are 'turned on' by processes initiated by the recognition of antigen. A further group of CD4[+] T-cells known as T-regulatory cells (Tregs), which appear to be characterized by expression of the intracellular molecule *Foxp3*, are responsible for 'turning off', i.e. preventing the continuation of potentially harmful immune responses by shutting down T-cell-mediated immunity towards the end of an immune reaction.

Because antibodies and T-cells recognize particular microbial antigens, these responses are

(Continued)

(Continued)

described as 'adaptive' immune responses. However there are also 'innate' immune responses: aspects of host defence which are key for defence in the initial stages of infection and do not require specific recognition of the invading microbe; these include antimicrobial defensins, the neutrophil response, activation of complement and attack by **natural killer (NK) lymphocytes**. Our understanding of which of these mechanisms are actually important in trachoma, and the extent to which variations in this host immune response might be important in explaining why some people but not others develop trachomatous scarring or intense trachoma, is incomplete, and an area of active research.

Immune responses in trachoma

Why do persons in trachoma endemic communities suffer repeated episodes of ocular infection with *C. trachomatis*, even with the same genovar? The acquisition of repeated infections suggests the absence of any long-lasting protective immunity. Neutralizing antibodies against MOMP have been shown to protect against infection in the laboratory, but the extent of a natural protective immune response is not clear.[32] However, there is evidence that an immune response to *C. trachomatis*, expressed through either partial resistance to, or resolution of, infection, is induced. This evidence comes from the epidemiological pattern of trachoma and the results of human vaccine trials.

Studies of trachoma have universally found that signs of active disease and evidence of ocular chlamydial infection are more common in children than in adults in trachoma-endemic settings. Adults may have less exposure to infection, or they could be protected, at least partially, from re-infection by prior exposure. A longitudinal study suggested that, in the absence of treatment, adults had fewer episodes

(Continued)

(Continued)

and also resolved their disease episodes more quickly compared with children.[33] Such spontaneous healing in the absence of treatment, presumably due to immune mechanisms, has long been observed.

Experiments in which volunteers were re-challenged with *C. trachomatis* strains, with a six-month interval between priming and challenge, suggested that time-limited resistance to re-infection occurred but was strain-specific.[34] In the trachoma vaccine trials of the 1960s, short-term, partial protection from incident disease or re-infection was produced by vaccination with whole inactivated Chlamydia.[35] In animal models, immunity was shown to be short-lived, and serotype-specific.[36–37] A better understanding of host defence mechanisms that underlie resistance to re-infection with *C. trachomatis* will be essential for the design of an effective vaccine.

Innate immunity

Both innate and adaptive immune responses are invoked during *C. trachomatis* infection. Chlamydia-infected cells produce a number of cytokines and chemokines including interleukin-8, a powerful neutrophil attractant.[38] As Chlamydiae are susceptible to neutrophil inactivation *in vitro*, the recruitment of neutrophils is probably important in host defence. The role of natural killer (NK) cells and natural killer T (NKT) cells in chlamydial infection have not been well studied. Limited data suggest that chlamydial infection of epithelial cells induces a down-regulation of surface molecules involved in recognition by NKT cells,[39] and that persons with ocular *C. trachomatis* infection may have reduced NK cell function.

Antibody responses

Antibodies are produced in response to ocular chlamydial infection, with MOMP being the immunodominant antigen in this response.

(Continued)

(Continued)

Neutralizing antibodies against MOMP have been shown to protect against infection in the laboratory, but the extent to which antibodies generated during natural infection produce protection is not well clarified.[32] Re-infection with a different serovar tends to raise antibody responses to the previous serovar. Though antibody responses are found in ocular secretions, there is no evidence that they confer protection against chlamydial infection.[40–41] Studies have been conducted in trachoma to characterize trafficking **antibody secreting cells (ASCs)**. ASCs were readily detectable in subjects with trachoma, but there were relatively few **IgA**-secreting ASCs in subjects with intense trachoma.[42] The explanation for this altered ASC trafficking is unclear, but it might indicate that the normal tightly regulated mucosal immune response is dysregulated in intense disease.

Because of the importance of MOMP in the antibody response, genetic variation in the *ompA* gene has been studied in ocular chlamydial infection. One hypothesis for recurrent disease and re-infection is that immune pressure in populations selects for MOMP variants that can escape immune surveillance. If so, this would have implications for vaccine development using MOMP as a candidate. In two villages in the Gambia, genotype variants of *C. trachomatis* were established; four genotypes accounted for 89% of infections, and although the introduction of novel genotypes was observed, none became established in the population.[43] Moreover, individuals within these trachoma endemic communities appeared to be often or repetitively infected with the same *ompA* genotype, as 70% of subjects infected at both the baseline and at subsequent follow-up were infected with the same genotype. Similar studies on samples from Tunisia and from Tanzania have shown *ompA* variants in those populations.[44–45] These studies have generally found an excess of rare *ompA* mutations, which does not support the

(Continued)

(Continued)

hypothesis that *ompA* polymorphism is maintained within these populations by immune selection pressure. This conclusion has been supported by the few studies which have applied population genetic methods to *ompA* sequence data in trachoma[44,46] and cast doubt on the primacy of MOMP as a vaccine candidate.

Cellular responses

Lymphocyte proliferative responses, reflecting class-II restricted CD4[+] memory or effector T-cell responses to chlamydial antigens, are readily demonstrable in humans with trachoma. Subjects who spontaneously cleared their disease had enhanced lymphoproliferative responses to chlamydial antigens compared with those with persistent disease whose responses were reduced.[47] In animal models the CD4[+] response is of central importance in the resolution of *C. trachomatis* infection, and the ability to clear infection can be restored by adoptive transfer of CD4[+] cells of Th1 phenotype.[48–49] In these models, the Th1 cytokine gamma interferon also partially restores the ability to clear infection. Thus there is some evidence to support the idea that Th1 responses to chlamydial antigens, including gamma interferon production, may be important in resolving ocular chlamydial infection. However, little is known about the antigenic targets that elicit these responses.

Conversely the cellular immune response may contribute to the serious clinical manifestations of trachoma. Peripheral blood lymphocyte proliferative responses were reduced in scarred subjects compared with controls in the Gambia and showed a predominantly Th2 type response to a range of chlamydial antigens.[50] Together with observations that scarred subjects may be more likely to be infected, this suggests that some chronic sequelae of infection occur in individuals who have an immune response that fails to

(Continued)

(Continued)

clear infection. In support of this, studies of host genetic susceptibility to scarring trachoma have suggested that one **haplotype** spanning the gamma-interferon locus, which may be associated with reduction or delay in the gamma-interferon response, and another spanning the *IL10* locus, which was shown to be associated with increased transcription of IL-10, both independently increased the risk of scarring.[51–52] Subjects with scarring trachoma have been found to have increased **mRNA** transcripts of TGF-beta,[53] a fibrogenic cytokine which may induce polarization towards Th2 responses. A study of gene expression during active trachoma episodes found evidence of sustained expression of matrix metalloprotease 9, (MMP-9) a mediator which links inflammation to fibrosis.[54]

Cytotoxic lymphocyte (CTL) responses have been found at low level in trachoma subjects using autologous Chlamydia-infected fibroblasts (which express HLA class I antigens) as targets. As described above, the recent demonstration that apoptosis is inhibited in Chlamydia-infected cells may indicate why such responses are difficult to demonstrate. However, CD8[+] cells could still be important in human immunity through cytokine secretion. Increased conjunctival expression of perforin, one of the molecular effectors of the CTL response, was found during ocular *C. trachomatis* infection.[54]

The role for T-regulatory (Treg) cells in trachoma has been little studied, but the finding of increased Foxp3 expression associated with resolution of infection in subjects with trachoma is consistent with their involvement in turning off the adaptive immune response in the conjunctiva when it is no longer needed.[55]

Hypersensitivity and chlamydial persistence

It has been proposed that severe inflammation in trachoma may be the result of a delayed

(Continued)

(Continued)

hypersensitivity response in ocular tissues elicited by the 57 kD chlamydial heat shock protein (hsp 60).[56] This protein is a 'chaperonin' whose relative expression is increased under stress, particularly in the conditions of arrested chlamydial development induced by gamma interferon.[57] This may be why serological studies have consistently demonstrated serological responses to Hsp 60 in subjects with damaging sequelae of chlamydial infection, including trachomatous scarring.[58]

There is controversy over the role of persistent infection as a factor in the spread of infection further and the pathogenesis of trachoma. Electron micrographic studies have shown that, in cell culture systems, some epithelial cells contain aberrant, non-culturable, reticulate body-like structures that may represent persistent or latent infection.[57] Such forms may play a role in heightened hypersensitivity to infection, or explain why conjunctival scarring should proceed in the absence of demonstrable infection. Many researchers have found that in those with no inflammatory disease, scarring was associated with chlamydial antigen positivity, which tends to support this conjecture. Infection was a strong predictor of progression to scarring and trichiasis in cohorts followed in Tanzania.[25,59] The finding of genotypic evidence for the same organism in women who were infected at time points years apart is additional evidence for a role of persistent infection in the pathogenesis of trachoma.[60] While a study of migrant Sikh Indians showed that those with previous trachoma who moved to Canada (an area with no trachoma) had no further cases of disease, cases of scarring and trichiasis continue to occur in areas where active trachoma has been eliminated.[61-62] Further work on characterizing persistent infection, and its role in driving the progression of trachoma, needs to be done.

17.4 EPIDEMIOLOGY OF TRACHOMA

17.4.1 Prevalence

Since 1999, when renewed efforts at trachoma control worldwide were undertaken, trachoma has declined in many areas, notably in the Middle East, India, Latin America and Asia. It continues to be a major cause of ocular morbidity in Africa, the Pacific Islands, and Aboriginal communities in Australia.[2]

The overall prevalence of trachoma globally is somewhat difficult to determine, as many of the studies have been carried out in areas of countries known to be at high risk. Extrapolation to the entire country or even region may not be justified. While most recent data suggest trachoma is no longer a problem in India,[63] there are scant data on trachoma prevalence from China, and even low prevalence in such very large populations could alter any estimate of the global burden of trachoma. The WHO estimates that 40.6 million persons suffer from active trachoma and 8.2 million have trichiasis, a decline from the 2003 estimate of 84 million with active trachoma.[2] However, the data may over-represent the status in some countries, like Ghana, which is applying for certification of elimination of trachoma, and under-represent some areas because it reports from only 42 of 57 endemic countries with extrapolation to others. A summary of trachoma prevalence surveys demonstrates that the burden of disease is primarily in Africa, but due to the large population sizes, many cases of active trachoma are estimated to be in China and India, despite low prevalence estimates (Table 17.2).

Where still endemic, trachoma is more often found in rural, economically under-developed areas, where good water supplies and basic sanitation services are lacking. Even within hyper-endemic areas, trachoma clusters both at the neighbourhood and at the household level.[64-67] Trachoma is an infectious disease and transmission can occur by sharing clothes, towels or sleeping quarters. Following mass treatment of trachoma in a hyperendemic community, infection and trachoma re-emerged within six months in

Table 17.2 Available studies on the prevalence of trachoma: 1996 to 2007 (Reproduced with permission from Mariotti S, Pascolini D, Rose-Nussbaumer J. Trachoma: Global magnitude of a preventable cause of blindness. Br J Ophthalmol 2009: 93;563–568.[2])

Country	Date of survey	Location	Type of survey	Age group	Sources
Afghanistan	2006	Four provinces	Door-to-door assessment	All ages	Comprehensive Eye Care Program, Ministry of Public Health Afghanistan
Australia	1997–2003	Aboriginal and Torres Strait Islander communities	Screening in schools and in remote communities, clinical assessments	All ages	Mak DB, et al. The Office for Aboriginal and Torres Strait Islander Health, Australian Government Department of Health
Brazil	2003–2006	Thirteen states	School screening	1–9	Trachoma Control Program, Health Surveillance Secretariat, Brazil Ministry of Health
Burkina Faso	2005	Budondè, Diapaga districts	Population-based survey	1–9, 15 and older	Programme National de Prévention de la Cécité, Ministry of Health, Burkina Faso
Cambodia	2000	Six endemic regions	Trachoma rapid assessment	0–14, 40 and older	National Prevention of Blindness Program, National Program for Eye Health, Ministry of Health, Cambodia
Cameroon	2006	Kolofata district, far north Province	Population-based survey	1–10, women over 14	Einterz EM, et al. 2008
Chad	2001–2005	Eight provinces	Population-based survey	1–10, women over 14	Dézoumbé D, et al. 2007, Programme national de lutte contre la cécité, Ministry of Health, Republic of Chad
China	2003–2006	Ten provinces	Trachoma rapid assessment	1–9, 40 and older	National Programme for Prevention of Blindness, Ministry of Health, China
Egypt	2001	Menofiya Governorate	Population-based survey	2–6, 50 and older	Gamal Ezz al Arab, et al. 2001
Eritrea	2006	Three endemic regions: North Red Sea, Debub, Gash Barka	Population-based survey	1–9, 15 and older	Blindness Prevention Program, Ministry of Health of the State of Eritrea
Ethiopia	2005–2006	All regions of the country	Population-based survey	All ages	Berhane Y, et al. 2006, Federal Ministry of Health of Ethiopia
Gambia	2006	North bank, lower river	Population-based survey	0–9	Prevention of Blindness Program, Ministry of Health, the Gambia
Ghana	2000–2003	Northern region, upper west region	Population-based survey	1–10, 40 and older	National Eye Care Programme, Ministry of Health, Ghana
Guinea	2001–2002	Upper and Middle Guinea	Population-based survey and assessment	0–10, women over 14	Programme de lutte contre la cécité, Ministry of Health, Guinea
Guinea-Bissau	2005	Whole country	Population-based survey	All ages	Prevention of Blindness and Deafness, Ministry of Public Health, Republic of Guinea-Bissau
India	2006	Punjab, Rajasthan, Uttar Pradesh, Uttarakhand, Haryana, Gujarat	Trachoma rapid assessment	< 10, 15 and older	Directorate General of Health Services, Ministry of Health and Family Welfare, India

(Continued)

Table 17.2 (Continued)

Country	Date of survey	Location	Type of survey	Age group	Sources
Iran (Islamic Republic of)	2002	Four provinces in the south	Trachoma rapid assessment	All ages	Ministry of Health and Education
Kenya	2004	Five endemic districts in Rift Valley province and one in eastern province	Population-based survey	1–9, 15 and older	Karimurio J, et al. 2006
Malawi	2002–2003	Salima and Chikwawa districts (central and south provinces)	Trachoma rapid assessment	5–9, and 0–9	National Programme for Prevention of Blindness, Ministry of Health, Malawi
Mali	1996 and 2005–2006	All endemic regions	Population-based survey	0–9, 15 and older	Programme national de lutte contre la cécité, Ministry of Health, Mali
Mauritania	2004	National survey	Population-based survey	1–9, 14 and older	Programme national de lutte contre la cécité, Ministry of Health, Mauritania
Mexico	2006	Chiapas	Surveillance house to house	All ages	State Institute of Health, Chiapas, Mexico
Morocco	2004	Five endemic regions	Community-based surveillance	All ages	Programme national de lutte contre la cécité, Ministry of Health, Kingdom of Morocco
Mozambique	2002	Northern Manica province	Population-based survey	1–9, 40 and older	National Programme for Prevention of Blindness, Ministry of Health, Mozambique
Myanmar	2006	Meiktila district	Population-based survey	40 and older	Durkin SR, et al. 2007
Nepal	1996–2002, 2003, 2006	Several endemic districts	Population-based survey and trachoma rapid assessment	All ages	National Trachoma Program, Ministry of Health and Population, Nepal
Niger	2001–2006	Several districts in the Zinder, Maradi and Diffa regions	Population-based survey	1–9, 15 and older	Programme national de lutte contre la cécité, Ministry of Public Health, Republic of Niger, and Abdou A, et al. 2007
Nigeria	2005–2006	Eight endemic regions	Population-based survey	1–9, 15 and older	National Programme for Prevention of Blindness, Ministry of Health, Nigeria
Oman	2005	Three regions: Dhakhiliya, North Sharqiya, South Batinah	Population-based survey	1–5	Khandekar R, et al. 2006
Pacific Islands Sub-region	1996–2002, 2003, 2006	Kiribati, Nauru, Solomon Islands, Vanuatu, Fiji	Trachoma rapid assessment	1–10, 40 and older	Mathew A, et al. 2007
Pakistan	2004	All four provinces and in the northern area	Door-to-door assessment	All ages	Prevention and Control of Blindness Programme, Ministry of Health, Government of Pakistan
Senegal	2000–2004	Whole country and Thiès region	Population-based survey	1–9, women over 14	Saal MB, et al. 2003; and Programme national de lutte contre la cécité, Ministry of Health, Senegal

(Continued)

Table 17.2 (*Continued*)

Country	Date of survey	Location	Type of survey	Age group	Sources
Sudan	2003, 2005–2006	Eastern Equatoria, Upper Nile, Unity, Northern, Kassala and Khartoum states	Population-based survey	1–9, 15 and older	Ngondi J, *et al.* 2005, 2006; and Prevention of Blindness Administration Federal Ministry of Health, Sudan
Tanzania (United Republic of)	2004–2006	Fifty districts in endemic regions	Population-based survey	1–9, 15 and older	National Eye Care Program, Ministry of Health and Social Welfare, United Republic of Tanzania
Uganda	2006	Three districts in the Northern and Eastern regions	Population-based survey	1–9, 15 and older	National Programme for Prevention of Blindness, Ministry of Health, Uganda
Vietnam	2001, 2006	Districts in the northern provinces	School-based assessment and population-based survey	1–5, 35 and older	National Programme for Prevention of Blindness, Ministry of Health Vietnam, Khandekar R, *et al.* 2006
Yemen	2004	Nine Governorates and Socotra Island	Trachoma rapid assessment	1–9	Al Khatib TK, *et al.* 2006
Zambia	2001–2003	Gwembe district, southern region	Exhaustive screening of population in chosen villages	All ages	Astle WF, *et al.* 2006

household members, and across neighbouring households before one year.[68]

The age distribution of the different signs of trachoma depends in part on the stability and endemicity of the disease in the community. In hyper-endemic areas, active disease is most common in preschool children, with prevalences as high as 60% to 90%.[64,69–70] The prevalence of infection, and the greatest infectious load, is found in pre-school children as well.[71] The prevalence of active trachoma decreases with increasing age, with less than 5% of the adults showing signs of active disease, and the infectious load in cases is also lower.[64,71] In areas where trachoma has been endemic for a long period of time, the presence of conjunctival scars increases with age, and the prevalence in those 25 and older could be as high as 90%.[72] Although similar rates of active disease are observed in male and female children, the later sequelae of trichiasis and entropion, and corneal opacities due to trachoma are more common in women than in men.[64,72] A typical pattern of the age distribution of active and chronic trachoma for a hyper-endemic area can be illustrated by the data from a survey of 20 villages in Tanzania (Fig. 17.2).

However, the prevalence of the signs of active trachoma reflects both the incidence and duration of disease and the duration of disease has been shown to decline strongly with increasing age.[33] Thus, while the incidence rate of disease is lower in adults compared with children, the much lower prevalence rate is also a function of the much shorter duration of disease in this age group.

In areas where active trachoma has largely disappeared, a different pattern of the presentation of trachoma is observed. Lid scarring and chronic sequelae are more common than active disease, and trachoma is present only in adults.[62,73–74] The prevalences of trichiasis and corneal opacities due to trachoma in adults largely reflect past episodes of disease when this cohort was young, and likely also represent some persistent infection in the adults. While the blinding complications may continue to be a problem, the low or absent incidence of active disease in children is a good indicator of the future absence of blinding disease as a public health problem.

The WHO has developed a rapid assessment methodology for use by health officials within countries to identify regions and districts where

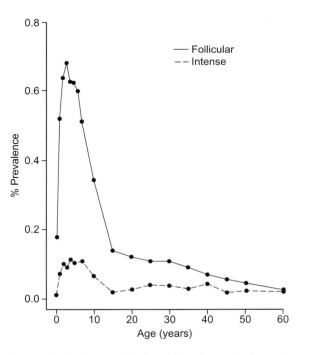

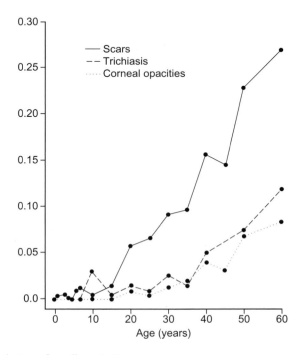

Figure 17.2 *Age distribution of trachoma in the entire population of a village in Tanzania.*

trachoma is a public health problem, and rank the priority of districts for trachoma control activities. This technique, while valuable for assigning health priorities, has been mistakenly used in place of true prevalence surveys to provide estimates of prevalence of trachoma. Validation of the rapid assessment technique against true prevalence surveys even for ranking villages has shown about 60% agreement,[75] with correlations of 0.58.[76]

17.4.2 Risk factors for active disease

Trachoma remains a blinding disease in communities where *C. trachomatis* persists and the living conditions facilitate continuous transmission. Research into specific factors which increase the risk of trachoma have guided the current recommendations for intervention strategies to control the disease, and so we concentrate the review on some of these personal and environmental factors.

17.4.2.1 *Personal factors*

Age is a predictor of the signs of trachoma. In hyper-endemic areas, preschool children are the main reservoir of active disease and infection. A significant decline in the prevalence of active trachoma is observed after the age of ten for both males and females. The prevalence of chronic trachoma (scars, trichiasis and corneal opacities) increases with age and reflects the accumulated experiences with re-infection.

Children with active ocular Chlamydia infection may also have extraocular Chlamydia infections.[77-78] Auto-reinfection from extra-ocular sources of Chlamydia infection may be one source of transmission, and may explain why treatment with topical antibiotic ointment is effective for only a short time. However, there are conflicting data on the possible role of extra-ocular sites in re-infection following treatment, with some studies finding no evidence for this as a source of auto-re-infection or re-emergence,[78-79] and another suggesting an increased risk with a nasal positive swab for infection following treatment.[80]

While research has not found trachoma associated with evidence of acute malnutrition in children, a detailed study in Ethiopia found that children with signs of chronic malnutrition (low height for age or stunting and low weight for age) were more likely to have active trachoma compared with children who did not have signs of chronic malnutrition.[81] There was no relationship of chronic malnutrition with infection. However, the authors found that children with chronic malnutrition were more likely to manifest infection as severe trachoma, and to have severe trachoma with absence of infection, compared with children without chronic malnutrition. This suggests differences in disease manifestation with nutritional status.

In trachoma hyper-endemic areas, there is a subgroup of children, about 8–10%, who appear to have constant infection,[59,82] and respond to infection by consistently mounting a severe, inflammatory response.[83] Moreover, the seven-year incidence of scarring in those with constant, severe trachoma was almost five times greater than in children without constant severe trachoma (but who had episodes of trachoma).[84] The incidence of scarring in children with constant infection, regardless of clinical signs, was equivalent to those with constant severe trachoma, although most children with either constant infection or trachoma had both.[59] The differing immune responses to chlamydial infection that may explain why these children manifest severe, constant, disease is an active area of research, and likely relates to their increased risk of early scarring.

17.4.2.2 *Environmental factors*
Water

Trachoma occurs in communities or households without adequate water supply, although the data are inconsistent. Several studies have found a positive association between the distance from the household to the water source and the prevalence of active trachoma. In Tanzania, the water allocated to be used for hygiene purposes was the link between trachoma and water at the household level.[85] Clearly, the distance to water can place constraints on the amount of water brought to the house, and water becomes a scarce resource whose use for hygiene purposes may be limited. However, the provision of water to communities does not necessarily ensure that infection or trachoma rates will decline. The decision to use water to improve hygienic conditions is very complex in these communities, and is clearly an important factor.[86]

Personal hygiene

In general, poor hygienic conditions favour the transmission of *C. trachomatis* through contact with ocular and other secretions, which are clearly a potential source of infection. Improving facial cleanliness, while not affecting the course of disease itself, may decrease the likelihood of transmission. Research in Tanzania determined the specific elements of an unclean face that were related to the risk of trachoma in children. Four elements were studied: flies, nasal discharge, food on the face and dust. Children having flies on the face and nasal discharge simultaneously had a two-fold increased risk of active trachoma compared with children without these signs.[87]

However, ascertaining the frequency of face washing among children is difficult and prone to reporting bias, since in most cultures mothers are aware that face washing is a desirable activity, regardless of their actual practices. The use of observational data is also prone to bias, as a recent study showed that data from observing children's faces at a central examination site led to higher prevalence rate of clean faces compared with data from the same child when observed at home.[88]

Numerous cross-sectional and longitudinal studies have linked clean faces to a decreased risk of trachoma or severe trachoma compared with children with unclean faces. A randomized, community-based intervention trial was conducted in Tanzania to test the effectiveness of face washing following mass topical antibiotic treatment in reducing active trachoma in children. An intensive, participatory face-washing campaign that involved the entire community was implemented over several weeks.[89] Children who kept their faces clean were about half as likely to have trachoma at the end of the one-year follow-up, and a third as likely to have severe trachoma as children who did not

have clean faces.[90] The difficulties of carrying out a behavioural intervention were evident, but such an approach is likely to result in more sustainable reduction of disease than the constant provision of antibiotic treatment.

Poor hygienic conditions also favour transmission in crowded living conditions. The number of persons per sleeping room[67] showed a positive association with the prevalence of active trachoma. The increasing risk with increasingly crowded conditions is logical, as there is more exposure to infection via close contact with infected persons and **fomites,** which can be numerous.[91,b] A large family *per se* is not necessarily a risk factor for trachoma in children; rather the risk appears to be related to the likelihood of contact with an infected individual. Thus, for example, mothers of children with trachoma are more likely themselves to have active disease, compared with women who either did not take care of children or whose children did not have trachoma.[92]

Flies

One of the earliest risk factors noted for trachoma was the presence of eye-seeking flies.[93] Studies in Tanzania have found an association between fly density in the household or the presence of flies on children's faces and presence and severity of trachoma and infection with *C. trachomatis*.[87,94–96] Flies are presumed to act as physical vectors for transmission of *C. trachomatis*, and the presence of *C. trachomatis* in flies caught in villages with trachoma has been demonstrated,[97,98] although it is not known if they are capable of transmitting an infective dose.

Two clinical trials on the value of fly control have reported different results. In the Gambia, a cluster randomized trial of villages was conducted where one arm received six months of intense space-spraying with permethrin to control flies.[99] Muscid flies were the targets of the intervention, especially *Musca sorbens*, the fly most commonly found in contact with eyes. After six months, the

---

b Nanji A, Mkocha H, Munoz B *et al*. Not just flies. Multiple sources of infection with *C. trachomatis* in Kongwa Tanzania. *PLoS NTD*, submitted 2010.

continual spraying resulted in significantly fewer fly–eye contacts in the intervention villages, and significant reduction in trachoma, from 7.18% to 3.69%, compared with control villages. In this study, trachoma graders were not masked to intervention status of the villages.

A clinical trial in Tanzania, using exactly the same fly-control methodology but over a one-year period, and following mass treatment with antibiotic, found a significant reduction in flies in the intervention communities but no significant difference in either trachoma or infection between intervention and control communities.[100] In this study, space-spraying followed mass treatment with oral azithromycin. Trachoma went from 63% to 43% in the intervention communities, and from 68% to 44% in the control communities. Infection was 9% in the intervention communities compared with 6% in the control communities. The authors speculated that, because communities in Tanzania were more hyper-endemic for trachoma than in the Gambia, many routes of transmission may have been operating so that alleviation of just one route would have no effect. Flies may play a more important role in transmission in the Gambia.

Flies are not the only source of transmission, as others have found trachoma where the fly populations are absent[97] or less intense.[101–102] Numerous fomites such as skirts, bedposts, etc. have been reported from Tanzania, although whether they contribute to transmission of infection is unknown.[c]

Latrines

The presence of a functional latrine near the house has been associated with lower trachoma prevalence in several different countries. The mechanism by which the presence of a latrine would decrease trachoma is not entirely clear, but presumably results, in part, by removing breeding sites for the eye-seeking fly, *M. sorbens*.[103] However, a clinical trial to test the effect of provision of latrines was not associated with a significant reduction in trachoma.[99]

The latrine may also be a marker for families who have better hygiene practices overall. In Egypt, presence of a latrine was related to other measures of higher socio-economical status, such as more professional occupation and more education of the head of the household, numerous and larger farm animals and bigger farming plots.[104]

17.4.3 Risk factors for scarring and trichiasis/entropion

The sequelae of active trachoma (trichiasis, entropion and corneal opacities) appears in young adulthood and in middle-aged persons. In some hyper-endemic areas, severe scarring and even trichiasis can appear in children, but the prevalence of severe scarring is usually low in children and increases with age. Because of the long time from repeated or prolonged active infection in childhood to the development of blinding sequelae in middle-aged adults, there are few good longitudinal studies of risk factors for scarring or trichiasis/entropion. This area is of considerable interest because, although the majority of children in trachoma endemic areas have active disease, only a small percentage go on to develop the blinding complications, and there are limited data to suggest who is at risk.

Clearly, long-term exposure to infection that is characteristic of residence in hyper-endemic communities is the major risk for scarring and trichiasis. Risk factor studies in hyper-endemic communities in Sudan and Ethiopia have associated an increased risk of trichiasis, even trichiasis in children, with increasing prevalence of trachoma in the children in the household.[105–106] Incidence rates of scarring in children in hyper-endemic communities in Tanzania were around 1% to 4% per year.[28,84]

Within these trachoma endemic communities, there are those who are at greater risk of scarring and adverse sequelae than others. A cohort study of preschool children in Tanzania found that 29% of children with constant severe trachoma at baseline developed incident scarring, compared

---

[c] Nanji A, Mkocha H, Munoz B *et al*. Not just flies. Multiple sources of infection with *C. trachomatis* in Kongwa Tanzania. *PLoS NTD*, submitted 2010.

with 9.6% of children with trachoma, but not constant severe trachoma (constant severe trachoma was defined as the presence of TI or severe trachoma on three–four of four examinations over a one-year period).[84] Constant infection and constant severe trachoma have also been linked to increased risk of early scarring.[59] These children appear to have an inappropriate response to *C. trachomatis*, one that does not result in clearance of infection or disease and can lead to scarring. The reasons for this heterogeneity in susceptibility to infection, disease phenotype, and progression are complex, and under investigation.

Clinically inapparent infection with *C. trachomatis* has been found in adults with conjunctival scarring living in hyper-endemic communities.[15,91] This infection is suspected to play an active role in the continued pathogenesis of scarring.[107] In a follow-up study of women with *C. trachomatis* infection three years after baseline, 47% of the women who had infection at both time points had no obvious household source of infection.[60] The fact that 73% were infected with the same *ompA* genotype at follow-up as at baseline suggests that most of the infections were persistent. An estimated one third of women with infection had no sign of clinical disease. The women who had infection at both time points were also five times as likely to have trichiasis compared with women with no, or sporadic, infection.

Scarring of the conjunctiva is an obvious risk factor for trichiasis. The seven-year incidence rate in women with scars was 9.2%, and virtually none of the women without scars at baseline developed trichiasis (0.6%).[25] Incident trichiasis was also associated with having active trachoma at baseline, and infection at follow-up was associated with a 2.5-fold increased risk of trichiasis, lending further support for the role of infection and immune response in the development of trichiasis. In the Gambia, where trachoma rates are substantially lower, the 12-year progression from scarring to trichiasis in a cohort of 326 persons, including men, was 6.4%, about half that of Tanzania.[108]

Evidence implicating immune responses in scarring derives largely from animal models and work in sexually transmitted Chlamydia. Case-control studies of the association between ocular scarring, trichiasis and immunogenetic polymorphisms affecting host responses to infection has been carried out in the Gambia as described in the section above. At least four cytokines or enzymes and genetic variation at the locus have been routinely implicated: **tumour necrosis factor (TNF)**, which may be a key mediator for the fibrotic response to chlamydia infection; matrix metalloproteinase (MMP9), which can degrade structural proteins in the extra-cellular matrix and is regulated in response, in part, to TNF; interleukin-10 (IL-10), a cytokine associated with susceptibility and persistence of infection; and interferon gamma (IFNγ), a cytokine shown in animal models to inhibit chlamydial replication, but has also been implicated in inducing chlamydial persistence that may also result in tissue damage.[52,109–110] Natividad and colleagues have identified **single nucleotide polymorphisms (SNPs)** that define a risk haplotype which was associated with a modest increase in IL-10 expression during infection and associated with an increased risk of scarring.[51]

Women are at much greater risk of developing the blinding complications of trachoma than are men.[111] This increased risk has been explained by the women's close contact with small children, who are the main reservoir of infection, and active disease in adults is highly associated with being caretakers of children with trachoma.[92] However, a case-control study of risk factors for trichiasis in women did not find any association with years of exposure to childcare activities,[112] although exposure to children with infection could not be ascertained retrospectively. Women with trichiasis were more likely to have mothers (but not fathers) with trichiasis, which could be a marker for a home environment in childhood with high transmission rates of Chlamydia infection but could also be a marker of a female familial tendency to trichiasis. Research in animal models and human cell lines of genital chlamydia suggest that female hormones may influence or modulate infection, specifically implicating a role of oestrogen in enhancing attachment and infectivity. Using reverse-transcriptase-polymerase chain reaction (RT-PCR) technology, oestrogen receptors have been detected in the conjunctiva and cornea of female ocular samples.[113] Taken together, these data suggest at least in part a biological explanation for the excess risk in females beyond greater exposure to infection sources.

The progression of trichiasis and progression to corneal opacity were studied in trichiasis cases in the Gambia examined four years apart.[114] The four-year incidence rate of new trichiasis was 29%, and 37% had trichiasis progression. New corneal opacification developed in 10% of eyes with five or more lashes touching the globe, and in 5% of eyes with fewer than five lashes touching the globe. Unfortunately, the graders at baseline and follow-up were different, and unexpected regression was also observed: 8.5% of eyes with trichiasis at baseline had no trichiasis at follow-up, and 40% of eyes with corneal opacity at baseline had none at follow-up. While infection with *C. trachomatis* was rare, bacterial infection was common, and more frequent with increasing severity of trichiasis. Conjunctival inflammation was associated with progression of trichiasis, possibly reflecting an active scarring process. Of interest are the relatively high progression rates, given the decline in prevalence of trachoma in the Gambia.

With continued efforts to eliminate active trachoma, scarring will also decrease and trichiasis will no longer be a public health problem. At present there is no clear intervention that can be used to interrupt the scarring process.

17.5 CONTROL STRATEGY: SURGERY/ANTIBIOTICS/ FACE-WASHING/ENVIRONMENTAL CHANGE (SAFE)

In line with the Vision 2020 initiative (see Chapter 24), the World Health Organization has recommended the use of the **SAFE** strategy for countries implementing trachoma control programmes. This multifaceted approach includes **S**urgery for trichiasis cases, **A**ntibiotics to treat the community pool of infection, **F**ace-washing to reduce transmission, and **E**nvironmental change

to sustain reduction in transmission. There is epidemiological evidence to support each component of the SAFE strategy, which must be implemented on a community-wide basis. The implementation is critically important, as the temptation is strong to follow a more medically oriented model of concentration on provision of surgery and antibiotics, with less attention to the hygiene and environmental components. The part of the strategy involving motivating significant behaviour change on a community level is not easy, and involves training and experience that is not traditionally part of an eye care worker's job. Research is still needed on optimal implementation of SAFE, and how long control strategies must be in place to reduce blinding trachoma so that it is no longer a public health problem. Nevertheless, there are data from uncontrolled surveys following large-scale SAFE implementation showing that, even without full penetration of all elements of SAFE, there is reduction in active trachoma in the most endemic environments.[70,115] Below, each component is described more fully.

17.5.1 Surgery

Even if current control strategies are effective in reducing active trachoma in children, trichiasis will continue to occur in the adult population as a result of previous years of exposure to trachoma, and many will progress to corneal opacification and blindness without surgical intervention.[114] On the basis of a clinical trial carried out by ophthalmologists, the WHO recommends **bilamellar tarsal–rotation BLTR procedure (BTRP)** for the correction of entropion and trichiasis.[116] However, in areas in which trachoma is endemic, patients with trichiasis often have very limited, if any, access to an ophthalmologist. Eye nurses and integrated eye care workers can be successfully trained to perform this surgery.[117-118]

Some reports from trachoma programmes based on outcomes after follow-up of trichiasis surgery patients paint a dismal picture. One study of trichiasis surgery cases with follow-up of at least two years, done in several districts of Tanzania, found a recurrence rate of trichiasis of 28%, varying by district from 16% to 38%.[119] In the Gambia, trichiasis recurrence rates at one year were 41%, and varied among surgeons from 0% to more than 80%.[120] Yet, in controlled clinical trials under strict surgical conditions, adverse outcomes following surgery are low. In a clinical trial of BTRP, the adverse outcome rate (including recurrent trichiasis) at 18 months was 18%.[121] In another large clinical trial using integrated eye care workers in Ethiopia, recurrence of trichiasis was only 10% at 12 months, and 30% lower if azithromycin was used post-surgery.[122] Clearly, the variable rate of adverse outcomes following trichiasis surgery suggests factors that could be altered to improve outcomes.

One factor is the severity of the trichiasis at time of surgery. Patients who present with more severe trichiasis, as quantified by increasing number of lashes touching the globe or severe entropion, are at greater risk of recurrence.[120,122,123] These findings argue for an earlier presentation of trichiasis for surgery, to ensure a more successful outcome. If the patient has had previous lid surgery, risk of recurrence is higher.[121,124] Thus, from a programme perspective it is even more critical to have low recurrence rates following the first surgery, as the risk of adverse outcomes following repair of recurrent trichiasis is so much greater.

It is clear that the skill of the surgeon is an important component of the outcome of the surgery. No other explanations can possibly account for the wide variation in recurrence rates between 0% and 80% in the study reported from the Gambia.[120] West *et al.* found significant differences in recurrence rates between districts in Tanzania, where specific surgeons were assigned to a district and all were using the same surgical technique.[119]

Surgeon factors can be somewhat ameliorated by proper training. In the Ethiopian clinical trial of antibiotic use post-surgery, extensive use was made of the certification of the surgeons manual.[122,125] There was no difference in the very low recurrence rates between one surgeon and another. The trial found that use of azithromycin post-surgery reduced recurrence by 30%, but the authors also speculated on other factors that might have reduced recurrence rates overall: the surgeons were especially trained in sterile techniques, and strict procedures for preserving a sterile field were in place during the trial. More effort by country programmes to improve surgeon technique is needed. Ongoing surgical audit has been proposed, and the need to de-certify surgeons who cannot perform to standard must be considered.[126–127]

Two clinical trials have now evaluated the effect of using a single dose of azithromycin immediately post-operatively to reduce recurrence. One trial showed no benefit, but the surgeons were not standardized, and some had extremely high recurrence rates.[120] It is not reasonable to expect added benefit from azithromycin where surgeon skill factors overwhelm the outcome. The other trial, with greater numbers of cases and standardization of surgeons, showed no difference in outcome by surgeon and the recurrence rate was low.[122] A single dose of azithromycin postoperatively reduced recurrence rates by 30% up to one year post-surgery, compared with provision of topical tetracycline, suggesting added benefit in improved outcomes. However, there was no added benefit to treating the entire family of the case with azithromycin, compared with treating the case alone.

While it is clear that risk of trichiasis is greatest for those living in trachoma hyper-endemic communities, and at risk of multiple bouts of infection, it is not clear that recurrent trichiasis post-surgery is due to ongoing bouts of *C. trachomatis*. It is possible that the wider systemic protection afforded by azithromycin's broad spectrum of activity prevented other infections from contributing to recurrence. In a longitudinal study of trichiasis cases in the Gambia, bacterial infection at follow-up was associated with three-fold higher risk of recurrence.[128]

Availability of trained personnel does not necessarily ensure that patients will use the surgical services. In a cohort of Tanzanian patients with trichiasis, only 27% had surgery within seven years after diagnosis; patients were aware that surgery was available and could prevent vision loss, and the main barriers were perceived cost and lack of accessibility to the health facilities.[129] In this environment, cost includes cost of transport, food, and costs of an accompanying person who acts as a caretaker. Similar barriers were reported in a study of trichiasis cases in Nigeria, of whom 9% had had surgery.[130]

The introduction of surgery at the village level, as opposed to requiring patients to present at a hospital or health centre, should reduce these barriers. A randomized trial of several villages in the Gambia found that acceptance of surgery was higher when surgery was offered in the village compared with the health centre.[131] In the Gambia, Frick and colleagues have shown that the productivity gains from the additional surgeries done because the surgeries were carried out in the village exceed the costs of moving the surgery to the local level.[132] However, surgical acceptance drops off markedly with the institution of cost recovery schemes, which increases the cost barrier, regardless of location.

Corneal transplantation is not an option for most areas with blinding trachoma, and even if it were, corneas blind from trachoma are not good candidates for transplant because of the extensive neo-vascularization and poor state of the conjunctiva.

17.5.2   Antibiotics

The use of 1% topical tetracycline eye ointment, once a day for four to six weeks, is one alternative for treating active trachoma, but far superior in terms of compliance is a single oral dose of azithromycin at 20 mg/kg up to 1 g. The WHO recommends mass treatment of the entire village when the prevalence of TF is more than 10% in children aged under ten years.[133] Mass treatment changes to targeted treatment when prevalence is between 5% and 10%; when TF rates are less than 5%, the ultimate intervention goal is achieved and antibiotic treatment, whether targeted or mass treatment, can cease. Current WHO guidelines suggest mass treatment of communities for three years, then re-evaluation to determine continued need, although this guideline was based on expert opinion in the absence of data.

Most trachoma control programmes offer mass treatment to communities once per year, and data from Tanzania on speed of re-emergent infection suggest annual treatment may be adequate.[68] Mass treatment with azithromycin has a profound effect on decreasing chlamydial load.[134–135] In a hyper-endemic community, 90% of those with a modest load of infection at baseline had no evidence of infection two months after treatment, and 74% of those with a greater load (> 20 copies) had no infection.[135]

There are several key operational research questions that must be addressed for optimal but realistic use of azithromycin in programme settings. Can we target treatment, or is mass treatment most appropriate? In a mesoendemic area of Nepal, where the prevalence of trachoma in children was about 16%, mass treatment with azithromycin of children only was slightly more effective in reducing infection and disease at six months compared with targeting children with trachoma and their families; mass treatment was also significantly more cost-effective.[136–137] This in part stems from the costs of having to screen households for presence of a person with trachoma, and as the prevalence decreases, it becomes more labour intensive to ensure all household members are free of disease before not treating. Treatment of children is essential, as they are reservoirs of infection, but the added advantage of treating adults in terms of re-emergent infection is not clear, especially in low prevalence areas. There is infection in adults, and treatment for them is likely important.

How often should communities be treated? In hyper-endemic villages in Ethiopia, biannual mass treatment with azithromycin reduced infection from 32% to 0.9% at 24 months, compared with annual treatment, which reduced infection from 43% to 7%; the lower prevalence for biannual treatment was statistically significant.[138] In a mesoendemic community in Tanzania, a single mass treatment with azithromycin at very high coverage plus intense follow-up and treatment of trachoma cases with topical tetracycline virtually eliminated infection in the community at 24 months.[134] Similarly, in low prevalence communities (average 8% TF) in the Gambia, a single mass treatment with modestly high coverage cleared all baseline infections and only isolated cases re-emerged.[31] In summary, starting prevalence clearly influences the frequency of treatment, but more often than twice a year is unlikely to be programmatically feasible. A trial is under-way in hyper-endemic communities in Ethiopia to compare the cost-effectiveness of biannual treatment of children only, with annual mass treatment of all persons in reducing trachoma and infection.

A key question is what happens once mass treatment is stopped. Re-emergence of infection with cessation of mass treatment does occur, and has been reported primarily from hyper-endemic communities.[31,135] Despite high coverage with mass treatment in a Tanzanian hyper-endemic community, infection at two months post-treatment was 12% and came primarily from those who had been treated.[135] The strongest predictor of infection post-treatment was having infection prior to treatment. Interestingly, transmission of infection to susceptible family members six months after mass treatment was significant only if a household member had at least 20 organisms or more per ocular swab at two months. In this community, infection began to increase again 18 months after mass treatment. Return of infection 18 months following cessation of treatment in Ethiopian hyper-endemic communities has also been reported.[139] However, where trachoma rates are very low (the Gambia), and after a single mass treatment, infection was largely gone over the follow-up period of 17 months, except in two villages where residents had extensive contact with untreated villages in neighbouring Senegal.[31] However, even these imported infections did not lead to re-emergence to the baseline level, as infection declined without treatment from 30% post-reinfection to 11% at 17 months in these two villages.

What is the source of infection following mass treatment? First, non-compliance with treatment was a main predictor of infection and disease at follow-up in studies in three different settings.[79] Infected persons, especially with heavy loads of organisms, are a clear source of re-emergence. Very young children, less than one year of age who are not eligible for azithromycin, may have very high chlamydial burdens and are potential sources of re-infection. Infection in communities is less related to how many rounds of mass treatment the community has received, than to the coverage of the community during the last round.[d] The association with non-compliance argues for striving

to achieve very high coverage; community trials are underway in Ethiopia, the Gambia and Tanzania to determine the added benefit on infection and disease of increasing coverage beyond 80%.

However, even with high coverage, infection does remain following mass treatment, and most infected persons are those who were, in fact, treated. The persons at greatest risk of infection following treatment are those who had infection prior to treatment, and who had the greatest infectious burden.[135,140] Resistance of Chlamydia to azithromycin has not been reported, so this is likely due to an insufficient dose of azithromycin for those with heavy infection. However, increasing the dose from 20 to 30 mg/kg in children with infection did not result in significantly less infection six weeks post-treatment, but the load of infection was not measured, so it is not known if there was a difference in the load of infection between the two groups after treatment.[141]

Another source of infection is re-introduction of *C. trachomatis*, with immigration of individuals who can bring in infection, and returning community members who acquire infection outside. While travel outside the community was a not risk factor for incident infection in Tanzania,[140] it was the primary explanation in the Gambia.[31] The importance of travel reflects local conditions, the nature of the travel, and the likelihood of close contact with infected persons.

Thus, questions still remain regarding how long to treat communities in order to achieve infection levels where re-emergence does not become an issue. The WHO recommends treatment of districts for three years, then a re-survey to see if further mass treatment is warranted. Unfortunately, irresponsible interpretation of this guideline has resulted in thinking that countries can stop after three rounds, which is clearly not the case in most hyper-endemic communities. Misinterpretation of research findings has also led to the thinking that, with high coverage alone, communities can stop after one round. While this may be true where districts have low starting endemicity, it is clearly not the case where districts have high prevalence at the start.[142] Empirical data from Tanzania in 71 communities where the

---

[d] West SK, Munoz B, Mkocha H *et al*. Number of years of annual mass treatment with azithromycin needed to control trachoma in hyper-endemic communities in Tanzania. *J Infect Dis*, submitted 2010.

average prevalence of trachoma was 50% suggest that, even after seven rounds of mass treatment, disease and infection are still high enough to warrant continued treatment.[d] The authors suggested that up to ten years of annual mass treatment under programme conditions would be necessary to achieve 5% prevalence of disease or less. Clinical trials currently underway will help address the number of rounds of mass treatment needed, depending on starting endemicity, and the target infection rate at which re-emergence is not a problem.

Despite potential concerns for *S. pneumoniae* resistance developing with mass treatment, research has not found persistent or clinically significant resistance.[143,144] Studies are ongoing of the effect of multiple rounds or more frequent rounds of treatment on resistance, but in many trachoma endemic areas, azithromycin is not available to treat acute lower respiratory tract infections. Others suggest that resistance can be avoided with use of topical formulations, but one study showed that use of topical tetracycline can induce carriage of tetracycline resistant strains of *S. pneumoniae* in the nasopharynx six months after treatment.[145]

Operational research on different strategies to distribute azithromycin in trachoma endemic communities have focused on the effectiveness and cost-effectiveness of various alternatives for improving coverage.[146] Programmes are largely devolving control of mass distribution to the communities. A pilot study in Ghana demonstrated the competency of trained community volunteers to diagnose trachoma and to properly treat cases with azithromycin.[147] A comparison of using community volunteers versus village government leaders to recruit families for mass treatment in communities in Tanzania showed higher coverage rates for women and children in villages under the community volunteer programme.[148] Research has shown that, for children over age six months, height can be used as a proxy for weight in dosing azithromycin, which also simplifies the logistics of providing treatment.[149]

Trachoma has been included in new initiatives on **Neglected Tropical Diseases (NTDs)**, where considerable resources are being directed at infections that respond to mass drug administration.[150] Theoretically, there are opportunities to bundle control of trachoma with other diseases where there is geographical overlap, in order to realize cost savings. To date, the effort has proved less than ideal for the trachoma community, for several reasons: first, the emphasis on preventive chemotherapy ignores the need for surgery and the hygiene and environmental components that must also accompany trachoma control; second, early implementation efforts do not clearly show that the integration at the country level that is needed for this approach is valuable. For example, teams working in other NTDs in Niger ignored the needs of country trachoma programmes, literally hijacking resources away from priority trachoma endemic areas to treat districts where trachoma rates were low but overlapped with other NTDS, for the sake of 'integration'. Finally, while there is overlap of some of the NTDs at the country level, at the level of district or community implementation, trachoma is a disease of water-poor areas and is not likely to be a problem where onchocerciasis or shistosomiasis is hyper-endemic. While some integration and coordination of drug management at a national level may be realized, the extent of programme integration at the implementation level within country should reflect careful mapping and evidence of geographical overlap of the diseases at priority levels, true integration of programme approaches that meet all the needs of all NTDS, and better appreciation by partners that trachoma control is not simply about delivering antibiotics.

17.5.3 Face-washing and environmental change

Trachoma disappeared in many countries prior to the advent of antibiotic use. The disappearance is attributed to improvements in socioeconomic conditions, better hygiene and environmental sanitation. Without the inclusion of hygiene and environmental behaviour changes as part of trachoma control within trachoma endemic communities, it is unlikely that antibiotics alone will create a long-term solution to the reduction of the level of disease. The challenge for trachoma control programme managers will be to resist the lure of an antibiotic siren, and to integrate persons skilled in community development for water and sanitation into the country strategy.

Country programmes that use a strategy of antibiotics, hygiene promotion, and some form of environmental improvement are reporting either elimination of active trachoma[151] or substantial reductions in disease[30,69,115,152,153] in non-randomized designs. Arguments can be made that secular trends could explain the reduction, although in highly endemic areas, like Sudan, it seems unlikely. Secular trends do not always favour reduction in trachoma either.[28] Data from Sudan suggest independent benefits of azithromycin, facial cleanliness and use of a pit latrine in protecting against severe trachoma, although only 6.3% of households had pit latrines, so the attributable protective effect of this intervention was modest. In a community randomized trial of alternative approaches to health education messages, compared with no health education, a modest, non-significant effect on trachoma was seen after one year; but the interventions (radio programmes, videos and unspecified activities) appeared to have no effect on observed hygiene practices.[154]

17.5.4   Vaccine

Efforts to create a vaccine against chlamydial infection have been unsuccessful to date. Attempts were made to develop chlamydial vaccines by using killed elementary bodies, but their use resulted in even more severe disease than naturally acquired infection, thus arguing against the use of either inactivated or live-attenuated vaccines. Most of the effort has focused on sub-unit candidates that would result in protective immunity without evoking a damaging pathological response.

In a mouse model, systemic immunization with MOMP purified in its native conformation induced a protective immune response against a genital challenge.[155] Use of a similar vaccine in a non-human primate model resulted in a significant decrease in infectious burden on primary ocular challenge, but at later time points showed no difference from controls in either the burden or

duration of infection; immunization had no effect on the ocular disease.[156] The authors concluded that effective vaccines for trachoma will probably have to target regional ocular immune induction sites. At present, control of trachoma through a vaccine strategy appears to be several years away.

17.6   FUTURE RESEARCH

Basic and applied research into chlamydial ocular infection and trachoma is essential for the elimination of blinding trachoma as a public health problem. Trachoma is an ancient disease and, despite its disappearance from much of the world, is tenacious and persistent; it is not liable to vanish completely without a sustained effort. This chapter has focused on the epidemiologic aspects of trachoma, and this section on future research needs will continue that focus. However, the strides made by basic science into the molecular biology and immunology of *C. trachomatis* are prodigious, and findings from these disciplines will greatly inform the future directions of the epidemiological investigations. Any ophthalmologist or epidemiologist interested in trachoma should be aware of literature in the basic science field as well.

Epidemiological investigations into trachoma should provide knowledge that contributes to the prevention, treatment and control of this blinding disease. Priorities include the following:

1. Further work is indicated to determine the host and Chlamydia interactions and factors that predict chronic infection and drive scarring and trichiasis in these communities. Such research is invaluable for vaccine development. In particular, an explanation is needed for why a subgroup of children in hyper-endemic trachoma areas manifest severe, constant disease.
2. How can we improve trichiasis surgery in order to avoid recurrence and other adverse outcomes? Current clinical trials are investigating different types of sutures, a new tool to aid trichiasis surgeons, and alternative approaches to suturing.
3. A rapid, point-of-care diagnostic test that is affordable, sensitive, specific and robust for field use in detecting infection is urgently

needed. Such a test would help communities to determine that transmission of infection had been interrupted, even in the face of residual follicular trachoma, that would otherwise suggest that ongoing mass treatment was needed.

4. In the past, research has focused on hyperendemic countries where the burden of trachoma is great. However, many countries are now mesoendemic or hypoendemic, and the burden of surveys to determine prevalence or target areas of an increasingly rare disease is growing. New survey methodologies, using tools such as a rapid field test for infection, that will help low prevalence districts determine if they have reached target, or identify 'hot spots', are urgently needed.

5. Operational research on implementation of the SAFE strategy, with appropriate evaluation, is critically important for the design of alternative cost-effective strategies for trachoma control programmes. Data are needed on optimal, but feasible, coverage rates for antibiotic treatment of communities, and the number of years that mass treatment must be included in programmes; this is likely to depend on the starting trachoma prevalence. Of critical importance is information on the community level of infection at which re-emergence of blinding trachoma will have ceased.

6. In this era of control of NTDs, further work on models of successful integration of trachoma with other NTDS is needed. This starts with the WHO, whose production of suitable materials for country programmes must include trachoma, and teams at the country level for whom breaking the silos of vertical programmes to achieve integration may also mean relinquishing resources. Most importantly, integration of preventive chemotherapy may be efficient, but for trachoma will not be effective without the other components of SAFE.

REFERENCES

1. World Health Organization. Global elimination of blinding trachoma. In: World Health Assembly (ed). WHA51.11; 1998.

2. Mariotti S, Pascolini D, Rose-Nussbaumer J. Trachoma: Global magnitude of a preventable cause of blindness. *Br J Ophthalmol* 2009; 93:563–568.

3. Frick KD, Hanson CL, Jacobson GA. Global burden of trachoma and economics of the disease. *Am J Trop Med Hyg* 2003; 69:1–10.

4. Al-Rifai K. Trachoma throughout history. *Int Ophthalmol* 1998; 12:9–14.

5. Duke-Elder S (ed). *Diseases of the Outer Eye, Part I. System of Ophthalmology*. London: Henry Kempton; 1977. pp. 249–307.

6. MacCallan A. The epidemiology of trachoma. *Br J Ophthalmol* 1931; 15:370–411.

7. Mettler C. History of medicine. In: Mettler F (ed). *History of Medicine*. Philadelphia: Blakiston Co.; 1947. pp. 1005–1023.

8. Wyman WS. Letter from Dr. Walter S. Wyman to Frank H. Larned, Acting Commissioner General of Immigration, 30 October 1897. In: *Letters Sent by the Office of the Surgeon General 1872–1918*. College Park, MD: National Archives; 1897. pp. 303–304.

9. Markel H. 'The Eyes Have It': Trachoma, the perception of disease, the United States Public Health Service, and the American Jewish Immigration Experience 1897–1924. *B Hist Med* 2000; 74:525–560.

10. Taylor HR (ed). *Trachoma: A Blinding Scourge from the Bronze Age to the Twenty-First Century*. East Melbourne: Centre for Eye Research Australia; 2004. pp. 1–272.

11. Elliot RH. *Tropical Ophthalmology*. London: Oxford University Press; 1920. p. 300.

12. Stephens RS. Genome sequence of an obligate pathogen of humans: Chlamydia trachomatis. *Science* 1998; 282:754–759.

13. Sharma M, Rudel T. Apoptosis resistance in Chlamydia-infected cells: a fate worse than death? *FEMS Immunol Med Microbiol* 2009; 55:154–161.

14. Zhang J, Lietman T, Olinger L, *et al*. Genetic diversity of Chlamydia trachomatis and the prevalence of trachoma. *Pediatr Infect Dis J* 2004; 23:217–220.

15. Taylor HR, Rapoza PA, West S, *et al*. The epidemiology of infection in trachoma. *Invest Ophthalmol Vis Sci* 1989; 30:1823–1833.

16. Schachter J, Moncada J, Dawson CR, et al. Nonculture methods of diagnosing chlamydial infection in patients with trachoma: a clue to the pathogenesis of the disease? J Infect Dis 1988; 158:1347–1352.

17. An Q, Radcliffe G, Vassallo R, et al. Infection with a plasmid-free variant Chlamydia related to Chlamydia trachomatis identified by using multiple assays for nucleic acid detection. J Clin Microbiol 1992; 30:2814–2821.

18. Yang JL, Schachter J, Moncada J, et al. Comparison of an rRNA-based and DNA-based nucleic acid amplification test for the detection of Chlamydia trachomatis in trachoma. Br J Ophthalmol 2007; 91:293–295.

19. Diamant J, Benis R, Schachter J, et al. Pooling of Chlamydia laboratory tests to determine the prevalence of ocular Chlamydia trachomatis infection. Ophthalmic Epidemiol 2001; 8:109–117.

20. Bobo L, Munoz B, Viscidi R, et al. Diagnosis of Chlamydial trachomatis eye infection in Tanzania by polymerase chain reaction/enzyme immunoassay. Lancet 1991; 338:847–850.

21. Bailey RL, Hampton TJ, Hayes LJ, et al. Polymerase chain reaction for the detection of ocular chlamydial infection in trachoma-endemic communities. J Infect Dis 1994; 170:709–712.

22. Michel CE, Solomon AW, Magbanua JP, et al. Field evaluation of a rapid point-of-care assay for targeting antibiotic treatment for trachoma control: a comparative study. Lancet 2006; 367:1585–1590.

23. Grayston J, Yeh L, Kuo C. Importance of reinfection in the pathogenesis of trachoma. Rev Infect Dis 1985; 7:717–725.

24. Taylor HR, Johnson SL, Prendergast RA, et al. An animal model of trachoma: the importance of repeated reinfection. Invest Ophthalmol Vis Sci 1982; 23:507–515.

25. Munoz B, Bobo L, Mkocha H, et al. Incidence of trichiasis in a cohort of women with and without scarring. Int J Epidemiol 1999; 28:1167–1171.

26. Thylefors B, Dawson CR, Jones BR, et al. A simple system for the assessment of trachoma and its complications. Bull World Health Organ 1987; 65:477–483.

27. Dawson C, Jones BR, Tarizzo ML. Guide to Trachoma Control. Geneva: WHO; 1981.

28. Wolle MA, Munoz B, Mkocha H, et al. Age, sex, and cohort effects in a longitudinal study of trachomatous scarring. Invest Ophthalmol Vis Sci 2009; 50:592–596.

29. Melese M, Alemayehu W, Bejiga A, et al. Modified grading system for upper eyelid trachomatous trichiasis. Ophthalmic Epidemiol 2003; 10:75–80.

30. Mkocha H, Munoz B, West S. Trachoma and ocular chlamydia trachomatis rates in children in trachoma-endemic communities enrolled for at least three years in the Tanzania National Trachoma control program. Tanz J Health Res 2009: II.

31. Burton MJ, Holland MK, Makalo P, et al. Re-emergence of Chlamydia trachomatis infection after mass antibiotic treatment of a trachoma-endemic Gambian community: a longitudinal study. Lancet 2005; 365:1321–1328.

32. Zhang YX, Stewart S, Joseph T, et al. Protective monoclonal antibodies recognize epitopes located on the major outer membrane protein of chlamydia trachomatis. J Immunol 1987; 138:575–581.

33. Bailey R, Duong T, Carpenter R, et al. The duration of human ocular Chlamydia trachomatis infection is age dependent. Epidemiol Infect 1999; 123:479–486.

34. Jawetz E, Rose L, Hanna L, et al. Experimental inclusion conjunctivitis in man: measurements of infectivity and resistance. JAMA 1965; 194:620–632.

35. Grayston T, Wang SP. The potential for a vaccine against infection of the genital tract by chlamydia trachomatis. Sex Transm Dis 1987; 5:73–77.

36. Murray ES, Charbonnet LT, MacDonald AB. Immunity to chlamydial infection of the eye. The role of circulatory and secretory antibodies in resistance to reinfection with guinea pig conjunctivitis. J Immunol 1973; 110:1518–1525.

37. Wang SP, Grayston J, Alexander ER. Trachoma vaccine studies in monkeys. Am J Ophthalmol 1967; 63:1615–1630.

38. Rasmussen SJ, Eckmann L, Alison J, et al. Secretion of proinflammatory cytokines by epithelial cells in response to Chlamydia infection suggests a central role for epithelial cells in chlamydial pathogenesis. J Clin Invest Med 1997; 99:77–87.

39. Kawana K, Ficarra M, Ibana JA, et al. CD1d degradation in Chlamydia trachomatis-infected epithelial cells is the result of both cellular and

chlamydial proteasomal activity. *J Biol Chem* 2007; 282:7368–7375.

40. Treharne JT, Dwyer RS, Darougar S, *et al*. Antichlamydial antibody in tears and sera and serotypes of chlamydia trachomatis isolated from school children in Southern Tunisia. *Br J Ophthalmol* 1978; 62:509–515.

41. Bailey RL, Kajbaf M, Whittle HC, *et al*. The influence of local antichlamydial antibody on the acquisition and persistence of human ocular chlamydial infection: IgG antibodies are not protective. *Epidemiol Infect* 1993; 111:315–324.

42. Ghaem-Maghami S, Bailey RL, Mabey DC, *et al*. Characterization of B-cell responses to Chlamydia trachomatis antigens in humans with trachoma. *Infect Immun* 1997; 65:4958–4964.

43. Hayes LJ, Pecharatana S, Bailey RL, *et al*. Extent and kinetics of genetic change in the omp1 gene of Chlamydia trachomatis in two villages with endemic trachoma. *J Infect Dis* 1995; 172:268–272.

44. Hseih YH, Bobo LD, Quinn TC, *et al*. Determinants of trachoma endemnicity using chlamydia trachomatis ompA DNA sequencing. *Microbes Infect* 2001; 3:447–458.

45. Dean D, Schachter J, Dawson JR, *et al*. Comparison of the major outer membrane protein sequence variant regions of B/Ba isolates: a molecular epidemiological approach to chlamydial trachomatis infections. *J Infect Dis* 1992; 116:383–392.

46. Andreasen AA, Burton MJ, Holland MJ, *et al*. Chlamydia trachomatis ompA Variants in Trachoma: What Do They Tell Us? *PLoS Negl Trop Dis* 2008; 2:e306.

47. Bailey RL, Holland MJ, Whittle HC, *et al*. Subjects recovering from human ocular chlamydial infection have enhanced lymphoproliferative responses to chlamydial antigens compared with those of persistently diseased controls. *Infect Immun* 1995; 63:389–392.

48. Igietseme J, Ramsey KH, Magee DM, *et al*. Resolution of murine chlamydial genital infection by the adoptive transfer of a biovar-specific, Th-1 lymphocyte clone. *Reg Immunol* 1993; 5:317–324.

49. Morrison RP, Feilzer K, Tumas DB. Gene knockout mice establish a primary protectvie role for major histocompatibility complex class II-restricted

responses in chlamydia trachomatis genital tract infection. *Infect Immun* 1995; 63:4661–4668.

50. Holland MJ, Bailey RL, Hayes LJ, *et al*. Conjunctival scarring in trachoma is associated with depressed cell-mediated immune responses to chlamydial antigens. *J Infect Dis* 1993; 168:1528–1531.

51. Natividad A, Holland MJ, Rockett KA, *et al*. Susceptibility to sequelae of human ocular chlamydial infection associated with allelic variation in IL10 cis-regulation. *Hum Mol Genet* 2008; 17:323–329.

52. Natividad A, Wilson J, Kock O, *et al*. Risk of trachomatous scarring and trichiasis in Gambians varies with SNP haplotypes at the interferon-gamma and interleukin-10 loci. *Genes Immun* 2005; 6:332–340.

53. Bobo L, Novak N, Mkocha H, *et al*. Evidence for a predominant proinflammatory conjunctival cytokine response in individuals with trachoma. *Infect Immun* 1996; 64:3273–3279.

54. Burton MJ, Bailey RL, Jeffries D, *et al*. Cytokine and fibrogenic gene expression in the conjunctivas of subjects from a Gambian community where trachoma is endemic. *Infect Immun* 2004; 72:7352–7356.

55. Faal N, Bailey RL, Jeffries D, *et al*. Conjunctival FOXP3 expression in trachoma: do regulatory T cells have a role in human ocular Chlamydia trachomatis infection? *PLoS Med* 2006; 3:e266.

56. Morrison RP, Lyng K, Caldwell HD. Chlamydial disease pathogenesis. Ocular delayed hypersensitivity elicited by a genus specific 57kD protein. *J Exp Med* 1989; 169:3023–3027.

57. Beatty WL, Byrne GI, Morrison RP. Morphological and antigenic characteristics of interferon gamma mediated persistent C. trachomatis infection *in vitro*. *Proc Natl Acad Sci* 1993; 90:3998–4002.

58. Peeling RW, Bailey RL, Conway DJ, *et al*. Antibody response to the 60-kDa chlamydial heat-shock protein is associated with scarring trachoma. *J Infect Dis* 1998; 177:256–259.

59. Wolle MA, Munoz BE, Mkocha H, *et al*. Constant ocular infection with Chlamydia trachomatis predicts risk of scarring in children in Tanzania. *Ophthalmology* 2009; 116:243–247.

60. Smith A, Munoz B, Hsieh YH, *et al*. OmpA genotypic evidence for persistent ocular Chlamydia

trachomatis infection in Tanzanian village women. *Ophthalmic Epidemiol* 2001; 8:127–135.

61. Detels R, Alexander ER, Dhir SP. Trachoma in Punjab Indians in British Columbia. A prevalence study with comparisons to India. *Am J Epidemiol* 1966; 84:81–91.

62. Khandekar R, Mohammed AJ. The prevalence of trachomatous trichiasis in Oman (Oman eye study 2005). *Ophthalmic Epidemiol* 2007; 14:267–272.

63. Uzma N, Kumar BS, Khaja Mohinuddin Salar BM, *et al*. A comparative clinical survey of the prevalence of refractive errors and eye diseases in urban and rural school children. *Can J Ophthalmol* 2009; 44:328–333.

64. West SK, Munoz B, Turner VM, *et al*. The epidemiology of trachoma in Central Tanzania. *Int J Epidemiol* 1991; 20:1088–1092.

65. Katz J, Zeger S, Tielsch L. Village and household clustering of xerophthalmia and trachoma. *Int J Epidemiol* 1988; 17:865–869.

66. Blake IM, Burton MJ, Bailey RL, *et al*. Estimating household and community transmission of ocular chlamydia trachomatis. *PLoS Negl Trop Dis* 2009; 3: e401.

67. Bailey R, Osmond C, Mabey DC, *et al*. Analysis of the household distribution of trachoma in a Gambian village using a Monte Carlo simulation procedure. *Int J Epidemiol* 1989; 18: 944–951.

68. Broman AT, Shum K, Munoz B, *et al*. Spatial clustering of ocular chlamydial infection over time following treatment, among households in a village in Tanzania. *Invest Ophthalmol Vis Sci* 2006; 47:99–104.

69. Ngondi J, Onsarigo A, Adamu L, *et al*. The epidemiology of trachoma in Eastern Equatoria and Upper Nile States, southern Sudan. *Bull World Health Organ* 2005; 83:904–912.

70. Ngondi J, Gebre T, Shargie EB, *et al*. Evaluation of three years of the SAFE strategy (Surgery, Antibiotics, Facial cleanliness and Environmental improvement) for trachoma control in five districts of Ethiopia hyperendemic for trachoma. *Trans Roy Soc Trop Med Hyg* 2009; 103:1001–1010.

71. Solomon AW, Holland MJ, Burton MJ, *et al*. Strategies for control of trachoma: observational study with quantitative PCR. *Lancet* 2003; 362:198–204.

72. Courtright P, Sheppard J, Schachter J, *et al*. Trachoma and blindness in the Nile Delta: Current patterns and projections for the future in the rural Egyptian population. *Br J Ophthalmol* 1989; 73:536–540.

73. Tabbara K, al-Omar O. Trachoma in Saudi Arabia. *Ophthalmic Epidemiol* 1997; 4:117–118.

74. Khandekar R, Mohammed AJ, Al Raisi A, *et al*. Prevalence and distribution of active trachoma in children of less than five years of age in trachoma endemic regions of Oman in 2005. *Ophthalmic Epidemiol* 2006; 13:167–172.

75. Rabui M. Alhassan MB, Abiose A. Trial of trachoma rapid assessment in a subdistrict of Northern Nigeria. *Ophthalmic Epidemiol* 2001; 8:263–272.

76. Paxton ASTST. Rapid assessment of trachoma prevalence – Singida, Tanzania: a study to compare assessment methods. *Ophthalmic Epidemiol* 2001; 8:87–96.

77. Malaty R, Zaki S, Said ME, *et al*. Extraocular infections in children in areas with endemic trachoma. *J Infect Dis* 1981; 143:853–853.

78. West SK, Munoz B, Bobo L, *et al*. Nonocular chlamydial infection and risk of ocular reinfection after mass treatment in a trachoma hyperendemic area. *Invest Ophthalmol Vis Sci* 1993; 34: 3194–3198.

79. Schachter J, West SK, Mabey D, *et al*. Azithromycin in control of trachoma. *Lancet* 1999; 354:630–635.

80. Gower EW, Solomon AW, Burton MJ, *et al*. Chlamydial positivity of nasal discharge at baseline is associated with ocular chlamydial positivity 2 months following azithromycin treatment. *Invest Ophthalmol Vis Sci* 2006; 47:4767–4771.

81. Smith AG, Broman AT, Alemayehu W, *et al*. Relationship between trachoma and chronic and acute malnutrition in children in rural Ethiopia. *J Trop Pediatr* 2007; 53:308–312.

82. Bobo LD, Novak N, Munoz B, *et al*. Severe disease in children with trachoma is associated with persistent Chlamydia trachomatis infection. *J Infect Dis* 1997; 176:1524–1530.

83. West SK, Munoz B, Lynch M, *et al*. Risk factors for constant, severe trachoma in pre-school children in Kongwa, Tanzania. *Am J Epidemiol* 1996; 143:73–78.

84. West SK, Munoz B, Mkocha H, *et al.* Progression of active trachoma to scarring in a cohort of Tanzanian children. *Ophthalmic Epidemiol* 2001; 8:137–144.

85. Polack S, Kuper H, Solomon AW, *et al.* The relationship between prevalence of active trachoma, water availability and its use in a Tanzanian village. *Trans Roy Soc Trop Med Hyg* 2006; 100: 1075–1083.

86. McCauley AP, Lynch M, Pounds MB, *et al.* Changing water-use patterns in a water-poor area: lessons for a trachoma intervention project. *Soc Sci Med* 1990; 31: 1233–1238.

87. West SK, Congdon N, Katala S, *et al.* Facial cleanliness and risk of trachoma in families. *Arch Ophthalmol* 1991; 109:855–857.

88. Zack R, Mkocha H, Zack E, *et al.* Issues in defining and measuring facial cleanliness for national trachoma control programs. *Trans Roy Soc Trop Med Hyg* 2008; 102:426–431.

89. Lynch M, West SK, Munoz B, *et al.* Testing a participatory strategy to change hygiene behaviour: face washing in central Tanzania. *Trans Roy Soc Trop Med Hyg* 1994; 88:513–517.

90. West S, Munoz B, Lynch M, *et al.* Impact of face-washing on trachoma in Kongwa, Tanzania. *Lancet* 1995; 345:155–158.

91. Mabey DC, Bailey RL, Ward ME, *et al.* A longitudinal study of trachoma in a Gambian village: implications concerning the pathogenesis of chlamydial infection. *Epidemiol Infect* 1992; 108:343–351.

92. Congdon N, West S, Vitale S, *et al.* Exposure to children and risk of active trachoma in Tanzanian women. *Am J Epidemiol* 1993; 137:366–372.

93. Wilson RP. Ophthalmia Aegyptiaca. *Am J Ophthalmol* 1932; 15:397–406.

94. West SK, Rapoza P, Munoz B, *et al.* Epidemiology of ocular chlamydial infection in a trachoma-hyperendemic area. *J Infect Dis* 1991; 163: 752–756.

95. Taylor HR, West SK, Mmbaga BB, *et al.* Hygiene factors and increased risk of trachoma in central Tanzania. *Arch Ophthalmol* 1989; 107:1821–1825.

96. Brechner RJ, West S, Lynch M. Trachoma and flies. Individual vs environmental risk factors. *Arch Ophthalmol* 1992; 110:687–689.

97. Emerson PM, Bailey RL, Mahdi OS, *et al.* Transmission ecology of the fly Musca sorbens, a putative vector of trachoma. *Trans Roy Soc Trop Med Hyg* 2000; 94:28–32.

98. Miller K, Pakpour N, Yi E, *et al.* Pesky trachoma suspect finally caught. *Br J Ophthalmol* 2004; 88:750–751.

99. Emerson PM, Lindsay SW, Alexander N, *et al.* Role of flies and provision of latrines in trachoma control: cluster-randomised controlled trial. *Lancet* 2004; 363:1093–1098.

100. West SK, Emerson PM, Mkocha H, *et al.* Intensive insecticide spraying for fly control after mass antibiotic treatment for trachoma in a hyperendemic setting: a randomised trial. *Lancet* 2006; 368:596–600.

101. Taylor HR, Velasco FM, Sommer A. The ecology of trachoma: an epidemiological study in southern Mexico. *Bull World Health Organ* 1985; 63:559–567.

102. Reinhards J, Weber A, Nizetic B, *et al.* Studies in the epidemiology and control of seasonal conjunctivitis and trachoma in southern Morocco. *Bull World Health Organ* 1968; 39:497–545.

103. Emerson PM, Bailey RL, Walraven GE, *et al.* Human and other faeces as breeding media of the trachoma vector Musca sorbens. *Med Vet Entomol* 2001; 15:314–320.

104. Courtright P, Sheppard J, Lane S, *et al.* Latrine ownership as a protective factor in inflammatory trachoma in Egypt. *Br J Ophthalmol* 1991; 75:322–325.

105. Ngondi J, Gebre T, Shargie EB, *et al.* Risk factors for active trachoma in children and trichiasis in adults: a household survey in Amhara Regional State, Ethiopia. *Trans Roy Soc Trop Med Hyg* 2008; 102:432–438.

106. Ngondi J, Reacher MH, Matthews FE, *et al.* Risk factors for trachomatous trichiasis in children: cross-sectional household surveys in Southern Sudan. *Trans Roy Soc Trop Med Hyg* 2009; 103: 305–314.

107. Ward M, Bailey R, Lesley A, *et al.* Persisting inapparent chlamydial infection in a trachoma endemic community in The Gambia. *Scand J Infect Dis Suppl* 1990; 69:137–148.

108. Bowman RJ, Jatta B, Cham B, *et al.* Natural history of trachomatous scarring in The Gambia: results

of a 12-year longitudinal follow-up. *Ophthalmology* 2001; 108:2219–2224.

109. Natividad A, Cooke G, Holland MJ, *et al.* A coding polymorphism in matrix metalloproteinase 9 reduces risk of scarring sequelae of ocular Chlamydia trachomatis infection. *BMC Med Genet* 2006; 7:40.

110. Natividad A, Hanchard N, Holland MJ, *et al.* Genetic variation at the TNF locus and the risk of severe sequelae of ocular Chlamydia trachomatis infection in Gambians. *Genes Immun* 2007; 8:288–295.

111. Cromwell EA, Courtright P, King JD, *et al.* The excess burden of trachomatous trichiasis in women: a systematic review and meta-analysis. *Trans Roy Soc Trop Med Hyg* 2009; 103:985–992.

112. Turner VM, West SK, Munoz B, *et al.* Risk factors for trichiasis in women in Kongwa, Tanzania: a case-control study. *Int J Epidemiol* 1993; 22:341–347.

113. Fuchsjäger-Mayrl G, Nepp J, Schneeberger C, *et al.* Identification of estrogen and progesterone receptor mRNA expression in the conjunctiva of premenopausal women. *Invest Ophthalmol Vis Sci* 2002; 43:2841–2844.

114. Burton MJ, Bowman RJ, Faal H, *et al.* The long-term natural history of trachomatous trichiasis in the Gambia. *Invest Ophth Vis Sci* 2006; 47:847–852.

115. Ngondi J, Onsarigo A, Matthews F, *et al.* Effect of 3 years of SAFE (surgery, antibiotics, facial cleanliness, and environmental change) strategy for trachoma control in southern Sudan: a cross-sectional study. *Lancet* 2006; 368:589–595.

116. Reacher MH, Munoz B, Alghassany A, *et al.* A controlled trial of surgery for trachomatous trichiasis of the upper lid. *Arch Ophthalmol* 1992; 110:667–674.

117. Bog H, Yorston D, Foster A. Results of community-based eyelid surgery for trichiasis due to trachoma. *Br J Ophthalmol* 1993; 77:81–83.

118. Alemayehu W, Melese M, Bejiga A, *et al.* Surgery for trichiasis by ophthalmologists versus integrated eye care workers: a randomized trial. *Ophthalmology* 2004; 111:578–584.

119. West ES, Mkocha H, Munoz B, *et al.* Risk factors for postsurgical trichiasis recurrence in a trachoma-endemic area. *Invest Ophth Vis Sci* 2005; 46:447–453.

120. Burton MJ, Kinteh F, Jallow O, *et al.* A randomised controlled trial of azithromycin following surgery for trachomatous trichiasis in the Gambia. *Br J Ophthalmol* 2005; 89:1282–1288.

121. Reacher MH, Munoz B, Alghassany A, *et al.* A controlled trial of surgery for trachomatous trichiasis of the upper lid. *Arch Ophthalmol* 1992; 110:667–674.

122. West SK, West ES, Alemayehu W, *et al.* Single-dose azithromycin prevents trichiasis recurrence following surgery: randomized trial in Ethiopia. *Arch Ophthalmol* 2006; 124:309–314.

123. West S, Alemayehu W, Munoz B, *et al.* Azithromycin prevents recurrence of severe trichiasis following trichiasis surgery: STAR trial. *Ophthalmic Epidemiol* 2007; 14:273–277.

124. Thanh TT, Khandekar R, Luong VQ, *et al.* One year recurrence of trachomatous trichiasis in routinely operated Cuenod Nataf procedure cases in Vietnam. *Br J Ophthalmol* 2004; 88:1114–1118.

125. West SK, Bedri A, *et al. Final Assessment of Trichiasis Surgeons.* Geneva: WHO/PBD/GET; 2006.

126. West, SK. Blinding trachoma: prevention with the safe strategy. *Am J Trop Med Hyg* 2003; 69:18–23.

127. Wright HR, Turner A, Taylor HR. Trachoma. *Lancet* 2008; 371:1945–1954.

128. Burton MJ, Bowman RJ, Faal H, *et al.* Long term outcome of trichiasis surgery in the Gambia. *Br J Ophthalmol* 2005; 89:575–579.

129. Oliva MS, Munoz B, Lynch M, *et al.* Evaluation of barriers to surgical compliance in the treatment of trichiasis. *Int Ophthalmol* 1997; 21:235–241.

130. Rabiu MM, Abiose A. Magnitude of trachoma and barriers to uptake of lid surgery in a rural community of northern Nigeria. *Ophthalmic Epidemiol* 2001; 8:181–190.

131. Bowman RJ, Soma OS, Alexander N, *et al.* Should trichiasis surgery be offered in the village? A community randomised trial of village vs. health centre-based surgery. *Trop Med Int Health* 2000; 5:528–533.

132. Frick KD, Keuffel EL, Bowman RJ. Epidemiological, demographic, and economic analyses: measurement of the value of trichiasis surgery

in The Gambia. *Ophthalmic Epidemiol* 2001; 8:191–201.

133. WHO Working Group. *Report of the Eighth Meeting of the WHO Alliance for the Global Elimination of Blinding Trachoma.* Geneva: WHO/PBD/GET/04.2; 2004.

134. Solomon AW, Holland MJ, Alexander ND, *et al.* Mass treatment with single-dose azithromycin for trachoma. *N Engl J Med* 2004; 351: 1962–1971.

135. West ES, Munoz B, Mkocha H, *et al.* Mass treatment and the effect on the load of Chlamydia trachomatis infection in a trachoma-hyperendemic community. *Invest Ophthalmol Vis Sci* 2005; 46:83–87.

136. Holm SO, Jha HC, Bhatta RC, *et al.* Comparison of two azithromycin distribution strategies for controlling trachoma in Nepal. *Bull World Health Organ* 2001; 79:194–200.

137. Frick KD, Lietman TM, Holm SO, *et al.* Cost-effectiveness of trachoma control measures: comparing targeted household treatment and mass treatment of children. *Bull World Health Organ* 2001; 79:201–207.

138. Melese M, Alemayehu W, Lakew T, *et al.* Comparison of annual and biannual mass antibiotic administration for elimination of infectious trachoma. *JAMA* 2008; 299:778–784.

139. Lakew T, House J, Honk KC, *et al.* Reduction and return of infectious trachoma in severely affected communities in ethiopia. *PLoS Negl Trop Dis* 2009; 3: e376.

140. West SK, Munoz B, Mkocha H, *et al.* Infection with Chlamydia trachomatis after mass treatment of a trachoma hyperendemic community in Tanzania: a longitudinal study. *Lancet* 2005; 366:1296–1300.

141. Campbell JP, Mkocha H, Munoz B, *et al.* Randomized trial of high dose azithromycin compared with standard dosing for children with severe trachoma in Tanzania. *Ophthalmic Epidemiol* 2009; 16:175–180.

142. West SK, Munoz B, Mkocha H, *et al.* Trachoma and ocular Chlamydia trachomatis were not eliminated three years after two rounds of mass treatment in a trachoma hyperendemic village. *Invest Ophthalmol Vis Sci* 2007; 48:1492–1497.

143. Batt SL, Charalambous BM, Solomon AW, *et al.* Impact of azithromycin administration for trachoma control on the carriage of antibiotic-resistant Streptococcus pneumoniae. *Antimicrob Agents Chemother* 2003; 47:2765–2769.

144. Gaynor BD, Holbrook KA, Whitcher JP, *et al.* Community treatment with azithromycin for trachoma is not associated with antibiotic resistance in Streptococcus pneumoniae at 1 year. *Br J Ophthalmol* 2003; 87:147–148.

145. Gaynor BD, Chidambaram JD, Cevallos V, *et al.* Topical ocular antibiotics induce bacterial resistance at extraocular sites. *Br J Ophthalmol* 2005; 89:1097–1099.

146. Frick KD, West SK. The SAFE strategy for trachoma control: planning a cost-effectiveness analysis of the antibiotic component and beyond. *Ophthalmic Epidemiol* 2001; 8:205–214.

147. Solomon AW, Akudibillah J, Abugri P, *et al.* Pilot study of the use of community volunteers to distribute azithromycin for trachoma control in Ghana. *Bull World Health Organ* 2001; 79:8–14.

148. Lynch M, West S, Munoz B, *et al.* Azithromycin treatment coverage in Tanzanian children using community volunteers. *Ophthalmic Epidemiol* 2003; 10:167–175.

149. Basilion EV, Kilima PM, Mecaskey JW. Simplification and improvement of height-based azithromycin treatment for paediatric trachoma. *Trans Roy Soc Trop Med Hyg* 2005; 99:6–12.

150. Hotez PJ, Molyneux DH, Fenwick A, *et al.* Control of neglected tropical diseases. *N Engl J Med* 2007; 357:1018–1027.

151. Yayemain D, King JD, Debrah O, *et al.* Achieving trachoma control in Ghana after implementing the SAFE strategy. *Trans Roy Soc Trop Med Hyg* 2009; 103:993–1000.

152. Khandekar R, Ton TK, Do TP. Impact of face washing and environmental improvement on reduction of active trachoma in Vietnam — a public health intervention study. *Ophthalmic Epidemiol* 2006; 13:43–52.

153. Astle WF, Wiafe B, Ingram AD, *et al.* Trachoma control in Southern Zambia — an international team project employing the SAFE strategy. *Ophthalmic Epidemiol* 2006; 13:227–236.

154. Edwards T, Cumberland P, Hailu G, *et al.* Impact of health education on active trachoma in hyperendemic rural communities in Ethiopia. *Ophthalmology* 2006; 113:548–555.

155. Pal S, Peterson EM, de ka Maza LM. Vaccination with Chlamydia trachomatis major outer membrane protein can elicit an immune response as protective as that resulting from inoculation with live bacteria. *Infect Immun* 2005; 73:853–860.

156. Kari L, Whitemire WM, Crane DD, *et al.* Chlamydia trachomatis native major outer membrane protein induces partial protection in nonhuman primates: implication for a trachoma transmission-blocking vaccine. *J Immunol* 2009; 182:8063–8070.

Onchocerciasis

ADRIAN HOPKINS

18.1	Introduction and history	487
18.2	The parasite and vector	488
18.3	Clinical description	491
18.4	Prevalence and geographical distribution	493
18.5	Control strategies	495
18.6	Research priorities	503
	References	505

18.1 INTRODUCTION AND HISTORY

Onchocerciasis, a disease caused by the filaria parasite *Onchocerca volvulus*, is found alongside many rivers flowing through Sub-Saharan Africa, particularly in the Sahel and savannah areas. It has had a major impact on the health of the communities, provoking blindness (hence the name 'river blindness') as well as severe skin disease, epilepsy and even growth retardation. The disease is also found in forest areas in Central Africa and along its West coast, but the forest form provokes less blindness. Although 99% of the disease is found in Africa it is also found in the Americas and in Yemen.

The adult form of *Onchocerca volvulus* is found in fibrous nodules, mostly present in the subcutaneous tissues, particularly over bony prominences. The female worms produce thousands of larvae, or **microfilariae (mfs)**, each day. These migrate principally to the skin, the site necessary for the transmission of the disease, but also to other tissues, including the eye. The vector is a small blackfly of the family Simuliidae and the genus *Simulium* of which *Simulium damnosum* complex is the most common

in Africa. It is the microfilariae, mainly when dying, that provoke the typical signs and symptoms.

The disease involves complex and fascinating relationships between host, parasite and vector, including population factors and ecology. Unfortunately, the disease mostly affects people living 'at the end of the road' in remote villages. In fact, personal experience in many conflict and post-conflict areas has shown that these populations are often beyond the end of the road where they seek to eke out an existence away from the areas of instability. These populations carry no economic or political weight.

The disease was first described by O'Neil in 1875[1] as the skin disease 'craw-craw' in the former Gold Coast (now Ghana). Robles in Guatemala associated the subcutaneous nodules with the eye lesions in 1893.[2] The life cycle involving the Simulium was described by Blacklock in 1926.[3] In 1932 Hissette, working in the Belgian Congo, described the pathology in the eye, which Ridley confirmed and described more fully from his studies in the Gold Coast (Ghana).[4,5] In 1947 it was found that **Diethylcarbamazine (DEC)** was an effective microfilaricide. However, DEC provokes massive destruction of the microfilariae, creating severe inflammatory reactions, including blinding lesions, in the eye.

The first effective control measures were directed against the vector and the **Onchocerciasis Control Programme (OCP)** of West Africa initially used vector control alone as the strategy.[6] The OCP was also involved in the trials of a medication called ivermectin. When it was approved for use in humans in 1987, Merck committed to donate Mectizan® (ivermectin Merck) to as many people as needed it for as long as it was needed,[7] and has expanded the donation for the elimination of lymphatic filariasis where it is co-endemic with onchocerciasis.[8]

The use of ivermectin has led to important developments in onchocerciasis control. Ministries of Health outside West Africa, working mostly with **Non-Governmental Development Organizations (NGDOs)**, were able to begin control measures. These efforts led to the creation of the **African Programme for Onchocerciasis Control (APOC)**. In the Americas, programmes were coordinated to create a new activity under the **Pan-American Health Organization (PAHO)**, the **Onchocerciasis Elimination Programme in the Americas (OEPA)**.

Due to the impact of these various control and/or elimination programmes, onchocerciasis, which was once the fourth major preventable blinding disease, will probably be the first to actually be eliminated worldwide, providing the current momentum is maintained.

18.2   THE PARASITE AND VECTOR

The relationship of parasite, host and vector is demonstrated in the life cycle shown in Fig. 18.1.

18.2.1   The parasite

Onchocerca volvulus is one of the nematodes of the super-family Filaroidea, which has a complex life cycle both in the human host and in the vector. The female adult worms are much bigger than the males (50–70 cms and 3–5 cms long respectively). The adults are found in nodules, the majority of

which are located in the subcutaneous tissues, but are also found in the deeper tissues.[9] The adults are entwined around each other and enmeshed in fibrous tissue. Male worms are less frequent in nodules and sometimes not found at all, and they migrate between nodules. The adult females live for around ten years (range 9–15). The subcutaneous nodules are relatively easy to palpate, being mobile in the tissues, with a rubbery consistency but firmer in the middle. With practice, they can be distinguished from other subcutaneous masses but, as prevalence declines, so does the number of nodules, and there is risk of confusion with other masses, such as small lipomas, lymph nodes and even cysticercosis.

The adult female produces many (up to 1,600) larvae every day. These L1 stage larvae, or **microfilariae (mf)**, which measure 300–320 μm in length, migrate particularly to the skin but also to other tissues. If the mf are not ingested by the vector they begin to die off after six months (6–30 months). The death of each microfilaria in the tissues provokes a mild inflammatory reaction. However, the massive numbers of mf that die in the skin each day provoke a considerable reaction leading to the typical skin manifestations. In the eye, the inflammatory reaction around the dying mf can also produce considerable damage. It depends on which structure of the eye is involved as to what the final eye pathology might be (See 18.3.1).

Microfilariae (L1 larvae) are ingested by the Simulium. Some of the mf are destroyed in the process of ingestion by some Simulium species; some will also be lost in the stomach and mid-gut. Some survive and migrate out of the stomach and into the thoracic muscles of the fly. In the muscles of the thorax there is a moult into the L2 larva. The larvae increase in size before undergoing a further moult into longer and much more active infective L3 larvae. The cycle in the fly lasts from 6–12 days. The L3 stage larvae actively penetrate the body of the host through the wound created by the bite of the fly. Two to seven days later they moult into the L4 larvae, which live in the tissues for a further 6–12 weeks before the final change into the juvenile adult stage. These juvenile larvae migrate through the tissues towards nodules, mature to become full adults, and eventually

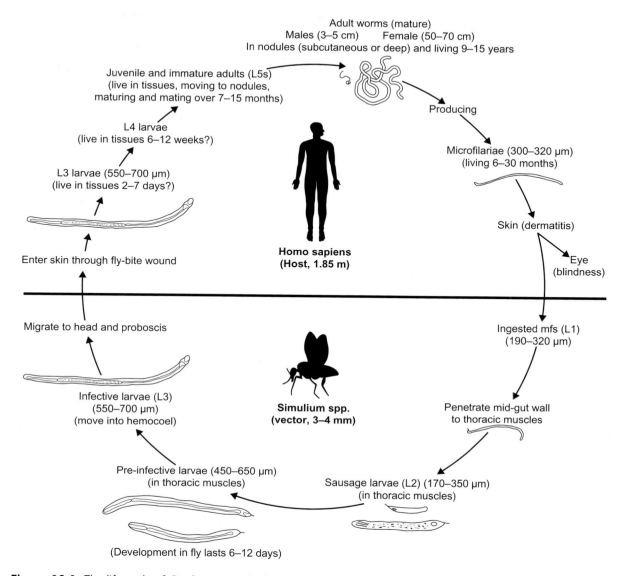

Adult worms (mature)
Males (3–5 cm) Female (50–70 cm)
In nodules (subcutaneous or deep) and living 9–15 years

Juvenile and immature adults (L5s)
(live in tissues, moving to nodules,
maturing and mating over 7–15 months)

Producing

L4 larvae
(live in tissues 6–12 weeks?)

Microfilariae (300–320 μm)
(living 6–30 months)

L3 larvae (550–700 μm)
(live in tissues 2–7 days?)

Skin (dermatitis)

Enter skin through fly-bite wound

Eye
(blindness)

Homo sapiens
(Host, 1.85 m)

Migrate to head and proboscis

Ingested mfs (L1)
(190–320 μm)

Simulium spp.
(vector, 3–4 mm)

Penetrate mid-gut wall
to thoracic muscles

Infective larvae (L3)
(550–700 μm)
(move into hemocoel)

Pre-infective larvae (450–650 μm)
(in thoracic muscles)

Sausage larvae (L2) (170–350 μm)
(in thoracic muscles)

(Development in fly lasts 6–12 days)

Figure 18.1 *The life cycle of Onchocerca volvulus*

produce microfilariae, which appear in the skin after around one year (7–15 months).

The **polymerase chain reaction (PCR)** can be used to identify different species and strains of onchocerciasis based on DNA patterns. The larvae of *O. ochengi* from cattle can be transmitted by the same Simulium species as *O. volvulus*. Differences between savannah and forest strains can also be identified. The savannah strain of West Africa is by far the most blinding whereas eye pathology in the forest areas is relatively infrequent. These different strains are also adapted to the local vector, those of

the savannah strains being adapted to the savannah strains of Simulium and the forest strains adapted to the forest vectors.[10,11,12] *Onchocerca volvulus* in the Americas also provokes considerable eye pathology, which is consistent with the theory that it may have been imported with slaves from West Africa.[13]

18.2.2   The vector

The Simulium species are small black flies 3–4 mm in length that are found in many parts of the world. The

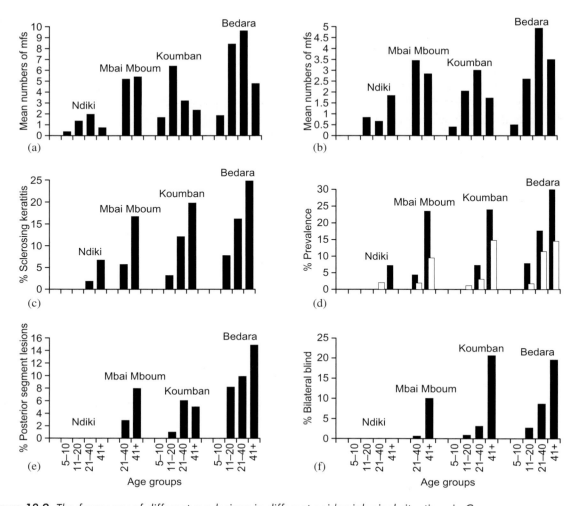

Figure 18.2 *The frequency of different eye lesions in different epidemiological situations in Cameroon*

Histograms comparing, by age groups, the populations of four villages in the savannah zone of Cameroon, having different onchocerciasis endemicity levels with regard to (a) mean number of microfilariae in the cornea; (b) mean number of microfilariae in the anterior chamber; (c) prevalence of sclerosing keratitis; (d) prevalence of iridocyclitis (black columns) and posterior synechiae (white columns); (e) prevalence of choroido-retinitis and/or optic atrophy; and (f) prevalence of bilateral blindness caused by onchocerciasis. (Adapted from Duke BOL, Anderson J, Fuglsang H. Tropenmen Parasit 1975; 26:143–154.)

female Simulium needs a blood meal for the development of her eggs. The black flies breed in well-oxygenated water and so are found often in areas where there are cataracts or waterfalls, or where fast-flowing water swirls around vegetation in the river. People living near these areas are the most affected.

Simulium species also feed on animals. The vectors of *O. volvulus* are preferentially anthropophilic although some will also feed on cattle. Initially the main vector in West Africa was identified as *Simulium damnosum* but ongoing

studies have identified many subspecies of *S. damnosum*. Whereas different subspecies may respond differently to vector control, where this control strategy is no longer being carried out the distinction between sub-species is not so important. Vector biology will, however, remain important as programmes move towards elimination and risks of reinvasion have to be considered. In general, in West Africa there are three main groups of the *S. damnosum* complex (*Simulium damnosum* **sensu lato or s.l.**): the *S. damnosum* subcomplex, the *S. sanctipauli* subcomplex and the *S. squamosum* subcomplex. There are also *S. mengense* in the Cameroon and *S. kilibanum* in Burundi and East Africa. Also in East Africa there are subspecies of the *S. neavei* complex. These are interesting species in that the Simulium larvae are found attached to Potamonautes crabs, and so remain in highly oxygenated water. Although *S. neavei* is a very efficient vector, it is easy to eliminate by eliminating the crabs. The crabs, which live in shady forest streams, are also disappearing in some areas due to deforestation. In some areas of Uganda, *S. neavei* is being replaced with *S. damnosum*. In the Congo basin there is yet another adaptation with *S. albivirgulatum*, which is attached to the underside of leaves floating on the surface of relatively slow moving streams.

The vectors in the Americas are different Simulium species and in general are not as efficient as vectors as *Simulium damnosum* (i.e. the number of larvae transmitted by each bite of the fly is lower than in most of the African species). Although the vectors are not as effective in transmitting the disease as in Africa, the **Annual Biting Rates (ABRs)** are usually higher. The main vectors are *S. ochraceum* s.l. and *S. exiguum* s.l.

18.3   CLINICAL DESCRIPTION

The clinical picture of onchocerciasis is mostly created by inflammatory reactions around dying microfilariae, whether in the eye, the skin or elsewhere in the body. The savannah species of onchocerciasis are much more dangerous than the forest species for the anterior segment of the eye, although this is also related to the intensity of infection.[14,15] This has been shown experimentally in the rabbit eye when inoculation into the eyes of mf of the savannah strains produced considerable invasion and subsequent severe lesions similar to sclerosing keratitis, whereas mf from forest strains produced much less reaction.[16] The differences in severity were less marked in the choroid and optic nerve.[17] The effects on the eye are also cumulative and therefore the more and longer the exposure the higher the risk of eye damage. One other important point related to blindness from onchocerciasis is the impact on mortality, with a significantly shortened expectation of life.[18]

18.3.1   Signs and symptoms of eye disease

Microfilariae are found in all the tissues of the eye from the conjunctiva to the optic nerve.

Conjunctiva

Microfilariae in the conjunctiva have been reported to produce mild pruritis and occasional mild pigmentation changes. In view of the many other causes of similar symptoms in the tropical, dusty climate where the disease is common these are often too non-specific to have much clinical significance.

Cornea

The degree of corneal damage depends on the degree of microfilarial invasion and the time the cornea has been exposed. Microfilariae are mobile and they can penetrate the stroma. If a microfilaria dies in the cornea the inflammatory reaction provokes an area of oedema around the microfilaria. Initially the shape of the microfilaria is visible, but the form is eventually lost as it is destroyed. These areas of punctuate keratitis have been variously described as 'snowflake' or 'cotton wool' keratitis. Once a microfilaria has been absorbed the area of punctuate keratitis resolves, so at this stage lesions are reversible and, if treatment is instituted, more permanent lesions can be avoided. Microfilariae are also found, often in groups, sticking to the corneal endothelium. Some of these may penetrate the cornea but will most probably swim in the anterior chamber. With repeated infection of the cornea, changes become more permanent and lead to sclerosing keratitis. This begins as white sclerotic areas found mostly at around the three and nine o'clock areas of the cornea towards the limbus. These areas spread inferiorly and often join together, creating a white band of sclerotic cornea that, because of its shape, is often called semi-lunar keratitis. As the condition evolves, the space inferiorly also begins to sclerose and the optical axis is at risk of being compromised. Eventually the whole cornea becomes a dense white scar with, occasionally, a small clearer area at 12 o'clock.

Anterior chamber

Microfilariae are found swimming in the anterior chamber. They are seen on high-magnification slit-lamp examination like small mobile threads reflecting the light in a focused beam. Microfilariae also fall to the bottom of the anterior chamber and, if sufficient in number, form a mass in the angle creating a pseudohypopyon. Some microfilariae are still alive on the surface of this pseudohypopyon, creating a mobile shimmering appearance. Secondary glaucoma is also common. The blockage of the trabecular meshwork with microfilariae is one possible mechanism, although glaucoma is also often associated with chronic anterior uveitis.

Iris (anterior uveitis)

Microfilariae dying in the ciliary body provoke an anterior uveitis, which is usually chronic, low grade and asymptomatic. The patients usually present late when posterior synechiae are already well established. In fact the iris is often stuck down around most of its circumference but with the pupil sometimes drawn down inferiorly. Secondary cataract and glaucoma are common. Great care has to be taken in the management of cataract in onchocercal eye disease. Although some cases are due to age-related changes, many cases are secondary cataracts and often associated with posterior uveitis and choroido-retinitis, leading to poor surgical outcomes. Chronic anterior uveitis leads to iris atrophy.

Posterior segment

Microfilariae are found in the vitreous but the most serious problem in the posterior segment of the eye is choroido-retinitis. Lesions often appear in the periphery of the fundus. There may be an early retinal oedema but the classical changes are of a disruption of the retinal pigment epithelium, leading to clumping of pigment, with some areas almost devoid of pigment. This is usually associated with a disruption of the choroid. The appearance on looking at the fundus in the later stages of the disease is one of clumps of pigment surrounded by de-pigmented white areas. The lesions tend to start in the periphery and the effects are often to reduce the peripheral visual fields before the macula is eventually involved with total loss of vision.

Optic nerve

Optic neuritis is a common finding. The active stages of infiltration by microfilariae are rarely seen, but the optic atrophy which follows is very common and seen particularly in posterior segment disease.[19,20]

The frequency of different eye lesions in different epidemiological situations in Cameroon is presented in Fig. 18.2.

18.3.2 Skin disease

Nodules

These cause little in the way of symptoms. The majority are found subcutaneously over bony prominences and are mobile, easily moveable over the underlying structures. Nodules are also present in the deeper tissues. The presence of nodules is a useful sign for the community diagnosis of the disease.

Acute onchocercal papillo-dermatitis

This acute stage of skin disease is seen in early infections. The microfilariae in the skin provoke an acute inflammation which causes severe pruritis. This can be so severe that patients scratch constantly, sometimes using sticks or stones, which are more aggressive than their fingernails, in order to gain some relief. This constant scratching provokes skins abrasions, secondary infections, localized oedema of the skin (peau d'orange) and can progress to a lymphadenitis. This is described by the name 'craw-craw'. In northern Sudan and in the Yemen, the disease is modified and called 'sowda'. As well as severe itching this presents with swelling and hyper-pigmentation of the whole limb.

Chronic skin changes

In some patients the acute phase is followed by lichenoid skin changes, with drier scaly skin, often called 'lizard skin dermatitis'. In most patients the chronic skin changes provoke changes in pigmentation with areas of hypopigmentation, 'leopard skin dermatitis', typically present on the shins but which can be found elsewhere.

18.3.3 Other systemic manifestations of onchocerciasis

Epilepsy

This has remained controversial for some time; however, a recent meta-analysis has shown the connection between epilepsy and onchocerciasis.[22,23]

There have also been reports of growth disorders, 'the Nakalanga Syndrome'.[24]

18.4 PREVALENCE AND GEOGRAPHICAL DISTRIBUTION

The last WHO estimates of prevalence of onchocerciasis, made in 1993,[25] estimated 17.6 million people infected and almost 300,000 blind (Table 18.1). These were based on figures submitted from endemic countries and from studies with OPC. It is estimated that for every person infected approximately seven others are at risk of getting the disease; hence there were 123 million at risk.

Following the donation and massive distribution of Mectizan, and the success of the OCP programme, these figures are being reviewed. Although no accurate estimates are available at the current time the total of people infected is now considerably less. Until transmission has been fully eliminated the risk of recrudescence remains and constant vigilance is required.

Africa

The original distribution of the disease in the 1970s is reflected in the map (Fig.18.3), which also shows the small foci of infection in the Yemen.

The OPC original area included Benin, Burkina Faso, Côte d'Ivoire, Ghana, Mali, Niger and Togo and the extensions included Guinea, Guinea Bissau, Senegal and Sierra Leone. In most of the original area there is no further transmission. The non-OCP area includes Angola, Burundi, Cameroon, Central African Republic, Chad, Congo, Democratic Republic of Congo, Equatorial Guinea, Ethiopia, Gabon, Liberia, Malawi, Nigeria, Sudan, Uganda, and the United Republic of Tanzania. There are hypo-endemic areas in Rwanda and in Mozambique (Fig. 18.3).

Table 18.1 *Global estimates of the population at risk, infected and blind from onchocerciasis in 1993*

Region	Population at risk of infection (millions)	Population infected	Number blind as a result of onchocerciasis
Africa			
OCP area:			
Original area	17.6[a]	10,032	17,650
Extensions	6.0	2,230,000	31,700
Non-OCP area	94.5	15,246,800	217,850
African subtotal	118.1	17,486,832	267,200
Yemen	0.1	30,000	0
Americas	4.7	140,455	750
Total	122.9	17,657,287	267,950

[a] The population given is that which would have been at risk had the OCP not existed.

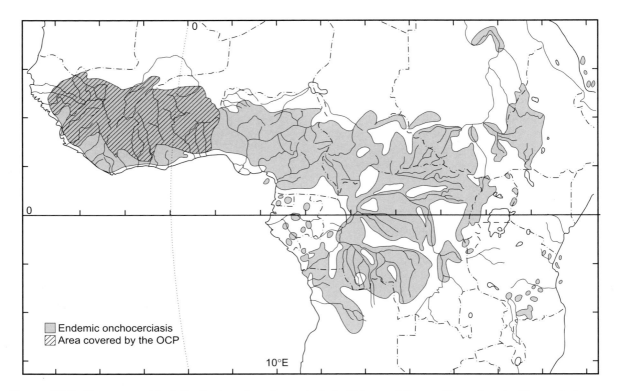

Figure 18.3 *The geographical distribution of onchocerciasis in Africa and Yemen (Reproduced with permission from WHO Technical Report Series No. 582, Fig.1, p. 26).*

In West Africa the disease is now largely controlled, although ivermectin distribution is continuing in some foci in a few of these countries, as there is some ongoing transmission. Not all these areas had been under vector control and so ivermectin distribution alone has been the strategy adopted in some of the extension areas. In some of these places, studies in 2007–2009 have shown that transmission has been interrupted; strategies are now being developed for stopping ivermectin mass treatment and continuing surveillance.

Liberia was never included in the OCP programme due to political instability and the fact that most of the onchocerciasis is in forest areas. Due to conflict, control strategies in Sierra Leone, Ivory Coast and Guinea Bissau have been interrupted. The situation in Sierra Leone was the most serious, with prevalence of the disease remaining high and this, potentially, threatened areas already cleared of the disease. Ivermectin distribution has recommenced in almost all of

Sierra Leone to try to control the problem. However, recent studies in neighbouring Guinea Bissau have shown no sign of recurrence. In Ivory Coast control measures are continuing in the south of the country, where the disease is still present.

The 19 countries in the APOC programme include Kenya,[26] where onchocerciasis was eliminated pre-independence by vector control and where some new cases were reported amongst refugees from Sudan. In Rwanda and Mozambique there are isolated foci shown to be hypo-endemic and so they are not eligible for treatment with mass drug administration. The APOC programme also includes Liberia.[27]

It must be emphasized that, although new evidence indicates elimination of transmission in some areas in West Africa and Uganda, the potential for recrudescence is always present until elimination of transmission is achieved and until the risk of re-invasion from neighbouring areas has also been eliminated.[28]

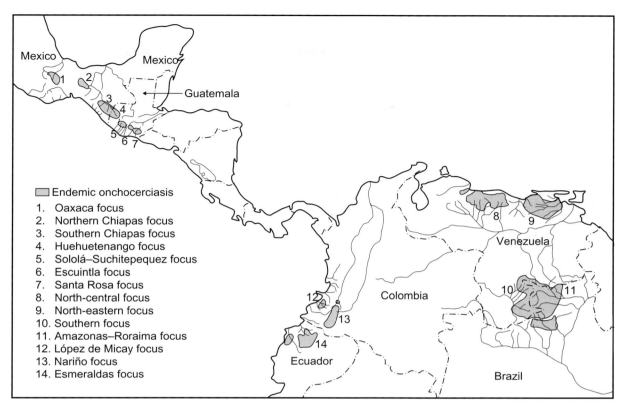

Figure 18.4 *The geographical distribution of endemic onchocerciasis in Latin America (Reproduced with permission from WHO Technical Report Series No. 582, Fig. 2, p. 27).*

The Americas

The disease in the Americas requiring treatment (Fig. 18.4) was confined to 12 foci in six countries, and in 1993 was estimated to affect a total of half a million people. The largest of these foci crosses the Venezuela–Brazil border, so is counted as two foci, making a total of 13. Numerically these foci are small but affect the mobile Yanomami Indians, making them difficult to treat. The treatment strategy was based on treating every case in a closed transmission zone twice yearly. This has resulted in dramatic improvement and has already eliminated transmission in some foci and is now on the verge of elimination in the remainder.[29] The Narino focus in Fig. 18.4 was found not to need treatment.

Yemen

The disease is present in the modified skin form called 'sowda'[30] and affects those living up in the valleys; it is not present in the plains. It was thought that infection was found in approximately 30,000 people but studies have shown the presence of disease in many asymptomatic people living in these areas, and probably around 300,000 to half a million are at risk.

18.5   CONTROL STRATEGIES

To appreciate the various control strategies for the disease it is necessary to understand the life cycle and at what point it can be broken. Methods exist to control the vector, kill the adult worm and kill the microfilariae. Killing the adult worm in the human host would be the best form of control. Unfortunately this is not easy and a suitable macrofilaricide for mass distribution has not yet been found. The most effective programme in West Africa relied initially entirely on the destruction of the vector by regular larviciding of the Simulium breeding sites. This proved to be a very effective but expensive control programme. With the introduction of Mectizan (ivermectin Merck), a safe microfilaricide, the way was opened for a mass treatment programme with the hope that following repeated distribution there would eventually be a reduction in transmission.

18.5.1   Mapping the disease

Mapping of onchocerciasis is necessary, not only to know where the disease is found, but also to decide on strategies for control or elimination of the disease. As mentioned above, the parasite exists in savannah strains that are much more blinding than the forest strains, so various factors have to be taken into consideration involving both the parasite and the vector in order to decide on strategies.

Skin snip surveys

Early mapping of the disease was done by skin snip surveys in affected populations. Prevalence of the disease was determined traditionally by taking skin from the iliac crest (in Africa countries) or scapular skin (in some Latin American countries). This was done either using a needle and fine scalpel blade to remove a small piece of skin avascularly, or by using a corneo-scleral punch, which gave a snip of approximately the same size. Sometimes the result was measured as the percentage of positive cases. A more accurate assessment, but more time consuming if done correctly, is to measure the **Community Microfilarial Load (CMFL).** The CMFL is the geometric mean of the number of microfilariae per mg of skin in a population aged 20 years or over.

However the CMFL has to be interpreted with care in terms of symptoms. In the savannah strain of onchocerciasis a CMFL above four may indicate high levels of blindness, whereas the CMFL can be more than 20 times that level with little blindness in the forest strain.

Mapping using rapid epidemiological assessment (REA)

Subcutaneous nodules are found in somewhere between 35% and 50% of positive cases. This fact has been used to develop non-invasive methods of mapping. Initially nodules were counted in a random sample of 30–50 adults over 20 years old who had been living in the community for at least ten years. The prevalence of nodules is between 30–50% of the prevalence of onchocerciasis measured by skin snip. This simple, non-invasive epidemiological tool is accurate enough for decisions to be made on whether to do mass treatment in that community.[31] Below 20% nodules (40% estimated skin snip prevalence) severe skin disease and blindness are very rare events and therefore these 'hypo-endemic' areas can be classed as not needing treatment for control purposes. This situation could change if the programme changes to one of elimination. Meso-endemic and hyper-endemic areas need mass treatment with Mectizan, with hyper-endemic (>40% nodules) being the priority areas.

Mapping using rapid epidemiological mapping of onchocerciasis (REMO)

Ngoumou and Walsh[32] developed a method of **rapid epidemiological mapping of onchocerciasis (REMO)** using REA data from specifically targeted villages. Using knowledge of the Simulium and of the human population, it is possible to predict which communities are most at risk. The Simulium prefers to feed close to the breeding sites and therefore the communities close to the river are the most at risk. The vector can, however, fly up to 15 km for a blood meal and so secondary communities can be identified up to this distance. Using local knowledge of the terrain, the limits of river basins, the flow of the river, the presence of rapids or waterfalls, the knowledge of the communities and their location and habits, it is possible to target only certain villages for REA in a biased selection.

The REMO map of APOC countries is seen in Plate 18.1. The REMO map, when fully refined, identifies areas of meso- and hyper-endemic onchocerciasis targeted for mass treatment (in red) and other areas of hypo-endemic disease or sporadic cases where clinic-based treatment of patients with symptoms is sufficient (in green). Some areas remain yellow where ongoing refinement is necessary.

Limitations of rapid mapping

It must be understood that REA and REMO are very useful for making decisions about mass treatment for onchocerciasis control. As annual treatment continues most nodules will get smaller as the worms inside die, and some nodules may disappear. This means REA or REMO is only useful for an initial diagnosis and not as a means of deciding when to stop treatment or if transmission is continuing. Moving from control to the elimination of transmission, use must be made of other techniques. Even the use of skin snips becomes less sensitive as numbers of microfilariae in the skin are reduced as a result of treatment. Cheap diagnostic tests, with a high specificity and sensitivity, are still required to evaluate the disease where prevalence is low and where control is developing into elimination.

18.5.2 Control measures

18.5.2.1 Vector control/elimination

If the Simulium can be controlled or eliminated beyond the life span of the adult parasites in the human host in the community then, even if the fly returns and begins biting again, the disease will not be transmitted. Insecticides have been developed with little impact on the flora and fauna of the rivers, but often need to be used weekly on breeding sites. Knowledge of the vector and its movements is fundamental to this approach. Although the fly does not travel far to feed,[33] it can make use of prevailing winds and has been recorded as flying up to 500 km. S. neavei is, however, much more localized and very susceptible to vector control, e.g. Uganda, where elimination of foci has been demonstrated.

18.5.2.2 Control of the parasite; destruction of adult worms

There are two approaches to the control of the adult parasite:

a) *Nodulectomy*: Surgery has been done to excise nodules but this has limited effect as many of the nodules remain deep in the tissues.
b) *Medication*: Although Suramin is effective against the adult worms, unfortunately it is far too toxic for mass drug administration. Research continues for a safe macrofilaricide including Moxidectin (Milbemycin B) which, although similar to ivermectin, has a longer half-life. There is increasing evidence that Mectizan is macrofilaricidal after several doses within a closed system, where there is no further re-infection.

18.5.2.3 Control/elimination of the parasite (microfilaricide)

Another approach to the control of the parasite is to destroy the larvae (microfilariae), thus reducing and, hopefully, eventually interrupting transmission.

a) *Diethylcarbamazine (DEC)* is a very effective medication for destroying the microfilariae, but it can create major reactions. Symptoms include intense pruritis, fever and joint pains due to massive destruction of microfilariae. Major sight threatening inflammation occurs in both the anterior and the posterior segment of the eye. DEC is therefore contra-indicated for the treatment of onchocerciasis. DEC prepared as a lotion has been used as a skin 'patch test', applying the lotion on a dressing and reviewing the patient 24 hours later to see if there is any inflammatory reaction.
b) *Mectizan*® (ivermectin Merck) was licensed for use in onchocerciasis control in 1987. It is an effective microfilaricide and, although it does provoke some Mazzotti reactions in heavily infected individuals, it is much less 'toxic' than DEC. It also does not provoke inflammatory reactions in the eye. Another advantage of ivermectin is a temporarily inhibiting effect on the release of larvae by the adult female worms. After a treatment with ivermectin, skin microfilariae drop almost to zero after 48 hours and only begin to reappear in the skin after four to six months. After one year the microfilariae in the skin are at around 20% of the previous pre-treatment level. Ivermectin can be therefore be given as an annual or six-monthly dose of 150 μg/kg. Height is usually used in the community-setting as a proxy for weight since the margins between therapeutic dose and toxic dose is very large, and therefore it is very safe for community distribution. Children under five years

(<90 cm) are excluded from treatment, as are women who are pregnant or in the first week of lactation. Patients with other serious chronic disease, particularly of the central nervous system, are also excluded.

Treatment of patients with *Loa loa* (another filarial infection) must be carried out with extreme caution with either of the microfilaricides, as death of these blood-borne mf can cause major problems for the circulation, principally in the brain, leading to confusion and coma.

The development of ivermectin was the first major breakthrough in the treatment and prevention of the disease itself, and opened the way for new control strategies rather than the expensive and therefore limited approach with pure vector control. It has also led to new integrated approaches to other neglected tropical diseases, using mass drug administration as the principal strategy.

18.5.3   Control programmes

18.5.3.1   *The Onchocerciasis Control Programme*

The FAO/UNDP/World Bank/WHO Onchocerciasis Control Programme for West Africa (OCP) began in 1972 before Mectizan was available, and diethylcarbamazine was too dangerous to give as a mass treatment. The only strategy was therefore one of vector control. This very effective programme was, however, a very costly one, so it was confined to the worst areas of blinding savannah onchocerciasis. Initially the control strategy was in eight countries but, due to the migration of flies, it was eventually extended to 11 countries.

Comparing the two maps in Figs. 18.5 and 18.6 it can be seen that there was dramatic improvement in the prevalence in most of the area; although in 2002 there remained a few areas where there were still problems in Guinea, Ghana, Togo and Benin. These were treated as Special Intervention Zones, where residual vector control and Mectizan distribution was continued for a further five years. These areas now receive regular Mectizan distribution only and the prevalence has fallen almost to zero. As previously discussed, Sierra Leone stands out as a failure since activities were halted due to civil war. However, mass drug administration with Mectizan is now under way. It is important that this focus does not spread to recently cleared areas. No prevalence studies were done in Liberia during the life of OCP as it is mostly forest area and there was ongoing instability and war. Liberia is now being treated within APOC.[34] Some forest areas were not

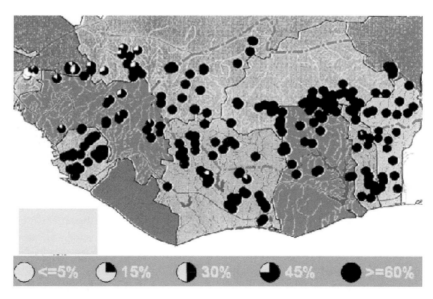

Figure 18.5 *Prevalence of onchocerciasis in Sub-Saharan West Africa in 1974 (Reproduced with permission of the African Programme for Onchocerciasis Control (APOC))*

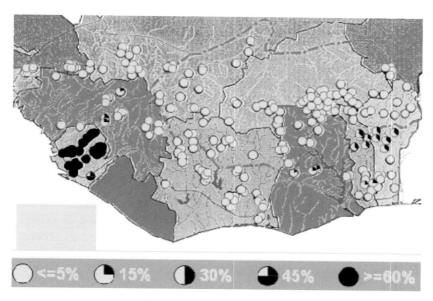

Figure 18.6 *Prevalence of onchocerciasis in Sub-Sahara West Africa in 2002, showing the efficacy of the interventions introduced by the Onchocerciasis Control Programme. (Reproduced with the permission of APOC)*

included in OCP activities and Mectizan distribution continues in these areas.

18.5.3.2 The African Programme for Onchocerciasis Control (APOC)

With the introduction of Mectizan, NGDOs had been in the forefront of developing strategies with national governments to undertake mass treatment with ivermectin and integrate these activities into primary healthcare. During early studies in OCP some of these programmes were carried out by mobile teams, but it was soon found that this was not only uneconomical and unsustainable but also did not really get 'buy-in' from local communities. Thus community involvement became the cornerstone of the treatment strategies in the early 1990s, although the programmes were still run by ministries and NGDOs together in a fairly top-down approach.

APOC was inaugurated in December 1995 with the objective of eliminating onchocerciasis as a public health problem in 19 countries not covered by OCP. As this was planned as a long-term control programme, it involved developing and implementing sustainable strategies to ensure continued treatment by the endemic countries when the APOC programme finished. There was also a policy of

eliminating the vector in a few sites where this was considered possible. Two main problems remained to be solved. The first problem was how to map the disease in a way that was non-invasive and acceptable to the communities, while giving accurate enough data to make decisions on treatment. This led to the REA and later the REMO mapping, described above. The second problem was how to put in place sustainable strategies that could continue for what was thought initially to be ten years, and after using simulation models, was shown to be necessary for 25 years or more, if coverage was not more than 65% of the total population.

18.5.3.3 Community-directed treatment with ivermectin

Work done by TDR (WHO/World Bank/UNDP Tropical Disease Research) further developed strategies that put communities in the driving seat of the programme, and developed what is now called the **community-directed treatment with ivermectin**, or **CDTI** strategy.[35]

Where communities within the APOC areas are fully informed of the disease, its consequences and the means to prevent or avoid its more sinister consequences, they are able to take charge of all the administrative and logistical needs to run the programme. Ownership of the programme only comes about after considerable sensitization and involvement of the whole community in decision-making, not just by local health teams or village elders, although they must also be fully involved in the process. The community can also be sensitized to run its own supervision programme. However, it is vital that a community-directed programme is not run independently of or parallel to the national health system, nor be a programme that does not involve the whole community at all levels.

Once the community is involved and has taken ownership of the programme they will choose key players to work for the community. This will chiefly be the distributors, but will also include other helpers who may work with the community to undertake the tasks below after suitable information, education and communication (IEC):

1. Choose a distributor for training.
2. Do a census to calculate Mectizan requirements.
3. Organize the collection of Mectizan from a health centre or other distribution point.
4. Organize a distribution method (house to house, fixed point in village etc.).
5. Help the distributor calculate the dose and distribute the Mectizan.
6. Organize transfer of patients with adverse events if required.
7. Note the treatment statistics and report to the health authorities.
8. Participate in community supervision.
9. Arrange appropriate recognition at the community level of those who have given their time to work for the distribution.

After five years communities should be ready to continue treatment alone with minimal supervision from the primary health care services.

Community-directed treatment has been one of the striking achievements of the APOC programme. Many NGDOs have also used the system to add on other interventions such as integrated eye care, vitamin A distribution and treatment for other NTDs, such as schistosomiasis and lymphatic filariasis, and even malaria control. These activities have now been categorized as 'community-directed interventions' and have been well tested in a multi-country study by TDR.[36]

18.5.4　A paradigm shift from control to elimination in Africa

At a meeting in 2005 it was decided that elimination was not possible in Africa.[37,38] Following the excellent results of the studies done on the Senegal, Mali and Guinea borders, and in some areas of Nigeria and Uganda, there has been a change in thinking about the control of onchocerciasis in Africa.[37] At a meeting of experts in Ouagadougou in February 2009, it was decided to move towards strategies for elimination. It was recognized that initially this would be a shrinking of the map of endemic onchocerciasis, particularly in West and East Africa. In those countries of Central Africa, where there has been considerable political instability, and also where *Loa loa* is endemic, elimination is feasible but is some way off and will probably need other tools to finish the task.

Initial studies in West Africa were done after 16–18 years of ivermectin treatment, some twice a year and some once a year. These studies so far have been done in savannah areas and the application to a different geographical setting may not be appropriate. There is now a considerable research agenda to identify where Mectizan treatment can be stopped; where it may be better to increase the frequency of treatment (to two or four times a year) to prevent any possible skin repopulation and therefore stop all transmission of the disease; and also whether it may be necessary to treat populations living in hypo-endemic areas.

Uganda has been the first APOC country to create a national onchocerciasis elimination committee advising the government on strategies leading to elimination. Uganda is unique, in that there are many small foci of the disease. In many cases the vector is *S. neavei*, allowing for easier vector elimination, and in others the system is closed, and twice-yearly ivermectin treatment is proving effective in reducing and eliminating transmission.[39]

18.5.4.1 The Onchocerciasis Elimination Programme of the Americas (OEPA)

The OEPA has an ambitious programme for the elimination of transmission of onchocerciasis, by treating every known case. In 1995 a twice-yearly treatment strategy was adopted, and major efforts were made to scale up treatment. Since 2000 coverage has significantly increased so that, in some areas, following seven years of treatment, there are no further signs of ongoing transmission. In some areas treatment has been increased to four times a year to try to achieve elimination by 2012.[40] Four-times-a-year treatment may have an increased impact on adult worms and it is also hoped that by doing so there will be an increase in coverage.

Treatment has already been suspended in Colombia, Mexico and Ecuador (Plate 18.2). One small focus remains in Guatemala. Before WHO will certify the elimination of transmission, each country has to continue post-treatment surveillance for three years. The remaining treatment areas are in central Guatemala, Venezuela and Brazil. The focus on the Venezuela–Brazil border will be the most difficult to treat, as it is deep in the Amazon jungle and the people infected are the highly mobile Yanomami Indians.

Plate 18.3 shows how the number of treatments within OEPA reached a peak in 2005 and is now being scaled back.

18.5.4.2 The elimination of transmission of onchocerciasis

In order to understand elimination of transmission of the disease it is important to have a clear definition. At the informal meeting to discuss the elimination of onchocerciasis in Africa using current tools, the following definition of 'elimination' was suggested:

'Reduction of *O. volvulus* infection and transmission to the extent that interventions can be stopped, but post-intervention surveillance is still necessary.'[42]

This definition involves four critical steps:

➢ Interventions have reduced *O. volvulus* infection and transmission below the point where the parasite population is believed to be irreversibly moving to its demise/extinction in a defined geographical area (the break point in modelling).
➢ Interventions have been stopped.
➢ Post-intervention surveillance for an appropriate period has demonstrated no recrudescence of transmission to a level suggesting recovery of the *O. volvulus* population.
➢ Additional surveillance is still necessary for timely detection of recurrent infection, if a risk of reintroduction of infection from other areas remains.

These steps are illustrated in Fig. 18.7.

The four phases shown are critical periods in the progress of elimination. In Phase 1 there is ongoing transmission but the **Annual Transmission Potential (ATP)** is gradually reduced due to an appropriate intervention (ivermectin treatment, vector control or both). The ATP is the number of infective larvae that could be transmitted to an individual if all the flies biting him during one year were able to transfer all their load of L3s. Two to five percent of flies are infected and the mean infection is 2.2–2.6 in savannah areas, but may increase to 4–6 in forest areas. ATPs have been reported as high as 90,000 in forest areas, but in savannah areas the maximum is around 3,000. An ATP of less than 100 is considered to be safe for eye manifestations of the disease but must be brought down much lower to eliminate transmission. As this strategy continues there will be no more transmission, either due to no flies because of vector control or no infected bites if ivermectin treatment is used.

In Phase 2, because there is no more transmission, the adult worm population will age and die off. However, not all the adults will have died by the end of Phase 1, and if treatment is stopped at this phase the disease will recur. The length of this period will vary. Fourteen years was used in OCP using vector control. A similar period is proposed for ivermectin, but if multiple treatments per year are used, the adult worms will age and die much more quickly, and this period could be shortened to six or seven years. It must be noted that these periods of 14 or seven years will only begin when transmission has been suppressed because, until that is achieved, there is always the possibility of new filariae entering into the system.

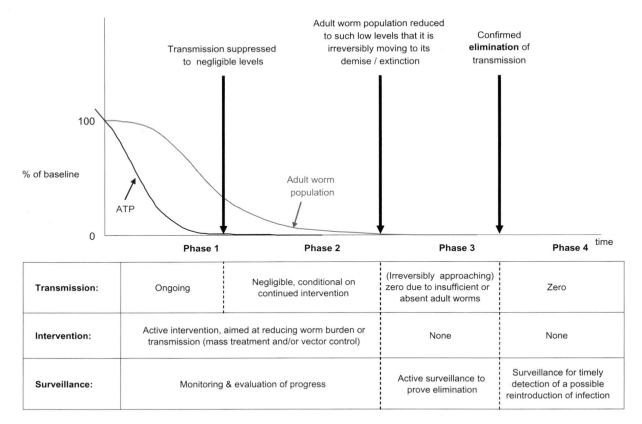

Figure 18.7 *Schematic representation of the phases in programmes for elimination of onchocerciasis transmission, in relation to the theoretical fall-off of the adult worm population and annual transmission potential (ATP). Vertical arrows mark major achievements, which indicate the transition between phases and changes in required interventions or surveillance activities as described*

In Phase 3 treatment is stopped. The numbers of adult worms do not have to be zero but close to it so that the disease will die out naturally. It is important that during this phase regular surveillance is carried out. This is sometimes difficult to fund if donors consider the disease eliminated.

Phase 4 covers a period when there are no signs of infection in the focus concerned but a risk remains that flies will invade from another focus or because massive population movements (e.g. refugees in a war situation) may introduce the infection from elsewhere.

18.5.4.3   *Criteria for elimination*[43]

The WHO has produced guidelines to certify elimination. The criteria are applicable to a country and not a focus of infection; for certification each focus

must be monitored for three years; when the last focus meets the criteria, an application to the WHO can be made. Although the preparation for these criteria was pushed by OEPA, they were intended for widespread use. However, these criteria are not entirely satisfactory in all circumstances; for example, where the vector has been eliminated (e.g. *S. neavei*), or where there are few eye manifestations of the disease as in forest onchocerciasis.

➢ Elimination of morbidity:
  • Prevalence of microfilariae (mfs) in the cornea or anterior chamber of the eye <1%.
➢ Elimination of transmission:
  • L3 in flies <0.05% (0.1% in parous flies).
  • ATP lower than 5–20 L3 per season.
  • Absence of detectable infection in school children and antibody prevalence of <0.1%.

18.5.4.4 Transmission zones

In the Americas, the small, well-defined and widely separated foci of infection are called 'closed transmission zones'. Elimination using ivermectin is easier as there is no risk of importing the disease from another area.

In Africa, the foci are much larger and may overlap. Populations and flies may migrate, bringing the infection from outside the area, and so prevent elimination. The potential source of these re-infections outside these 'open transmission zones' must also be treated to achieve full elimination.

Treatment to date in APOC has been based on a control strategy that identifies high priority areas where blindness or severe skin disease is a problem. The hypo-endemic areas around these foci have not been treated. Hypo-endemic foci in the APOC programme are defined as foci with less than 20% prevalence of nodules. This could equal as much as 40% prevalence of the disease. It is clear that transmission continues in some of these foci. Some foci, however, may not be important for transmission if neighbouring meso- and hyper-endemic areas are controlled.

18.5.4.5 Challenges to control and elimination[44]

Co-endemicity with Loa loa (the eye worm)

Adult Loa loas are sometimes seen crossing the eye in the subconjuctival space and can sometimes be removed. The dying adult also causes swellings, typically over the wrist (Calabar swellings), but also occasionally in the orbit. Mectizan is active against *Loa loa* and unfortunately with massive infections, more than 8000 mf per ml, the destruction can create an encephalopathy that can lead to death. *Loa loa* is found in forest areas, and particularly in some areas of southern Nigeria close to the coast, southern Cameroon, Democratic Republic of Congo, northern Angola, southern Central African Republic and Sudan. Where onchocerciasis is found to be meso- or hyper-endemic, it has been considered justifiable to take the risk of treatment with ivermectin, providing the Mectizan Expert Committee/APOC Technical Consultative Committee guidelines are followed and patients are identified early and receive appropriate supportive therapy. Because of these extra precautions, which are difficult to implement in the poorest and post-conflict Africa countries, these areas are slow to scale up treatment.

Post-conflict countries

Many countries in Central Africa have experienced conflict, from the Sudan to Angola. Conflict has destroyed infrastructure, and caused the breakdown of primary healthcare and migration of qualified personnel to more stable regions. These factors have led to a slow scale up of treatment and poor geographical coverage.

Sustainability

Many programmes will have to continue beyond the life of APOC in 2015. APOC has been working at the district level to try to ensure continued distribution, but as the symptoms and signs of the disease gradually disappear it will be more difficult to maintain interest and financial support at the district level. Vital Mectizan distribution and the post-treatment surveillance necessary are at risk of losing support during a critical period. All that has been gained so far must not be lost at the last hurdle.

Integration with neglected tropical diseases

Onchocerciasis has been labelled as one of the **neglected tropical diseases (NTDs)**. Focus on the disease, however, must not be lost. It is important for elimination that 80% of the total population get regular treatment. Where lymphatic filariasis (LF) and onchocerciasis are co-endemic, both programmes will probably benefit, especially as Mectizan will be distributed more widely, including in hypo-endemic areas.

18.6 RESEARCH PRIORITIES

18.6.1 Ideal treatment frequency

There is still discussion on the ideal frequency of treatment with ivermectin. OEPA adopted the twice-yearly regime. This rapidly eliminates microfilariae from the skin on a permanent basis, and therefore interrupts transmission quickly, as foci are small and the systems closed. The effect on female worms is greater where people are treated twice a year. Recent work shows that viable worms in nodules removed after ivermectin treatment could represent re-infection. It is important to be able to distinguish re-infections, particularly if using a macrofilaricide; otherwise finding live adult worms might be wrongly diagnosed as resistance.[45] This is a further argument for two- or even four-times-a-year treatment as is now the treatment strategy in the remaining sites in OEPA.[46]

As control moves to elimination in Africa, research is necessary to clarify the best frequency of treatment, as well as what would be the best strategy operationally, as changes in strategy are likely to be needed in some sites already on the verge of elimination after more than 15 years of treatment.

18.6.2   Hypo-endemic zones/transmission zones

Hypo-endemic zones as defined by REMO are below 20% nodule prevalence, which could equal 40% mf prevalence. Transmission certainly occurs in some hypo-endemic zones, for example in Gabon. It remains to be decided whether, once the meso- and hyper-endemic zones are treated, the hypo-endemic zones will die out. Research is needed to define transmission zones in varied circumstances.

18.6.3   Other drug combinations (particularly for Loa loa areas)

There are three avenues for research into alternative drug therapies:

➢ A macrofilaricide, suitable for mass distribution, which could eliminate onchocerciasis much more rapidly.
➢ Anti-filarial drugs that are safe to use in the presence of *Loa loa*.

➢ Potential second line drugs should resistance to ivermectin develop on a large scale.

Potential drugs:

➢ *Doxycycline*. Doxycycline acts on *Wolbachia* infections. *Wolbachia* is an endosymbiotic bacterial infection in several species of filariae, including onchocerciasis. When this bacterium is destroyed by suitable antibiotics the adults cease production of larvae and eventually die. Doxycycline could be used in the possible case of resistance and could also be useful in *Loa loa* areas as there is no *Wolbachia* infection in *Loa loa*. There are two main drawbacks. First, the drug has to be given daily for six weeks and second, the drug cannot be given to persons under 12 years old. This means that there is a risk that, even with the best coverage possible, it would not be enough to eliminate the disease from the community.[47] Operational research is needed to determine its effectiveness at the community level.

➢ *Moxidectin*. Moxidectin is undergoing trials to test its efficacy as a macrofilaricide.[48] Although its structure is very similar to ivermectin, its half-life in the human host is considerably longer. This may make the adult worms more vulnerable to treatment. Its similarity to ivermectin will probably mean that it is not effective in potential resistance and its effect on microfilariae will probably rule out its use in *Loa loa*. Both these effects need to be researched.

➢ *Flubendazole* has shown to be effective against adult filariae.[49] Unfortunately, when taken orally, it remains in the intestine with little absorption, effective against intestinal worms but not effective for filariae. Injectable forms have been tried but they are associated with painful sterile abscesses. Research is needed to develop bioavailable forms for filariasis control and then to test the drug for use as a macrofilaricide.

18.6.4   Diagnostic tools

To confirm elimination it is necessary to have reliable diagnostic tools to verify the absence of disease.

In flies

Where ivermectin alone has been used, the flies remain. Dissection of flies to look for larval forms of *Onchocerca* is a long and tedious task. Pool screening using the polymerase chain reaction (PCR) looking for onchocercal DNA has been used with good results. However, flies still have to be collected and using human volunteers is becoming problematic. There is an urgent need to develop fly-traps so that sufficient flies can be examined to confirm the absence of disease.

In the host

The classical method has relied on skin snips. There are two problems: first, the act of snipping is invasive and therefore this has to be done with great care for the large numbers surveyed. Second, the test becomes less sensitive as the numbers of microfilariae decrease. Suitable tests need to be developed to detect antigens of the parasite even in the presence of small numbers of worms. The DEC patch test is one possibility but its specificity needs to be determined in the presence of other filarial worms. The OV16 antigen test, which can be done with blood spots on paper, is probably the most accurate, but it needs more sophisticated laboratories than those available in the field.[50] This could be developed into a card test, if there is general agreement on its use, in order to maintain its production.

18.6.5 Modelling

Modelling (ONCHOCIM) has been largely based on OCP strategies.[51] These need to be adapted, as most strategies now rely solely on mass distribution of ivermectin. Earlier studies predicted at least 20–25 years of annual treatment if coverage was adequate, but longer still with low coverage. Studies on the Senegal–Mali border have shown elimination of the parasite after 16 years. The model needs to be further developed, taking into account results of current strategies as well as modelling for multiple treatments per year and treatment in hypo-endemic areas.

18.6.6 Combinations of vector control and mass drug administration (MDA)

An understanding of the different Simulium vectors can help in planning further elimination activities. Where *S. neavei* is the vector, it may be possible to eliminate the vector and halt transmission. However, it must not be forgotten that patients with the disease will still need ivermectin on a regular basis until the adult worms die. It has also been postulated that if the vectors are kept under control for a few years, particularly with twice-yearly treatment, the period of treatment with Mectizan could be considerably shortened. This hypothesis needs further work in the field.

18.6.7 Combination with other NTD programmes

In spite of all the efforts in developing strategies, and the funding available for onchocerciasis, it has been labelled as one of the neglected tropical diseases, suitable for rapid impact interventions with **mass drug administration (MDA)**.[52] While it is logical to combine treatments where they fit well together, e.g. onchocerciasis and lymphatic filariasis, care must be taken not to lose the focus on onchocerciasis control/elimination. This is especially true where other treatment strategies such as maternal and child health weeks are proposed for MDA, and where Mectizan is targeted to the whole population up to four times a year. For sustainability it is also vital that Mectizan distribution is fully integrated into the primary healthcare system[53] rather than being a parallel activity.

REFERENCES

1. O'Neil J. On the presence of filaria in 'craw-craw'. *Lancet* 1875; 1:265–266.
2. Robles R. Enfermedad nueva in Guatemala. *Juventud Med* 1917; 17:97–115.
3. Blacklock DB. The development of *Onchocerca Volvulus* in *Simulium Damnosum. Ann Trop Med Parasitol* 1926; 20:1–48.

4. Hissette J. Mémoire on *Onchocerca volvulus* and ocular manifestations in the Belgian Congo. *Ann Soc Belge Med Trop* 1932: 12:433–529.

5. Ridley H. Ocular Onchocerciasis, including an investigation in the Gold Coast. *Br J Ophthalmol* 1945; 10:1–58.

6. Samba EM. *The Onchocerciasis Control Programme in West Africa. An Example of Effective Public Health Management.* Geneva: WHO; 1994.

7. Collatrella B. The Mectizan Donation Program: 20 years of successful collaboration. *Ann Trop Med Parasitol* 2008; 2:S7–S11.

8. Gustavsen KM, Bradley MH, Wright AL. GlaxoSmithKline and Merck: private-sector collaboration for the elimination of lymphatic filariasis. *Ann Trop Med Parasitol* 2009; 103: S11–S15.

9. Duke BOL. The population dynamics of *Onchocerca volvulus* in the human host. *Trop Med Parasitol* 1993; 44:61–68.

10. Duke BOL, Lewis DJ, Moore PJ. Onchocerca — Simulium complexes I. Transmission of forest and Sudan-savannah strains of *Onchocerca volvulus* from Cameroon, by *Simulium damnosum* from various West Africa bioclimatic zones. *Ann Trop Med Parasitol* 1996; 60:318–316.

11. Lewis DJ, Duke BOL. Onchocerca — Simulium complexes II. Variation in West African *Simulium damnosum*. *Ann Trop Med Parasitol* 1996; 60:318–316.

12. Anderson, Fuglsang H, Hamilton PJS, *et al.* Studies on Onchocerciasis in the United Cameroon Republic II. Comparison of onchocerciasis in rainforest and Sudan Savannah. *Trans Roy Soc Trop Med Hyg* 1974; 68:209–222.

13. Zimmerman PA, Katholi CR, Wooten MC, *et al.* Recent evolutionary history of American Onchocerca volvulus, based on analysis of a tandemly repeated DNA sequence family. Mol Bio Evo 1994; 11:384–392.

14. Remme J, Dadzie KY, Rolland A, *et al.* Ocular onchocerciasis and intensity of infection in the community I. West African Savannah. *Ann Trop Med Parasitol* 1989; 40:340–347.

15. Dadzie KY, Remme J, Rolland A, *et al.* Ocular onchocerciasis and intensity of infection in the community II. West African Savannah. *Ann Trop Med Parasitol* 1989; 40:348–354.

16. Duke BOL, Anderson J. A comparison of the lesions produced in the cornea of the rabbit eye by microfilaria of the forest and Sudan-Savannah strains of *Onchocerca volvulus* from Cameroon. *Trop Med Parasitol* 1972; 23:354–368.

17. Duke BOL, Garner A. Fundus lesions in the rabbit eye following inoculation of *Onchocerca volvulus* in the posterior segment. *Tropenmed Parasitol* 1976; 27:3–17.

18. Prost A, Vaugelade J. The excess mortality of blind people in the savannah zone of West Africa [Article in French]. *Bull World Health Organ* 1981; 59:773–776.

19. Cousens SN, Yahaya H, Murdoch I, *et al.* Risk factors for optic nerve disease in communities mesoendemic for savannah onchocerciasis, Kaduna State, Nigeria. *Trop Med Int Health* 1997; 2:89–98.

20. Abiose A, Jones B, Murdoch I, *et al.* Reduction in incidence of optic nerve disease with annual ivermectin to control onchocerciasis. *Lancet* 1993; 341:130–134.

21. Murdoch ME, Hay RJ, Mackenzie CD, *et al.* A clinical classification and grading system of the cutaneous changes in onchocerciasis. *Br J Dermatol* 1993; 129:260–269.

22. Druet-Cabanac M, Preux PM, Bouteille B, *et al.* Onchocerciasis and epilepsy: a matched case-control study in the Central African Republic. *Am J Epidemiol* 1999; 149:565–570.

23. Pion SDS, Kaiser C, Boutros-Toni F, *et al.* Epilepsy in onchocerciasis endemic areas: systematic review and meta-analysis of population-based surveys. *PLoS Negl Trop Dis* 2009; 3:e461.

24. Kipp W, Burnham G, Bamuhiiga J, *et al.* Syndrome in Kabarole District, Western Uganda. *Am J Trop Med Hyg* 1996; 54:80–83.

25. Onchocerciasis and its Control. Report of a WHO Expert Committee on Onchocerciasis Control. WHO Technical report series 852. Geneva: WHO; 1995.

26. Roberts JMD, Neumann E, Guckel CW, *et al.* Onchocerciasis in Kenya, 9, 11 and 18 years after elimination of the vector. *Bull World Health Organ* 1986; 64:667–681.

27. Amazigo U. The African Programme for Onchocerciasis Control (APOC). *Ann Trop Med Parasitol* 2008; 102:S19–S22.

28. Hopkins AD. Onchocerciasis control: impressive achievements not to be wasted. *Can J Ophthalmol* 2007; 42:13–15.

29. Sauerbrey M. The Onchocerciasis Elimination Program for the Americas. *Ann Trop Med Parasitol* 2008; 102:S25–S29.

30. Anderson J, Fuglsang H, al-Zubaidy A. Onchocerciasis in Yemen with special reference to sowda. *Trans Roy Soc Trop Med Hyg* 1973; 67:30–31.

31. Taylor HR, Duke BOL, Munoz B. The selection of communities for treatment of onchocerciasis with ivermectin. *Trop Med Parasitol* 1992; 43:267–270.

32. Ngoumopu P, Wash JF. A manual for rapid epidemiological mapping of onchocerciasis. Doc. No. TDR/TDE/ONCHO/93.4. Geneva: WHO; 1993.

33. Thompson BH. Studies on the flight range and dispersal of *Simulium damnsosum* (*Diptera Simuliidae*) in the rain forest of Cameroon. *Am Trop Med Parasitol* 1976; 70:343–354.

34. Boatin B. The Onchocerciasis Control Program in West Africa (OCP). *Ann Trop Med Parasitol* 2008; 102:13–17.

35. Community Directed Treatment with Ivermectin (CDTI) 2009. www.who.int/apoc/cdti/en.

36. Community Directed Interventions for major health problems in Africa — a multi-country study: final report 2008. who.int/tdr/publications.

37. Final Report of the Conference on the Eradicability of Onchocerciasis. www.cartercenter.org/news/documents/doc1172.html.

38. Diawara L, Traoré MO, Badji A, *et al.* Feasibility of onchocerciasis elimination with ivermectin treatment in endemic foci in Africa: first evidence from studies in Mali and Senegal. *PLoS Negl Trop Dis* 2009; 3:e497.

39. Ndyomugyenyi R, Lakwo T, Habomugisha P, *et al.* Progress towards the elimination of onchocerciasis as a public-health problem in Uganda: opportunities, challenges and the way forward. *Ann Trop Med Parasitol* 2007; 101:323–333.

40. Pan-American Health Organization 48th Directing Council (CD48-10-e). PAHO 2008. www.paho.org/English/GOV/CD/cd48-10-e.pdf.

41. OEPA website. http://www.oepa.net/ OEPA 2009.

42. Informal consultation on elimination of onchocerciasis transmission using current tools in Africa 'Shrinking the Map'. WHO/APOC/2009.

43. WHO Certification of elimination of human onchocerciasis criteria and procedures. WHO/CDS/CPE/CEE/2001.18a. http://whqlibdoc.who.int/hq/2001/WHO_CDS_CPE_CEE_2001.18b.pdf.

44. Hopkins AD. Ivermectin and onchocerciasis: is it all solved? *Eye* 2005; 19:1057–1066.

45. Specht S, Hoerauf A, Adjei O, *et al.* Newly acquired *Onchocerca volvulus* filariae after doxycycline treatment. *Parasitol Res* 2009; 106:23–31.

46. Cupp EW, Cupp MS. Short report: impact of ivermectin community-level treatments on elimination of adult *Onchocerca volvulus* when individuals receive multiple treatments per year. *Am J Trop Med Hyg* 2005; 73:1159–1161.

47. Wanji S, Tendongfor N, Nji T, *et al.* Community-directed delivery of doxycycline for the treatment of onchocerciasis in areas of co-endemicity with loiasis in Cameroon. *Parasites and Vectors* 2009; 2:39.

48. TDR press release. http://apps.who.int/tdrsvc/news-events/news/phase3-trial-moxidectin 2009.

49. Dominguez-Vazquez A, Taylor HR, Greene BM, *et al.* Comparison of flubendazole and diethylcarbamazine in treatment of onchocerciasis. *Lancet* 1983; 22:139–143.

50. Lipner EM, Dembele N, Souleymane S, *et al.* Field applicability of a rapid-format anti-ov-16 antibody test for the assessment of onchocerciasis control measures in regions of endemicity. *J Infect Dis* 2006; 194:216–221.

51. Plaisier AP, van Oortmarssen GJ, Habbema JD, *et al.* ONCHOSIM: a model and computer simulation program for the transmission and control of onchocerciasis. *Comput Methods Programs Biomed* 1990; 31:43–56.

52. Molyneux DH, Hotez PJ, Fenwick A. 'Rapid impact interventions': How a policy of integrated control for Africa's neglected tropical diseases could benefit the poor. *PLoS Med* 2; e336.

53. Hopkins AD. Challenges for the integration of mass drug administrations against multiple 'neglected tropical diseases'. *Ann Trop Med Parasitol* 2009; 103:S23–S31.

19

The epidemiology of uveitis

JENNIFER THORNE AND DOUGLAS JABS

19.1	Introduction	509
19.2	Definition	509
19.3	Classification and grading systems	509
19.4	Prevalence and incidence of uveitis	511
19.5	Management	512

19.6	Complications of uveitis	512
19.7	Visual loss attributable to uveitis	513
19.8	Ongoing and future research in uveitis	513
	References	514

19.1 INTRODUCTION

Uveitis refers to a set of diseases characterized by intraocular inflammation that vary by clinical presentation, severity, course and mode of treatment. Severe, non-infectious uveitis is often associated with an increased risk of vision loss and typically requires long-term therapy with oral cortico-steroids, and, when indicated, supplementing with immunosuppressive drugs.[1] The visual loss associated with uveitis is caused by structural ocular complications, including cataract, glaucoma, macular oedema, choroidal neovascularization and epiretinal membrane formation. Approximately 50–60% of patients with posterior uveitis or panuveitis will develop visual impairment to a visual acuity of 20/60 or worse.[2] As such, it is estimated that uveitis is the fifth to sixth leading cause of visual impairment and blindness in the USA.[3] Because uveitis is a disease that often affects the young to middle-aged, the cost to productivity associated with blindness attributed to uveitis is probably higher than that observed with age-related eye disease.[4] Thus management of patients with uveitis is aimed not only at suppression of the inflammation, but also treatment of its attendant structural complications in order to prevent visual loss.

19.2 DEFINITION

The term 'uveitis' refers to a group of approximately 25–30 diseases characterized by inflammation inside the eye. Uveitis may be infectious or non-infectious; however, the majority of cases (approximately 80% in most series) presenting for care to uveitis practices in the USA are presumed to be 'autoimmune' or 'autoinflammatory', based upon the absence of evidence for infection and the response to corticosteroid and immunosuppressive drug therapies. Non-infectious uveitides encompass a variety of specific syndromes, each with specific diagnostic features. A sample of these uveitic syndromes is listed in Table 19.1.[5–17]

19.3 CLASSIFICATION AND GRADING SYSTEMS

Although some forms of uveitis remit spontaneously, have a good prognosis and do not require

509

Table 19.1 *Select uveitic syndromes*

Anterior and intermediate uveitis

Fuch's heterochromic iridocyclitis
Herpetic anterior uveitis
HLA-B27-associated anterior uveitis
Juvenile idiopathic arthritis (JIA)-associated chronic anterior uveitis
Tubulointerstitial nephritis with uveitis
Intermediate uveitis, pars planitis type
Intermediate uveitis, non-pars planitis type
Multiple sclerosis-associated intermediate uveitis

Posterior

Birdshot chorioretinitis
Multifocal choroiditis with panuveitis
Punctate inner choroiditis
Acute posterior multifocal placoid pigment epitheliopathy
Serpiginous choroiditis
Ampiginous choroiditis
Multiple evanescent white dot syndrome

Panuveitis

Vogt–Koyanagi–Harada syndrome
Sympathetic ophthalmia
Behçet disease
Retinal vasculitis
Sarcoidosis-associated uveitis

Infectious Uveitis

Syphilitic uveitis
Lyme uveitis
Bartonella neuroretinitis
Acute retinal necrosis
Progressive outer retinal necrosis
Cytomegalovirus retinitis
Toxoplasmic retinitis
Tuberculous uveitis

In anterior uveitis, inflammation primarily effects the anterior chamber; in intermediate uveitis, primarily the vitreous (often called 'vitritis'); in posterior uveitis, the choroid or retina primarily is affected, often with an overlying vitritis; and in panuveitis, all parts of the eye are affected, without any one predominant location, and typically there is significant anterior chamber and vitreous inflammation. The course of uveitis may be characterized as acute (either monophasic or recurrent) or chronic. The key distinction is that acute uveitis typically has episodes of remission (i.e. inactive disease without therapy). Monophasic anterior uveitis has only one episode, whereas recurrent acute uveitis will have recurrent periods separated by periods of inactive disease without therapy. Chronic disease typically persists for longer than three months and requires chronic suppressive therapy because the uveitis will relapse once therapy is discontinued. The anatomic location of the inflammation, the disease course (including onset and duration of inflammation), and the findings observed on clinical examination typically are used to diagnose a specific uveitic syndrome. However, despite the fact that the majority of uveitic syndromes are diagnosed clinically, only a few have published classification criteria, and none of them have been independently validated.[18–22] A lack of validated classification criteria and the relative rarity of specific uveitic syndromes makes assessing the prevalence and incidence of specific syndromes particularly difficult, and thus most of the available data combine all forms of uveitis in the reporting of epidemiologic data.

Multiple grading systems to quantify the degree of inflammation have been published for grading the cellular inflammation in the anterior chamber, the proteineous material in the anterior chamber known as 'flare', and the cellular inflammation and haze in the vitreous.[23–28] The SUN Working Group ratified grading systems for anterior chamber cell and flare, and for vitreous haze, and a separate group reported good 'inter-rater' (inter-observer) reliability for the grading of anterior chamber cells.[5,29] These reports have helped to standardize the reporting of response of intraocular inflammation to treatment in clinical studies and clinical trials, but are not helpful in classifying

therapy, the majority of cases of uveitis require medical treatment. Because arriving at the appropriate diagnosis, and subsequently, the appropriate treatment approach, depends upon the anatomic location and the course of the uveitis, these characteristics are used to classify various types of uveitis. The anatomic location of the inflammation is determined by clinical examination. According to the **standardization of uveitis nomenclature (SUN)** method for anatomical classification, uveitis may be classified into anterior, intermediate, posterior uveitis or panuveitis, depending upon the primary location of the inflammation.[5]

or diagnosing specific uveitic diseases. Severity scales that grade the severity of inflammation at presentation of the patient to the clinic have been proposed for uveitis associated with juvenile idiopathic arthritis and for retinal vasculitis, but have yet to be commonly accepted.

19.4 PREVALENCE AND INCIDENCE OF UVEITIS

Estimated as the fifth or sixth leading cause of blindness, uveitis has become an important cause of visual loss in the USA. However, because uveitis was believed to be an uncommon ocular disease, classic population-based, epidemiologic studies of uveitis have been limited. Estimates of the prevalence and incidence rates of uveitis reported in the literature over the past 50 years are summarized in Table 19.2. Incidence estimates of uveitis range from 17–52/100,000 per year, and prevalence estimates from 52–204/100,000 population.[30–39] There is a single report by Reeves and colleagues[40] that reported dramatically higher incidence and prevalence rates of uveitis in the Medicare population, but the diagnosis of uveitis was not confirmed by

medical chart review, and therefore these data are discussed separately below. It has been estimated that there are 30,000 new cases of uveitis diagnosed in the USA each year. The Research to Prevent Blindness annual report of 1993 estimated that approximately 1% of the USA population was affected by uveitis.[39] These estimates are based on studies that rely on the assumption that a relatively isolated population would be seen at the most convenient ophthalmic centre, so that the prevalence and incidence rates can be calculated by dividing the number of cases from the region seen at the centre by the regional population. Such estimates are likely to underestimate prevalence and incidence rates (see Chapter 1), as it is unlikely that all cases would be captured.

Reports in the 1990s have suggested that the incidence and prevalence are higher than in previous reports.[31,40] In the **Northern California Epidemiology of Uveitis** (**NCEU**) Study published in 2004,[31] Gritz and Wong found a significantly higher incidence (52 cases per 100,000 person-years or approximately double previous estimates) and a higher annual prevalence than any previous USA or European study. It is possible that, because the NCEU study was more ethnically diverse than other studies of predominantly

Table 19.2 *Estimated incidence and prevalence rates for uveitis as reported in the literature*

Author and publication date	Population location and criteria	Population size	Dates of study	Incidence per 100,000 population	Prevalence per 100,000 population
Mann 1955	Papua and New Guinea	13,717	1954		146
Oskala 1960	Hospital reports of patients from Central Hospital in Finland	250,000			52
Darrell 1962	Residents of Rochester, Minnesota	29,885	1945–1954	17	204
Freedman 1974	South Africa	652,259	1971–1973	27.2	
Miettinen 1977	North-western Finland	613,426	1969	19.6	
Saari 1995	South-western Finland	459,515	1980–1982	22.6	75.4
Saari 1997*	South-western Finland	472,540	1988		
Gritz 2004	Six medical communities in Northern California	731,898	1998–1999	52.4	115.3
Reeves 2006	Random sample of US Medicare beneficiaries in the National Long Term Care Survey, 65 and older	21,644	1991–1999	340.9	511
Suhler 2008	Six VA medical centres in Washington and Oregon	152,267	2003–2004	25.6	69

*Second population study confirmed the findings of the first study (Saari).

European ancestry, the pattern and course of uveitis among non-Europeans patients may be different; therefore the prevalence and incidence of uveitis in these populations could be higher. The NCEU study also reported the highest incidence and prevalence rates of uveitis among the oldest age groups in their population sample. These findings of higher incidence and prevalence rates among older age groups contrast with the findings of all of the previously published studies, which have reported a peak in incident and prevalent uveitis in young adulthood that diminishes with age. Reeves and colleagues,[40] using Medicare data from 1991 to 1999, also reported higher incidence and prevalence rates of uveitis in a random sample of Medicare beneficiaries aged 65 and older. The incidence of uveitis was 340.9 cases per 100,000 person-years and the prevalence 511 cases per 100,000 population.[40] However, the cases of uveitis in this report were not confirmed by medical record review, which has been reported to lead to significant overestimation of the number of cases of uveitis in a population.[32] The majority of studies have found that the distribution of uveitis cases by gender has a slight female preponderance, although typically the difference has not been statistically significant. Lastly, the location, pattern, severity and course of uveitis tend to be different among different referral populations.[15] For example, McCannel and colleagues reported on the frequencies of various forms of uveitis diagnosed in two different clinic settings. Two-hundred and thirteen consecutive uveitis patients examined by a group of general ophthalmologists in practice in Southern California were compared with 213 uveitis patients who were examined by a uveitis specialist in a tertiary care centre in the same community. Although the majority of uveitis cases were anterior uveitis for both settings, approximately 40% of cases in the tertiary setting were more severe, sight-threatening forms.[15]

19.5   MANAGEMENT

The anatomic location of the uveitis determines the primary approach to therapy. Corticosteroids are the mainstay of treatment of the various uveitic syndromes. Anterior uveitis typically requires only topical corticosteroids. However, other forms of uveitis will require either regional (also known as local) corticosteroid injections or systemic corticosteroids because topical corticosteroids do not penetrate well into the posterior part of the eye. Because of the need for chronic treatment and the inability to adequately suppress the disease on tolerably low doses of oral corticosteroids on a chronic basis, many types of posterior uveitis and panuveitis require chronic immunosuppression as a corticosteroid-sparing approach.[1,41]

19.6   COMPLICATIONS OF UVEITIS

Patients with uveitis are subject to a variety of structural complications, including posterior synechiae, peripheral anterior synechiae, ocular hypertension and glaucoma, cataracts, macular oedema, also known as cystoid macular oedema (CME), retinal infarction in patients with retinal vasculitis, retinal neovascularization, epiretinal membrane formation, and choroidal neovascularization. Many of these structural complications are associated with visual morbidity, and both reversible and permanent visual loss may be observed.[2,4] The risk of developing structural complications appears to be associated with ongoing active inflammation in a dose-dependent fashion.[42–46] Therefore aggressive treatment of uveitis, including the use of topical, periocular or systemic therapies up to and including immunosuppressive drugs, is aimed at completely controlling the intraocular inflammation in order to avoid these ocular complications in the long term.[44–48] Cystoid macular oedema is the most frequently encountered structural complication resulting in visual loss. In a retrospective study from two uveitis referral centres in the Netherlands in the early 1990s, 40% of patients with intermediate uveitis, posterior uveitis or panuveitis had CME, and it was the most common cause of visual loss among all patients with uveitis, accounting for 41% of visual impairment.[2] In the **Multicenter Uveitis Steroid Treatment** (**MUST**) Trial, CME was present in 36% of eyes with uveitis with a similar frequency for patients with intermediate uveitis, posterior uveitis and panuveitis.[49] If left untreated or undertreated over a period of years, chronic macular oedema may result in destruction of the central portion of the retina and permanent loss of central vision, the vision that is required to read.[50] Although this type of 'retina rot' may occur in the peripheral retina when oedema persists throughout the retina (e.g. as is a typical finding in birdshot chorioretinitis),[51] the resultant visual loss may not be as damaging to the patient's overall quality of vision and quality of life until the disease is advanced, as is often the case with the natural history of primary open-angle glaucoma. Further, some structural complications of uveitis, such as macular oedema or choroidal neovascularization, may occur, recur or persist in the setting of controlled uveitis (e.g. no cells observed inside the eye) and therefore treatment over and above that required for suppression of the uveitis is required to prevent further visual loss.

19.7 VISUAL LOSS ATTRIBUTABLE TO UVEITIS

In 1990, uveitis was estimated to be responsible for approximately 10% of the visual impairment in the USA, with approximately 30,000 new cases of legal blindness.[52] A review of blind registry data in the United Kingdom found that approximately 10% of cases of blindness were attributed to uveitis.[a] Combining these data with the most recent estimates of the incidence and prevalence of uveitis in the USA[32,33] and the projected USA population data for the beginning of 2010, the incidence of blindness attributed to uveitis would be three to five cases per 100,000 population per year or approximately 9,300 to 15,500 new cases of blindness per year. The prevalence of blindness attributable to uveitis in the USA is estimated at 7–12 cases per 100,000 population or approximately 22,000 to 37,000 people.

Vision loss secondary to uveitis and its complications is likely to have a greater economic impact per case than vision loss from age-related eye diseases, because uveitis, as stated, most commonly occurs in middle-aged adults, resulting in disability during the working years and loss of work productivity.[53] In addition, chronic uveitis may require a higher average health professional (and patient) effort and cost per case, with more clinical visits over longer periods of time as compared with other conditions.[54] In their report *Vision Research: A National Plan 1999 to 2003*,[55] the National Advisory Eye Council identified the development of improved therapeutic approaches for uveitis as a priority due to the high risk of visual impairment and blindness in patients with intermediate uveitis, posterior uveitis or panuveitis. The available data are limited but support this risk even among tertiary care centres with uveitis specialists. For example, a retrospective study from two Dutch uveitis centres in the early 1990s reported that 48% of patients with intermediate uveitis, posterior uveitis or panuveitis suffered vision loss to a level of 20/60 or worse within a median observation of 4.3 years. CME was the most common structural complication observed and the most frequent cause of vision loss (approximately 40% of all vision loss reported in the cohort).[2,4] In the MUST Trial, decreased vision at enrolment of worse than 20/40 (visual impairment), which included worse than 20/200 (legal blindness), was present respectively in 50% and in 15% of eyes with intermediate uveitis, posterior uveitis or panuveitis.[49] Approximately 30% of patients had a bilateral visual impairment, and 5% of patients had bilateral blindness.[49] These data support the view that substantial visual impairment may occur among patients with uveitis.

19.8 ONGOING AND FUTURE RESEARCH IN UVEITIS

➢ Historically, the absence of standardization of terminology in the field of uveitis has hampered research in the discipline. An international group of uveitis specialists (the SUN Working Group) has begun this process of standardizing the terminology.[5] Efforts are focused on developing classification criteria for the major uveitic syndromes, which are validated and internationally accepted; and completing the process of standardizing grading schemes for intraocular

---

[a] S Lightman, personal communication, 2002.

inflammation and reporting of clinical research data related to uveitis and its complications.[b] The results of this work are critical for future patient-oriented research in the field of uveitis, including laboratory studies relating to pathogenesis, epidemiologic studies, genetic studies of complex disorders, and clinical trials.

➤ To date, there has been one multicentre randomized clinical trial, funded by the National Institutes of Health in the field of uveitis. The MUST Trial compares the effectiveness of the sustained-release intraocular fluocinolone acetonide implant (Retisert®, Bausch and Lomb, Tampa, FL) with systemic therapy with oral corticosteroids and immunosuppressive drugs when indicated (administered according to published guidelines) for patients with vision-threatening uveitis.[49] The rationale for the MUST Trial is to provide an evidence-based guide to management of intermediate, posterior and panuveitis. Given the lack of existing high-quality trial-based evidence to guide clinicians and patients in the management of uveitis, it is hoped that the MUST trial will lead to additional clinical trials of the treatments of uveitis and its complications.

REFERENCES

1. Jabs DA, Rosenbaum JT, Foster CS, *et al.* Guidelines for the use of immunosuppressive drugs in patients with ocular inflammatory disorders: recommendations of an expert panel. *Am J Ophthalmol* 2000; 130:492–513.

2. Rothova A, Suttorp-van Schluten MSA, Treffers WF, *et al.* Causes and frequency of blindness in patients with intraocular inflammatory disease. *Br J Ophthalmol* 1996; 80:332–336.

3. Nussenblatt RB. The natural history of uveitis. *Int Ophthalmol* 1990; 14:303–308.

4. Suttorp-van Schulten MSA, Rothova A. The possible impact of uveitis in blindness: a literature survey. *Br J Ophthalmol* 1996; 80:844–848.

5. Jabs DA, Nussenblatt RB, Rosenbaum JT. Standardization of uveitis nomenclature for reporting clinical data. Results of the First International Workshop. *Am J Ophthalmol* 2005; 140:509–516.

6. Perkins ES, Folk J. Uveitis in London and Iowa. *Ophthalmologica* 1984; 189:36–40.

7. Henderly DE, Genstler AJ, Smith RE, *et al.* Changing patterns of uveitis. *Am J Ophthalmol* 1987; 103:131–136.

8. Palmares J, Coutinho MF, Castro-Correia J. Uveitis in northern Portugal. *Curr Eye Res* 1990; 9 Suppl: 31–34.

9. Santin M, Badrinas F, Mascaro J, *et al.* Uveitis: an etiological study of 200 cases following a protocol. *Med Clin (Barc)* 1991; 96:641–644.

10. Rothova A, Buitenhuis HJ, Meenken C, *et al.* Uveitis and systemic disease. *Br J Ophthalmol* 1992; 76:137–141.

11. Smit RL, Baarsma GS, de Vries J. Classification of 750 consecutive uveitis patients in the Rotterdam Eye Hospital. *Int Ophthalmol* 1993; 17:71–76.

12. Tran VT, Auer C, Guex-Crosier Y, *et al.* Epidemiological characteristics of uveitis in Switzerland. *Int Ophthalmol* 1994; 18:293–298.

13. Pivetti-Pezzi P, Accorinti M, La Cava M, *et al.* Endogenous uveitis: an analysis of 1,417 cases. *Ophthalmologica* 1996; 210:234–238.

14. Rodriguez A, Calonge M, Pedroza-Seres M, *et al.* Referral patterns of uveitis in a tertiary eye care center. *Arch Ophthalmol* 1996; 114:593–599.

15. McCannel CA, Holland GN, Helm CJ, *et al.* Causes of uveitis in the general practice of ophthalmology. UCLA Community-Based Uveitis Study Group. *Am J Ophthalmol* 1996; 121:35–46.

16. Merrill PT, Kim J, Cox TA, *et al.* Uveitis in the southeastern United States. *Curr Eye Res* 1997; 16: 865–874.

17. Mercanti A, Parolini B, Bonora A, *et al.* Epidemiology of endogenous uveitis in northeastern Italy. Analysis of 655 new cases. *Acta Ophthalmol Scand* 2001; 79:64–68.

18. Holland GN, the Executive Committee of the American Uveitis Society. Standard diagnostic criteria for the acute retinal necrosis syndrome. *Am J Ophthalmol* 1994; 117:663–666.

19. Engstrom RE Jr, Holland GN, Margolis TP, *et al.* The progressive outer retinal necrosis syndrome. A variant of necrotizing herpetic retinopathy in patients with AIDS. *Ophthalmology* 1994; 101: 1488–1502.

---

[b] D Jabs, personal communication, 2010.

20. Read RW, Holland GN, Rao NA, *et al.* Revised diagnostic criteria for Vogt-Koyanagi-Harada disease; report of an international committee on nomenclature. *Am J Ophthalmol* 2001; 131:647–652.

21. Mandeville JT, Levinson RD, Holland GN. The tubulointerstitial nephritis and uveitis syndrome. *Surv Ophthalmol* 2001; 46:195–208.

22. Levinson RD, Brezin A, Rothova A, *et al.* Research criteria for the diagnosis of birdshot chorioretinopthy: results of an international consensus conference. *Am J Ophthalmol* 2006; 185–187.

23. Hogan MJ, Kimura SJ, Thygeson P. Signs and symptoms of uveitis: I. Anterior uveitis. *Am J Ophthalmol* 1964; 47:155–170.

24. Schlaegel TF. *Essentials of Uveitis.* Boston: Little, Brown, Inc.; 1967.

25. Nussenblatt RB, Whitcup SM. *Uveitis: Fundamentals and Clinical Practice*, 3rd Edition. Philadelphia: Mosby; 2004.

26. Foster CS, Vitale AT. *Diagnosis and Treatment of Uveitis.* Philadelphia: WB Saunders Company; 2002.

27. Kimura SJ, Hogan MJ. Signs and symptoms of uveitis: II. Classification of the posterior manifestations of uveitis. *Am J Ophthalmol* 1964; 47:171–176.

28. Nussenblatt RB, Palestine AG, Chan CC, *et al.* Standardization of vitreal inflammatory activity in intermediate and posterior uveitis. *Ophthalmology* 1985; 92:467–471.

29. Kempen JH, Ganesh SK, Sangwan VS, *et al.* Interobserver agreement in grading activity and site of inflammation in eyes of patients with uveitis. *Am J Ophthalmol* 2008; 146:813–818.

30. Darrell RW, Wagener HP, Kurland LR. Epidemiology of uveitis: incidence and prevalence in a small urban community. *Arch Ophthalmol* 1962;68: 502–514.

31. Gritz DC, Wong IG. Incidence and prevalence of uveitis in Northern California; the Northern California Epidemiology of Uveitis Study. *Ophthalmology* 2004; 111:491–500; discussion 500.

32. Suhler EB, Lloyd MJ, Choi D, *et al.* Incidence and prevalence of uveitis in veterans affairs medical centers of the pacific northwest. *Am J Ophthalmol* 2008; 146:890–896.

33. Oskala A. Atiologie der uveitis in mittel-Finnland. *Docum Ophthalmol* 1960; 14:399.

34. Mann I. *Ophthalmic Survey of the Territories of Papua and New Guinea*, 1955. Port Moresby: Government Printing Office; 1956.

35. Saari KM, Paivonsalo-Heitanen T, Vaahtoranta-Lehtonen H, *et al.* Epidemiology of endogenous uveitis in south-western Finland. *Acta Ophthalmol Scan* 1995; 73:345–349.

36. Paivonsalo-Hietanen T, Tuominen J, Vaahtoranta-Lehtonen H, *et al.* Incidence and prevalance of different uveitis entities in Finland. *Acta Ophthalmol Scan* 1997; 75:76–81.

37. Miettinen R. Incidence of uveitis in Northern Finland. *Acta Ophthalmologica* 1977; 55:252–260.

38. Freedman J. Incidence of uveitis in Bantu-speaking Negroes of South Africa. *Br J Ophthalmol* 1974; 58:595–599.

39. Research to Prevent Blindness. Annual Report 1993. New York: RTB; 1993.

40. Reeves SW, Sloan FA, Lee PP, *et al.* Uveitis in the elderly: epidemiological data from the National Long-term Care Survey Medicare Cohort. *Ophthalmology* 2006; 113:302–307.

41. Jabs DA. Treatment of ocular inflammation. *Ocul Immunol Inflamm* 2004; 12:163–168.

42. Kaçmaz RO, Kempen JH, Newcomb C, *et al.* for the Systemic Immunosuppressive Therapy for Eye Diseases Cohort Study Group. Ocular inflammation in Behçet disease: Incidence of ocular complications and of loss of visual acuity. *Am J Ophthalmol* 2008; 146:828–836.

43. Thorne JE, Woreta F, Kedhar SR, *et al.* Juvenile idiopathic arthritis (JIA)-associated uveitis: Incidence of ocular complications and visual acuity loss. *Am J Ophthalmol* 2007; 143:840–846.

44. Thorne JE, Woreta FA, Dunn JP, *et al.* Risk of cataract development among children with juvenile idiopathic arthritis-related uveitis treated with topical corticosteroids. *Ophthalmology* 2010; 117:1436–1441.

45. Sijssens KM, Rothova A, Van de Vijver DA, *et al.* Risk factors for the development of cataract requiring surgery in uveitis associated with juvenile idiopathic arthritis. *Am J Ophthalmol* 2007; 144:574–579.

46. Thorne JE, Wittenberg S, Jabs DA, *et al.* Multifocal choroiditis with panuveitis incidence of ocular complications and of loss of visual acuity. *Ophthalmology* 2006; 113:2310–2316.

47. Thorne JE, Jabs DA, Peters GB, *et al.* Birdshot retinochoroidopathy: ocular complications and visual impairment. *Am J Ophthalmol* 2005; 140:45–51.

48. Dana MR, Merayo-Lloves J, Schaumberg DA, *et al.* Prognosticators for visual outcome in sarcoid uveitis. *Ophthalmology* 1996; 103:1846–1853.

49. The Multicenter Uveitis Steroid Treatment Trial Research Group. The Multicenter Uveitis Steroid Treatment (MUST) Trial: rationale, design, and baseline characteristics. *Am J Ophthalmol* 2010: in press.

50. Lardenoye CW, van Kooij B, Rothova A. Impact of macular oedema on visual acuity in uveitis. *Ophthalmology* 2006; 113:1146–1149.

51. Thorne JE, Jabs DA, Kedhar SR, *et al.* Loss of visual field among patients with birdshot chorioretinopathy. *Am J Ophthalmol* 2008; 145:23–28.

52. Nussenblatt RB. The natural history of uveitis. *Int Ophthalmol* 1990; 14:303–308.

53. Michel SS, Foster CS. Definition, Classification, Etiology and Epidemiology. Philadelphia: WB Saunders Company; 2002.

54. Watson SL, Edelsten C, Kanski JJ. The incidence of visual loss from uveitis. In: *Joint European Research Meeting in Ophthalmology and Vision*. Montpellier, France: Poster presentation; 1994.

55. National Advisory Eye Council. A National Plan: 1999–2003. In: *Vision Research*. Bethesda, MD: National Eye Institute, National Institutes of Health, Public Health Service, US Department of Health and Human Services; 1999–2003.

20

Ocular complications of human immunodeficiency virus infection

JOHN KEMPEN

20.1	Introduction	517	20.3	Ocular complications of HIV infection	524
20.2	Acquired immune deficiency syndrome (AIDS)	517	20.4	Priorities for future research	536
				References	538

20.1 INTRODUCTION

Ocular complications of **human immunodeficiency virus (HIV)** infection are integrally related to the underlying HIV disease itself. Biomarkers indicating the stage and progression rate of HIV infection are indicators of the risk of ocular complications, and treatments for HIV infection greatly influence the clinical course of ocular complications of HIV infection. Likewise, secular trends in the epidemiology of HIV disease drive the epidemiology of ocular complications of HIV infection. Therefore, this chapter will begin with a detailed discussion of HIV disease, after which the epidemiology of its ocular complications will be addressed.

20.2 ACQUIRED IMMUNE DEFICIENCY SYNDROME (AIDS)

20.2.1 History

Human immunodeficiency virus infection, an unknown disease prior to 1981, now affects approximately 33.4 million people worldwide,

causing two million deaths per year.[1] The first report of what would ultimately prove to be HIV disease was published in 1981.[2] Several other reports of opportunistic complications indicating an acquired cellular immune deficiency, called the **'Acquired Immune Deficiency Syndrome' (AIDS)**, appeared shortly thereafter. Once the syndrome was recognized, many series of large numbers of cases from geographically diverse locations throughout the USA — and then throughout the world — were reported,[3-6] indicating that HIV/AIDS had a worldwide pandemic before it was recognized.

20.2.2 Epidemiology

By December 2008, an estimated 33.4 million people worldwide (plausible range 31.1–35.8 million) were thought to be alive and infected with HIV (Plate 20.1), with approximately two thirds of cases in Sub-Saharan Africa.[1] Both HIV transmission and mortality have slightly declined from their peaks, near 1996 and 2005 respectively; however, because transmission exceeds mortality, the prevalence of

Global estimates 1990–2008

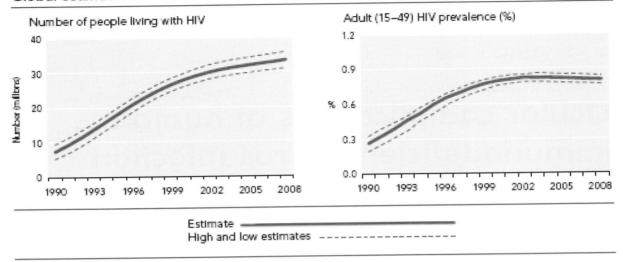

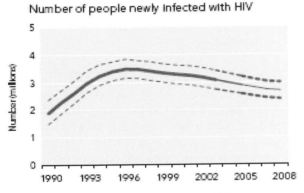

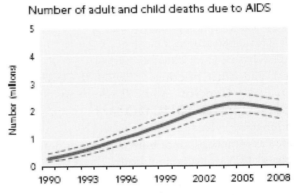

Figure 20.1 *Global estimates 1990–2008*
(*Source*: UNAIDS/WHO)

HIV/AIDS continues to rise each year (Fig. 20.1).[1] Improved methodology for estimating the prevalence of HIV infection has resulted in a reduction in prevalence estimates as compared with early reported estimates this decade, but it is thought that HIV prevalence has in fact continually risen throughout the pandemic.

Based on the UNAIDS AIDS Epidemic Update (December 2008),[1] of the estimated 33.4 million cases of HIV infection in the world, the large majority are concentrated in Sub-Saharan Africa (22.4 million); Southern and South East Asia (3.8 million), Latin America (2.0 million), Eastern Europe/Central Asia (1.5 million) and North America (1.4 million) (Plate 20.1). Sub-Saharan Africa continues to have the world's highest

incidence rate for new HIV infections (1.9 million/year). Earlier reports indicated that in the Sub-Saharan African countries with a high prevalence of HIV infection, life expectancy had reverted to its level in 1950 as a result of HIV/AIDS, eliminating the gains realized in the second half of the 20th century.[7] Greater coverage with antiretro-viral therapy is improving this situation, but the effects on life expectancy still are profound.[1] Fortunately, the incidence of new HIV infections has been declining slightly in recent years in most parts of the world (Fig. 20.1).[1] The prevalence of HIV infection in the highest risk group, adults ages 15–49, appears to be stabilizing (Fig. 20.1), suggesting that new infections and deaths in this age range are becoming balanced, an indicator that some measure of success in containing the epidemic is being achieved.

20.2.3   Definition and classification

The initial definition of AIDS was descriptive, based on the occurrence of a characteristic set of 'opportunistic' infections, tumours and other conditions, which were rarely seen in other circumstances, and were indicative of a cellular immune deficiency. The list of 'AIDS-defining' opportunistic complications has been increased over time, as more associations with AIDS were recognized.[8,9] These complications, affecting virtually all organ systems, have been the principal cause of morbidity and mortality in patients with HIV/AIDS.

As understanding of the clinical manifestations of HIV infection has evolved, the definition of AIDS has been modified to suit public health, clinical, and other priorities. The 2008 **Centers for Disease Control and Prevention (CDC) 'Surveillance case definition for human immunodeficiency virus (HIV) infection among adults and adolescents'**[8] is a widely accepted system for classifying cases of HIV infection and AIDS. This definition requires that patients have confirmed, laboratory evidence of HIV infection, and classifies the stage of HIV/AIDS into three categories based on immunologic status and history of opportunistic complications. Using this classification system, any patient who manifests an AIDS-defining opportunistic complication, or who is observed to have an absolute CD4+ T-lymphocyte count less than 200 cells/μL at any point in time, is counted ever after as having AIDS. The 2007 Revised WHO approach is similar, but subdivides patients into four categories, dividing CDC Stage 2 into two groups, at the threshold of an absolute CD4+ T cell count of 350 cells/μL or lower, corresponding to the recommended threshold for initiating antiretroviral treatment, and does not take into account CD4+ T-lymphocyte percentages.[8] The two systems are compared in Table 20.1. In settings where laboratory testing is less available, the provisional 'Bangui' case definition of the World Health Organization was previously used instead

of the CDC definition.[10] However, now that HIV testing is widely available, such an approach is not recommended for epidemiological studies and reports.

20.2.4   Pathogenesis

The '**human immunodeficiency virus**', a previously unknown virus, was first isolated in 1983; its role as the aetiologic agent of the acquired immune deficiency syndrome is well established.

The human immunodeficiency virus is a retrovirus, a member of the subfamily *lentivirinae*, a group of double-stranded RNA viruses. Lentiviruses typically cause slowly progressive diseases of the immune, neurologic and other organ systems. Clinically important characteristics of HIV include its surface glycoprotein **gp120**, which has specificity for the **CD4** molecule. Binding of gp120 to the CD4 molecule enables virus–cell fusion, providing the mechanism of entry of HIV into cells. This specificity restricts the number of cells susceptible to HIV infection, with T-helper lymphocytes and monocytic cells being the primary targets.

Once inside the cell, HIV releases its **reverse transcriptase** enzyme, which creates a DNA template from the viral RNA genome. Reverse transcriptase, an RNA-dependent DNA polymerase, has low fidelity, giving rise to approximately one mutation per replication cycle.[11] Because billions of replication cycles occur, this property gives rise to enormous viral genetic heterogeneity in infected individuals, allowing rapid development of resistance to antiretroviral agents. The high mutation rate of HIV and its consequent genetic heterogeneity dictate that antiretroviral therapy must attack multiple targets at once, and must suppress replication almost completely, in order to prevent the rapid development of drug-resistant strains.

The linear DNA copy of viral genes created from the viral RNA template is integrated into the host cell's genome by the viral **integrase** enzyme, where it remains inserted in the host DNA for the remainder of the cell's life as a '**provirus**'. Integration allows the proviral genes to direct the

Table 20.1 *Comparison of World Health Organization (WHO) and CDC stages of human immunodeficiency virus (HIV) infection,* by CD4+ T-Lymphocyte count and percentage of total lymphocytes*

WHO stage**	WHO T-lymphocyte count and percentage***	CDC stage****	CDC T-lymphocyte count and percentage
Stage 1 (HIV infection)	CD4+ T-lymphocyte count of ≥ 500 cells/μL	Stage 1 (HIV infection)	CD4+ T-lymphocyte count of ≥ 500 cells/μL or CD4 + T-lymphocyte percentage of ≥ 29
Stage 2 (HIV infection)	CD4+ T-lymphocyte count of 350–499 cells/μL	Stage 2 (HIV infection)	CD4+ T-lymphocyte count of 200–499 cells/μL or CD4 + T-lymphocyte percentage of 14–28
Stage 3 (advanced HIV disease [AHD])	CD4+ T-lymphocyte count of 200–349 cells/μL	Stage 2 (HIV infection)	CD4+ T-lymphocyte count of 200–499 cells/μL or CD4 + T-lymphocyte percentage of 14–28
Stage 4 (acquired immunodeficiency syndrome [AIDS])	CD4+ T-lymphocyte count of ≤ 200 cells/μL or CD4+ T-lymphocyte percentage of < 15	Stage 3 (AIDS)	CD4+ T-lymphocyte count of ≤ 200 cells/μL or CD4+ T-lymphocyte percentage of < 14

* For reporting purposes only; ** among adults and children aged ≥ five years; *** percentage applicable for stage 4 only; **** among adults and adolescents (aged ≥ 13 years). CDC also includes a fourth stage, stage unknown: laboratory confirmation of HIV infection but no information on CD4+ T-lymphocyte count or percentage and no information on AIDS-defining conditions.

cellular machinery to create new HIV virions, and ensures that the provirus will be propagated along with cellular DNA to the progeny of each infected cell. Because memory T-lymphocytes with a life expectancy of many decades are infected, the mechanism of integration assures a perpetual supply of virus in infected individuals, defeating early hopes that antiretroviral therapy would cure HIV infection,[12] although many continue to work toward this goal. Thus, the property of integration into the host cell genome renders HIV disease incurable by currently available treatment strategies.

The HIV **protease** enzyme, which is involved in packaging new infectious virions, and is required for the release thereof, is especially important because it can be successfully targeted in antiretroviral therapy.

Two subtypes of human immunodeficiency viruses exist, designated **HIV-1** and **HIV-2**. Compared with HIV-1, HIV-2 is less likely to be transmitted, gives rise to lower viral load in peripheral blood, and results in slower progression to AIDS (as indicated by CD4+ T-lymphocyte counts or clinical staging). Most cases of HIV-2 arise from West Africa; HIV-1 is responsible for most HIV disease throughout the rest of the world.[13]

20.2.5 Transmission and prevention of HIV infection

Infection with HIV is acquired by three principal routes: sexual exposure, parenteral exposure and vertical transmission. Vertical transmission to the offspring of an infected mother primarily occurs at the time of delivery or through breast milk. Although the HIV/AIDS epidemic initially appeared in western countries among men who had sex with men and injection drug users, the most frequent mechanism of transmission worldwide is through heterosexual intercourse. Preexisting infection with other sexually transmitted diseases facilitates sexual transmission of HIV, by damaging mucosal barriers. Therefore, HIV prevention efforts have focused on postponing the onset of sexual intercourse in young people, promotion of marital fidelity, use of barrier methods of contraception, and treatment of sexually transmitted diseases. Efforts to develop antiretroviral microbicides for use during sexual intercourse have not succeeded,[14] but it is hoped this approach will prove useful as technology improves. Recently it has been demonstrated that male circumcision reduces HIV infection risk in the male by approximately 60%[15] (but not in the female);[16] this approach may be useful in prevention efforts.

As with several infectious diseases, HIV is potentially preventable by vaccination. Because vaccination would provide a prevention strategy that could be readily implemented, development of an HIV vaccine has been targeted for a massive research effort. However, the challenges are formidable,[17] so that it is unclear when the effort will succeed in developing a useful product.

20.2.6   Clinical course of HIV infection

A schematic of the natural history of HIV infection is given in Fig. 20.2. The natural history of HIV infection often begins with an acute clinical syndrome resembling mononucleosis, called 'acute retroviral syndrome', although often no illness can be recalled by the patient. Acute infection is followed by a long asymptomatic interval lasting approximately eight years,[13] during which an estimated ten billion new virions are produced daily.[18] Although CD4+ T-lymphocytes are produced at a similar rate, destruction of these cells via HIV-mediated cell lysis and syncytium formation, immunologic destruction of infected cells, and perhaps other mechanisms,[19] ultimately

results in progressive depletion thereof. As a result, the number of circulating CD4+ T-lymphocytes progressively declines, which is the characteristic immunologic feature of HIV disease. Loss of CD4+ T-lymphocyte function as a result of depletion and of gp120 blockade of the CD4+ receptors (wherein gp120 on circulating virions binds the CD4+ receptor, inhibiting its immunologic function)[19] results in clinically evident disease, manifesting as progressive cellular immunodeficiency, the occurrence of opportunistic complications, and eventually death.

Susceptibility to the characteristic opportunistic complications of HIV infection is strongly related to the level of CD4+ T-lymphocytes in peripheral blood. Therefore, the **CD4+ T-lymphocyte count** can be used to 'stage' HIV infection,[20] enabling the clinician to predict what opportunistic infections a patient is likely to be susceptible to. The CD4+ T-lymphocyte percentage conveys similar information.[8] This predictability allows the use of specific primary antimicrobial prophylaxis in some instances (see below).[21,22] Unfortunately, no cost-effective strategy exists for the primary prevention of **cytomegalovirus (CMV)** retinitis,[23] the most important ocular complication of HIV/AIDS in most settings.

Measurement of the number of copies of HIV RNA in peripheral blood (**HIV 'viral load'**) also

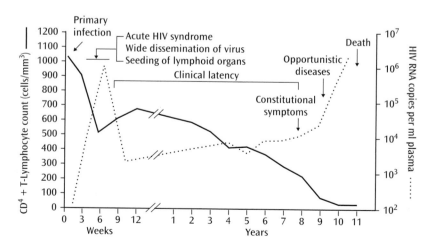

Figure 20.2 *Natural history of human immunodeficiency virus (HIV) infection in an average patient. (Reproduced from Fauci AS. Pantaleo G, Stanley S, Weissman D. Immunopathogenic mechanisms of HIV infection. Ann Intern Med 1996; 124:654–663, with permission.) (Fig 19.4 in 2nd edition)*

has become an important biomarker used in the management of HIV infection. High levels are predictive of more rapid progression to advanced stages of HIV infection, and of higher risk of opportunistic complications and mortality, over and above what would be predicted based on CD4+ T-lymphocyte levels alone.[24] Infectious disease clinicians now primarily rely on the viral load in assessing response to therapy. In settings where measurements of CD4+ T-lymphocyte count and HIV viral load are not economically or technically feasible, clinical staging of HIV/AIDS has been used;[10] the rapid development of laboratory support for HIV treatment programmes makes the need for such an approach unusual now.

20.2.7   Antiretroviral therapy

The first clinical trial demonstrating efficacy of an antiretroviral agent, **zidovudine (AZT)**, was published in 1987, just over three years after HIV was first identified.[25] Subsequently, a large number of antiretroviral agents have been developed and demonstrated to be effective.[26] Currently available agents inhibit either the HIV reverse transcriptase or HIV protease enzymes. Reverse transcriptase inhibitors are divided into competitive and non-competitive inhibitors. **Nucleoside reverse transcriptase inhibitors (NRTI)** are competitive inhibitors of reverse transcriptase. These agents, when used as monotherapy, typically reduce the HIV RNA load by approximately a half to one $\log_{10}$ unit, though newer agents may have higher potency. **Non-nucleoside reverse transcriptase inhibitors (NNRTIs)** covalently bond to reverse transcriptase, causing non-competitive inhibition. Both non-nucleoside reverse transcriptase inhibitors and **protease inhibitors (PIs)** are designated 'highly potent', because monotherapy with these agents results in an initial reduction in the HIV viral load of one to two $\log_{10}$ units. In addition, a **nucleotide reverse transcriptase inhibitor**, tenofovir, has a highly potent antiretroviral effect via competitive inhibition of reverse transcriptase. Three new classes of antiretroviral agents have been developed recently, including an **integrase inhibitor**, raltegravir, a **fusion inhibitor**, enfuvirtide, and a **CCR5 antagonist**, maraviroc.

Early antiretroviral therapy strategies, which involved treatment with one or two NRTIs, typically resulted in the rapid evolution of resistant HIV strains, with loss of benefit within approximately one year. Strains of HIV resistant to nearly all agents have been identified.[27] However, combination treatment with multiple antiretroviral agents, including one or more of the highly potent antiretroviral agents, provided a major breakthrough in treatment of HIV/AIDS. This strategy, so-called **'highly active antiretroviral therapy'** **(HAART)**, was introduced in western countries in the mid-1990s. On average, HAART reduces HIV viral load, increases CD4+ T-lymphocyte counts,[28,29] reduces the risk of opportunistic infections and mortality,[30] and improves quality of life measures.[31] The success of this strategy appears to depend on suppression of HIV replication to extremely low levels. Suppression of replication reduces the number of mutations occurring by reducing the number of replication events, making spontaneous development of a resistant strain less likely. In order to replicate in the presence of several agents with different mechanisms of action, HIV would need to develop several high-level resistance mutations simultaneously, while preserving sufficient enzymatic function to maintain virulence, an unlikely event. Application of antiretroviral therapy is now a specialty of medicine unto itself; regularly updated recommendations are available at http://www.aidsinfo.nih.gov/Guidelines/Default.aspx.

Clinical trials in which patients were treated with HAART have demonstrated that 60% to 90% of patients previously untreated with antiretroviral agents had reduction of the HIV RNA level in peripheral blood to levels below the limits of detection using conventional viral load assays.[28,29] However, in settings where patients' adherence to the often complicated HAART regimen is less complete, substantially lower levels of success may be achieved.[32] Thus, optimizing adherence to HAART regimens is a primary goal of any treatment programme that provides these drugs.

The introduction of HAART has caused a dramatic change in the clinical course of HIV/AIDS

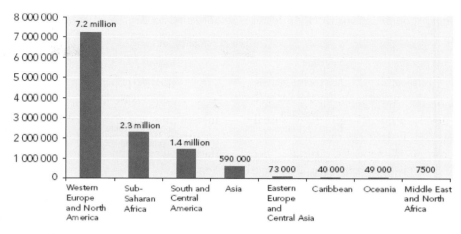

Figure 20.3 *Estimated number of life years added due to antiretroviral therapy, by region, 1996–2008*

everywhere it has been introduced.[1] Efforts by governmental and non-governmental organizations to extend HIV treatment coverage have now increased the proportion of those needing treatment who actually get treated to 42% as of 2008, with the benefits of such therapy now beginning to be enjoyed worldwide (Fig. 20.3). Given that a minority of patients are receiving this life-saving therapy, further work in extending programmes remains a global health priority.

20.2.7.1 Opportunistic infection risk in patients receiving HAART

As noted previously, highly active antiretroviral therapy often reduces the level of HIV RNA in peripheral blood, and increases the CD4+ T-lymphocyte count. The CD4+ T-lymphocyte count is strongly associated with the current risk for opportunistic complications, and therefore serves as the basis for decisions regarding opportunistic infection prophylaxis and treatment. For patients receiving HAART, even those who at one time had severe immunodeficiency, an increase in the CD4+ T-lymphocyte count to levels associated with low risk of an opportunistic infection typically indicates recovery of specific immunity to that pathogen,[33,34] with rare exceptions.[35] The recovery of specific immunity to opportunistic pathogens is gradual, lagging behind the observed CD4+ T-lymphocyte count by as much as three to six months. Therefore, both the extent of the rise in CD4+ T-lymphocyte

count and the duration of the rise need to be considered in deciding when prophylaxis or treatment for opportunistic infections may be discontinued. Comprehensive recommendations regarding these decisions have been provided by an expert panel,[21] and are regularly updated (available at: http://www.aidsinfo.nih.gov/Guidelines/Default.aspx).

20.2.7.2 Complications of antiretroviral therapy

Although the benefits of HAART greatly outweigh the risks in most cases, drug toxicity is a frequent problem, often requiring adjustment of therapy, and sometimes resulting in substantial morbidity. This difficulty requires that providers of care for HIV disease have a high degree of sophistication and laboratory support. The need for sophisticated management presents a substantial logistical problem for the development of antiretroviral therapy programmes in resource-poor settings, because availability of the necessary infrastructure is often limited. Nevertheless, the large amount of effort and resources being expended on programmes to provide antiretroviral treatment are making remarkable progress in overcoming these challenges.

In addition, new disorders, termed '**immune recovery phenomena**' or '**immune recovery inflammatory syndromes**' (IRIS), have been observed in some patients who gain immunologic benefit from HAART after suffering an opportunistic infection

Table 20.2 *Ocular complications of HIV infection: relationship to degree of immunodeficiency**

CD4+ count	Type of complication			
	Vascular	**Infection**	**Tumour**	**Neuro-ophthalmological**
Any (or uncertain)	Large vessel vaso-occlusion	Acute retinal necrosis Disseminated molluscum contagiosum	Squamous cell carcinoma of the conjunctiva	Direct complications of HIV infection
≤ 500 cells/μl		Herpes zoster ophthalmicus	Kaposi's sarcoma Lymphoma	
≤ 200 cells/μl		*Pneumocystis* choroidopathy Ocular tuberculosis Microsporidial keratoconjunctivitis		PML-related complications
≤ 100 cells/μl	HIV retinopathy Conjunctival vasculopathy	CMV retinitis Toxoplasmic retinitis Progressive outer retinal necrosis MAC choroidopathy Cryptococcal choroidopathy		Complications of cryptococcal meningitis (e.g. optic neuropathy)

HIV = human immunodeficiency virus; CMV = cytomegalovirus; MAC = Mycobacterium avium complex.

(which may or may not previously have been recognized). These inflammatory disorders, presumably resulting from immunologic attack on residual pathogens or antigen present in tissue, were first described in the setting of CMV retinitis (see below),[36,37] but have now been described in association with a broad array of HIV-associated co-infections. Such cases can be severe and vision-threatening (Plate 20.2).[38] The topic has been reviewed recently.[39]

20.3   OCULAR COMPLICATIONS OF HIV INFECTION

Ocular complications of AIDS were first reported in 1982,[40] one year after the first report of AIDS. It soon became clear that, at some time during their clinical course, ocular complications of HIV infection occur in the majority of patients. Although only HIV retinopathy and CMV retinitis occur commonly (in most parts of the world), a broad range of ocular complications can occur. The ocular complications of HIV/AIDS can be divided into the following four categories: vascular diseases, ocular opportunistic infections, ocular and adnexal tumours and neuro-ophthalmological lesions (Table 20.2). Some patients also suffer from ocular complications of medical therapies for HIV/AIDS and associated conditions. The clinical presentation

of the various ocular conditions arising in patients with HIV/AIDS is described below according to this categorization scheme (Table 20.2).

20.3.1   Vascular diseases

20.3.1.1   *Human immunodeficiency virus retinopathy*

The most common ocular complication of HIV/AIDS is a retinal microvasculopathy called **HIV retinopathy** (also known as AIDS retinopathy, AIDS-related retinal microvasculopathy, and HIV-related non-infectious vasculopathy). In the pre-HAART era, this condition affected approximately 50% of patients with AIDS as defined using the 1987 CDC revised surveillance case definition.[41] The prevalence has not been reported in the HAART era. HIV retinopathy is characterized by the presence of multiple retinal cotton wool spots and/or dot-blot intraretinal hemorrhages (Plate 20.3, Plate 20.4 — central part of picture). Fluorescein angiographic studies have demonstrated microvascular abnormalities in these areas.[42] Pathological study has demonstrated the typical histological findings of cotton wool spots, without evidence of the presence of viral antigen.[42] Patients with more advanced immunodeficiency, as indicated by the current CD4+ T-lymphocyte count, are more likely to have this complication.[41,43] HIV retinopathy typically does not affect vision to a degree that the patient will notice. Its primary clinical importance is as a sign suggesting that HIV infection may be present, and/or that HIV infection is at an advanced stage. However, there is some evidence to suggest that the cumulative effects of HIV retinopathy lesions might be the cause of subclinical visual deficits that are not infrequent among HIV/AIDS patients.[44] Also, some have suggested that HIV retinopathy may facilitate seeding of the retina by CMV because of breakdown of the blood-retina barrier,[42] which would make the condition important in terms of pathogenesis.

20.3.1.2 Conjunctival vasculopathy

A **conjunctival vasculopathy** has also been described in occasional reports. This condition is described as affecting a large proportion of HIV-infected persons. Findings include segmental vascular dilation, microaneurysms, 'sludging' of the small vessels, and the appearance of comma-shaped blood vessel fragments.[41] The condition seems to have no adverse effects on the eye.

20.3.1.3 Pathogenesis of microvasculopathy in patients with HIV infection

Conjunctival vasculopathy and HIV retinopathy are associated, and might be a manifestation of the same underlying process. Potential mechanisms by which microvasculopathy may occur in patients with HIV infection include deposition of HIV-related immune complexes in vessels, vascular injury caused by direct infection of the vascular endothelium by HIV, increased plasma viscosity leading to rheologic abnormalities, and/or combinations thereof.[45] In one study, the presence and severity of conjunctival vasculopathy and of retinal cotton wool spots were each associated with higher levels of fibrinogen in peripheral blood, manifesting a dose-response relationship.[45] As patients with advanced HIV survive longer in the era of HAART, it is conceivable that a larger number could develop clinically important complications of

microvascular disease, as occurs in other chronic diseases, such as diabetes mellitus.

20.3.1.4 Large-vessel vaso-occlusive disease

Retinal vascular occlusions, primarily venous occlusions, were observed in 1.3% of a series of approximately 2,500 patients with HIV infection sent for ophthalmic screening. Typical complications included retinal neovascularization, vitreous haemorrhage and optic atrophy, with approximately 40% of eyes losing vision to the level of 20/200 or less. HIV retinopathy was a strong risk factor for occurrence of retinal vascular occlusions (OR 5.76, 95% CI 2.59–12.80).[46] Further work is needed to confirm whether retinal vascular occlusions occur at higher rates in patients with HIV infection, and if so, by what pathogenic mechanism.

20.3.2 Opportunistic infections of the eye and ocular adnexae

20.3.2.1 Anterior segment and adnexal diseases

Herpes zoster ophthalmicus

Varicella zoster virus (VZV) is a member of the *Herpesviridae* family, subclass alpha, the same group as the herpes simplex viruses. Alpha herpes viruses characteristically reproduce quickly, destroying infected cells in the process.[47] For VZV, latency — characteristic of all herpes viruses — develops in nerve ganglia, from which the virus may re-emerge under favourable conditions. Infection with VZV is ubiquitous, probably affecting the majority of persons in most populations. Infection is acquired through contact with an active lesion or via inhalation. Infection is preventable by a live, attenuated vaccine, licensed for use in immunocompetent persons.[48]

Varicella zoster virus causes varicella (chickenpox), a self-limiting exanthem that typically resolves without sequelae, and rarely involves the eye. However, approximately 20% of infected persons will develop **herpes zoster** years later, most typically characterized by a unilateral dermatomal rash similar to that of chickenpox, often followed by neuralgia. The duration and/or severity of the clinical symptoms of herpes zoster are reduced, on average, by therapy using the antiviral agents acyclovir (aciclovir), valacyclovir (valaciclovir) or famciclovir.[48] A vaccine to prevent occurrence of herpes zoster is now available, and was shown to be safe, but only modestly immunogenic among HIV-infected patients with CD4+ T-cell counts ≥ 400 cells/μL.[49]

Because varicella is typically acquired in childhood, primary VZV infection rarely complicates HIV/AIDS. However, herpes zoster occurs with high frequency in patients with HIV infection. It tends to occur relatively early in the course of HIV infection, often when the CD4+ T-lymphocyte count is higher than 200 cells/μL. Hence, herpes zoster is not considered an AIDS-defining opportunistic infection, even though its higher rate of occurrence in patients with HIV infection strongly suggests a causal relationship. Occurrence of herpes zoster in a middle-aged or younger person is interpreted by many as an indication for HIV testing, and may precipitate the initial diagnosis of HIV infection.

Ocular complications are amongst the most frequent major sequelae of herpes zoster in patients with HIV infection.[50] Involvement of the first division of the trigeminal nerve is a frequent presentation of herpes zoster, known as **herpes zoster ophthalmicus (HZO)**, in both HIV-positive and HIV-negative individuals. Approximately 3–4% of HIV-infected patients develop HZO,[41,51] with a similar frequency of occurrence in patients with AIDS and earlier stages of HIV disease. The high frequency of HZO makes it a leading ocular complication of HIV/AIDS in the parts of the world where its incidence has been evaluated, although with more widespread availability of HAART — which reduces the risk of herpes zoster[52] — it is likely that the incidence has declined. Ocular complications of HZO occur in one half to two thirds of cases of HZO in HIV-infected patients, including stromal and neurotrophic keratitis, chronic infectious pseudodendritic keratitis, anterior uveitis, scleritis, ocular hypertension and, less commonly, retinitis.[41,51] Post-herpetic neuralgia seems to be less frequent in HIV-infected patients, but is still an important problem. Infectious retinitis caused by VZV can present as two distinct syndromes, acute retinal necrosis and progressive outer retinal necrosis (see Section 20.3.2.2).

Molluscum contagiosum

Molluscum contagiosum is an exanthem caused by a poxvirus, *Molluscum contagiosum*. Infection is transmitted sexually, or through direct contact. Classically, molluscum contagiosum infection presents as a small number of painless, elevated, round, pearly-white lesions about 2–4 mm in size, with central umbilication. When located around the eyes, a follicular conjunctivitis, or less frequently a superficial keratitis, may occur. In HIV-infected persons, but not in immunologically normal persons, molluscum contagiosum lesions can become large and disseminated, in some cases leading to cosmetic disfigurement. Therefore, widespread molluscum contagiosum suggests the possibility of HIV infection. Individual molluscum contagiosum lesions usually are cleared easily by currettage, excision, cryotherapy or other techniques. However, the disseminated presentation occasionally occurring in HIV-infected persons is difficult to clear by conventional techniques. Presently, treatment with HAART is the mainstay of therapy for disseminated molluscum contagiosum.

Infectious keratoconjunctivitis

Infections of the cornea are unusual in patients with HIV infection, except in the context of HZO (see above). However, some HIV-related anterior segment infections occur.

Microsporidial keratoconjunctivitis, although rare, appears to be related to HIV infection, based on a report of spontaneous clearance of the condition in a patient receiving HAART who had immunologic improvement.[53] Symptoms of ocular surface infection with this obligate intracellular protozoan include redness, mild pain, photophobia and foreign body sensation. Diagnosis is based on light and electron microscopy of conjunctival scrapings. Successful treatment with corneal debridement and oral itraconazole, topical fumigillin, or topical propamidine isethionate, and albendazole has been reported, but it is unclear whether all cases are cured — some may require suppressive therapy.[54]

Herpes simplex keratitis does not appear to occur with higher frequency in patients with HIV infection.[55] However, some evidence suggests that the clinical course of herpes simplex keratitis may be altered by HIV, in that severe or atypical presentations may occur.[56]

Although bacterial and fungal infections of the cornea do not appear to occur with higher frequency among patients with HIV infection living in temperate countries unless local predisposing factors are present, fungal corneal infections have been associated with HIV infection in Africa.[57]

20.3.2.2 *Posterior segment diseases*

20.3.2.2.1 *Cytomegalovirus retinitis*

i) *Virology of cytomegalovirus*

Cytomegalovirus (CMV) is an enveloped, double-stranded DNA virus, which is a member of the *Herpesviridae* family, subfamily beta. It is the largest known virus to infect humans. After entry into the cell, its genome is transported to the cell nucleus, where activity of the viral molecular machinery creates the characteristic intranuclear inclusions that are visible histopathologically. The virus reproduces by budding from infected cells.

Latency allows CMV infection to persist in an infected host until death. The site of CMV latency is not well characterized. Viral genes directly code for proteins that down-regulate the human immune system, which may be an important mechanism permitting latency,[58] and may have other immunologic effects that are adverse to the host. Most CMV disease in patients with HIV/AIDS is thought to arise from reactivation of latent virus from a previous infection.

Cytomegalovirus is ubiquitous, with 40–100% rates of seroprevalence at sites throughout the world.[59] Cytomegalovirus can be transmitted in semen, cervical secretions, saliva, infected blood products, transplanted organs and perhaps through other pathways. Patients with HIV/AIDS have been found to have higher seroprevalence of CMV than comparison groups,[60] probably because both CMV and HIV are often sexually transmitted infections.

ii) *Epidemiology and regional variation*

In the absence of HAART, cytomegalovirus disease is one of the leading opportunistic complications of HIV/AIDS.[30] The presentation of CMV disease includes retinitis in 71–85% of cases,[61,62] making **CMV retinitis** the most common opportunistic ocular infection, and the most common intraocular infection among patients with AIDS, even in the HAART era.[63] Because of its profound effects on vision[64] and strong association with early mortality,[65] CMV retinitis is the clinically most important ocular complication of HIV/AIDS in nearly all regions of the world.

Cytomegalovirus retinitis occurs most frequently in patients with very advanced immunodeficiency. In industrialized Western countries in the pre-HAART era, the incidence rate for CMV retinitis was estimated to be 10% per year for patients with CD4+ T-lymphocyte counts $\leq$ 100 cells/μL, and 20% per year for those with CD4+ T-lymphocyte counts $\leq$ 50 cells/μL.[62] Therefore, CMV retinitis is an indicator of advanced AIDS. However, the occurrence of CMV retinitis is associated with a substantially increased risk of mortality with respect to that observed in patients with advanced AIDS who otherwise have similar clinical characteristics.[66] Recent data have demonstrated that treatment of patients with CMV retinitis and AIDS using systemic anti-CMV medication reduces mortality.[65,67] This observation suggests that CMV disease itself directly or indirectly increases mortality risk. Potential mechanisms of this effect include transactivation of HIV by CMV,[68] and direct pathological effects of extraocular CMV disease, which is often present, but not recognized, in patients with AIDS and CMV retinitis.[69]

In the pre-HAART era, it was estimated that 30% of patients with HIV/AIDS would develop CMV retinitis during their lifetime.[61] The incidence of CMV retinitis in the USA in the HAART era has declined to approximately 5.6 cases/100 person-years among patients with AIDS.[63] However, new cases continue to occur in patients who are HAART-naive (who still constitute the majority of patients with HIV infection for whom treatment is indicated) or who respond poorly to antiretroviral therapy. Even though it appears the lifetime incidence of CMV retinitis will drop in patients who receive HAART, the number of cases is likely to rise as the prevalence of HIV/AIDS continues to rise.

In most parts of the world where HAART is (or was) not in use, the risk of CMV retinitis appears to be similar to that reported in the pre-HAART era in the USA.[70–76] Early reports from Sub-Saharan Africa, where the majority of HIV-infected persons live, indicated relatively few cases of CMV retinitis, possibly because HIV-infected persons in Sub-Saharan Africa were dying at earlier stages of HIV disease, with few reaching the advanced state of immunodeficiency at which CMV retinitis occurs.[77] However, as conditions improve, anecdotal and published[78–81] reports suggest that the number of CMV retinitis cases in Sub-Saharan Africa is substantial in places where ophthalmic evaluations are performed in patients with advanced AIDS, suggesting that failure to make the diagnosis is also a factor in the putatively lower incidence of CMV retinitis in this region.[80]

iii) *Clinical characteristics of CMV retinitis*
CMV retinitis may be reliably diagnosed by an experienced observer using indirect ophthalmoscopy through a dilated pupil. Diagnosis is based on the characteristic picture of necrotizing retinitis with or without intraretinal hemorrhage, with either granular or oedematous white borders (Plate 20.4 [left side], Plate 20.5).[41] In the absence of immune recovery or successful anti-CMV therapy, relentless progression occurs along the leading edge of retinal necrosis over several weeks to months, eventually leading to total retinal destruction and blindness.[82]

iv) *Anti-CMV therapy*
The several effective treatments for CMV retinitis (Table 20.3) may be categorized as systemic and local treatments respectively. Agents approved for by the United States Food and Drug Administration (**FDA**) for systemic treatment of CMV retinitis include intravenous **ganciclovir**, **foscarnet**, **cidofovir**, oral ganciclovir and

valganciclovir (a pro-drug of ganciclovir with higher oral bioavailability). Each is effective in suppressing cytomegalovirus replication and arresting progression of the retinitis. However, in the absence of immune recovery, suspension of suppressive anti-CMV therapy results in reactivation of CMV and progression of retinitis, leading to the concept that lifelong 'maintenance' suppressive anti-CMV therapy is needed. Furthermore, even with continued systemic maintenance therapy, progression of retinitis typically occurs, in the absence of immune recovery, often after a two to three month interval. The oral formulation of ganciclovir, which is approved only for maintenance therapy after induction with intravenous ganciclovir, appears to be associated with a shorter time to progression of retinitis than intravenous ganciclovir, presumably because of lower bioavailability.[83]

It appears that most progressions of CMV retinitis occur because relatively low levels of the drugs are achieved in the retina with systemically administered maintenance therapy after the blood–retina barrier has been restored by healing of the CMV retinitis lesion(s). This theory is supported by evidence that the level of anti-CMV medication achieved in the vitreous is near the inhibitory dose, 50% (IC_{50}) for CMV,[84] and by the observation that progression of retinitis typically can be controlled by 'reinduction' (temporarily doubling the frequency of dosage) using the same systemic anti-CMV agent.[85] However, resistance to anti-CMV agents, which occurs in about one fourth of cases within nine months' treatment,[86] appears to play an important role in progressions occurring later in the course of disease (Table 20.3).

In addition to the problem of progression after increasingly shorter intervals, each of the systemic anti-CMV agents has the potential for systemic side effects (Table 20.3). Furthermore, because intravenous ganciclovir and foscarnet require daily intravenous therapy through an indwelling central venous catheter, they are associated with increased risk of life-threatening catheter infections.[87] The extent of expertise and supervision required to use these agents, along with their high costs, limits their use in many countries. Valganciclovir, the most attractive drug from a health systems perspective due to its oral administration, remains

Table 20.3 *Anti-cytomegalovirus therapies**

	Induction dose	Maintenance dose	Price**	Major side effects
Systemic				
Intravenous				
Ganciclovir	5 mg/kg i.v. bid × 2–3 weeks	5 mg/kg qd	$927.43	Bone marrow suppression, line infection
Foscarnet	60 mg/kg i.v. tid × 2–3 weeks	90–120 mg/kg qd	$1,818.52	Nephrotoxicity, line infections
Cidofovir	5 mg/kg i.v. weekly × 2 weeks	5 mg/kg qowk	$804.00	Nephrotoxicity, uveitis, hypotony
Oral				
Ganciclovir	—	1,000 mg tid	$1,541.58	Bone marrow suppression
Valganciclovir	900 mg bid	900 mg qd	$1,438.80	Bone marrow suppression
Local				
Intravitreous, surgical				
Ganciclovir implant	Placement	Placement q6–8 mo	$1,072.43	Surgical complications
Intravitreous, injections				
Ganciclovir***	2000 μg, 2/week × 3 weeks	2000 μg weekly	NA	Procedural complications
Foscarnet***	2400 μg, 2/week × 3 weeks	2400 μg twice weekly	NA	Procedural complications
Cidofovir***	(?)15 μg	?	NA	Procedural complications, uveitis, hypotony
Fomivirsen	330 μg qowk × 2	330 μg q4wk	$1607.14	Procedural complications, pigmentary retinal degeneration, uveitis

* i.v. = intravenous; bid = twice daily; qd = once daily; tid = three times daily; qowk = every other week; q4wk = every four weeks; q6–8 mo = every 6–8 months; Price = US average wholesale price (2001 US dollars) for 30 days' therapy (as of Nov 15, 2001); NA = not available.

** The price given includes only acquisition costs for drug. Local therapy costs are calculated assuming 1.5 eyes require treatment per patient.

*** Intravitreous use of ganciclovir, foscarnet and cidofovir, except for the ganciclovir implant, is not approved by the US Food and Drug Administration, and is therefore investigational therapy.

Source: *2001 Drug Topics Red Book. Medical Economics*. Montvale, NJ: Thomson Healthcare; 2001. (Except valganciclovir pricing: http://www.rocheusa.com/programs/TradeNews/Valcyteintroductionwholesaler.doc [accessed 11-15-01].)

exceptionally expensive, but will go off patent in 2014, after which pricing will likely change so as to permit more widespread use.

An alternative to systemic therapy for CMV retinitis is the use of local anti-CMV therapy. Local therapy was proposed for CMV retinitis based on the assumption that few patients have extraocular activity of CMV disease, and also because of recognition that low intravitreous drug levels are obtained with systemic therapy. However, the recent emergence of evidence that systemic anti-CMV therapy improves survival[65,67] suggests that systemic therapy also should be used, even if local therapy is being used. **Intravitreous injection** of each of the agents approved for intravenous anti-CMV therapy has been reported, though none is approved by regulatory agencies for that purpose. Intravitreous ganciclovir (2 mg/0.1 mL, two doses weekly for three weeks then weekly)[88] and foscarnet (2.4 mg/0.1 mL two doses weekly for three weeks then weekly)[89] usually succeed in controlling retinitis. However, repetitive injections are required, each with the risk of endophthalmitis and of other local ocular complications, and progressions may occur despite maintenance intravitreous therapy. Intravitreous cidofovir is similarly effective in controlling retinitis, and has the attractive properties of a long duration of action (one injection appears to work for several weeks), and long-term stability in cold storage.[90] These properties might make intravitreous cidofovir an attractive form of anti-CMV therapy in resource-limited countries. However, the high risk of uveitis and hypotony,[91] which also occur with systemically administered cidofovir (see below),[92] have limited use of this therapy by most (but not all) clinicians. Fomivirsen, an antisense compound that was FDA-approved for intravitreous treatment of CMV retinitis in practice, was rarely used and is no longer available.

Although intravitreous injections are used widely for immediate treatment of vision-threatening CMV retinitis, they seldom are used in the USA for long-term maintenance therapy. In contrast, in developing countries, and even in South Africa and Singapore, repetitive intravitreous injection is the standard of care for CMV retinitis on the basis of cost considerations.

A **ganciclovir implant** — a reservoir of ganciclovir surrounded by a semi-permeable membrane, which is surgically implanted through the pars plana into the posterior segment of the eye — is also available for CMV retinitis. As long as drug remains in the implant, ganciclovir in solution filters out of the implant, maintaining nearly constant intravitreous levels of ganciclovir that is four to five times higher than the level obtained with systemic therapy.[93,94] The time to progression of retinitis in eyes treated with ganciclovir implants is similar to the expected duration of effect of the implant, i.e. about six to eight months.[95] Implant therapy is sometimes effective for management of retinitis that has progressed under systemic ganciclovir therapy, presumably because higher intravitreous and intraretinal ganciclovir levels are obtained.[96] However, this therapy is now infrequently used due to preference for valganciclovir in developed countries and high expense in developing countries.

Local therapy for CMV retinitis is associated with a higher rate of second eye and visceral CMV disease than occurs among patients treated with systemic therapy. In the pre-HAART era, the estimated rates of second eye retinitis and of visceral disease within six months among patients treated

with local therapy alone were 50% and 30% respectively,[94] about double that in patients receiving systemic anti-CMV therapy.[97] The higher rate of mortality observed in patients not receiving systemic anti-CMV therapy[65,67] provides another strong indication for use of systemic anti-CMV therapy in conjunction with local therapy. Given that valganciclovir is likely a superior therapy for CMV disease vis-à-vis intravitreous injections, taking into account its systemic and preventive benefits, efforts should be made to reduce its cost so that it could be made widely available in HIV programmes, as has been done with some other HIV-related drugs.

v) *Retinal detachment in CMV retinitis*

Rhegmatogenous **retinal detachment** is a common complication of CMV retinitis in patients who continue to have severe immunodeficiency, occurring during the pre-HAART era in about one third of eyes with CMV retinitis per year.[41] Risk factors for retinal detachment include involvement of the anterior retina in the area of the vitreous base, large lesion size, lower CD4+ T-lymphocyte count, current activity of retinitis, lack of current anti-CMV treatment, and lack of use of HAART (see below).[98,99] Retinal breaks leading to retinal detachment in eyes with CMV retinitis tend to be posteriorly located, difficult to visualize and numerous. The breaks are often located at the junction of 'healed' and actively inflamed retina. As a result of these characteristics, management using conventional retinal detachment repair methods often fails, in the absence of immune recovery. Therefore, for patients expected to have persistent severe immunodeficiency, repair of retinal detachments in eyes with CMV retinitis is typically approached by vitrectomy techniques using silicone oil tamponade. Although this method of repair typically succeeds in re-attaching the retina, visual outcomes often deteriorate over a period of months after an initial improvement. Factors that contribute to this deterioration include the rapid development of cataract after silicone oil placement[100] and refractive disturbances at oil interfaces.[101] Optic atrophy in eyes filled with silicone oil has been reported,[102] but no mechanism by which silicone oil might cause such optic atrophy is known.

The high incidence of retinal detachment in patients with CMV retinitis who continue to have severe immunodeficiency, combined with poor outcomes and high management costs, make retinal detachment a major clinical problem in this setting.

vi) *Clinical outcomes of CMV retinitis*

Cytomegalovirus retinitis is the leading cause of vision loss among patients with HIV/AIDS in most settings. Vision loss may occur as a result of full-thickness retinal necrosis affecting the macula and/or optic nerve,[41] retinal detachment[99] and, in the HAART era, immune recovery uveitis[103] (see below). In one series, visual acuity was found to be at or below the level of 6/15 and 6/60 by the time CMV retinitis was diagnosed in 33% and 17% of eyes respectively with retinitis.[64] Even in eyes receiving anti-CMV treatment that present with preserved visual acuity, the incidence of vision loss is high. Approximately one third of eyes with CMV retinitis will lose visual acuity to a level of 6/15 or worse, and one fourth to a level of 6/60 or worse, by one year after CMV retinitis diagnosis.[41,64] Risk factors for loss of visual acuity include large initial lesion size (i.e. more advanced disease at the time of diagnosis), posterior lesion location (near the optic nerve and macula) and non-use of HAART.[64] As mentioned previously, retinal detachment occurs at a high rate in this setting, and often has a poor visual outcome.[98]

Fortunately, outcomes of CMV retinitis have improved with the introduction of HAART. Restoration of specific immunity to CMV in patients receiving HAART, which has been directly demonstrated,[34] is presumably the major factor underlying improved outcomes, though other factors may also contribute. It is now well established that most patients who experience a sustained rise in the CD4+ T-lymphocyte count to a level of 100 to 150 cells/μL, in response to HAART for a period of three to six months, can discontinue anti-CMV maintenance therapy without experiencing retinitis relapse, as long as the CD4+ T-lymphocyte count remains above 50–100 cells/μL.[104] (In practice, most clinicians managing CMV retinitis with repetitive intravitreous injections stop treatment much sooner than this.) Risk of loss of visual acuity

is reduced by approximately one half in eyes of patients who receive HAART but do not have immune recovery, and by 80–90% in eyes of patients with immune recovery.[64] Use of HAART is also associated with a reduction by approximately one half in the risk of retinal detachment for eyes of patients on HAART but without immune recovery, and by approximately two thirds in those with immune recovery.[98]

In addition to improved outcomes, effective antiretroviral therapy has given rise to the syndrome of **immune recovery uveitis (IRU)**. IRU presumably results from immune responses to residual CMV antigen remaining in the retina,[37] causing symptoms of floaters and decreased vision in a subset of patients with CMV retinitis who experience immune recovery in response to HAART. Patients are only at risk of IRU in the eye with retinitis; eyes without CMV retinitis are rarely if ever affected. In a multicentre study, the point prevalence of IRU in patients with CMV retinitis was 15.5%.[105] Reported complications of IRU include macular oedema, epiretinal membrane formation, neovascularization and vitreous haemorrhage, papillitis, posterior subcapsular cataract, posterior synechiae, and intraocular lens deposits.[103,106,107] Of these, only macular oedema, epiretinal membrane formation, and cataract seem to occur commonly. Although severe vision loss has been reported,[103] most patients have mild to moderate vision loss. Treatment with multiple sub-Tenon injections of methylprednisolone in polyethylene glycol was associated with improvement of vision by at least two lines in four of five eyes in one, small series.[36] Unfortunately, recurrence of vision loss is frequent after the depot of corticosteroid dissipates.

20.3.2.2.2   *The acute retinal necrosis and progressive outer retinal necrosis syndromes*

Varicella zoster virus and, less commonly, **herpes simplex viruses (HSV)**, are capable of causing necrotizing retinitis in immunocompetent persons, which manifests as the **acute retinal necrosis syndrome (ARN)**.[108] This syndrome is characterized by one or more foci of discretely bounded necrotizing retinitis in the retinal periphery, associated with arteriolar occlusion and a prominent vitreous and anterior chamber inflammatory reaction (Plate 20.4 [left side]). Rapid spread, at least partly in a circumferential pattern, should be observed for the diagnosis to be confirmed.[109] The diagnosis can occur in immunocompetent patients, but the syndrome is more frequent in immunodeficient persons, including patients with HIV/AIDS. However, it seems to occur in fewer than 1% of patients, much less frequently than CMV retinitis.[41] Patients with HIV/AIDS suffering from herpes zoster ophthalmicus appear to have higher risk of necrotizing retinitis during the several months following the onset of the exanthem.[110]

Patients with HIV/AIDS are also at risk for **progressive outer retinal necrosis syndrome (PORNS)**, which is characterized by multifocal areas of opacification that appear to be located deep in the retina; lack of granular borders such as seen in CMV retinitis; minimal inflammatory reaction; and rapid progression.[111] In one study, VZV was identified in 13 out of 16 cases, suggesting that VZV is the predominant cause of this syndrome.[112] While acute retinal necrosis syndrome seems to occur at a variety of CD4+ T-lymphocyte levels in patients with HIV/AIDS, PORN syndrome occurs in patients with advanced AIDS, typically with a CD4+ T-lymphocyte count less than 50 cells/μL.

The ARN syndrome usually is clinically responsive to acyclovir therapy.[41] The progressive outer retinal necrosis syndrome is often non-responsive to single agent anti-herpetic therapy, rapidly progressing to confluent retinal necrosis with blindness.[111] However, small case series have suggested that control of PORN syndrome can sometimes be achieved with combination antiviral therapy, usually with foscarnet combined with acyclovir or ganciclovir.[113] For both syndromes, discontinuation of suppressive therapy in patients with HIV/AIDS may result, in the absence of immune recovery, in reactivation of retinitis. Both conditions are associated with a 50% or greater retinal detachment risk,[108,111] even higher than the very high level of risk observed with CMV retinitis.

It is unclear what factors determine the phenotype of necrotizing retinitis that is manifested in a given patient with VZV or HSV retinitis, though immunologic factors seem likely candidates. One report, in which the ARN syndrome was present in one eye, and PORN syndrome was simultaneously present in the fellow eye,[114] suggests that the syndromes may overlap. The question as to why PORN syndrome occurs exclusively in patients with HIV/AIDS remains to be explained, but perhaps severe immunodeficiency interferes with the inflammatory reaction to retinal necrosis, resulting in the less inflammatory phenotype of PORN instead of classic ARN syndrome.

20.3.2.2.3 Toxoplasmic retinitis

Chronic infections with *Toxoplasma gondii*, an obligate intracellular protozoan, occur throughout the world. Few extra-ocular infections are serious in immunocompetent adults. However, retinitis — though usually self-limiting in immunocompetent individuals — can cause clinically important ocular morbidity.

In contrast, toxoplasmosis may be a life-threatening infection in patients with HIV/AIDS. Seropositivity for *T. gondii* has been observed in a high proportion of patients with HIV/AIDS at locations throughout the world. Among patients with advanced AIDS who are seropositive for *T. gondii*, **central nervous system** (**CNS**) toxoplasmosis is a common cause of space-occupying brain lesions.[115] Prophylaxis against toxoplasmosis is recommended for patients with AIDS and a CD4+ T-lymphocyte count of less than 100 cells/μL who are seropositive for *T. gondii*.[104]

Toxoplasmic retinitis is less common than toxoplasmic encephalitis among patients with HIV/AIDS, but it is perhaps the second most common intraocular infection in this group, affecting about 1% of patients with AIDS in the USA.[41] Reports from France[116] and Brazil[117] suggest that the proportion affected may be higher in more highly endemic settings (3% and 4.4% in these sites respectively). A recent report from Uganda found toxoplasmic retinitis to be as common a cause of vision loss as CMV retinitis among patients with HIV/AIDS presenting for anti-retroviral therapy.[78] Radiological imaging of the head is indicated when diagnosis of toxoplasmic retinitis is made in a patient with HIV/AIDS, because a high proportion of these patients will have concurrent CNS toxoplasmosis (56% in one series).[41]

The clinical presentation of toxoplasmic retinitis in patients with HIV/AIDS may appear similar to that in non-HIV infected patients, most commonly manifesting as a focal necrotizing retinitis with overlying vitreous inflammation. However, patients with HIV may have diffuse or multifocal lesions, involvement of both eyes, and relatively little vitreous inflammation, features that are atypical in immunocompetent patients.[118] Such variations in the clinical presentation can make diagnosis of toxoplasmic retinitis challenging in the setting of HIV/AIDS, particularly advanced AIDS. However, conventional combination antibiotic therapy is typically successful once the diagnosis has been made.[41,118] Chronic suppressive secondary prophylaxis for toxoplasmosis appears to be indicated in patients with HIV/AIDS who do not experience substantial immune recovery after diagnosis of ocular toxoplasmosis, because reactivation of retinitis may occur when therapy for toxoplasmosis is withdrawn.[118] Oral corticosteroid therapy, sometimes used as an adjunctive treatment in immunocompetent patients with toxoplasmic retinitis to reduce 'innocent bystander damage' to the retina, appears to be unnecessary in patients with HIV/AIDS.

20.3.2.2.4 Ocular syphilis

The incidence of syphilis is expected to be higher in patients with HIV infection than in persons without HIV infection, because both syphilis and HIV disease often are sexually transmitted. Therefore, it is difficult to evaluate whether syphilitic eye disease is opportunistic in patients with HIV infection. One series, from an HIV/AIDS ophthalmology clinic located in a community with a relatively high prevalence of syphilis, diagnosed ocular syphilis in 1% of patients with HIV infection in the pre-HAART era.[41] Among those diagnosed with ocular syphilis, ten had uveitis and five had optic neuropathy. However, in another large series of patients with

and without HIV infection, ocular syphilis was similarly rare in both groups.[55] Because a high proportion of HIV-infected patients with ocular syphilis have neurosyphilis,[119] and because of the blood–ocular barrier, patients with ocular syphilis require neurosyphilis-dose antibiotic therapy, and serial follow-up to ensure an adequate and sustained clinical response.

20.3.2.2.5 Infectious choroidopathy

Clinically manifest infections of the choroid are rare in patients with AIDS (< 1%),[41] but are important because they serve as indicators of disseminated opportunistic infections, which are often fatal in the absence of treatment.[120] Choroidal granulomas in a patient with AIDS due to *Mycobacterium avium* **complex (MAC)** were first reported in 1983.[42] However, despite the relatively high prevalence of disseminated *M. avium* disease in patients with AIDS, choroidal manifestations have only been reported occasionally.

Tuberculosis, probably the most common opportunistic infection in patients with HIV disease worldwide, nevertheless seems to manifest itself in the eye rarely among patients with HIV/AIDS, affecting 1.95% in one tertiary series, with the most common presentations being choroidal granulomas (53%) and subretinal abscesses (37%).[121]

Leprosy is another mycobacterial disease that frequently affects the eye. However, reports of an increased incidence of ocular complications of leprosy in patients with HIV infection are rare in the literature, perhaps because the slow rate of reproduction of *M. leprae* does not allow it to be as effective an opportunistic pathogen as organisms with shorter generation times.

More common, but still rare, has been *Pneumocystis jirovecii* **choroidopathy** (formerly known as *Pneumocystis carinii*), which presents with multiple round or oval yellow-white, plaque-like choroidal lesions, without associated intraocular inflammation. These lesions are 300–3,000 μm in size, usually increasing in number until effective treatment is initiated, after which they decrease in size and number, or disappear entirely.[122] Most cases have been observed in patients receiving inhaled pentamidine rather than systemic medication as prophylaxis against *Pneumocystis* pneumonia, providing evidence that a systemic pneumocystosis was present despite the absence of pneumonia symptoms.[122] The worldwide effort to implement systemic *Pneumocystis* prophylaxis for patients with advanced immunodeficiency appeared to reduce the number of *Pneumocystis* choroidopathy cases, which became even rarer in developed countries following the widespread adoption of HAART.

Another infectious agent which rarely causes choroidopathy is *Cryptococcus neoformans*.[41,123] The few reports of **cryptococcal choroidopathy** have usually been on patients known to have cryptococcal meningitis. The choroidopathy does not usually give rise to symptoms, but the associated systemic disease is life-threatening.

20.3.3   Tumours of the eye and ocular adnexae

20.3.3.1   *Kaposi's sarcoma*

Kaposi's sarcoma (KS), a vascular tumour, was one of the earliest identified complications of AIDS. The epidemiology of KS resembles that of a sexually transmitted disease, which gave rise to the hypothesis that KS is a complication of an infectious disease. There is now strong evidence that KS is caused by **Human Herpesvirus 8 (HHV-8)**: HHV-8 can be isolated from KS tissue;[124] seroconversion precedes the occurrence of KS;[125] and seroconversion is highly predictive of development of KS.[126] As a result, HHV-8 sometimes is called the Kaposi's sarcoma-associated virus.

In the pre-HAART era, ocular adnexal Kaposi's sarcoma was found in 2% of patients with HIV infection presenting to an AIDS ophthalmology clinic (16% of those with HIV infection and a diagnosis of KS at any site).[41] Ocular adnexal KS is typically manifested as a discrete violaceous subconjunctival lesion, or as a similarly coloured eyelid nodule (Plate 20.6).[42] The clinical course is often minimally symptomatic, and slowly progressive. Symptoms, if they occur, may include irritation, trichiasis, obstruction of the visual axis by the tumour, and recurrent haemorrhages. Treatment is

indicated when lesions interfere with vision or cause cosmetic deformity. Radiation therapy,[127] excision,[128] and cryotherapy[128] appear to be successful treatment strategies, although recurrences sometimes occur. Lesions may also regress with systemic chemotherapy or immune recovery resulting from HAART.[129]

The incidence of KS among patients with HIV infection appears to have declined substantially since 1990 in developed countries, even before the introduction of HAART.[130] Clinical impression suggests that the frequency of ocular KS has similarly declined. The explanation for these declines in incidence is uncertain, because the prevalence of HHV-8 infection does not seem to have declined during this period.[131] Perhaps strains prone to induce KS became less common after that point.

20.3.3.2   *Lymphoma*

Although central nervous system lymphoma is an important opportunistic complication of HIV infection, often related to Epstein–Barr virus infection,[132] **ocular** and **orbital lymphomas** are very rare in patients with HIV infection,[41] so that it is unclear whether such tumours do or do not constitute opportunistic complications of HIV/AIDS.[55]

20.3.3.3   *Squamous neoplasia of the conjunctiva*

An epidemic of **ocular surface squamous neoplasia**, including its most extreme form **squamous cell carcinoma of the conjunctiva**, has been described in parts of Africa, coincident with the HIV epidemic, so that this condition has become the most common ocular tumour in Africa.[133] Over 70% of patients with this condition were found to be HIV positive, as opposed to 16% of controls (OR 13 at the Uganda site, risk attributable to HIV = 66%).[134]

One potential explanation of this outbreak is that **human papillomavirus infection (HPV)** and/or other viruses may be causing opportunistic squamous neoplasia in the setting of HIV infection. Advanced HIV infection (CD4+ T-lymphocyte count of less than 200 cells/μL) has been shown to be associated with high HPV viral load and a ten-fold higher risk of cervical intraepithelial neoplasia in HIV-infected women.[135] In Uganda, infection of conjunctival squamous neoplastic tissue with cutaneous forms of human papillomaviruses (most commonly types 5 and 8) was observed in 45% of specimens, supporting a potential role of HPV in the aetiology of this condition for some, but apparently not all, cases.[136] A recent study also identified a range of other potentially oncogenic viruses in squamous cell carcinoma specimens from HIV/AIDS patients.[133] Squamous cell carcinoma of the conjunctiva is rare in developed countries, all of which are located in temperate zones. This gives rise to the hypothesis that the higher degree of irradiance in the tropics is a risk factor for squamous conjunctival neoplasia.[133] However, there has not been a description of an epidemic of similar extent in tropical regions outside of Africa, and the way in which HIV infection and the irradiance would interact is unclear.

20.3.4   Neuro-ophthalmological lesions

Patients with HIV/AIDS are at risk of opportunistic infections and neoplasms affecting the central nervous system and meninges, and of direct neurologic injury from HIV itself. These conditions can cause damage to the optic nerve, other cranial nerves, motor centres and visual pathways, resulting in **neuro-ophthalmological** complications. In one USA AIDS ophthalmology clinic series, neuro-ophthalmological lesions were observed in 6% of patients with AIDS (1987 CDC definition). Such lesions were present in a substantially larger percentage of patients with AIDS than in those with less advanced HIV disease (p = 0.008).[41] In addition, subclinical abnormalities of saccades and, less frequently, smooth pursuits, have been noted in a large proportion of HIV-infected patients. These abnormalities correlated with the degree of cognitive impairment but not the clinical stage or CD4+ T-lymphocyte level.[137] These **subclinical neuro-ophthalmological abnormalities** may result from a direct HIV infection, perhaps arising from the same process that gives rise to HIV-related dementia. It is unclear whether similar mechanisms give rise to detectable visual function disturbances in patients with HIV/AIDS who appear free of retinal diseases,[44] whether episodes of HIV retinopathy cause cumulative injury, or both.

In the series described above, approximately one half of the clinically evident neuro-ophthalmological lesions in patients from AIDS arose from **cryptococcal meningitis**, and one fourth of patients, with AIDS and cryptococcal meningitis presenting to the eye clinic, had ophthalmic complications.[41] A study of patients with cryptococcal disease in Rwanda found that about one third had ocular complications thereof.[123] The most common ophthalmic complication of cryptococcal meningitis is **papilloedema**, attributable to elevated intracranial pressure. Other complications include **sequential optic atrophy**, **optic neuropathy** due to direct invasion of the nerve or perhaps other mechanisms, **cranial nerve palsies** (most commonly of the abducens nerve), **cortical blindness** and **supranuclear eye movement disorders**.[41,123] The Rwandan study found that use of amphotericin B was associated with worse visual outcomes in these patients than was use of alternative anti-fungal agents; however, because this study was not randomized, selection bias may explain this observation (i.e. patients with worse disease may have received amphotericin B).[123]

Progressive multifocal leukoencephalopathy has also been reported to have a high rate of visual and oculomotor complications, primarily arising from cortical injury.[137] Other reported causes of neuro-ophthalmological lesions in patients with AIDS include CNS toxoplasmosis, CNS lymphoma, other viral encephalitides and meningitides, syphilis, and optic nerve lesions due to medication toxicities (see below).[41]

20.3.5   Ophthalmic toxicity of medications for HIV and opportunistic infections

Cidofovir, an anti-CMV agent, has been associated with the occurrence of anterior uveitis and hypotony (as well as severe renal disease). The risk of uveitis in patients receiving systemic cidofovir is approximately 35% per person-year.[92] The risk with intravitreous therapy, using a 20 μg dose, appears to be similar.[91] The risk of uveitis with cidofovir is positively associated with the degree of rise in the CD4+ T-lymphocyte count during therapy,[138] and also with the use of protease inhibitor therapy (a surrogate for HAART in this study); however, cases have been observed in the absence of protease inhibitors as well.[139] If the risk of uveitis with intravitreous cidofovir proves to be low in patients not receiving HAART, or if complications could somehow be avoided, use of intravitreous cidofovir would have appeal as a useful and relatively affordable treatment for CMV retinitis in resource-limited settings where HAART cannot be used.

Therapy with **rifabutin**, a medication used for prophylaxis and treatment of *Mycobacterium avium* complex (MAC) infections, is occasionally associated with an anterior uveitis in patients with HIV/AIDS. The risk increases with factors expected to increase blood levels of rifabutin, including low body weight,[140] concomitant therapy with clarithromycin or fluconazole, and higher dosage.[141] Reports from studies of treatment for MAC bacteraemia have reported a higher risk of uveitis[141] than is thought to occur in patients taking rifabutin for MAC prophylaxis.[142] The uveitis ranges from a mild-to-moderate anterior uveitis to hypopyon uveitis. It responds to conventional topical corticosteroid and mydriatic therapy, and usually remits after discontinuation of rifabutin or a decrease in the dose.

Drug-induced **Stevens–Johnson syndrome** and **toxic epidermal necrolysis** — each of which can produce a cicatrizing conjunctivitis with goblet cell destruction followed by a chronic, severe ocular surface disease — appear to occur with higher frequency in patients with HIV/AIDS. A recent report documented an association of Stevens–Johnson syndrome and toxic epidermal necrolysis with use of nevirapine (infinite odds ratio, lower bound of 95% confidence interval on OR = 10.4).[143] Cases also have been reported in patients with HIV infection in association with sulfa drugs, such as trimethoprim-sulfamethoxazole, which is recommended worldwide when *Pneumocystis* prophylaxis is indicated, and with thiacetazone, a medication for tuberculosis.[144]

Ethambutol, sometimes used to treat tuberculosis in the setting of HIV/AIDS, is known to cause optic neuropathy in a small number of patients, which is often — but not always — reversible with prompt cessation of therapy.[145]

Most other ocular complications of pharmacologic therapy that occur in patients with HIV infection appear to be uncommon, or else reports of such complications have been inconsistent. In a study of the antiretroviral agent **didanosine (DDI)**, three of 43 children (7%) were noted to develop peripheral retinal atrophy, a finding which has not been reported in adults.[146] **Clofazamine**, used for MAC therapy, has been reported to be associated with a bullseye maculopathy and retinal degeneration in a single patient with AIDS.[147] Vortex keratopathy has been reported in a patient receiving **atovaquone** for *Pneumocystis* pneumonia.[148]

20.4   PRIORITIES FOR FUTURE RESEARCH

Following the HAART-induced declining incidence and improved clinical course of CMV retinitis in countries able to pay large amounts of money for the treatment, the market for anti-CMV therapy contracted substantially, except that valganciclovir is still widely used in transplant patients. As a result, development of new treatments for ocular complications of HIV/AIDS has been sharply curtailed. The most promising existing treatments for CMV retinitis remain financially out of reach in even middle-income countries. Because HIV in most patients in wealthy countries can be controlled with the existing treatments, most of the management questions that need to be addressed by future research relate to ocular complications of HIV/AIDS in the resource-limited setting.

20.4.1   Monitoring of secular trends in prevalence and incidence

All complications of HIV infection have been subject to secular trends as conditions change, and as new developments in the management of

HIV/AIDS come into use. In countries with wide-spread use of HAART, many patients with advanced AIDS have enjoyed sustained immuno-logic benefit for many years now, with diminished risk of ocular and other complications. This has led to the assumption by clinicians in developed countries that ocular complications of HIV/AIDS are now rare. The resulting level of complacency means that ocular complications are rarely considered as a possibility, even in highly immunodeficient patients. The massive expansion of HIV/AIDS treatment has rarely included ocular complications as an important aspect of programming. However, because CMV infection is widespread globally and CMV retinitis typically affects a large proportion of patients with advanced AIDS in areas where HAART is not in widespread use, there is little reason to think the problem should have gone away in the majority who today still do not receive anti-retroviral therapy. Continuing monitoring of the prevalence and incidence of CMV retinitis and other ocular complications in resource-limited settings is needed to determine the magnitude of this problem over time. Such monitoring would probably lead to recognition that ocular complications of HIV/AIDS should be diagnosed and managed as part of HIV/AIDS treatment programmes.

As mentioned previously, Sub-Saharan Africa historically has been viewed as an outlier in reports on the prevalence of CMV retinitis in series of patients with HIV/AIDS. However, more recent studies and clinical impression suggest that CMV retinitis is not uncommon in Sub-Saharan Africa among patients naive to HAART. Because approximately two thirds of HIV-infected persons are African,[1] and information regarding the risk of ocular complications of HIV/AIDS is still sparse and sometimes suffers from under-ascertainment, high quality studies on the risk of ocular complications in this region are needed. Studies involving dilated retinoscopy of the whole population at risk are particularly needed, so as to avoid missing retinal complications. Such studies should also document the immune status of patients, and patients with more advanced immunodeficiency should be the ones studied.

Should other discrepancies in the epidemiology of ocular complications of HIV/AIDS between different regions arise, they should be studied, because understanding of the mechanisms underlying such differences may lead to improvements in treatment strategies or public health interventions. The discovery of a viral contribution to squamous cell carcinoma of the conjunctiva in Sub-Saharan Africa[134] is an example of the information that can be gained from studies of this nature.

20.4.2 Treatment of CMV retinitis in resource-limited settings

Treatment of CMV retinitis in resource-limited settings is rarely available, primarily because of the high acquisition costs of anti-CMV medications and limited human resources trained in the management of such therapy. Because the largest numbers of cases of CMV retinitis are likely present in regions with these limitations, strategies that are cost-effective and feasible are needed urgently. Because of the mortality benefit of systemic anti-CMV therapy,[67] such therapy would ideally be systemic, inexpensive and associated with low complication rates. Such agents are not currently available. However, generic valganciclovir (expected to become available in 2014) could be such an agent, particularly if advocacy efforts and more widespread use were to lead to lower pricing, both of which depend in turn on a more widespread appreciation of the problem of ocular complications of HIV/AIDS. It is desirable to evaluate the cost-effectiveness of valganciclovir therapy in such a way as to identify a cost threshold that would make widespread use justified, and that might provide information needed for subsequent advocacy.

For many patients in resource-limited settings, the treatment burden of weekly intravitreous therapy and the costs of alternative anti-CMV therapies, make the existing conservative guidelines[21] regarding when to stop suppressive anti-CMV therapy following immune recovery untenable. Studies of the clinical course of patients with CMV retinitis with small peripheral lesions, who are treated with HAART alone because of resource limitations, could help determine whether there are situations in which anti-CMV therapy could be safely omitted. Studies of the recurrence risk associated with earlier cessation of suppressive anti-CMV therapy following immune recovery are needed to provide guidance regarding such decision-making. Work to provide an inexpensive test to evaluate the status of CMV-specific immunity would be an especially promising approach. Because intravitreous cidofovir is relatively inexpensive and long-lasting treatment for CMV retinitis (see above), but is subject to a high rate of adverse effects, studies of ways to prevent such side effects while maintaining the therapeutic effect of the drug could be useful. As with many other questions regarding treatment of HIV/AIDS and its complications in resource-limited settings, such studies pose difficult ethical dilemmas, which must be considered carefully in the design of prospective studies.

20.4.3 Ocular opportunistic complications of HIV/AIDS other than CMV retinitis

As mentioned previously, squamous cell carcinoma of the conjunctiva seems to represent a common ocular complication of HIV/AIDS in parts of Sub-Saharan Africa, but not elsewhere, and appears to be associated with certain infectious agents in at least some cases. Evaluation of optimal methods for the management of this condition and others of the more common ocular complications of HIV/AIDS in resource-limited (and in some cases worldwide) settings is needed. Study of such local ocular complication epidemics are likely to be fruitful for the identification of novel pathogens, and, it is to be hoped, will lead to effective and affordable management strategies over time.

20.4.4 Operations research regarding ocular complication detection and management

One of the reasons why ocular complications tend to be overlooked is that symptoms can be subtle

and diagnosis difficult without extensive, specialized ophthalmic training. Regarding improved diagnosis, some studies involving use of telemedicine approaches or non-ophthalmologist screeners trained in indirect ophthalmoscopy have been initiated,[80] and may provide useful results. Solutions to the treatment problem are complex because of the requirement for potentially toxic systemic therapy or intraocular injections (aside from issues of cost and supply), both of which can be argued to require considerable sophistication. Efforts to develop more feasible approaches for the detection and management of ocular complications of HIV/AIDS are clearly needed, and represent one of the most practical opportunities for research which will lead to improved outcomes for these patients.

REFERENCES

1. UNAIDS. AIDS Epidemic Update: November 2009. Geneva: UNAIDS; 2009.
2. Centers for Disease Control. Pneumocystis pneumonia — Los Angeles. *MMWR Morb Mortal Wkly Rep* 1981; 30:250–252.
3. World Health Organization. Acquired immune deficiency syndrome (AIDS). *Weekly Epidemiological Record* 1983; 58:227–228.
4. Centers for Disease Control. Current Trends Update: Acquired Immunodeficiency Syndrome. *MMWR Morb Mortal Wkly Rep* 1988; 37:286–295.
5. Update on acquired immune deficiency syndrome (AIDS) — United States. *MMWR Morb Mortal Wkly Rep* 1982; 31:507–514.
6. Update on acquired immunodeficiency syndrome (AIDS) — United States. *MMWR Morb Mortal Wkly Rep* 1983; 32:465–467.
7. UNAIDS. AIDS Epidemic Update: Special Report on HIV/AIDS: December 2006. Geneva: UNAIDS; 2006.
8. Schneider E, Whitmore S, Glynn KM, *et al.* Revised surveillance case definitions for HIV infection among adults, adolescents, and children aged < 18 months and for HIV infection and AIDS among children aged 18 months to < 13 years — United States, 2008. *MMWR Recomm Rep* 2008; 57:1–12.

9. Centers for Disease Control and Prevention. 1993 revised classification system for HIV infection and expanded surveillance case definition for AIDS among adolescents and adults. *Morb Mortal Wkly Rep* 1992; 41:1–19.

10. Acquired immunodeficiency syndrome AIDS: provisional WHO clinical case definition for AIDS. *Wkly Epidemiol Rec* 1986; 61:72–73.

11. Lukashov VV, Goudsmit J. HIV heterogeneity and disease progression in AIDS: a model of continuous virus adaptation. *AIDS* 1998; 12:S43–S52.

12. Finzi D, Hermankova M, Pierson T, *et al.* Identification of a reservoir for HIV-1 in patients on highly active antiretroviral therapy. *Science* 1997; 278:1295–1300.

13. Bartlett JG, Gallant JE. *2001–2002 Medical Management of HIV Infection.* Baltimore, MD: H&N Printing & Graphics; 2001. pp. 1–372.

14. Morris GC, Lacey CJ. Microbicides and HIV prevention: lessons from the past, looking to the future. *Curr Opin Infect Dis* 2010; 23:57–63.

15. Gray RH, Kigozi G, Serwadda D, *et al.* Male circumcision for HIV prevention in men in Rakai, Uganda: a randomised trial. *Lancet* 2007; 369:657–666.

16. Wawer MJ, Makumbi F, Kigozi G, *et al.* Circumcision in HIV-infected men and its effect on HIV transmission to female partners in Rakai, Uganda: a randomised controlled trial. *Lancet* 2009; 374:229–237.

17. Bradac J, Dieffenbach CW. HIV vaccine development: Lessons from the past, informing the future. *IDrugs* 2009; 12:435–439.

18. Ho DD, Neumann AU, Perelson AS, *et al.* Rapid turnover of plasma virions and CD4 lymphocytes in HIV-1 infection. *Nature* 1995; 373:123–126.

19. Pantaleo G, Graziosi C, Fauci AS. New concepts in the immunopathogenesis of human immunodeficiency virus infection. *N Engl J Med* 1993; 328:327–335.

20. Stein DS, Korvick JA, Vermund SH. CD4+ lymphocyte cell enumeration for prediction of clinical course of human immunodeficiency virus disease: a review. *J Infect Dis* 1992; 165:352–363.

21. Kaplan JE, Benson C, Holmes KH, *et al.* Guidelines for prevention and treatment of opportunistic infections in HIV-infected adults and adolescents: recommendations from CDC, the National Institutes of Health, and the HIV Medicine Association of the Infectious Diseases Society of America. *MMWR Recomm Rep* 2009; 58:1–207.

22. Mofenson LM, Brady MT, Danner SP, *et al.* Guidelines for the Prevention and Treatment of Opportunistic Infections among HIV-exposed and HIV-infected children: recommendations from CDC, the National Institutes of Health, the HIV Medicine Association of the Infectious Diseases Society of America, the Pediatric Infectious Diseases Society, and the American Academy of Pediatrics. *MMWR Recomm Rep* 2009; 58:1–166.

23. Kempen JH, Frick KD, Jabs DA. Incremental cost effectiveness of prophylaxis for cytomegalovirus disease in patients with AIDS. *Pharmacoeconomics* 2001; 19:1199–1208.

24. Mellors JW, Rinaldo CR Jr, Gupta P, *et al.* Prognosis in HIV-1 infection predicted by the quantity of virus in plasma. *Science* 1996; 272:1167–1170.

25. Fischl MA, Richman DD, Grieco MH, *et al.* The efficacy of azidothymidine (AZT) in the treatment of patients with AIDS and AIDS-related complex. A double-blind, placebo-controlled trial. *N Engl J Med* 1987; 317:185–191.

26. Panel on Antiretroviral Guidelines for Adults and Adolescents. Guidelines for the use of antiretroviral agents in HIV-1-infected adults and adolescents. Department of Health and Human Services. http://www.aidsinfo.nih.gov/ContentFiles/AdultandAdolescentGL.pdf, 2009:1–161.

27. Mayers DL. Prevalence and incidence of resistance to zidovudine and other antiretroviral drugs. *Am J Med* 1997; 102:70–75.

28. Gulick RM, Mellors JW, Havlir D, *et al.* Treatment with indinavir, zidovudine, and lamivudine in adults with human immunodeficiency virus infection and prior antiretroviral therapy. *N Engl J Med* 1997; 337:734–739.

29. Hammer SM, Squires KE, Hughes MD, *et al.* A controlled trial of two nucleoside analogues plus indinavir in persons with human immunodeficiency virus infection and CD4 cell counts of 200 per cubic millimeter or less. AIDS Clinical Trials Group 320 Study Team. *N Engl J Med* 1997; 337:725–733.

30. Palella FJ Jr, Delaney KM, Moorman AC, *et al.* HIV Outpatient Study Investigators. Declining morbidity and mortality among patients with advanced human immunodeficiency virus infection. *N Engl J Med* 1998; 338:853–860.

31. Nieuwkerk PT, Reijers MH, Weigel HM, *et al.* Quality of life in maintenance vs prolonged induction therapy for HIV. *JAMA* 2000; 284:178–179.

32. Lucas GM, Chaisson RE, Moore RD. Highly active antiretroviral therapy in a large urban clinic: risk factors for virologic failure and adverse drug reactions. *Ann Intern Med* 1999; 131:81–87.

33. 1999 USPHS/IDSA guidelines for the prevention of opportunistic infections in persons infected with human immunodeficiency virus. *Clin Infect Dis* 2000; 30:S29–S65.

34. Komanduri KV, Viswanathan MN, Wieder ED, *et al.* Restoration of cytomegalovirus-specific CD4+ T-lymphocyte responses after ganciclovir and highly active antiretroviral therapy in individuals infected with HIV-1. *Nat Med* 1998; 4:953–956.

35. Komanduri KV, Feinberg J, Hutchins RK, *et al.* Loss of cytomegalovirus-specific CD4+ T cell responses in human immunodeficiency virus type 1-infected patients with high CD4+ T cell counts and recurrent retinitis. *J Infect Dis* 2001; 183:1285–1289.

36. Karavellas MP, Azen SP, Macdonald JC, *et al.* Immune recovery vitritis and uveitis in AIDS: clinical predictors, sequelae, and treatment outcomes. *Retina* 2001; 21:1–9.

37. Otiti-Sengeri J, Meenken C, van den Horn GJ, *et al.* Ocular immune reconstitution inflammatory syndromes. *Curr Opin HIV AIDS* 2008; 3:432–437.

38. Rathinam SR, Lalitha P. Paradoxical worsening of ocular tuberculosis in HIV patients after antiretroviral therapy. *Eye* 2007; 21:667–668.

39. Dhasmana DJ, Dheda K, Ravn P, *et al.* Immune reconstitution inflammatory syndrome in HIV-infected patients receiving antiretroviral therapy: pathogenesis, clinical manifestations and management. *Drugs* 2008; 68:191–208.

40. Holland GN, Gottlieb MS, Yee RD, *et al.* Ocular disorders associated with a new severe acquired cellular immunodeficiency syndrome. *Am J Ophthalmol* 1982; 93:393–402.

41. Jabs DA. Ocular manifestations of HIV infection. *Trans Am Ophthalmol Soc* 1995; 93:623–683.

42. Holland GN, Pepose JS, Pettit TH, *et al.* Acquired immune deficiency syndrome. Ocular manifestations. *Ophthalmology* 1983; 90:859–873.

43. Freeman WR, Chen A, Henderly DE, *et al.* Prevalence and significance of acquired immunodeficiency syndrome-related retinal microvasculopathy. *Am J Ophthalmol* 1989; 107:229–235.

44. Plummer DJ, Sample PA, Freeman WR. Visual dysfunction in HIV-positive patients without infectious retinopathy. *AIDS Patient Care STDS* 1998; 12:171–179.

45. Engstrom RE Jr, Holland GN, Hardy WD, *et al.* Hemorheologic abnormalities in patients with human immunodeficiency virus infection and ophthalmic microvasculopathy. *Am J Ophthalmol* 1990; 109:153–161.

46. Dunn JP, Yamashita A, Kempen JH, *et al.* Retinal vascular occlusion in patients infected with human immunodeficiency virus. *Retina* 2005; 25:759–766.

47. Pavan-Langston D, Dunkel E. Varicella-zoster virus diseases: anterior segment of the eye. In: Pepose JS, Holland GN, Wilhelmus KR (eds). *Ocular Immunity and Infection.* St. Louis: Mosby; 1996. pp. 933–957.

48. Whitley RJ. Varicella-zoster virus. In: Mandell GL, Bennett JE, Dolin R (eds). *Principles and Practice of Infectious Diseases.* Philadelphia: Churchill Livingstone, Inc; 2000. pp. 1580–1586.

49. Weinberg A, Levin MJ, MacGregor RR. Safety and immunogenicity of a live attenuated varicella vaccine in VZV-seropositive HIV-infected adults. *Hum Vaccin* 2010; 6:318–321.

50. Glesby MJ, Moore RD, Chaisson RE. Clinical spectrum of herpes zoster in adults infected with human immunodeficiency virus. *Clin Infect Dis* 1995; 21:370–375.

51. Margolis TP, Milner MS, Shama A, *et al.* Herpes zoster ophthalmicus in patients with human immunodeficiency virus infection. *Am J Ophthalmol* 1998; 125:285–291.

52. Levin MJ, Anderson JP, Seage GR III, *et al.* Short-term and long-term effects of highly active antiretroviral therapy on the incidence of herpes zoster in HIV-infected children. *J Acquir Immune Defic Syndr* 2009; 50:182–191.

53. Martins SA, Muccioli C, Belfort R, Jr, *et al.* Resolution of microsporidial keratoconjunctivitis

in an AIDS patient treated with highly active anti-retroviral therapy. *Am J Ophthalmol* 2001; 131: 378–379.

54. Rastrelli PD, Didier E, Yee RW. Microsporidial keratitis. *Ophthalmology Clinics of North America* 1994; 7:617–633.

55. Hodge WG, Seiff SR, Margolis TP. Ocular opportunistic infection incidences among patients who are HIV positive compared to patients who are HIV negative. *Ophthalmology* 1998; 105: 895–900.

56. Pramod NP, Hari R, Sudhamathi K, *et al*. Influence of human immunodeficiency virus status on the clinical history of herpes simplex keratitis. *Ophthalmologica* 2000; 214:337–340.

57. Mselle J. Fungal keratitis as an indicator of HIV infection in Africa. *Trop Doct* 1999; 29: 133–135.

58. Beersma MF, Bijlmakers MJ, Ploegh HL. Human cytomegalovirus down-regulates HLA class I expression by reducing the stability of class I H chains. *J Immunol* 1993; 151:4455–4464.

59. Krech U. Complement-fixing antibodies against cytomegalovirus in different parts of the world. *Bull World Health Organ* 1973; 49:103–106.

60. Holland CA, Ma Y, Moscicki B, *et al*. Seroprevalence and risk factors of hepatitis B, hepatitis C, and human cytomegalovirus among HIV-infected and high-risk uninfected adolescents: findings of the REACH Study. Adolescent Medicine HIV/AIDS Research Network. *Sex Transm Dis* 2000; 27:296–303.

61. Gallant JE, Moore RD, Richman DD, *et al*. Incidence and natural history of cytomegalovirus disease in patients with advanced human immunodeficiency virus disease treated with zidovudine. The Zidovudine Epidemiology Study Group. *J Infect Dis* 1992; 166:1223–1227.

62. Hoover DR, Peng Y, Saah A, *et al*. Occurrence of cytomegalovirus retinitis after human immunodeficiency virus immunosuppression. *Arch Ophthalmol* 1996; 114:821–827.

63. Jabs DA, Van Natta ML, Holbrook JT, *et al*. Longitudinal study of the ocular complications of AIDS: 1. Ocular diagnoses at enrollment. *Ophthalmology* 2007; 114:780–786.

64. Kempen JH, Jabs DA, Wilson LA, *et al*. Risk of vision loss in patients with cytomegalovirus retinitis and the acquired immunodeficiency syndrome. *Arch Ophthalmol* 2003; 121:466–476.

65. Kempen JH, Jabs DA, Wilson LA, *et al*. Mortality risk for patients with cytomegalovirus retinitis and acquired immune deficiency syndrome. *Clin Infect Dis* 2003; 37:1365–1373.

66. Jabs DA, Holbrook JT, Van Natta ML, *et al*. Risk factors for mortality in patients with AIDS in the era of highly active antiretroviral therapy. *Ophthalmology* 2005; 112:771–779.

67. Binquet C, Saillour F, Bernard N, *et al*. Prognostic factors of survival of HIV-infected patients with cytomegalovirus disease: Aquitaine Cohort, 1986–1997. Groupe d'Epidémiologie Clinique du SIDA en Aquitaine (GECSA). *Eur J Epidemiol* 2000; 16:425–432.

68. Nardiello S, Digilio L, Pizzella T, *et al*. Cytomegalovirus as a co-factor of disease progression in human immunodeficiency virus type 1 infection. *Int J Clin Lab Res* 1994; 24:86–89.

69. Pepose JS, Holland GN, Nestor MS, *et al*. Acquired immune deficiency syndrome. Pathogenic mechanisms of ocular disease. *Ophthalmology* 1985; 92:472–484.

70. Biswas J, Madhavan HN, George AE, *et al*. Ocular lesions associated with HIV infection in India: a series of 100 consecutive patients evaluated at a referral center. *Am J Ophthalmol* 2000; 129:9–15.

71. Lim SA, Heng WJ, Lim TH, *et al*. Ophthalmic manifestations in human immunodeficiency virus infection in Singapore. *Ann Acad Med Singapore* 1997; 26:575–580.

72. Tanterdtam J, Suwannagool S, Namatra C, *et al*. A study of ocular manifestations in HIV patients. *Thai J Ophthalmol* 2002; 10:11–20.

73. Wong KH, Lee SS, Lo YC, *et al*. Profile of opportunistic infections among HIV-1 infected people in Hong Kong. *Zhonghua Yi Xue Za Zhi (Taipei)* 1995; 55:127–136.

74. Nagata Y, Fujino Y, Matsumoto S, *et al*. Ocular manifestations in Japanese patients with human immunodeficiency virus infection. *Jpn J Ophthalmol* 1993; 37:275–281.

75. Mesaric B, Begovac J, Ugrinovic N, *et al*. Cytomegalovirus retinitis in patients with human immunodeficiency virus infection. *Lijec Vjesn* 1998; 120:106–110.

76. Muccioli C, Belfort R Jr, Lottenberg C, *et al.* Ophthalmological manifestations in AIDS: evaluation of 445 patients in one year. *Rev Assoc Med Bras* 1994; 40:155–158.

77. Kestelyn P. The epidemiology of CMV retinitis in Africa. *Ocul Immunol Inflamm* 1999; 7:173–177.

78. Otiti-Sengeri J, Colebunders R, Kempen JH, *et al.* The prevalence and causes of visual loss among HIV-infected individuals with visual loss in Uganda. *J Acquir Immune Defic Syndr* 2009; 53:95–101.

79. Nkomazana O, Tshitswana D. Ocular complications of HIV infection in sub-Sahara Africa. *Curr HIV AIDS Rep* 2008; 5:120–125.

80. Heiden D, Ford N, Wilson DR, *et al.* Cytomegalovirus retinitis: the neglected disease of the AIDS pandemic. *PLoS Med* 2007; 4:e334.

81. Giorgis A, Melka F, Mariam A. Ophthalmic manifestation of AIDS in Armed Forces General Teaching Hospital, Addis Ababa. *Ethiop Med J* 2007; 45:327–334.

82. Bowen EF, Wilson P, Atkins M, *et al.* Natural history of untreated cytomegalovirus retinitis. *Lancet* 1995; 346:1671–1673.

83. Lalezari JP, Friedberg D, Bisset J, *et al.* A comparison of the safety and efficacy of 3 g, 4.5 g, and 6 g doses of oral ganciclovir vs. IV ganciclovir for maintenance treatment of CMV retinitis. *Abstracts of the Eleventh International Conference on AIDS* 1996; 2:226.

84. Arevalo JF, Gonzalez C, Capparelli EV, *et al.* Intravitreous and plasma concentrations of ganciclovir and foscarnet after intravenous therapy in patients with AIDS and cytomegalovirus retinitis. *J Infect Dis* 1995; 172:951–956.

85. Studies of Ocular Complications of AIDS Research Group in collaboration with the AIDS Clinical Trials Group. Combination foscarnet and ganciclovir therapy vs monotherapy for the treatment of relapsed cytomegalovirus retinitis in patients with AIDS. The Cytomegalovirus Retreatment Trial. *Arch Ophthalmol* 1996; 114:23–33.

86. Jabs DA, Enger C, Dunn JP, *et al.* CMV Retinitis and Viral Resistance Study Group. Cytomegalovirus retinitis and viral resistance: ganciclovir resistance. *J Infect Dis* 1998; 177:770–773.

87. Thorne JE, Jabs DA, Vitale S, *et al.* Catheter complications in AIDS patients treated for cytomegalovirus retinitis. *AIDS* 1998; 12:2321–2327.

88. Young S, Morlet N, Besen G, *et al.* High-dose (2000-microgram) intravitreous ganciclovir in the treatment of cytomegalovirus retinitis. *Ophthalmology* 1998; 105:1404–1410.

89. Diaz-Llopis M, Espana E, Munoz G, *et al.* High dose intravitreal foscarnet in the treatment of cytomegalovirus retinitis in AIDS. *Br J Ophthalmol* 1994; 78:120–124.

90. Kirsch LS, Arevalo JF, Chavez de la Paz E, *et al.* Intravitreal cidofovir (HPMPC) treatment of cytomegalovirus retinitis in patients with acquired immune deficiency syndrome. *Ophthalmology* 1995; 102:533–542.

91. Taskintuna I, Rahhal FM, Rao NA, *et al.* Adverse events and autopsy findings after intravitreous cidofovir (HPMPC) therapy in patients with acquired immune deficiency syndrome (AIDS). *Ophthalmology* 1997; 104:1827–1836.

92. Studies of Ocular Complications of AIDS Research Group in collaboration with the AIDS Clinical Trials Group. The ganciclovir implant plus oral ganciclovir versus parenteral cidofovir for the treatment of cytomegalovirus retinitis in patients with acquired immunodeficiency syndrome: The Ganciclovir Cidofovir Cytomegalovirus Retinitis Trial. *Am J Ophthalmol* 2001; 131:457–467.

93. Kuppermann BD, Quiceno JI, Flores-Aguilar M, *et al.* Intravitreal ganciclovir concentration after intravenous administration in AIDS patients with cytomegalovirus retinitis: implications for therapy. *J Infect Dis* 1993; 168:1506–1509.

94. Martin DF, Parks DJ, Mellow SD, *et al.* Treatment of cytomegalovirus retinitis with an intraocular sustained-release ganciclovir implant. A randomized controlled clinical trial. *Arch Ophthalmol* 1994; 112:1531–1539.

95. Musch DC, Martin DF, Gordon JF, *et al.* Treatment of cytomegalovirus retinitis with a sustained-release ganciclovir implant. The Ganciclovir Implant Study Group. *N Engl J Med* 1997; 337:83–90.

96. Marx JL, Kapusta MA, Patel SS, *et al.* Use of the ganciclovir implant in the treatment of recurrent cytomegalovirus retinitis. *Arch Ophthalmol* 1996; 114:815–820.

97. Martin DF, Kuppermann BD, Wolitz RA, *et al.* Roche Ganciclovir Study Group. Oral ganciclovir for patients with cytomegalovirus retinitis treated

with a ganciclovir implant. *N Engl J Med* 1999; 340:1063–1070.

98. Kempen JH, Jabs DA, Dunn JP, *et al*. Retinal detachment risk in cytomegalovirus retinitis related to the acquired immunodeficiency syndrome. *Arch Ophthalmol* 2001; 119:33–40.

99. Freeman WR, Friedberg DN, Berry C, *et al*. Risk factors for development of rhegmatogenous retinal detachment in patients with cytomegalovirus retinitis. *Am J Ophthalmol* 1993; 116:713–720.

100. Irvine AR, Lonn L, Schwartz D, *et al*. Retinal detachment in AIDS: long-term results after repair with silicone oil. *Br J Ophthalmol* 1997; 81:180–183.

101. Freeman WR. Retinal detachment in cytomegalovirus retinitis: should our approach be changed? *Retina* 1999; 19:271–273.

102. Dugel PU, Liggett PE, Lee MB, *et al*. Repair of retinal detachment caused by cytomegalovirus retinitis in patients with the acquired immunodeficiency syndrome. *Am J Ophthalmol* 1991; 112:235–242.

103. Karavellas MP, Song M, Macdonald JC, *et al*. Long-term posterior and anterior segment complications of immune recovery uveitis associated with cytomegalovirus retinitis. *Am J Ophthalmol* 2000; 130:57–64.

104. US Public Health Service, Infectious Diseases Society of America. 1999 USPHS/IDSA guidelines for the prevention of opportunistic infections in persons infected with human immunodeficiency virus. US Public Health Service (USPHS) and Infectious Diseases Society of America (IDSA). *MMWR Recomm Rep* 1999; 48:1–6.

105. Jabs DA, Van Natta ML, Kempen JH, *et al*. Characteristics of patients with cytomegalovirus retinitis in the era of highly active antiretroviral therapy. *Am J Ophthalmol* 2002; 133:48–61.

106. Karavellas MP, Plummer DJ, Macdonald JC, *et al*. Incidence of immune recovery vitritis in cytomegalovirus retinitis patients following institution of successful highly active antiretroviral therapy. *J Infect Dis* 1999; 179:697–700.

107. Nguyen QD, Kempen JH, Bolton SG, *et al*. Immune recovery uveitis in patients with AIDS and cytomegalovirus retinitis after highly active antiretroviral therapy. *Am J Ophthalmol* 2000; 129:634–639.

108. Fisher JP, Lewis ML, Blumenkranz M, *et al*. The acute retinal necrosis syndrome. Part 1: Clinical manifestations. *Ophthalmology* 1982; 89:1309–1316.

109. Holland GN, Executive Committee of the American Uveitis Society. Standard diagnostic criteria for the acute retinal necrosis syndrome. *Am J Ophthalmol* 1994; 117:663–667.

110. Sellitti TP, Huang AJ, Schiffman J, *et al*. Association of herpes zoster ophthalmicus with acquired immunodeficiency syndrome and acute retinal necrosis. *Am J Ophthalmol* 1993; 116:297–301.

111. Engstrom RE Jr, Holland GN, Margolis TP, *et al*. The progressive outer retinal necrosis syndrome. A variant of necrotizing herpetic retinopathy in patients with AIDS. *Ophthalmology* 1994; 101:1488–1502.

112. Short GA, Margolis TP, Kuppermann BD, *et al*. A polymerase chain reaction-based assay for diagnosing varicella-zoster virus retinitis in patients with acquired immunodeficiency syndrome. *Am J Ophthalmol* 1997; 123:157–164.

113. Spaide RF, Martin DF, Teich SA, *et al*. Successful treatment of progressive outer retinal necrosis syndrome. *Retina* 1996; 16:479–487.

114. Gariano RF, Berreen JP, Cooney EL. Progressive outer retinal necrosis and acute retinal necrosis in fellow eyes of a patient with acquired immunodeficiency syndrome. *Am J Ophthalmol* 2001; 132:421–423.

115. Montoya JG, Remington JS. Toxoplasma gondii. In: Mandell GL, Bennett JE, Dolin R (eds). *Principles and Practice of Infectious Diseases*. Philadelphia: Churchill Livingstone, Inc; 2000. pp. 2858–2888.

116. Cochereau-Massin I, LeHoang P, Lautier-Frau M, *et al*. Ocular toxoplasmosis in human immunodeficiency virus-infected patients. *Am J Ophthalmol* 1992; 114:130–135.

117. Matos KT, Santos MC, Muccioli C. Ocular manifestations in HIV infected patients attending the department of ophthalmology of Universidade Federal de São Paulo. *Rev Assoc Med Bras* 1999; 45:323–326.

118. Holland GN, Engstrom RE Jr, Glasgow BJ, *et al*. Ocular toxoplasmosis in patients with the acquired immunodeficiency syndrome. *Am J Ophthalmol* 1988; 106:653–667.

119. McLeish WM, Pulido JS, Holland S, *et al*. The ocular manifestations of syphilis in the human

immunodeficiency virus type 1-infected host. *Ophthalmology* 1990; 97:196–203.

120. Morinelli EN, Dugel PU, Riffenburgh R, *et al.* Infectious multifocal choroiditis in patients with acquired immunodeficiency syndrome. *Ophthalmology* 1993; 100:1014–1021.

121. Babu RB, Sudharshan S, Kumarasamy N, *et al.* Ocular tuberculosis in acquired immunodeficiency syndrome. *Am J Ophthalmol* 2006; 142:413–418.

122. Shami MJ, Freeman W, Friedberg D, *et al.* A multicenter study of Pneumocystis choroidopathy. *Am J Ophthalmol* 1991; 112:15–22.

123. Kestelyn P, Taelman H, Bogaerts J, *et al.* Ophthalmic manifestations of infections with Cryptococcus neoformans in patients with the acquired immunodeficiency syndrome. *Am J Ophthalmol* 1993; 116:721–727.

124. Chang Y, Cesarman E, Pessin MS, *et al.* Identification of herpesvirus-like DNA sequences in AIDS-associated Kaposi's sarcoma. *Science* 1994; 266:1865–1869.

125. Gao SJ, Kingsley L, Hoover DR, *et al.* Seroconversion to antibodies against Kaposi's sarcoma-associated herpesvirus-related latent nuclear antigens before the development of Kaposi's sarcoma. *N Engl J Med* 1996; 335:233–241.

126. Renwick N, Halaby T, Weverling GJ, *et al.* Seroconversion for human herpesvirus 8 during HIV infection is highly predictive of Kaposi's sarcoma. *AIDS* 1998; 12:2481–2488.

127. Shuler JD, Holland GN, Miles SA, *et al.* Kaposi's sarcoma of the conjunctiva and eyelids associated with the acquired immunodeficiency syndrome. *Arch Ophthalmol* 1989; 107: 858–862.

128. Dugel PU, Gill PS, Frangieh GT, *et al.* Treatment of ocular adnexal Kaposi's sarcoma in acquired immune deficiency syndrome. *Ophthalmology* 1992; 99:1127–1132.

129. Martellotta F, Berretta M, Vaccher E, *et al.* AIDS-related Kaposi's sarcoma: state of the art and therapeutic strategies. *Curr HIV Res* 2009; 7: 634–638.

130. Dore GJ, Li Y, Grulich AE, *et al.* Declining - incidence and later occurrence of Kaposi's sarcoma among persons with AIDS in Australia: the Australian AIDS cohort. *AIDS* 1996; 10: 1401–1406.

131. Osmond DH, Buchbinder S, Cheng A, *et al.* Prevalence of Kaposi's sarcoma-associated herpesvirus infection in homosexual men at beginning of and during the HIV epidemic. *JAMA* 2002; 287:221–225.

132. MacMahon EM, Glass JD, Hayward SD, *et al.* Epstein-Barr virus in AIDS-related primary central nervous system lymphoma. *Lancet* 1991; 338: 969–973.

133. Simbiri KO, Murakami M, Feldman M, *et al.* Multiple oncogenic viruses identified in ocular surface squamous neoplasia in HIV-1 patients. *Infect Agent Cancer* 2010; 5:6.

134. Waddell KM, Lewallen S, Lucas SB, *et al.* Carcinoma of the conjunctiva and HIV infection in Uganda and Malawi. *Br J Ophthalmol* 1996; 80:503–508.

135. Heard I, Tassie JM, Schmitz V, *et al.* Increased risk of cervical disease among human immunodeficiency virus-infected women with severe immunosuppression and high human papillomavirus load (1). *Obstet Gynecol* 2000; 96:403–409.

136. Teenyi-Agaba C, Franceschi S, Wabwire-Mangen F, *et al.* Human papillomavirus infection and squamous cell carcinoma of the conjunctiva. *Br J Cancer* 2010; 102:262–267.

137. Friedman DI. Neuro-ophthalmic manifestations of human immunodeficiency virus infection. *Neurol Clin* 1991; 9:55–72.

138. Ambati J, Wynne KB, Angerame MC, *et al.* Anterior uveitis associated with intravenous cidofovir use in patients with cytomegalovirus retinitis. *Br J Ophthalmol* 1999; 83: 1153–1158.

139. Studies of Ocular Complications of AIDS Research Group in collaboration with the AIDS Clinical Trials Group. Long-term follow-up of patients with AIDS treated with parenteral cidofovir for cytomegalovirus retinitis: the HPMPC Peripheral Cytomegalovirus Retinitis Trial. *AIDS* 2000; 14:1571–1581.

140. Shafran SD, Singer J, Zarowny DP, *et al.* Determinants of rifabutin-associated uveitis in patients treated with rifabutin, clarithromycin, and ethambutol for Mycobacterium avium complex bacteremia: a multivariate analysis. Canadian HIV Trials Network Protocol 010 Study Group. *J Infect Dis* 1998; 177:252–255.

141. Tseng AL, Walmsley SL. Rifabutin-associated uveitis. *Ann Pharmacother* 1995; 29:1149–1155.

142. Nichols CW. Mycobacterium avium complex infection, rifabutin, and uveitis — is there a connection? *Clin Infect Dis* 1996; 22: S43–S47.

143. Fagot JP, Mockenhaupt M, Bouwes-Bavinck JN, *et al.* Nevirapine and the risk of Stevens–Johnson syndrome or toxic epidermal necrolysis. *AIDS* 2001; 15:1843–1848.

144. Kestelyn PG, Cunningham ET Jr. HIV/AIDS and blindness. *Bull World Health Organ* 2001; 79:208–213.

145. Tsai RK, Lee YH. Reversibility of ethambutol optic neuropathy. *J Ocul Pharmacol Ther* 1997; 13:473–477.

146. Whitcup SM, Butler KM, Caruso R, *et al.* Retinal toxicity in human immunodeficiency virus-infected children treated with 2′,3′-dideoxyinosine. *Am J Ophthalmol* 1992; 113:1–7.

147. Cunningham CA, Friedberg DN, Carr RE. Clofazamine-induced generalized retinal degeneration. *Retina* 1990; 10:131–134.

148. Shah GK, Cantrill HL, Holland EJ. Vortex keratopathy associated with atovaquone. *Am J Ophthalmol* 1995; 120:669–671.

Diabetic retinopathy

BARBARA KLEIN AND RONALD KLEIN

21.1	Introduction	547
21.2	Description of diabetic retinopathy	548
21.3	Classification of diabetic retinopathy	549
21.4	Prevalence	549
21.5	Geographical distribution	551
21.6	Incidence	552
21.7	Changes in prevalence and geographical distribution with time	553
21.8	Risk factors for diabetic retinopathy	554
21.9	Genetic factors	561
21.10	Clincial trials	562
21.11	Summary of ophthalmic management	562
21.12	Other chronic ocular conditions associated with diabetes	563
21.13	Research priorities	563
	References	564

21.1 INTRODUCTION

This chapter provides an updated review of the epidemiology of **diabetic retinopathy (DR)** and the **visual impairment (VI)** associated with it. The chapter is only a summary of information available and we encourage the interested reader to access the literature to keep abreast of findings in the evolving picture of the epidemiology of diabetic retinopathy. The differences in the frequencies in various studies may be due to different study designs as well as differences in distributions of diabetes with regard to age, gender and type of diabetes. However, diabetic retinopathy is a common occurrence in any group of persons with diabetes. Until diabetes itself is prevented, this common complication will pose a risk of impaired vision. Medical intervention, primarily control of glycaemia, can decrease some of that risk. Although maintaining normal blood glucose level from the onset would be ideal, any improvement in glycaemic control at virtually any stage in the course of retinopathy seems to be associated with a decreased risk of progression of retinopathy. If proliferative retinopathy is present, timely detection and laser photocoagulation of the retina decrease the risk of a subsequent severe loss of vision. Thus, epidemiology can guide the development of healthcare policy that aims to decrease loss of vision and blindness from diabetic retinopathy. While diabetic retinopathy has always been of great importance, the burden may burgeon because it has been estimated that diabetes will increase in prevalence to about 300 million persons worldwide by 2025.[1]

Diabetic retinopathy is characterized by a group of lesions found in the retina or fundus of individuals who have had **type 1** or **type 2 diabetes** for several years. It has serious implications for the affected eye in that the functional ocular sequelae may include a blind, painful eye or enucleation. In addition, the presence and severity of diabetic retinopathy may parallel, in varying degrees, complications of diabetes in other organs.

The abnormalities that constitute diabetic retinopathy occur in predictable progression, with minor variations, in the order of their appearance.[2] The detection of their presence and the extent of involvement of the retina require a careful examination with an ophthalmoscope after dilation of the pupil. A trained observer who is determined to examine as much of the retina as possible will be the most desirable examiner, irrespective of academic degree. The best epidemiologic data are based on a careful examination of the fundus with high-quality standardized stereoscopic photographs of the retina.

21.2 DESCRIPTION OF DIABETIC RETINOPATHY

21.2.1 Non-proliferative retinopathy (See Plate 21.1)

Diabetic retinopathy is considered to be the result of vascular changes in the retinal circulation. In the early stages, vascular occlusion of the retinal arterioles and capillaries and dilation of the retinal venules may occur and there may be an increased permeability of the retinal blood vessels. Histologically, the earliest findings are usually a decrease in the number of capillary pericytes and a thickening of the basement membrane.

Some of the early vascular findings can be seen using fluorescein angiography. This may reveal leakage of the fluorescein dye as well as filling defects and the dilation of retinal vessels. However, early in the course of diabetes, fluorescein angiography is rarely justified because of its expense, inconvenience and potential side effects for little additional benefit. Thus, ophthalmoscopy is the most important clinical diagnostic tool for use in the detection of this complication.

The retinal microaneurysm is usually the first lesion to be detected. It appears as a red spot about 20–200 μm in diameter and can appear to be contiguous with a small blood vessel. It is lined with endothelium and appears to have an increased permeability. Microaneurysms rarely occur before at least three years of diabetes. Based on observations made in the 1980s, about 70% of persons with insulin-dependent diabetes (type 1) for ten years will have these lesions. In contrast, about 55% of persons with ten years of non-insulin dependent diabetes (type 2) will have retinal microaneurysms. Blot and

flame-shaped haemorrhages in the retinal nerve fibre layer may develop at about the same time. The haemorrhages tend to disappear. Thereafter, hard exudates begin to develop, appearing as yellow deposits, often larger than the microaneurysms. Their origin is thought to be 'leaky' capillary blood vessels and microaneurysms in the retina, and they are composed, in part, of lipid material. Soft exudates or cotton-wool spots (infarctions of the retinal nerve fibre layer) may occur at the same time as the appearance of hard exudates. These are white lesions, usually without discrete margins (hence the term 'soft'), and may be slightly elevated from the surface of the surrounding retina. They may disappear any time during the subsequent course of retinopathy.

21.2.2 Pre-proliferative retinopathy (See Plate 21.2)

The next lesions to appear after microaneurysms, small retinal haemorrhages, and exudates, are those associated with retinal ischaemia. There may be dilation of the retinal capillary bed, which sometimes appears as a mass of 'red threads' or may consist only of a few small dilated vessels in what appeared to be avascular areas of the retina. After this, abnormalities may be observed in the larger blood vessels. The retinal venules may develop segments that are dilated, alternating with segments that are constricted, resembling beading, and on occasion may look like strings of sausages. Duplications or loops of veins may develop so that there appear to be parallel veins in some areas. Segments of retinal arterioles may become constricted. Eyes with these lesions are at increased risk of progression to proliferative retinopathy and macular oedema.

21.2.3 Proliferative retinopathy (See Plates 21.3 and 21.4)

The subsequent lesions to appear are those of **proliferative diabetic retinopathy (PDR),** that is, the growth of retinal new blood vessels, which are thin-walled and fragile. The development and progression of diabetic retinopathy is often asymptomatic at this stage, and there are symptoms only if these new vessels bleed (which is a painless event), causing vision to be obscured. Later, contraction of the fibrovascular tissue that develops in the eye, often after a bleed, may result in traction and retinal detachment and, if this involves the macular area, will cause a decrease or distortion of vision. Although spontaneous regression may occur at this stage, it is uncommon.

21.2.4 Macular oedema

Macular oedema is the accumulation of fluid, leaking from retinal capillaries, within the layers of the retina; it causes thickening of the retina, a cystoid appearance and reduction of vision.

A codified system of grading macular oedema (Table 21.1), and its presence with regard to the specific anatomic feature of the macula, is used to define this lesion (Plate 21.5). Macular thickening can be detected in stereoscopic photography of the fundus and by Ocular Computerized Tomography (OCT) (See Plate 21.6).

Table 21.1 *Grading scheme for macular oedema*

Grading scheme for macular oedema	
Level 0	Absent at examination, no prior photocoagulation treatment
Level 1	Questionable at examination, no prior photocoagulation treatment
Level 2	Present (regardless of prior photocoagulation treatment)
Level 3	Absent at examination, prior history of macular oedema, prior photocoagulation treatment
Level 4	Absent at examination, no prior history of macular oedema, prior photocoagulation treatment
Level 5	Present but due to other non-diabetic condition (e.g. macular degeneration, central retinal vein occlusion, aphakic cystoid macular oedema, etc., in the absence of diabetic retinopathy)
Level 8	Cannot grade

21.3 CLASSIFICATION OF DIABETIC RETINOPATHY

The rationale for a classification scheme is to describe the severity of retinopathy using a simple, clinically relevant scale that is reproducible, enabling standardized descriptions across many studies. Scales are based on the observed course of the disease. The Airlie House Classification has been widely used. It describes the presence and severity of the major lesions of retinopathy.

In most epidemiologic studies of diabetic retinopathy, trained graders review stereoscopic photographs of seven standard photographic fields and assign a grade for each lesion seen. The severities of these lesions are summarized using a codified algorithm to assign a level for each eye. A summary classification for an individual in-coporates the severity level for each eye, as diabetic retinopathy is not an entirely symmetric phenomenon.

A grading scheme has also been developed to describe its severity (Table 21.2).

21.4 PREVALENCE

21.4.1 Description of diabetic retinopathy in population-based studies

Although there are specific situations when a computation of the (total) population prevalence of diabetic retinopathy is useful (e.g. to estimate the health costs due to this disease), it is prevalence among those with diabetes that is more germane. Much of the information provided in this chapter comes from the **Wisconsin Epidemiologic Study of Diabetic Retinopathy (WESDR)**,[3,4] a population-based study of people receiving care for diabetes from a well-defined geographical area in south central Wisconsin. In that study, at the baseline examination during 1980–1982, there were 996 persons whose onset of diabetes occurred before the age of 30 years and who were taking insulin (younger-onset group, virtually all had type 1 diabetes by C-peptide testing), and 1,370 people whose age of onset of diabetes was above 30 years (older-onset group includes persons with type 1 and type 2 diabetes). Duration of diabetes ranged from less than a year to more than 50 years in the entire sample. The nature of the lesions of diabetic retinopathy and their relationships to different risk factors did not differ materially from those found in other studies. Thus, inferences from the WESDR may be

Table 21.2 *Severity levels of diabetic retinopathy*

Severity levels of diabetic retinopathy

Level 10	No retinopathy
Level 21*	Microaneurysms (Ma) only or retinal haemorrhages (H) or soft exudates in the absence of microaneurysms
Level 31	Microaneurysms and one or more of the following: venous loops ≥ 31 μm; questionable soft exudate, intraretinal microvascular abnormalities (IRMA) or venous beading; and retinal H
Level 37	Microaneurysms and one or more of the following: hard exudate and soft exudate
Level 43	Microaneurysms and one or more of the following: H/Ma $\geq$ standard photo (SP) #1 in 4–5 fields; H/Ma $\geq$ SP #2A in 1 field; and IRMA in 1–3 fields
Level 47	Microaneurysms and one or more of the following: both IRMA and H/Ma characteristics from level 43; IRMA in 4–5 fields; H/Ma $\geq$ SP #2A in 2–3 fields; and venous beading in 1 field
Level 53	Microaneurysms plus one or more of the following: any 2–3 of level 47 characteristics; H/Ma $\geq$ SP #2A in 4–5 fields; IRMA $\geq$ SP #8A; venous beading in 2 or more fields
Level 60	Fibrous proliferations only
Level 61	No evidence of levels 60 or 65 but scars of photocoagulation either in 'scatter' or confluent patches, presumably directed at new vessels
Level 65	Proliferative diabetic retinopathy (PDR) less than Diabetic Retinopathy Study High-Risk Characteristics (DRS-HRC). Lesions as follows: new vessels elsewhere (NVE); new vessels on or within 1 disc diameter (NVD) of the disc graded less than SP #10A; or preretinal (PRH) or vitreous haemorrhage (VH) less than 1 disc area (DA)
Level 71	DRS-HRC. Lesions as follows: VH and/or PRH $\geq$ 1 DA; NVE $\geq$ 1/2 DA with VH and/or PRH; NVD < SP #10A with VH and/or PRH; and NVD $\geq$ SP 10A
Level 75	Advanced PDR. Lesions as follows: NVD $\geq$ SP #10A with VH and/or PRH
Level 85	End-stage PDR. Lesions as follows: macula obscured by VH and/or PRH; retinal detachment at centre of macula; phthisis bulbi; and enucleation secondary to complications of diabetic retinopathy

Modifications to this scheme were developed for use in the Early Treatment Diabetic Retinopathy Study (ETDRS). This was further elaborated for use in the Wisconsin Epidemiologic Study of Diabetic Retinopathy.[18]
* Lesions included in level 21 rarely occur in those without diagnosed diabetes.

referable to other populations. We draw heavily on the Wisconsin experience for two additional reasons. First, it was a population-based study. Second, the identification of the presence of diabetic retinopathy and the assessment of its severity (according to the scheme described in Table 21.2) was done in a uniform fashion using stereoscopic fundus photographs graded by trained observers who were **masked** as to the characteristics of study subjects. The uniformity of the evaluation and the standardized measures of risk and outcome characteristics give confidence in describing the stages of severity of retinopathy (and macular oedema) and their associations with personal and other risk characteristics.

The WESDR prevalence survey in 1980–1982 found that 71% of the younger-onset group had diabetic retinopathy. Of the older-onset persons who took insulin, 70% had retinopathy, while only 39% of those not taking insulin had retinopathy.

There was, in addition, a relationship of type of diabetes to the severity of retinopathy. In the younger-onset group, 23% had proliferative retinopathy, and in the two older-onset groups, proliferative retinopathy occurred in 14% of insulin takers and 3% of those not taking insulin. Given the projected increase in prevalence of type 2 diabetes,[5] the prevalence of retinopathy may increase as well.[6] However, Sloan and colleagues, using Medicare data, have shown that for older adults the six-year incidence of diabetes-related eye diseases (mostly diabetic retinopathy) decreased from 1994–1999 to 2000–2005.[7]

In the WESDR the prevalence of proliferative diabetic retinopathy (PDR) was significantly lower in persons more recently diagnosed compared with those diagnosed earlier who had similar duration of diabetes ($p < 0.001$). This difference remained while controlling for glycosylated haemoglobin, systolic or diastolic blood pressure and presence of proteinuria.[8] While these data were from those with type 1 diabetes, it is likely that the decrease resulted from changes in management of diabetes[7,9] and this is likely to have benefited those with type 2 diabetes as well.

Macular oedema (also called diabetic maculopathy), severe enough to be a likely cause of visual disturbance, occurred in 6% (younger-onset), 11% (older-onset insulin takers) and 4% (older-onset persons not taking insulin) at the WESDR baseline examination in 1980–1982.[10] Thus this lesion, while not considered in the classification scheme for diabetic retinopathy, is a significant diabetes-related retinal problem. At the moment it is not certain whether there has been a decline in this complication in recent years.

21.4.2 Prevalence of visual impairment related to diabetes

Impaired vision is a common complication in persons with diabetes, and because it affects function this makes it important to patients and eye care providers. In prevalence data from the WESDR, 1.4% of younger-onset persons had best corrected visual acuity of 20/80 (0.25; 6/24) to 20/160 (0.125; 6/48) and 3.6% had an acuity no better than 20/200 (0.1; 6/60) in the better eye. In persons with diabetes at an older age of onset, 3% had acuity of 20/80 to 20/160 and 1.6% had vision no better than 20/200 in the better eye. For those with more severely impaired acuity, diabetic retinopathy was at least partly responsible in 86% of younger-onset persons and in 33% of older-onset persons. Other causes for diminished vision in the older-onset group were cataract, glaucoma and age-related macular degeneration. There are recent data to suggest, however, that the impact of diabetes (mostly diabetic retinopathy) on vision may be diminishing. In the WESDR younger-onset group the prevalence of visual impairment (VI, vision of 20/40 or worse in the better eye) was lower in those persons diagnosed more recently than in those diagnosed earlier. For example, the prevalence of VI in people with 15–19 years of diabetes at the time of examination was 13% among persons diagnosed in 1960–1969 and 2% among those diagnosed in 1975–1979. The prevalence of VI in people with 30–34 years of diabetes was 16% among those diagnosed in 1922–1959, 15% among those diagnosed in 1960–1969, and 9% among those diagnosed in 1970–1974.[11] While these data reflect the experience of better diagnosis and management in persons with type 1 diabetes, it is likely that changes in healthcare will reap benefits for those with type 2 diabetes as well.

The estimates of the strength of the relationship of impaired vision related to retinopathy may be difficult to compare across studies because of inconsistency of measures of visual acuity, population differences in age, ethnicity, proportion of persons with type 1 and type 2 diabetes (as they are often combined), as well as differences in healthcare and other factors influencing this outcome. The WESDR provided long-term incidence data for those with type 1 diabetes. The overall 25-year incidence accounting for competing risk of death was 13% for incident visual impairment and 15% for incident doubling of the visual angle, a continuous measure of decline in visual acuity while controlling for relevant confounders.[12] From the population perspective, the Eye Disease Prevalence group reported that the percentage of persons with severe visual impairment that was attributable to diabetic retinopathy was 6.4% in whites, 26% in blacks and 28.6% in Hispanics.[13] While the percentages are lower for causes of less severe impairment attributable to diabetic retinopathy, there again appeared to be ethnic differences, with non-whites being more disadvantaged than whites in the USA. Some of this is likely to be attributable to differences in the distributions of risk factors and also in access to medical care. It is not clear whether the trends for decreased prevalence in the white persons found in the WESDR are occurring in non-whites as well.

21.5 GEOGRAPHICAL DISTRIBUTION

There have been many reports on populations of diabetic persons around the world giving data on the prevalence of diabetic retinopathy. Some of them are listed in Table 21.3. There is great variability in the reported frequencies of retinopathy,

Table 21.3 *Selected list of population-based studies of diabetic retinopathy*

Location	Selected list of population-based studies of diabetic retinopathy			
	Studied (n)	Duration of diabetes (years)	Prevalence (%)	Reference
Type 1 diabetes				
Perth, Australia	179	0–20+	33	91
Falster, Denmark	215	0–58	66	92
County of Fyn, Denmark	718	0–30+	48	93,94
Denmark	339	–	58	67
Switzerland	105	0–30+	51	95
Allegheny County, PA, USA	657	6–38	86	73
Seattle, WA, USA	78	0–10+	11.5	96
Central Wisconsin, USA	996	0–30+	71	3
Newark, NJ, USA	594	?	75	97,98
Type 2 diabetes				
Falster, Denmark	333	0–42	41	99
Nauru	343	0–10+	24	100
Gotland, Sweden	140	0–20+	17	101
Switzerland	94	–	9	95
Pima Indians, AZ, USA	339	0–10+	18	59
Oklahoma Indians, OK, USA	973	0–20+	24	60,102,103
Central Wisconsin, USA	1,370	0–30+	39	4
San Antonio, TX, USA	257	0–10+	45	61
Pima and Santa Cruz Counties, AZ, USA (Hispanic)	1,044	0–20+	48	104
Chennai, India	1,715	0–?	18	105
Los Angeles, CA, USA	1,217	?	47	106
Barbados, West Indies (black and mixed)	636	?	29	107
Handan, China	368	0–10+	43.1	108

and there are obvious reasons for some of the apparent disparities. For example, some studies are of persons with type 1 and some of persons with type 2 diabetes. These groups may have true differences in their prevalences of diabetic retinopathy. Other reasons include differences in duration of diabetes, age, gender and socio-economic status. Less obvious causes may be related to differences in the distributions of other risk factors. Table 21.3 is meant to be used as a quick reference source for a selected group of studies. It highlights the fact that diabetic retinopathy is a common complication in virtually all studies.

21.6 INCIDENCE

Incidence of retinopathy differs between those with type 1 and type 2 diabetes and is influenced by several characteristics and exposures within these groups. Even without knowing the specific effects of

these influential factors in each population, it is useful to know the incidence in different populations in order to plan for health services. However, the projections based on past experience may be somewhat higher than actually occur. In the WESDR, the overall incidence of any diabetic retinopathy was 40% over a four-year interval. In those with younger-onset diabetes the incidence was 59%. In those with older-onset diabetes, 47% of those taking insulin and 34% of those not taking insulin had developed retinopathy by the four-year follow-up. Progression of retinopathy to the proliferative stage, when the probability of severe loss of vision becomes substantial, differed among the three groups as well. In the younger-onset group such progression occurred in 11%, in the older-onset group taking insulin it occurred in 7%, and in the older-onset group not taking insulin it occurred in 2%.

This population was followed for an additional examination six years later. The adjusted average annual incidence of retinopathy varied little over the two intervals; it was about 20% in the younger-onset group, 15% in the older-onset group taking insulin, and about 10% in the older-onset group not taking insulin. Further follow-up of the younger-onset group for an additional four years indicated that nearly all persons had developed retinopathy and that the cumulative incidence of proliferative retinopathy was 37% in that group. The WESDR has continued longitudinal follow-up of the cohort. Because of the effect of mortality in the older-onset group, long-term follow-up of this group was not possible; however, it was done for the younger-onset group. The 25-year cumulative incidence of diabetic retinopathy in the population, accounting for the competing risk of death, was 97%. Thus, because diabetic retinopathy became so common in this group over the years, progression of relatively early lesions of diabetic retinopathy became the most meaningful retinal outcome. The 25-year cumulative rate of progression of DR was 83%, progression to PDR was 42%, and improvement of DR was 18%.

Of the 227 persons who were found to have PDR in at least one eye at baseline, 74% (n = 167) died during the 25-year follow-up. In the 103 persons with **Diabetic Retinopathy Study High Risk Characteristics (DRS-HRC)** or worse in at least one eye, 82% (n = 84) died by 25 years, significantly higher (P = 0.001) than in the 67% (n = 84) of 124 persons without DRS-HRC.

Of the 95 persons with active PDR without DRS-HRC in at least one eye (level 65) at baseline who were re-examined, 31% (n = 29) were found to have PDR with at least DRS-HRC (levels 71 and 75) in at least one eye, and 7% (n = 7) were found to have progressed beyond DRS-HRC and to have lost vision in at least one eye (level 85) by the 25-year follow-up. New panretinal photocoagulation treatment was observed in 90% (n = 26) and new vitrectomy treatment in 25% (n = 7) of this group. Of the 38 persons with DRS-HRC in at least one eye who were re-examined, 40% (n = 15) had progressed to level 85 in at least one eye and 13% (n = 5) in both eyes. New panretinal photocoagulation treatment was seen in 100% (n = 14) and vitrectomy procedures in 60% (n = 9).[8] Persons diagnosed most recently with similar duration of diabetes had lower prevalence of PDR independent of glycosylated

haemoglobin level, blood pressure level and presence of proteinuria.

Sloan and colleagues[7] reported on six-year cumulative incidence of diabetic retinopathy and macular oedema in two cohorts of persons with newly diagnosed type 2 diabetes in the US Medicare population. They found a 17% lower incidence of non-proliferative diabetic retinopathy in persons who had been diagnosed in 2000–2005 compared with those diagnosed in 1994–1999, a 9% lower incidence of proliferative diabetic retinopathy in the more recent cohort and a 23% lower incidence of macular oedema in the more recent cohort. Klein and colleagues reported a diminishing five-year incidence of diabetic retinopathy in persons more recently diagnosed to have type 1 diabetes.[8] In addition, Klein et al. reported a declining annualized incidence of macular oedema from 2.3% in the first follow-up period to 0.9% in the most recent follow-up period.[14] Hovind and colleagues also demonstrated a steady decrease in the cumulative incidence of PDR in those groups of persons with type 1 diabetes who had been diagnosed in more recent years.[15] These authors find data to suggest that this is related to better treatment of hypertension and glycaemia in those more recently diagnosed.

Based on WESDR data, it was estimated (as of 1993) that about 84,000 Americans of the approximately 7,800,000 people with diabetes would develop proliferative retinopathy and about 95,000 would develop macular oedema over a ten-year period. However, based on the work by Klein and colleagues,[14] Lecaire and colleagues[16] in those with type 1 diabetes and Sloan[7] in those with type 2 diabetes, the recent declines in prevalence and incidence of diabetic retinopathy and macular oedema suggest that despite an apparently growing burden of diabetes, previous forecasts may need to be readjusted.

21.7 CHANGES IN PREVALENCE AND GEOGRAPHICAL DISTRIBUTION WITH TIME

There are important temporal differences over the past two decades in diagnosis, reporting, medical care, socio-economic factors and other risk factors that influence the prevalence and geo-graphical distribution of diabetes and retinopathy as well as other complications of diabetes. For example, **maturity-onset diabetes of youth (MODY)** is a recently described syndrome, the recognition of which may lead to the diagnosis of retinopathy in a group of persons who had not necessarily been under care or surveillance in the past. The advent of more screening programmes for diabetes would likely result in identifying more persons at risk of retinopathy. On the other hand, in the USA, changes in healthcare delivery influ-ence access to care, and not always in a positive direction. Newer pharmacologic agents have become available, which may provide superior gly-caemic control. In addition, there has been greater emphasis on self-monitoring of blood glucose and more frequent dosing with insulin. The impor-tance of the latter in making a meaningful change in rates of complications of diabetes has yet to be documented, but the reports suggest that the need for panretinal photocoagulation for severe proliferative retinopathy has diminished in the USA. Whether reported increases in diabetes in India and islanders in the South Pacific represent true increases in incidence or improved reporting, they nevertheless have resulted in increased cases of complications related to diabetes. It seems that obesity or overweight is a problem not confined to any particular area on the globe and, ethnic differ-ences notwithstanding, appears to be in part related to increased rates of type 2 diabetes. It remains to be determined whether these trends are being balanced by better glycaemic and blood pressure control to offset the potential increase of all the known micro- and macro-vascular sequelae.

21.8 RISK FACTORS FOR DIABETIC RETINOPATHY

21.8.1 Duration of diabetes

In virtually every prevalence study of diabetic retinopathy, duration of diabetes is the most important characteristic associated with increased risk. Although not a 'causal' exposure in a way that is informative about the mechanisms of disease, it

is a convenient marker for the presence of most chronic complications seen in people with diabetes. Table 21.3 lists many of the studies in which the relation between duration of diabetes and the pres-ence or severity of retinopathy has been examined.

In the WESDR, frequency and severity of retinopathy were positively associated with the duration of diabetes.[3] The strength and time courses of the relationships between duration and prevalence or severity differed somewhat between the groups. In younger-onset persons, the preva-lence was about 20% in those with diabetes of three to four years' duration, but proliferative retinopa-thy was not found at this short duration (Fig. 21.1); whereas in those in the older-onset group, whether taking insulin or not, about 30% had any retinopa-thy after three years and about 2% had proliferative disease (Fig. 21.2).[4] Because duration of diabetes is often inaccurate in those with type 2, the age of onset often not being known with precision, the exact time course in this group is difficult to esti-mate. Using the presence and severity of retinopa-thy as a marker of established disease, Harris *et al.* estimated that the onset of diabetes in those with type 2 may occur four to seven years before it is usually diagnosed.[17]

Follow-up of the WESDR cohort has provided useful information about long-duration diabetes.[18] After ten years of follow-up of younger-onset

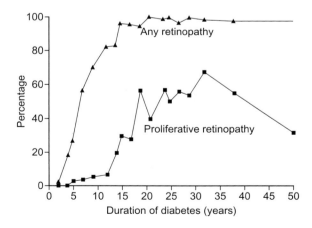

Figure 21.1 *Prevalence of any retinopathy and of pro-liferative retinopathy in persons diagnosed with dia-betes below 30 years of age, by duration of diabetes (from the Wisconsin Epidemiologic Study of Diabetic Retinopathy baseline examination 1980–1982)*

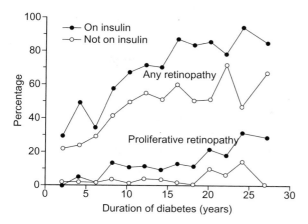

Figure 21.2 *Prevalence of any retinopathy and of proliferative retinopathy by persons diagnosed with diabetes at or above 30 years of age, by duration of diabetes (from the Wisconsin Epidemiologic Study of Diabetic Retinopathy baseline examination, 1980–1982)*

persons, there was little change in the incidence of retinopathy with increasing duration of diabetes. Duration did have a positive relation with progression of retinopathy to the proliferative stage, but the effect was not linear, levelling out after about ten (additional) years of diabetes. In those of the older-onset group using insulin, there was a decline in incident retinopathy with increasing duration and an increase in progression to proliferative disease. There was no consistent relationship of duration to incident retinopathy in those who did not use insulin. However, 15 or more years' duration was associated with an increase in frequency of progression to proliferative retinopathy in this group.

21.8.2 Glycaemic control

There is now strong epidemiologic evidence of a monotonic relation between the level of glycaemia and the severity of diabetic retinopathy from incidence data. This has been found in observational studies and in clinical trials. In the ten-year follow-up in the WESDR, each successively higher quartile of glycosylated haemoglobin at baseline was associated with a greater incidence and a greater risk of developing proliferative retinopathy.[19] The level of glycaemia was the strongest risk factor for predicting incidence in the WESDR.

In order to evaluate the findings from the observational studies, the **Diabetes Control and Complications Trial (DCCT)** was designed to test the effects of good glycaemic control in 1,441 patients with type 1 diabetes. This study assigned patients to either intensive treatment or usual care, and followed them for three to nine years with the outcome measure being the progression of diabetic retinopathy[20] of at least three steps on a codified scale of increasing severity of retinopathy. In the primary prevention group (no retinopathy at baseline), the frequency of progression of retinopathy was reduced by 76% in the intensive treatment group compared with those in the usual care group; in the secondary prevention group, the corresponding reduction in risk was 54%. A residual protective effect on retinopathy of this early tight control has become apparent from following this cohort for many years after the completion of the trial. Although the DCCT was performed in those with type 1 diabetes, data from the WESDR suggested that beneficial effects of good glycaemic control in those with type 2 diabetes could be expected as has been borne out in findings from the **United Kingdom Prospective Diabetes Study (UKPDS).**[21]

An important piece of evidence supporting the causal nature of the relationship of hyperglycaemia to diabetic retinopathy has been provided by the continued follow-up of the DCCT cohort after the constraints of the trial were terminated.[22] By the first post-trial year the glycosylated haemoglobin (HbA1c) of the intensive control group was still significantly lower than that of the conventional group, although the difference between the groups was smaller than at the trial close out. However, by the ten-year post-trial examination the level of HbA1c in the group originally assigned to conventional care was significantly lower than for the group initially assigned to intensive control; there had been no difference between the groups since the fourth post-trial examination. While the difference in cumulative incidence of retinopathy continued to be better in the intensive group, there is evidence that the effect of the earlier intensive control is waning as the level of glycaemia in that group is rising.

While the accumulated data show the clear benefit of intensive glycaemic control in reducing the risk of development and progression of retinopathy, there is a less consistent effect on macrovascular disease. The Finnish Diabetic Nephropathy Study and the DCCT as well as the UKPDS (type 2 diabetes) have reported beneficial effects of glycaemic control on macrovascular disease.[23–26] However, the results of three large randomized controlled clinical trials (Action to Control Cardiovascular Risk in Diabetes (ACCORD),[27] Action in Diabetes and Vascular Disease: Preterax and Diamicron Modified Release Controlled Evaluation (ADVANCE) trials[28] and the Veteran Administration Diabetes Trial (VADT)[29]) in persons with type 2 diabetes failed to find a beneficial effect on cardiovascular endpoints.

There are troublesome complications attendant upon rigorous glycaemic control. For example, weight gain and episodes of severe hypoglycaemia occurred more frequently in those in the intensively treated group in the DCCT.[30] These side effects may cause even more concern in those with type 2 diabetes who are usually older and whose risk of compromised cardiovascular status owing to age and diabetes may put them at greater risk of adverse sequelae associated with increased weight and hypoglycemia.[31]

21.8.3 Blood pressure

Anecdotal observations from clinical studies suggested an association between hypertension and the severity of retinopathy in people with diabetes.[32] While epidemiological data from cross-sectional studies suggested an association of hypertension with diabetic retinopathy, data from cohort studies have been inconsistent.[33] Epidemiological analyses from the UKPDS showed that the incidence of retinopathy was associated with systolic blood pressure. For each 10 mmHg decrease in mean systolic blood pressure, a 13% reduction was found for this microvascular complication and no threshold was found for any endpoint.[34] In the WESDR, diastolic blood pressure was a significant predictor of progression of diabetic retinopathy and the incidence of proliferative diabetic retinopathy in persons with younger-onset diabetes mellitus.[35] However, neither systolic nor diastolic blood pressure or hypertension status at baseline were

associated with the incidence and progression of retinopathy in people with older-onset diabetes.[33] Diastolic blood pressure, however, was found to be associated with a 330% increased four-year risk of developing macular oedema in those with younger-onset diabetes and a 210% increased risk in those with older-onset diabetes in the WESDR.

The EURODIAB Controlled Trial of Lisinopril in Insulin-Dependent Diabetes Mellitus (EUCLID) Study sought to examine the role of an **angiotensin-converting enzyme (ACE)** inhibitor in reducing the incidence and progression of retinopathy in a group of largely normotensive type 1 diabetic patients of whom 85% did not have microalbuminuria at baseline.[36] This study showed a statistically significant 50% reduction in the progression of retinopathy in those taking lisinopril over a two-year period after adjustment for glycaemic control. Progression to proliferative retinopathy was also reduced. There was no significant interaction with blood glucose control. It was postulated that ACE inhibitors might have an effect independent of blood pressure lowering.[37]

The UKPDS also sought to determine whether lower blood pressure achieved with either a beta blocker or an ACE inhibitor was beneficial in reducing macrovascular and microvascular complications associated with type 2 diabetes.[38] One thousand and forty-eight patients with hypertension (mean blood pressure 160/94 mmHg) were randomized to a regimen of tight control with either captopril or atenolol and another 390 patients to less tight control of their blood pressure. The aim in the group randomized to tight control was to achieve blood pressure values <150/<85 mmHg, a relatively high level by today's standard. If these goals were not met with maximal doses of a beta blocker or ACE inhibitor, additional medications were prescribed, including a loop diuretic, a calcium channel blocker and a vasodilator. The aim in the group randomized to less tight control was to achieve blood pressure values <180/<105 mmHg. Tight blood pressure control resulted in a 35% reduction in the number of persons requiring retinal photocoagulation compared with conventional control. After 7.5 years of follow-up, there was a 34% reduction in the rate of progression of retinopathy by two or more steps using the modified **Early Treatment Diabetic Retinopathy Study (ETDRS)** severity scale and a 47% reduction in the deterioration of visual acuity by three lines or more using the ETDRS charts (for example, a reduction in vision from 20/30 to 20/60 or worse on a Snellen chart). The effect was largely due to a reduction in the incidence of diabetic macular oedema. Atenolol and captopril were equally effective in reducing the risk of developing these microvascular complications. The effects of blood pressure control were independent of those of glycaemic control. These findings support the recommendations for tight blood pressure control in patients with type 2 diabetes as a means of preventing visual loss from diabetic retinopathy.

The **Appropriate Blood Pressure Control in Diabetes (ABCD) Trial** was a prospective randomized masked clinical trial comparing the effects of intensive (diastolic blood pressure goal of 75 mmHg) and moderate (diastolic blood pressure of 80 to 89 mmHg) blood pressure control in 470 hypertensive subjects (baseline diastolic blood pressure of 90 mmHg) with type 2 diabetes.[39] Persons were randomized to either nisoldipine 10 mg/day as needed (titrated up to 60 mg/day as needed) versus placebo or enalapril 5 mg/day (titrated up to 40 mg/day as needed), versus placebo as the initial hypertensive medication.[39] If singlestudy medication alone did not achieve the target blood pressure, then metoprolol followed by hydrochlorothiazide were added until the target blood pressure was achieved. The mean blood pressure achieved was 132/78 mmHg in the intensive group and 138/86 mmHg in the moderate control group. Over a five-year follow-up period, there was no difference between the intensive and moderate groups with regard to progression of diabetic retinopathy. There was no difference in nisoldipine versus enalapril in progression of retinopathy. The authors concluded that lack of efficacy in their study compared with the UKPDS might have resulted from the shorter time period of the ABCD (five years versus nine years on average for the UKPDS), lower average blood pressure control in the ABCD (144/82 mmHg versus 154/87 mmHg in the UKPDS), and poorer glycaemic control in the ABCD than the UKPDS. These data also suggest the possibility of a threshold effect below which

minimal efficacy for reducing the risk of progression of retinopathy is achieved by further reduction of blood pressure. Results from other clinical trials that are currently underway should provide more information regarding the relative efficacy of blood pressure control and specific antihypertensive medications in reducing the progression of retinopathy in persons with diabetes.

The Renin-Angiotensin System Study (RASS), a study of persons with type 1 diabetes who had neither hypertension nor albuminurea, reported that treatment with enalapril or losartan was associated with a reduction in the progression of diabetic retinopathy independent of blood pressure. While this is suggestive of a possible benefit of the two classes of drug — an angiotensin-converting enzyme inhibitor (ACE-I) and angiotensin receptor blockers (ARB) — the investigators could not determine whether this was due to the reduction of blood pressure.[40] Further, the Diabetic Retinopathy Candesartan Trials (DIRECT) study reported that there was a marginally significant effect of candesartan on incidence of retinopathy (p-value 0.0508). This effect was attenuated when adjusted for blood pressure, suggesting that blood pressure control is more important than the specific agent used to achieve it.[41] For those with type 1 and type 2 diabetes in this study with retinopathy present at baseline, there was no effect on progression of retinopathy in those taking candesartan compared with placebo. The medication appeared to have an effect on regression of retinopathy during the trial.[42] While this effect was attenuated when controlling for blood pressure during the trial, the medication effect was still statistically significant. Thus, blood pressure appears to have had an effect even on this secondary endpoint. It seems, in summary, that blood pressure is an important contributing cause of diabetic retinopathy and that controlling it is important in attempts to minimize the incidence and progression of retinopathy in diabetics.

21.8.4 Contraception and pregnancy

The question of which mode of contraception should be used in fertile women with diabetes has received some attention both from patients and from those caring for them. While oral contraceptives are relatively efficacious and convenient, they have been associated with elevated systemic blood pressure and with glucose intolerance in those who had gestational diabetes. Thus, because of the potential effects of these drugs on retinopathy and because of the noted effects on glycaemia and blood pressure, some investigators have studied the possibility of a relationship[43,44] of these drugs to worsening retinopathy. Neither Garg[43] nor Klein and co-workers[44] found any evidence of a harmful effect of oral contraceptive use on diabetic retinopathy.

Two recent large studies found that pregnancy in persons with type 1 diabetes increases the rate of progression of diabetic retinopathy,[45,46] although pre-existing risk factors such as level of glycaemia and severity of retinopathy prior to pregnancy influence the risk of progression.[47] The Diabetes Control and Complications Trial[48] reported that the probability of worsening of diabetic retinopathy was higher during pregnancy than in non-pregnant women followed over the same interval, but at the end of the study the women who had been pregnant fared no more poorly than their non-pregnant counterparts. Nevertheless, physicians may consider the use of oral (or other forms of) contraceptives for those fertile women who desire to limit the number of their pregnancies.

21.8.5   Insulin

Dependence upon insulin for glycaemic control has served as a useful marker in predicting the immediate and long-term course of diabetes, and of retinopathy in particular. Thus, the most useful epidemiological studies describe retinopathy findings separately for those with type 1 and type 2. Whether the differences in frequency and severity of retinopathy between type 1 and type 2 are related to endogenous insulin secretion is unclear. In the WESDR population, retinopathy was more frequent and severe in those with very low levels of plasma C-peptide (a measure of endogenous insulin secretion). However, after the level of glycaemia had been taken into consideration, C-peptide was found to be unrelated to the severity of retinopathy. As

regards the use of exogenous insulin, in the WESDR older-onset insulin-takers with at least 0.3 mM/dl of C-peptide, severity of retinopathy was unrelated to dosage or type of exogenous insulin. This finding supports the notion that the level of glycaemia is more important than the degree of endogenous insulin secretion in the aetiology of retinopathy.[49]

21.8.6   Serum lipids

Several investigators have reported a positive association between serum lipids and diabetic retinopathy, but the findings have not been universal or consistent.[50,51] Some have found positive associations between cholesterol and retinopathy, while others found a positive relationship between triglycerides and retinopathy, but not cholesterol and retinopathy. The WESDR examined the relationship between the severity of retinopathy and levels both of total and high-density lipoprotein (HDL) cholesterol.[49] In insulin-using persons, higher total-serum cholesterol was associated with increased odds of having retinal hard exudates. There was no relation between either of these lipid fractions and other retinopathy or retinal hard exudates in older-onset persons not taking insulin. The Early Treatment Diabetic Retinopathy Study (ETDRS)[52] reported a positive association between serum lipids and retinopathy. However, despite these associations, there are no clinical trial data to suggest that medical therapy to alter serum lipids would reduce the risk of any of the retinal findings. Moreover, there is some suggestive evidence that use of statin drugs may be harmful to microvascular epithelium.[53] The pleiotropic effects of simvastatin on retinal microvascular endothelium has important implications for ischaemic retinopathies.[54] Thus, until clinical trial data are available supporting the beneficial effects of lipid lowering drugs on retinopathy it would not be appropriate to institute lipid therapy based on the retinopathy status alone.

21.8.7   Ethnicity

Table 21.3 summarizes findings from studies of diabetic retinopathy of many ethnic groups from a variety of geographical locations. While the variability in frequency may reflect true differences in prevalence, lack of uniformity in study designs, protocols for examination and documentation may explain some of these differences. There are few studies in which the same techniques for population sampling and documentation of the severity of retinopathy are used in members of different ethnic groups. Harris and co-workers reported a higher prevalence of retinopathy in black men with type 2 than in other race-sex groups, although the difference did not reach statistical significance.[55] Roy has shown relatively high rates of retinopathy in blacks with type 1 diabetes.[56] Risk factors for retinopathy appear to be the same[57] as those found in WESDR, an essentially white population.

In the **National Health and Nutrition Examination Surveys (NHANES)** III, a national survey carried out periodically to ascertain health and nutritional status of the US population, retinopathy was more prevalent in black men than in non-Hispanic white men. There was no difference after control for glycaemia and blood pressure. Tielsch and co-workers found, in the Baltimore Nursing Home Eye Study, that diabetic retinopathy was responsible for 2.3% of blindness in black nursing-home residents, but retinopathy was the cause of blindness for only 0.4% of white nursing-home residents.[58]

Studies of various native American groups indicate that most have higher frequencies of diabetic retinopathy than white Americans with type 2, although there are differences in rates between the groups of native American peoples.[59,60] Mexican Americans also appear to be at greater risk for retinopathy than the white Americans who participated in the WESDR, although rates in Hispanics in Arizona were similar to early rates reported in WESDR.[61,104] No difference was found between Hispanic and non-Hispanic whites in the San Luis Valley Study.[62] A study of Japanese Americans found lower rates of retinopathy than in Japanese who reside in Japan.

Many difficulties are attendant upon comparisons of different studies. While differences in environmental and genetic risk factors as well as other co-variants may have a marked impact on frequency, there appear to be cohort effects, probably related to medical treatments for diabetes and specifically for retinopathy, that are now occurring and which will alter projections for incidence in most ethnic groups in the near future.

21.8.8 Age

Age at diagnosis has had meaning historically because it served as an indicator of the type of diabetes; that is, insulin-dependent or not. This is still a convenient marker, as most people who develop diabetes before 30 years of age are insulin-dependent. There may be some who are older than this when diabetes is diagnosed but who otherwise behave similarly to those of younger-onset, and who depend upon insulin for glycaemic control. In addition, there are some individuals who develop diabetes in their youth, but whose glycaemic control can be more easily influenced by weight reduction, diet and oral agents. Many of these individuals are now considered to have 'maturity-onset diabetes of the young' (MODY). Thus, using age of onset as the criterion for labelling may produce some spurious classifications.

Information concerning retinopathy in those who have MODY is limited. Despite the report in the literature of a single patient with this condition who developed proliferative diabetic retinopathy,[63] the estimated risk for patients in general with MODY is unknown. While persons with this condition seem to have signs of more typical type 2 diabetes it is unclear whether the age at onset of this syndrome is important in the severity of complications or the time it takes to develop these complications.

It is uncertain if age itself is an independent risk factor. In younger-onset persons in WESDR, prevalence of retinopathy was positively associated with age, although this is likely due to the high correlation between age and duration of diabetes. In those of older-onset, the association was less consistent, with a marked increase in frequency of retinopathy in those younger than 50 years of age, but little relationship between age and retinopathy thereafter. In the Framingham Eye Study (FES), the frequencies of those with retinopathy were 18.0% in those aged 52–65 years, 16.8% in those

65–74 years of age and 25.9% in those aged 75 or more.[64] It seems, however, that the relationship with age is more likely to be due to an association of retinopathy with the duration of diabetes.

Puberty is one particular biological transition that is related to age and that may affect the frequency of diabetic retinopathy. In the WESDR, diabetic retinopathy was uncommon before the age of 13. Children who were older than 13 years of age at diagnosis were more likely to have retinopathy than those who were younger even when the duration of diabetes was considered.[65] Two additional studies done on a large series of patients found evidence to suggest that years of diabetes before puberty does have some influence on increasing the risk of retinopathy.[66,67]

In the large population-based studies whose data are included in the collaborative Eye Disease Prevalence consortium, the prevalence by age group of any retinopathy in white, black and Hispanic persons with diabetes varied among the studies.[68] Type 2 is the most common type in these populations. The lack of consistency may reflect differences in the distribution of important risk variables, selective mortality, and possibly genetic factors that contribute to the age-related risk (and severity) of retinopathy in the groups.

21.8.9   Nutritional factors

Although many people are interested in the effects of diet on the development of complications of diabetes, there is little epidemiological data evaluating relationships between nutrition and complications. Aside from controlling glycaemia, in part through dietary limitation of glucose, regulation of more complex carbohydrates and other macronutrients appears to have little effect on retinopathy. Although one study suggested that α-tocopherol might have a beneficial effect on complications because it seemed to decrease glycaemia, no effect was found in the **Beaver Dam Eye Study (BDES)**. While there is experimental data suggesting that the **Age-Related Eye Disease (AREDS)** type supplements (antioxidants and zinc) in an animal model may decrease the risk of microvascular changes related

to diabetes,[69] there is no convincing data that specific dietary or supplement regimens influence the course of retinopathy in humans.

21.8.10   Cigarette smoking

The noxious effects of cigarette smoking, and possibly of passive smoking, have been well documented for cardiovascular disease in the general population. Thus one may anticipate that this behaviour would be associated with increased risk of retinopathy, which is a vascular phenomenon associated with ischemia and hypoxia. However, in the WESDR study,[70,71] and in others,[60,72] no such relationship has been found. It may be that the apparent lack of an association is due to altered smoking patterns prior to the evaluation for retinopathy and/or the competing morbidity and mortality attendant upon cigarette smoking. Cigarette smoking was associated with the incidence of diabetic macular oedema in univariate analyses but in multivariate analysis controlling for other relevant characteristics the effect of smoking was no longer significant.[14]

21.8.11   Alcohol

Potential effects of alcohol in any study are often difficult to evaluate. There is a particular scepticism regarding the accuracy of the self-reported quantities of intake in many studies. In those with diabetes, care-givers may admonish their patients not to imbibe. Therefore, reporting may be an especially imprecise measure of actual intake. That said, a few studies have examined this exposure. One study reported a protective,[73] while another reported a deleterious effect on retinopathy.[74] In the WESDR, alcohol consumption was associated cross-sectionally with a lower frequency of proliferative retinopathy in younger-onset persons, but there was no significant association with incidence or progression of retinopathy six years later.[75] Moderate alcohol consumption was associated with decreased risk of microvascular events in the EuroDiab study.[76] A protective association between alcohol intake and cardiovascular disease mortality in those with older-onset diabetes has been found.[77]

21.8.12 Other risk factors

Obesity

Obesity or body mass index has been investigated not only as a characteristic associated with the development of diabetes, but also as a risk factor for retinopathy once diabetes is present. There is little consistency in the studies regarding the effect of body mass on retinopathy. At the moment, it seems that the body mass index may reflect other factors that are more relevant to the risk of retinopathy (for example, level of glycaemia and insulin use).

Physical activity

Physical activity has been evaluated as a potentially protective factor in the WESDR. In that study, women diagnosed to have diabetes before 14 years of age who participated in team sports were less likely to have proliferative retinopathy than those who did not. However, there was no association between physical activity or leisure time energy expenditure and the presence or severity of diabetic retinopathy in men. Another epidemiological study in Pittsburgh found no relation between a history of participation in team sports in high school and a history of laser treatment or blindness.

Socio-economic status

Some studies have attempted to evaluate a relationship between **socio-economic status (SES)** and severity of retinopathy. Although educational attainment was inversely associated with retinopathy in women in the WESDR, most studies find no relation to a socio-economic index. It may be that once the level of glycaemia is accounted for, social factors have little or no influence on this complication of diabetes, suggesting that glycaemic control is the pathway by which socio-economic factors influence retinopathy. Thus, for example, barriers to care experienced by low SES may play a large role in the ability to control hyperglycaemia, and thus increase risk of complications.

Kidney disease

Kidney disease is a frequent concomitant of retinal manifestations of diabetes.[31,78] In the WESDR, microalbuminuria was associated with proliferative diabetic retinopathy in the younger-onset (type 1) group and with any retinopathy in those with older-onset diabetes,[79] and gross proteinuria was associated with the four-year incidence of PDR in both younger- and older-onset groups after adjusting for confounders.[80] While it may be best to describe renal disease in those with diabetes as a risk indicator, it seems reasonable that those caring for people with diabetes should seek eye care for those patients who have not previously been referred.

It has been suggested that markers of systemic inflammation and endothelial dysfunction may be associated with increased risk of diabetic retinopathy. Klein and colleagues, however, reported that selected risk factors were only associated with retinopathy outcomes in persons with kidney disease as well as diabetes; they found no independent association of the markers with retinopathy in the absence of kidney disease.[81]

21.9 GENETIC FACTORS

The susceptibility to diabetes may well depend upon genetic factors, as evidenced by significant family clustering of cases, but the pattern of inheritance is unlikely to conform to a straightforward Mendelian characteristic for either type 1 or type 2. The elusiveness of defining genetic influences extends to identifying genetic factors related to retinopathy in those with either type of diabetes. There have been reports of a positive relationship between the presence of some HLA antigens and the absence of others.

It seems likely that both genetic and environmental confounders exist for the expression of diabetic retinopathy. Data from the DCCT indicated significant correlations of the severity of diabetic retinopathy between family members.[82] Keeping in mind that several studies have found that there are genes associated with retinopathy distinct from those associated directly with diabetes, and that glycaemia and blood pressure also have an effect on retinopathy severity, it may be reasonable to approach retinopathy as a more typical quantitative trait.[83] Identifying genes that underlie susceptibility to the systemic microvascular vascular phenomena are currently under investigation.

21.10   CLINICAL TRIALS

PubMed, through ClinicalTrials.gov (www.clinical-trials.gov), lists registered trials and gives a description of their designs. Pertinent to this chapter, there are **primary**, **secondary** and **tertiary prevention** trials that are important. **Primary** prevention trials would be those aimed at preventing diabetes. An example of a primary prevention trial would be a trial aimed at preventing type 1 diabetes amongst youngsters who are thought to be at high risk by virtue of having a sibling or other first-degree family member who has manifest disease. Results of the trial to prevent type 2 diabetes (Diabetic Prevention Trial) have demonstrated some success. The study participants were a group at high risk of diabetes related to their weight, insulin resistance and hypertension. Weight reduction and physical activity levels were associated with decreased incidence of diabetes in the special intervention group.[84]

With respect to **secondary** prevention, there are many trials that are on the verge of enrolment or are in the active phase of recruitment. While most are trials designed to improve glycaemic control, there are some that are working on more basic mechanisms to decrease antibody formation in the causal pathway to islet cell destruction. Some are designed to decrease complications such as risk of retinopathy in persons with either type 1 or type 2, while some are specific to type of diabetes.[20,21] Zimmet has recently reviewed some of the **secondary** prevention strategies.[85]

Clinical trials of various interventions to prevent severe loss of vision from diabetic retinopathy (**tertiary** prevention) are numerous. The most successful include the Diabetic Retinopathy Study (DRS)[86] which showed that panretinal photocoagulation reduced the risk of severe loss of vision over a two-year follow-up in persons with proliferative retinopathy; the ETDRS,[87] which showed that focal photocoagulation of severe macular oedema decreased the risk of loss of vision from this cause; and the Diabetic Retinopathy Vitrectomy Study (DRVS),[88] which showed that in persons with type 1 diabetes who had sustained a vitreous haemorrhage, early vitrectomy significantly improved the chance for recovering vision compared with deferred surgery. Some countries are moving towards systematic screening programmes to detect retinopathy in the population that has diabetes. An example is the nationwide screening programme that has been introduced in the UK (see Chapter 8).

Tertiary prevention trials using medications have shown that, in general, these agents are not successful and/or are related to unacceptable side effects. An example was the use of sorbinil to decrease progression of retinopathy. Those on the treatment had a slightly slower rate of increase of microaneurysms than those in the control group, but had a higher rate of developing a hypersensitivity reaction in the first three months of treatment than controls.[89] There are other studies underway evaluating effects of protein kinase C, antagonists to epithelial growth factors, and others. Results of a recent clinical trial suggest that fibrates may decrease the risk of microvascular complication of diabetes.[90]

21.11   SUMMARY OF OPHTHALMIC MANAGEMENT

From the time of diagnosis, emphasis is now placed on intensive glycaemic and blood pressure control to prevent incidence and progression of retinopathy. This has been discussed above. The role of the ophthalmologist is to communicate his/her clinical findings to the primary care physician and inform the patient of the benefits of such care.

Philosophies of management, including diagnostic and treatment plans, vary from country to country and even in different communities within countries. The cornerstone of management is regular and thorough dilated eye examinations according to a schedule, which may be modified by symptoms of the patient and concerns of the diabetologist or other health providers caring for the general health of patients with diabetes. The physical examination may include fundus photography, angiography and ultrasonography as symptoms and signs warrant and as facilities to accomplish these are available. In general, fundus photography may be helpful in judging the rate of progression of diabetic retinopathy, in planning for panretinal photocoagulation if needed, in judging the adequacy of treatment and in evaluating the response to it. Usually, fluorescein angiography may be helpful in managing macular oedema and in identifying subtle neovascularization and areas of capillary non-perfusion in the retina. Ocular Coherence Tomography (OCT) is assuming a larger role in evaluating diabetic macular oedema (Plate 21.6). Contact B-scan ultrasonography is often helpful when vitreous haemorrhage or other media opacity obscure the fundus. The clinician may be able to detect retinal detachment which might otherwise be unobserved and treatment unadvisedly delayed. Both diagnostic and treatment modalities are in a constant state of change, especially in countries where technology is advanced. Nevertheless, careful dilated eye examinations (using ophthalmoscopy, fundus photography and fluorescein angiography and/or OCT) and laser treatment remain the mainstay of management once severe diabetic retinopathy is present.

21.12 OTHER CHRONIC OCULAR CONDITIONS ASSOCIATED WITH DIABETES

There are chronic ocular problems other than those affecting the retina that are more common in people with diabetes. In the Western countries, there are often conditions that occur with increasing frequency in older age groups.

Cataracts

Cataracts were responsible for more instances of decreased visual acuity than diabetic retinopathy in older-onset subjects in the WESDR. Data from the NHANES indicate that cataract is more common in those with diabetes than in those without diabetes in the United States. Cortical lens opacity is more frequent in those with diabetes in the BDES and the risk rises with the duration of diabetes. Cataract surgery is more common in diabetic persons, but the effect of diabetes diminishes with increasing age.

Glaucoma

Glaucoma, of at least two distinct types, is more frequent in people with diabetes. Called neovascular glaucoma, a very severe and relatively rare type (precise estimates are not available) can occur usually in eyes that have had proliferative retinopathy and in those that have had vitrectomy. There is a development of neovascularization in the anterior chamber angle leading to the occlusion of the aqueous outflow tract and subsequent dramatic increases in intraocular pressure. This usually leads to severe optic nerve damage and is usually accompanied by an inflammatory reaction which may also include bleeding into the anterior chamber. Although it may be possible to decrease the intraocular pressure with surgical and medical means, there is usually a marked decrease in visual function. The other form of glaucoma which is probably found in increased frequency among diabetic persons is open-angle glaucoma. In persons without diabetes, this is usually an age-related disorder, but it appears to occur earlier in people with diabetes. In the BDES, the increased risk associated with diabetes was about 60% compared with similarly aged persons without diabetes.

Infections

Diabetes may increase the risk of superficial or intraocular infections. Data regarding actual estimates of risk of these conditions are scarce.

21.13 RESEARCH PRIORITIES

The first priority in caring for persons with diabetes is, of course, preventing diabetic retinopathy and its complications. This implies high quality medical care with appropriate dietary counselling and availability of medications as needed. For secondary care, when microvascular complications appear, competent clinical examination and imaging, when adequate clinical examination capabilities are not at hand, is imperative.

There are many areas where further research is needed in order to better identify modes of prevention of eye diseases related to diabetes. These include basic sciences, clinical trials and modes of identifying persons with diabetes and patients at risk of vision loss due to diabetes. Further evaluation of the effects of these conditions on quality of life of patients with diabetes and development of modalities to improve the healthcare and well-being of these patients should be high research priorities.

Much future research will be in genetic epidemiology. Genetic make-up influences many of the phenotypes associated with anthropometry and, in general, phenotypes that characterize individuals and their predisposition to disease. Thus, there have been genes that are associated with the development of diabetes, both type 1 and type 2, and also probably for the complications of those diseases. However, there have been environmental factors that appear to influence expression of genetically influenced traits. For example, obesity appears to increase risk of diabetes in most populations.[84] In another setting, smoking influences the risk of cardiovascular disease. The mechanisms responsible for these increased risks are likely to be **epigenetic** phenomena such as methylation or histone acetylation of genes that modify their function and lead to diseases and their sequelae. Researchers hope to develop medications to correct disease caused by gene misregulation.

REFERENCES

1. King H, Aubert RE, Herman WH. Global burden of diabetes, 1995–2025: prevalence, numerical estimates, and projections. *Diabetes Care* 1998; 21:1414–1431.

2. Diabetic Retinopathy Study Research Group. Report Number 7. A modification of the Airlie House classification of diabetic retinopathy. *Invest Ophthalmol Vis Sci* 1981; 21210–21226.

3. Klein R, Klein BE, Moss SE, *et al*. The Wisconsin epidemiologic study of diabetic retinopathy. II. Prevalence and risk of diabetic retinopathy when age at diagnosis is less than 30 years. *Arch Ophthalmol* 1984; 102:520–526.

4. Klein R, Klein BE, Moss SE, *et al*. The Wisconsin epidemiologic study of diabetic retinopathy. III. Prevalence and risk of diabetic retinopathy when age at diagnosis is 30 or more years. *Arch Ophthalmol* 1984; 102:527–532.

5. Wild S, Roglic G, Green A, *et al*. Global prevalence of diabetes: estimates for the year 2000 and projections for 2030. *Diabetes Care* 2004; 27:1047–1053.

6. Saaddine JB, Honeycutt AA, Narayan KM, *et al*. Projection of diabetic retinopathy and other major eye diseases among people with diabetes mellitus: United States, 2005–2050. *Arch Ophthalmol* 2008; 126:1740–1747.

7. Sloan FA, Belsky D, Ruiz D, Jr., *et al*. Changes in incidence of diabetes mellitus-related eye disease among US elderly persons, 1994–2005. *Arch Ophthalmol* 2008; 126:1548–1553.

8. Klein R, Knudtson MD, Lee KE, *et al*. The Wisconsin Epidemiologic Study of Diabetic Retinopathy: XXII the 25-year progression of retinopathy in persons with type 1 diabetes. *Ophthalmology* 2008; 115:1859–1868.

9. Ong KL, Cheung BM, Wong LY, *et al*. Prevalence, treatment, and control of diagnosed diabetes in the U.S. National Health and Nutrition Examination Survey 1999–2004. *Ann Epidemiol* 2008; 18:222–229.

10. Klein R, Klein BE, Moss SE, *et al*. The Wisconsin epidemiologic study of diabetic retinopathy. IV. Diabetic macular edema. *Ophthalmology* 1984; 91:1464–1474.

11. Klein R, Klein BE, Lee KE, *et al*. Changes in visual acuity in a population over a 15-year period: the Beaver Dam Eye Study. *Am J Ophthalmol* 2006; 142:539–549.

12. Klein R, Lee KE, Gangnon R, *et al*. The 25-year Incidence of visual impairment in type 1 diabetes mellitus: the Wisconsin Epidemiologic Study of Diabetic Retinopathy. *Ophthalmology* 2010; 117: 63–70.

13. Congdon N, O'Colmain B, Klaver CC, *et al*. Causes and prevalence of visual impairment

among adults in the United States. *Arch Ophthalmol* 2004; 122:477–485.

14. Klein R, Knudtson MD, Lee KE. The Wisconsin Epidemiologic Study of Diabetic Retinopathy XXIII: the 25-year incidence of macular edema in persons with type 1 diabetes. *Ophthalmology* 2009; 116:497–503.

15. Hovind P, Tarnow L, Rossing K, *et al*. Decreasing incidence of severe diabetic microangiopathy in type 1 diabetes. *Diabetes Care* 2003; 26:1258–1264.

16. Lecaire T, Palta M, Zhang H, *et al*. Lower-than-expected prevalence and severity of retinopathy in an incident cohort followed during the first 4–14 years of type 1 diabetes: the Wisconsin Diabetes Registry Study. *Am J Epidemiol* 2006; 164:143–150.

17. Harris MI, Klein R, Welborn TA, *et al*. Onset of NIDDM occurs at least 4–7 years before clinical diagnosis. *Diabetes Care* 1992; 15:815–819.

18. Klein R, Klein BE, Moss SE, *et al*. The Wisconsin Epidemiologic Study of diabetic retinopathy. XIV. Ten-year incidence and progression of diabetic retinopathy. *Arch Ophthalmol* 1994; 112:1217–1228.

19. Klein R, Klein BE, Moss SE, *et al*. Relationship of hyperglycemia to the long-term incidence and progression of diabetic retinopathy. *Arch Intern Med* 1994; 154:2169–2178.

20. The effect of intensive diabetes treatment on the progression of diabetic retinopathy in insulin-dependent diabetes mellitus. The Diabetes Control and Complications Trial. *Arch Ophthalmol* 1995; 113:36–51.

21. UK Prospective Diabetes Study (UKPDS) Group. Intensive blood-glucose control with sulphonylureas or insulin compared with conventional treatment and risk of complications in patients with type 2 diabetes (UKPDS 33). *Lancet* 1998; 352:837–853.

22. White NH, Sun W, Cleary PA, *et al*. Prolonged effect of intensive therapy on the risk of retinopathy complications in patients with type 1 diabetes mellitus: 10 years after the Diabetes Control and Complications Trial. *Arch Ophthalmol* 2008; 126:1707–1715.

23. Waden J, Forsblom C, Thorn LM, *et al*. A1C variability predicts incident cardiovascular events, microalbuminuria, and overt diabetic nephropathy in patients with type 1 diabetes. *Diabetes* 2009; 58:2649–2655.

24. Carter RE, Lackland DT, Cleary PA, *et al*. Intensive treatment of diabetes is associated with a reduced rate of peripheral arterial calcification in the diabetes control and complications trial. *Diabetes Care* 2007; 30:2646–2648.

25. Cleary PA, Orchard TJ, Genuth S, *et al*. The effect of intensive glycemic treatment on coronary artery calcification in type 1 diabetic participants of the Diabetes Control and Complications Trial/Epidemiology of Diabetes Interventions and Complications (DCCT/EDIC) Study. *Diabetes* 2006; 55:3556–3565.

26. Holman RR, Paul SK, Bethel MA, *et al*. Ten-year follow-up of intensive glucose control in type 2 diabetes. *N Engl J Med* 2008; 359:1577–1589.

27. Gerstein HC, Miller ME, Byington RP, *et al*. Effects of intensive glucose lowering in type 2 diabetes. *N Engl J Med* 2008; 358:2545–2559.

28. Patel A, MacMahon S, Chalmers J, *et al*. Intensive blood glucose control and vascular outcomes in patients with type 2 diabetes. *N Engl J Med* 2008; 358:2560–2572.

29. Duckworth W, Abraira C, Moritz T, *et al*. Glucose control and vascular complications in veterans with type 2 diabetes. *N Engl J Med* 2009; 360:129–139.

30. Diabetes Control and Complications Trial Research Group. The effect of intensive treatment of diabetes on the development and progression of long-term complications in insulin-dependent diabetes mellitus. *N Engl J Med* 1993; 329:977–986.

31. UK Prospective Diabetes Study 6. Complications in newly diagnosed type 2 diabetic patients and their association with different clinical and biochemical risk factors. *Diabetes Res* 1990; 13:1–11.

32. Davis MD. Diabetic retinopathy, diabetic control, and blood pressure. *Transplant Proc* 1986; 18:1565–1568.

33. Klein R, Klein BE. Vision disorders in diabetes. In: Harris MI, Cowie CC, Stern MP, Boyko EJ, Reiber GE, Bennett PH (eds.). *Diabetes in America*, 2nd Edition. Bethesda, MD: National Institutes of Health. NIH Publication No. 95-1468; 1995; pp. 293–338.

34. Adler AI, Stratton IM, Neil HA, *et al*. Association of systolic blood pressure with macrovascular and microvascular complications of type 2 diabetes

(UKPDS 36): prospective observational study. *Br Med J* 2000; 321:412–419.

35. Klein R, Klein BE, Moss SE, *et al.* The Wisconsin Epidemiologic Study of Diabetic Retinopathy: XVII. The 14-year incidence and progression of diabetic retinopathy and associated risk factors in type 1 diabetes. *Ophthalmology* 1998; 105:1801–1815.

36. Chaturvedi N, Sjolie AK, Stephenson JM, *et al.* Effect of lisinopril on progression of retinopathy in normotensive people with type 1 diabetes. The EUCLID Study Group. EURODIAB Controlled Trial of Lisinopril in Insulin-Dependent Diabetes Mellitus. *Lancet* 1998; 351:28–31.

37. Chaturvedi N. Modulation of the renin-angiotensin system and retinopathy. *Heart* 2000; 84 Suppl:i29–i31.

38. UK Prospective Diabetes Study Group. Tight blood pressure control and risk of macrovascular and microvascular complications in type 2 diabetes: UKPDS 38. *Br Med J* 1998; 317:703–713.

39. Estacio RO, Jeffers BW, Gifford N, *et al.* Effect of blood pressure control on diabetic microvascular complications in patients with hypertension and type 2 diabetes. *Diabetes Care* 2000; 23:B54–B64.

40. Mauer M, Zinman B, Gardiner R, *et al.* Renal and retinal effects of enalapril and losartan in type 1 diabetes. *N Engl J Med* 2009; 361:40–51.

41. Chaturvedi N, Porta M, Klein R, *et al.* Effect of candesartan on prevention (DIRECT-Prevent 1) and progression (DIRECT-Protect 1) of retinopathy in type 1 diabetes: randomised, placebo-controlled trials. *Lancet* 2008; 372:1394–1402.

42. Sjolie AK, Klein R, Porta M, *et al.* Effect of candesartan on progression and regression of retinopathy in type 2 diabetes (DIRECT-Protect 2): a randomised placebo-controlled trial. *Lancet* 2008; 372:1385–1393.

43. Garg SK, Chase HP, Marshall G, *et al.* Oral contraceptives and renal and retinal complications in young women with insulin-dependent diabetes mellitus. *JAMA* 1994; 271:1099–1102.

44. Klein BE, Moss SE, Klein R. Oral contraceptives in women with diabetes. *Diabetes Care* 1990; 13:895–898.

45. Chew EY, Mills JL, Metzger BE, *et al.* Metabolic control and progression of retinopathy. The Diabetes in Early Pregnancy Study. National

Institute of Child Health and Human Development. *Diabetes Care* 1995; 18:631–637.

46. Klein BE, Moss SE, Klein R. Effect of pregnancy on progression of diabetic retinopathy. *Diabetes Care* 1990; 13:34–40.

47. Axer-Siegel R, Hod M, Fink-Cohen S, *et al.* Diabetic retinopathy during pregnancy. *Ophthalmology* 1996; 103:1815–1819.

48. Diabetes Control and Complications Trial Research Group. Effect of pregnancy on microvascular complications in the diabetes control and complications trial. *Diabetes Care* 2000; 23:1084–1091.

49. Klein R, Klein BE, Moss SE. The Wisconsin Epidemiologic Study of Diabetic Retinopathy. XVI. The relationship of C-peptide to the incidence and progression of diabetic retinopathy. *Diabetes* 1995; 44:796–801.

50. Raymond NT, Varadhan L, Reynold DR, *et al.* Higher prevalence of retinopathy in diabetic patients of South Asian ethnicity compared with white Europeans in the community: a cross-sectional study. *Diabetes Care* 2009; 32:410–415.

51. van Leiden HA, Dekker JM, Moll AC, *et al.* Risk factors for incident retinopathy in a diabetic and nondiabetic population: the Hoorn study. *Arch Ophthalmol* 2003; 121:245–251.

52. Chew EY, Klein ML, Ferris FL, III, *et al.* Association of elevated serum lipid levels with retinal hard exudate in diabetic retinopathy. Early Treatment Diabetic Retinopathy Study (ETDRS) Report 22. *Arch Ophthalmol* 1996; 114:1079–1084.

53. Medina RJ, O'Neill CL, Devine AB, *et al.* The pleiotropic effects of simvastatin on retinal microvascular endothelium has important implications for ischaemic retinopathies. *PLoS One* 2008; 3:e2584.

54. Boucher K, Siegel CS, Sharma P, *et al.* HMG-CoA reductase inhibitors induce apoptosis in pericytes. *Microvasc Res* 2006; 71:91–102.

55. Harris EL, Feldman S, Robinson CR, *et al.* Racial differences in the relationship between blood pressure and risk of retinopathy among individuals with NIDDM. *Diabetes Care* 1993; 16:748–754.

56. Roy MS. Diabetic retinopathy in African Americans with type 1 diabetes: the New Jersey 725: I. Methodology, population, frequency of

retinopathy, and visual impairment. *Arch Ophthalmol* 2000; 118:97–104.

57. Roy MS. Diabetic retinopathy in African Americans with type 1 diabetes: the New Jersey 725: II. Risk factors. *Arch Ophthalmol* 2000; 118:105–115.

58. Tielsch JM, Javitt JC, Coleman A, *et al.* The prevalence of blindness and visual impairment among nursing home residents in Baltimore. *N Engl J Med* 1995; 332:1205–1209.

59. Dorf A, Ballintine EJ, Bennett PH, *et al.* Retinopathy in Pima Indians. Relationships to glucose level, duration of diabetes, age at diagnosis of diabetes, and age at examination in a population with a high prevalence of diabetes mellitus. *Diabetes* 1976; 25:554–560.

60. West KM, Erdreich LJ, Stober JA. A detailed study of risk factors for retinopathy and nephropathy in diabetes. *Diabetes* 1980; 29:501–508.

61. Haffner SM, Fong D, Stern MP, *et al.* Diabetic retinopathy in Mexican Americans and non-Hispanic whites. *Diabetes* 1988; 37:878–884.

62. Hamman RF, Mayer EJ, Moo-Young GA, *et al.* Prevalence and risk factors of diabetic retinopathy in non-Hispanic whites and Hispanics with NIDDM. San Luis Valley Diabetes Study. *Diabetes* 1989; 38:1231–1237.

63. Tymms DJ, Reckless JP. Proliferative diabetic retinopathy in a patient with maturity-onset diabetes of the young (MODY). *Diabet Med* 1989; 6:451–453.

64. Leibowitz HM, Krueger DE, Maunder LR, *et al.* The Framingham Eye Study monograph: an ophthalmological and epidemiological study of cataract, glaucoma, diabetic retinopathy, macular degeneration, and visual acuity in a general population of 2631 adults, 1973–1975. *Surv Ophthalmol* 1980; 24:335–610.

65. Klein BE, Moss SE, Klein R. Is menarche associated with diabetic retinopathy? *Diabetes Care* 1990; 13:1034–1038.

66. Kostraba JN, Dorman JS, Orchard TJ, *et al.* Contribution of diabetes duration before puberty to development of microvascular complications in IDDM subjects. *Diabetes Care* 1989; 12:686–693.

67. Olsen BS, Sjolie A, Hougaard P, *et al.* A 6-year nationwide cohort study of glycaemic control in young people with type 1 diabetes. Risk markers for the development of retinopathy, nephropathy and neuropathy. Danish Study Group of Diabetes in Childhood. *J Diabetes Complications* 2000; 14:295–300.

68. Kempen JH, O'Colmain BJ, Leske MC, *et al.* The prevalence of diabetic retinopathy among adults in the United States. *Arch Ophthalmol* 2004; 122:552–563.

69. Kowluru RA, Kanwar M, Chan PS, *et al.* Inhibition of retinopathy and retinal metabolic abnormalities in diabetic rats with AREDS-based micronutrients. *Arch Ophthalmol* 2008; 126: 1266–1272.

70. Moss SE, Klein R, Klein BE. Association of cigarette smoking with diabetic retinopathy. *Diabetes Care* 1991; 14:119–126.

71. Klein R, Klein BE, Moss SE, *et al.* The Wisconsin Epidemiologic Study of Diabetic Retinopathy. IX. Four-year incidence and progression of diabetic retinopathy when age at diagnosis is less than 30 years. *Arch Ophthalmol* 1989; 107:237–243.

72. Kostraba JN, Klein R, Dorman JS, *et al.* The epidemiology of diabetes complications study. IV. Correlates of diabetic background and proliferative retinopathy. *Am J Epidemiol* 1991; 133:381–391.

73. Kingsley LA, Dorman JS, Doft BH, *et al.* An epidemiologic approach to the study of retinopathy: the Pittsburgh diabetic morbidity and retinopathy studies. *Diabetes Res Clin Pract* 1988; 4:99–109.

74. Young RJ, McCulloch DK, Prescott RJ, *et al.* Alcohol: another risk factor for diabetic retinopathy? *Br Med J* 1984; 288:1035–1037.

75. Moss SE, Klein R, Klein BE. The association of alcohol consumption with the incidence and progression of diabetic retinopathy. *Ophthalmology* 1994; 101:1962–1968.

76. Beulens JW, Kruidhof JS, Grobbee DE, *et al.* Alcohol consumption and risk of microvascular complications in type 1 diabetes patients: the EURODIAB Prospective Complications Study. *Diabetologia* 2008; 51:1631–1638.

77. Valmadrid CT, Klein R, Moss SE, *et al.* Alcohol intake and the risk of coronary heart disease mortality in persons with older-onset diabetes mellitus. *JAMA* 1999; 282:239–246.

78. Parving HH, Hommel E, Mathiesen E, *et al.* Prevalence of microalbuminuria, arterial hypertension, retinopathy and neuropathy in patients with

insulin dependent diabetes. *Br Med J* 1988; 296:156–160.

79. Cruickshanks KJ, Ritter LL, Klein R, *et al.* The association of microalbuminuria with diabetic retinopathy. The Wisconsin Epidemiologic Study of Diabetic Retinopathy. *Ophthalmology* 1993; 100:862–867.

80. Klein R, Moss SE, Klein BE. Is gross proteinuria a risk factor for the incidence of proliferative diabetic retinopathy? *Ophthalmology* 1993; 100:1140–1146.

81. Klein BE, Knudtson MD, Tsai MY, *et al.* The relation of markers of inflammation and endothelial dysfunction to the prevalence and progression of diabetic retinopathy: Wisconsin epidemiologic study of diabetic retinopathy. *Arch Ophthalmol* 2009; 127:1175–1182.

82. The Diabetes Control and Complications Trial Research Group. Clustering of long-term complications in families with diabetes in the diabetes control and complications trial. *Diabetes* 1997; 46:1829–1839.

83. Uhlmann K, Kovacs P, Boettcher Y, *et al.* Genetics of diabetic retinopathy. *Exp Clin Endocrinol Diabetes* 2006; 114:275–294.

84. Knowler WC, Barrett-Connor E, Fowler SE, *et al.* Reduction in the incidence of type 2 diabetes with lifestyle intervention or metformin. *N Engl J Med* 2002; 346:393–403.

85. Zimmet P. Preventing diabetic complications: a primary care perspective. *Diabetes Res Clin Pract* 2009; 84:107–116.

86. Preliminary report on effects of photocoagulation therapy. The Diabetic Retinopathy Study Research Group. *Am J Ophthalmol* 1976; 81:383–396.

87. Early Treatment Diabetic Retinopathy Study Research Group. Grading diabetic retinopathy from stereoscopic color fundus photographs — an extension of the modified Airlie House classification. ETDRS report number 10. *Ophthalmology* 1991; 98:786–806.

88. Diabetic Retinopathy Vitrectomy Study Research Group. Early vitrectomy for severe vitreous hemorrhage in diabetic retinopathy. Two-year results of a randomized trial. Diabetic Retinopathy Vitrectomy Study report 2. *Arch Ophthalmol* 1985; 103:1644–1652.

89. Sorbinil Retinopathy Trial Research Group. A randomized trial of sorbinil, an aldose reductase inhibitor, in diabetic retinopathy. *Arch Ophthalmol* 1990; 108:1234–1244.

90. Ansquer JC, Foucher C, Aubonnet P, *et al.* Fibrates and microvascular complications in diabetes — insight from the FIELD study. *Curr Pharm Des* 2009; 15:537–552.

91. Constable IJ, Knuiman MW, Welborn TA, *et al.* Assessing the risk of diabetic retinopathy. *Am J Ophthalmol* 1984; 97:53–61.

92. Nielsen NV. Diabetic retinopathy I. The course of retinopathy in insulin-treated diabetics. A one year epidemiological cohort study of diabetes mellitus. The Island of Falster, Denmark. *Acta Ophthalmol* 1984; 62:256–265.

93. Sjolie AK. Ocular complications in insulin treated diabetes mellitus. An epidemiological study. *Acta Ophthalmol Suppl* 1985; 1721–1777.

94. Grauslund J, Green A, Sjolie AK. Prevalence and 25-year incidence of proliferative retinopathy among Danish type 1 diabetic patients. *Diabetologia* 2009; 52:1829–1835.

95. Teuscher A, Schnell H, Wilson PW. Incidence of diabetic retinopathy and relationship to baseline plasma glucose and blood pressure. *Diabetes Care* 1988; 11:246–251.

96. Fujimoto W, Fukada M. Natural history of diabetic retinopathy and its treatment in Japan. In: Baba S, Goto Y, Fukui I, (eds). Amsterdam: Excerpta Medica; 1976; pp. 225–231.

97. Roy MS. Diabetic retinopathy in African Americans with type 1 diabetes: The New Jersey 725: I. Methodology, population, frequency of retinopathy, and visual impairment. *Arch Ophthalmol* 2000; 118:97–104.

98. Roy MS. Diabetic retinopathy in African Americans with type 1 diabetes: The New Jersey 725: II. Risk factors. *Arch Ophthalmol* 2000; 118:105–115.

99. Nielsen NV. Diabetic retinopathy II. The course of retinopathy in diabetics treated with oral hypoglycaemic agents and diet regime alone. A one year epidemiological cohort study of diabetes mellitus. The Island of Falster, Denmark. *Acta Ophthalmol* 1984; 62:266–273.

100. King H, Balkau B, Zimmet P, *et al.* Diabetic retinopathy in Nauruans. *Am J Epidemiol* 1983; 117:659–667.

101. Jerneld B. Prevalence of diabetic retinopathy. A population study from the Swedish island of Gotland. *Acta Ophthalmol* 1988; 1883–1832.

102. Lee ET, Lee VS, Lu M, *et al.* Development of proliferative retinopathy in NIDDM. A follow-up

study of American Indians in Oklahoma. *Diabetes* 1992; 41:359–367.

103. Lee ET, Lee VS, Kingsley RM, *et al.* Diabetic retinopathy in Oklahoma Indians with NIDDM. Incidence and risk factors. *Diabetes Care* 1992; 15:1620–1627.

104. West SK, Klein R, Rodriguez J, *et al.* Diabetes and diabetic retinopathy in a Mexican-American population: proyecto VER. *Diabetes Care* 2001; 24:1204–1209.

105. Rema M, Premkumar S, Anitha B, *et al.* Prevalence of diabetic retinopathy in urban India: the Chennai Urban Rural Epidemiology Study

(CURES) eye study I. *Invest Ophthalmol Vis Sci* 2005; 46:2328–2333.

106. Varma R, Torres M, Pena F, *et al.* Prevalence of diabetic retinopathy in adult Latinos: the Los Angeles Latino eye study. *Ophthalmology* 2004; 111:1298–1306.

107. Leske MC, Wu SY, Hyman L, *et al.* Diabetic retinopathy in a black population: the Barbados Eye Study. *Ophthalmology* 1999; 106:1893–1899.

108. Wang FH, Liang YB, Zhang F, *et al.* Prevalence of diabetic retinopathy in rural China: the Handan Eye Study. *Ophthalmology* 2009; 116:461–467.

22

Age-related macular degeneration

JENNIFER EVANS AND TIEN WONG

22.1	Introduction	571
22.2	Definition and diagnosis	571
22.3	Classification	572
22.4	Prevalence	572
22.5	Incidence and progression	574
22.6	Changes in incidence and prevalence with time	575

22.7	Geographical distribution	576
22.8	Aetiology and risk factors	576
22.9	Control and treatment strategies	580
22.10	Priorities for future epidemiological research	581
	References	582

22.1 INTRODUCTION

Age-related macular degeneration (AMD) is a condition of the central area of the retina (macula) in people aged 50 years and above with no obvious cause. It is the leading cause of blindness in older people in the USA, UK and in many industrialized countries.[1]

22.2 DEFINITION AND DIAGNOSIS

In the early stages of AMD, lipid-like material accumulates in deposits underneath the retinal pigment epithelium within Bruch's membrane. They are known as drusen, appearing as pale yellow spots on the retina, and consisting of an accumulation of material, probably waste products of cells of the **retinal pigment epithelium (RPE)**, between Bruch's membrane and the RPE. The pigment of the RPE is also commonly disturbed by areas of hyperpigmentation and hypopigmentation. In Caucasian populations, small, well-defined 'hard'

drusen are very common and may be considered an age-related condition. However, larger, ill-defined 'soft' drusen, which are less common (Plate 22.1), are associated with a higher risk of progression to later stages of AMD. The early stages of the disease are in general asymptomatic.

Late stage AMD includes geographic atrophy ('dry' AMD) and neovascular disease ('wet' AMD). Geographic atrophy is a sharply demarcated area of partial or complete depigmentation reflecting atrophy of the retinal pigment epithelium (Plate 22.2). Neovascular AMD occurs when new vessels grow under the retinal pigment epithelium and occasionally into the subretinal space, with leakage of fluid, blood and with subsequent scarring and fibrosis (Plate 22.3). At this stage, there is considerable distortion of vision or more severe loss of visual function, particularly in the central area of the visual field.

AMD can be identified and diagnosed in four ways:

➢ Clinical ophthalmoscopy — a clinician makes a direct examination of the retina.

➢ Retinal photographs — document changes seen in the photographs, usually undertaken after dilation of the pupil. Film-based, colour stereoscopic 30 degree photography centred on the maculae has been the recommended photographic method for many years, although digital, colour, non-stereoscopic, 45 or 60 degree photographs are now also used to document retinal pathology in clinical or research settings.

➢ Fundus Fluorescein Angiogram — this is an invasive investigation whereby a yellow dye (fluorescein) is injected into the circulation and the camera takes photographs to evaluate the blood flow through the choroidal and retinal vessels. In neovascular AMD, hyperfluorescence (relatively bright fluorescence) can be observed representing active focal leakage of fluorescein into the retinal tissues.

➢ **Optical coherence tomography (OCT)** is useful in the diagnosis and monitoring of treatment for neovascular AMD because it enables the measurement of the thickness of the retina and can quantify subtle fluid in the retina and subretinal space (see also Plate 21.6).

22.3   CLASSIFICATION

There are a number of classification schemes for AMD based on clinical examination and photographs. The aim of these schemes is to provide a common nomenclature so that the prevalence of AMD and its development over time can be compared between different studies and locations. The classification schemes share many similar features and are largely derived from the Wisconsin Age-Related Maculopathy Grading Scheme.[2] Colour fundus photographs or digitized images are graded for drusen characteristics (size, type, area), pigmentary abnormalities (increased pigment, depigmentation, geographic atrophy) and presence of abnormalities characteristic of neovascular AMD (RPE detachment, serous or haemorrhagic sensory retinal detachment, subretinal or sub-RPE, or subretinal fibrous tissue).

The four-stage classification of AMD from the **Age-Related Eye Disease Study (AREDS)**[3] has been widely adopted in recent years.

➢ *No AMD* (AREDS category 1): no or a few small drusen (<63 μm in diameter).

➢ *Early AMD* (AREDS category 2): any or all of the following: multiple small drusen, few intermediate drusen (63 μm to 124 μm in diameter), or RPE abnormalities.

➢ *Intermediate AMD* (AREDS category 3): any or all of the following: extensive intermediate drusen, and at least one large druse (≥125 μm in diameter), or **geographic atrophy** not involving the centre of the fovea.

➢ *Advanced AMD* (AREDS category 4): geographic atrophy involving the fovea and/or or any of the features of neovascular AMD.

In the AREDS study, the risk of developing advanced AMD in at least one eye in participants assigned to placebo five years after the start of the study was 1.3%, 18.3% and 43.9% in categories 2, 3 and 4. Only 5/1117 participants in category 1 developed AMD over the course of the study.

In neovascular AMD, the **choroidal neovascularisation (CNV)** lesion can be further classified using fluorescein angiography. CNV can be defined by location — extra-foveal, juxtafoveal or subfoveal — and whether classic, occult or mixed.[4] Classic CNV is characterized by an area of choroidal hyperfluorescence with well-demarcated boundaries seen in the early phase of the angiogram. Occult CNV (either pigment epithelial detachment or undetermined late leakage) is identified by late-phase leakage and poorly demarcated boundaries. These patterns have implications for prognosis and treatment (classic lesions tend to progress more rapidly and lead to sharper drops in central vision, but respond better to treatment).

22.4   PREVALENCE

Estimates of the prevalence of AMD depend both on the definition of the disease and age

Table 22.1 *Prevalence (%) of AMD from two meta-analyses*

Age group	*Friedman et al. (ref. 5)*						Age group	**Owen et al. (ref. 6)**	
	Any AMD		**Geographic atrophy**		**Neovascular AMD**			**Geographic atrophy**	**Neovascular AMD**
	Men	Women	Men	Women	Men	Women		Men and women	Men and women
50–54	0.34	0.20	0.15	0.11	0.23	0.14	50–54	0	0.06
55–59	0.41	0.22	0.22	0.12	0.28	0.16	55–59	0.07	0.03
60–64	0.63	0.35	0.37	0.19	0.42	0.26	60–64	0.03	0.26
65–69	1.08	0.70	0.66	0.37	0.73	0.51	65–69	0.24	0.33
70–74	1.98	1.52	1.19	0.81	1.33	1.09	70–74	0.46	0.85
75–79	3.97	3.44	2.16	1.85	2.49	2.40	75–79	1.26	2.29
80+	11.90	16.39	6.60	9.37	8.29	11.07	80–84	2.86	4.65
							85–89	6.02	6.99
							90+	10.56	11.27

AMD: geographic atrophy and/or neovascular AMD.
* Studies: Baltimore Eye Survey, Beaver Dam Eye Study, Blue Mountains Eye Study, Salisbury Eye Evaluation project, Melbourne Visual Impairment Project.
** Studies: Beaver Dam Eye Study, Blue Mountains Eye Study, Copenhagen City Study, Melbourne Visual Impairment Project, Rotterdam Eye Study.

group. The prevalence of the condition increases markedly with age; thus, prevalence estimates are meaningless unless it is clear to which age groups they refer.

There have been many population-based studies of AMD since the original Framingham Eye Study in the 1970s. Two reviews have pooled data from a selection of these studies to provide estimates of the prevalence of AMD (Table 22.1).[5,6]

There are some differences in the way that these data were reported in the two reviews which makes direct comparison problematic. However, we can summarize the overall prevalence of late AMD (neovascular disease and/or geographic atrophy) in Caucasian white people in industrialized countries as follows: between the ages of 50 and 70 the prevalence is low at less than 1%; between the ages of 70 and 80 the prevalence is higher and is in the order of 1–5%; from 80 onwards the prevalence increases steeply and is of the order of 10–20%. There is little evidence of any important difference between men and women in the prevalence of the disease. It is likely that the observed higher prevalence of AMD in older women is due to uncontrolled confounding by age.[7] In most age groups, for men and women,

the prevalence of neovascular AMD is higher than geographic atrophy.

A striking feature is the difference in the prevalence of the disease between black and Caucasian white people. Figure 22.1 shows the prevalence of late (advanced) AMD in population-based studies and compares white and black populations.

Although data from black populations are relatively sparse, there is some evidence that the steep rise in prevalence with increasing age, seen in white populations, is not evident in black ones. In the Salisbury Eye Evaluation Study (SEE), for example, the white participants had a non-significant higher prevalence of neovascular disease (1.7%) compared with black participants (1.1%), but white participants were much more likely to have bilateral involvement. White participants had a much higher prevalence of geographic atrophy compared with black participants (1.8% versus 0.3%).[8] However, signs of early AMD, such as drusen and pigmentary abnormalities, are commonly seen in the black population.[8,9] Some studies have reported a lower prevalence of AMD in Hispanic people but similar prevalence of early signs of the disease.[10]

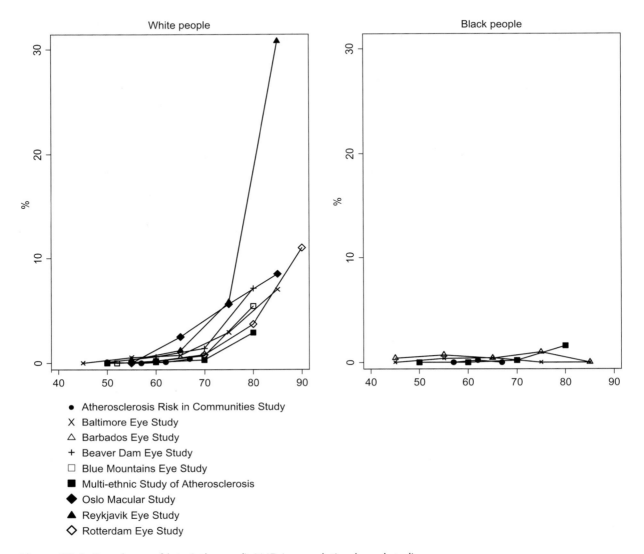

Figure 22.1 *Prevalence of late (advanced) AMD in population-based studies*

22.5 INCIDENCE AND PROGRESSION

In contrast to prevalence data, there are fewer studies on the incidence and progression of AMD.

Figure 22.2 summarizes the incidence of AMD in the general population, based on data from population-based studies in Australia, Europe and North America. Until now only one study[11] has reported 15-year incidence. The cumulative incidence for late AMD was 3.1% over 15 years. The incidence of earlier signs of the disease (soft, indistinct drusen or pigmentary abnormalities with

drusen) was higher at 14.3%. These data were reported using the 'competing risks approach', which estimates risk of developing AMD before death. This gives lower estimates than the **Kaplan–Meier method** that was used in previous reports on incidence in the same study (see Fig. 22.2). The Kaplan–Meier method assumes that people who died developed AMD at the same rate as people who lived and therefore estimates are higher.

Three ocular factors predict the progression of AMD: a presence of large drusen (≥125 μm, which approximates the diameter of a normal retinal vein at

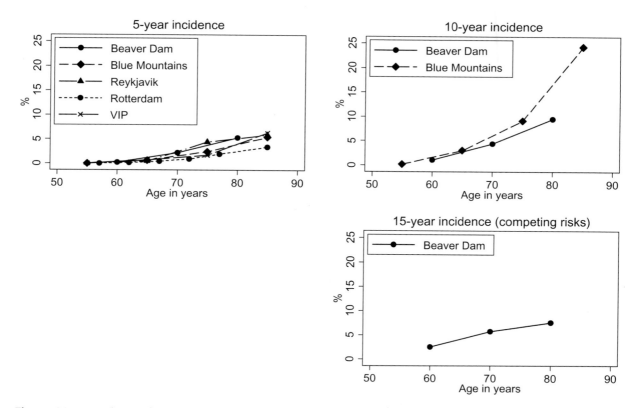

Figure 22.2 *Incidence of AMD*

the disc margin), RPE abnormalities and the bilaterality of the signs.[12] The resulting five-step score (0 to 4) can be used to identify the approximate five-year risk of developing advanced AMD (geographic atrophy or neovascular disease): 0–0.5%; 1–3%; 2–12%; 3–25%; 4–50%. For people who already have advanced AMD in one eye, the five-year risk of advanced AMD in the second eye can be estimated by assigning a score of two for the first eye and additional scores for the presence of large drusen and/or pigment abnormalities in the second eye.

Neovascular AMD and geographic atrophy progress at different rates. The progression of neovascular disease is particularly rapid. In an average cohort of people with neovascular AMD enrolled in clinical trials, 20% will have vision worse than 20/200 (6/60; 0.1) at baseline, and after three years this rises to 75% if untreated.[13] Approximately 20% of people with the disease will develop severe vision loss (that is, lose six or more lines of visual acuity, which is equivalent to a quadrupling of the visual angle) over six months, and this figure rises

to over 40% at three years. Geographic atrophy, in contrast, progresses more slowly, with 20% of people with the condition developing severe vision loss over two years.[14]

22.6   CHANGES IN INCIDENCE AND PREVALENCE WITH TIME

Because the classification of AMD has changed over time, it is difficult to assess temporal trends in the occurrence of the disease. Analysis of registration data, collected routinely over the course of the 20th century, suggested that the incidence of the disease has increased in England and Wales during that period.[15] However, more reliable survey data collected in three cross-sectional surveys in the Beaver Dam Eye Study (BDES) in Wisconsin, suggest that the opposite is the case; in that location more recent cohorts or generations appear to have a lower incidence of the disease compared with their predecessors,[16] possibly attributable to successful efforts in public health measures (for example, 'stop smoking' campaigns in recent years). Further research is clearly needed. However, given the ageing global population, it is undisputed that the number of people affected by the disease will increase markedly in the 21st century, even taking into account the development of new preventive and therapeutic strategies.[17]

22.7 GEOGRAPHICAL DISTRIBUTION

Along with cataract (see Chapter 10), AMD is the most frequently occurring cause of visual impairment and blindness among people 65 years and older in the USA, Australia and Europe.[1] It is, however, not yet an important cause of visual loss in other parts of the world. This is due partly to regional differences in population age structure. AMD predominantly affects the very old; populations with younger age-structures will be less affected, and due partly to the fact that other common causes of visual loss, such as cataract and corneal opacity, will mask the relative impact of AMD in developing countries.

There are increasing amounts of data from Asian countries such as India,[18] although these surveys are complicated in older people by high rates of age-related cataract, making it difficult to obtain clear fundus images. In one Indian population-based study, for example, nearly 30% of participants' photographs could not be graded because of the presence of cataract;[19] the observed prevalence of AMD of 1.2% (95% CI 0.8% to 1.5%) at ages 60–79 and 2.5% (0.4% to 4.7%) at ages 80 years and above was probably an underestimate.[20] Although there have been a number of population-based studies in mainland China, these data are difficult to interpret because they are reported for ages 50 and over only.[21]

In a recent meta-analysis, the prevalence estimates of early and late AMD in Asian populations aged 40–79 years were 6.8% (95% CI 4.6% to 8.9%) and 0.56% (0.3% to 0.81%) respectively, with corresponding prevalence estimates in white populations of 8.8% (3.8% to 13.8%) and 0.59% (0.35% to 0.84%), respectively.[22] These new data suggest that the prevalence of early and late AMD is of a similar order in Asian and white people,

although the possibility that early AMD signs are less frequent in Asian people compared with white people cannot be excluded.

22.8 AETIOLOGY AND RISK FACTORS

Historically it used to be believed that AMD arose as a result of degenerative changes in the choroidal vasculature which led to deterioration in the RPE, due either to ischaemia or an accumulation of waste products. This generated interest in the association between AMD and *cardiovascular disease* and its risk factors. AMD is also associated with *inflammation* (both genetic and physiological markers of inflammation) and this may be a shared common pathway for the development of both conditions. Research has also focused on the role of potentially damaging *oxidative processes* in the retina, generated as a result of absorption of light by the photoreceptors. Environmental factors that may affect these oxidative processes include those that may increase the level of oxidative activity in the retina, such as *light exposure* and *smoking*, and factors that might act to reduce the effect of damaging oxidative processes, such as dietary and blood plasma levels of *antioxidant micronutrients* and sex hormones (*oestrogen*). High levels of docosahexaenoic acid (DHA) in the retina, particularly in the disc membranes of the photoreceptors, and the possible role of eicosapentaenoic acid (EPA) in inflammation have also lead to interest in the possible protective effect of diets high in polyunsaturated fatty acids. Finally, there is now strong evidence for a *genetic* component to AMD.

22.8.1 Cardiovascular disease and its risk factors

AMD has been associated with an increased risk of cardiovascular disease in some but not all studies.[7] For example, in the Cardiovascular Health Study, people with AMD had a higher cumulative incidence of coronary heart disease with an adjusted hazard ratio of 1.57 (95% CI 1.17 to 2.22).[23] The number of cases of late AMD in this study, however, was small (n = 25). Participants with AMD were not at increased risk of stroke. In the Rotterdam Study, individuals with carotid artery plaques were four times more likely to have late AMD than those without plaque.[24] An association between hypertension and AMD has been observed in both cross-sectional and prospective data. In one case-control study, for example, people with hypertension had a three-fold increased chance of AMD.[25] In the Beaver Dam Eye Study, elevated systolic blood pressure at baseline was associated with an increased ten-year risk of AMD.[26] However, this association between raised blood pressure and AMD has not been reported consistently.[7]

High intakes of dietary fat have been linked in several studies to an increased risk of developing AMD; for example, in the Nurses' Health Study, a large prospective study, women with total fat intake in the highest quintile had a 50% increased risk of developing AMD.[27] Findings with plasma levels of cholesterol and other biochemical markers of dietary fat have been inconsistent,[7] and there is little evidence that reduction in levels of cholesterol, for example by use of statins, reduces the risk of AMD.[28]

Some limited research has been carried out on the relationship of obesity and physical activity to AMD. In one study, modest reductions in waist–hip ratio were associated with a reduced risk of AMD.[29] In the Beaver Dam Eye Study, after controlling for relevant confounders, people who were physically active at baseline were less likely to develop neovascular AMD 15 years later compared with people without an active lifestyle. Physical activity, however, was not associated with the incidence of early AMD or geographic atrophy.[30] There appears to be little relationship between diabetes, hyperglycaemia and AMD. If there is any association, it is probably weak. Studies of AMD and diabetic retinopathy are confounded by the difficulty of diagnosing AMD in the presence of diabetic retinopathy.

Finally, the data are most consistent as regards the effect of smoking, another major cardiovascular risk factor. There is also emerging evidence on the role of inflammation in the development of AMD (see below). Moreover, genes involved in the regulation of inflammatory processes have been identified as being factors in the aetiology of AMD.

22.8.2 Smoking

Smoking tobacco is associated with a wide range of harmful effects, largely mediated by the effect of nicotine, a highly toxic alkaloid that affects the autonomic and central nervous systems. There are two potential mechanisms by which smoking may lead to an increased risk of AMD: via direct effects on the choroidal circulation, or via a decrease in the blood plasma levels of antioxidant micronutrients.

The relationship between smoking and AMD has been investigated in many studies with different designs, with consistent results. In the majority of studies, a significantly increased risk of developing AMD has been found associated with smoking cigarettes.[31,32] Pooled analysis suggests that current smoking is associated with a two- to three-fold increased risk of AMD compared with never having smoked. Ex-smokers are at risk of AMD but their risk is lower at approximately 50%. There is evidence of a dose–response relationship with smoking, with people who smoke greater numbers of cigarettes per day being at increased risk. People who stop smoking reduce their risk of AMD but it may be up to 20 years of smoking cessation that is required to reduce the risk to that of non-smokers.

22.8.3 Inflammation

Systemic markers of inflammation such as raised levels of white blood cell counts, plasma fibrinogen and C-reactive protein have been associated with AMD in a number of new studies.[33–35]

Recently, an infective mechanism has been hypothesized as being the trigger, and associations of AMD with *Chlamydia pneumoniae* and *Cytomegalovirus* have been reported, although studies have been inconsistent. It remains unclear if the infective agent initiates the chronic inflammatory process which is then a risk factor for AMD, or if inflammation is a natural consequence of the development of AMD. It is interesting to note that smoking induces inflammation in the retina in mice.[36] Further research is needed to clarify the exact role of inflammation in AMD pathogenesis.

22.8.4 Diet

It has been suggested that antioxidant vitamins may prevent cellular damage in the retina by acting as singlet oxygen and free radical scavengers, mopping up reactive oxygen species produced in the process of light absorption.

They include carotenoids — lutein and zeaxanthin — which are present in the retina and dietary in origin. Two enzymes — superoxide dismutase and glutathione peroxidase — are present in the retina, and particularly in the RPE, along with the water-soluble antioxidant ascorbic acid (vitamin C) and lipid-soluble α-tocopherol (vitamin E). Retinol (vitamin A) is, as its name suggests, an important component of the retina, being present in the photoreceptors and RPE. Experimental evidence on the role of vitamin A is contradictory. It has been suggested that absorption in the visual pigments, retinal and retinol, may contribute to the damaging effects of visible radiation. Dietary restriction of retinol in rats results in photoreceptor outer segments becoming more resistant to radiation damage. Other animal studies have shown that vitamin A deficiency may lead to retinal degeneration.

Prospective studies and randomized controlled trials in humans, at least in well-nourished populations, do not provide convincing evidence to support the hypothesis that relatively high dietary intake of antioxidant micronutrients protects from the development of AMD;[37] there is, however, some evidence for the view that antioxidant vitamin supplementation in people with early/moderate AMD[38] is of benefit. The evidence comes mainly from one large trial in a relatively well-nourished American population that showed modest benefit in people with moderate to severe signs of the disease (AREDS).[39] There is no evidence at present that people with no AMD, or early signs of the disease, should take supplementation.

There is more evidence, although not conclusive, that omega-3 fatty acids may play a role in the primary prevention of AMD. Meta-analysis of nine studies providing data on nearly 90,000 people found that a high dietary intake of omega-3 fatty acids was associated with a 38% reduction in the risk of advanced AMD.[40] Fish intake at least twice a week was associated with a reduced risk of both early and advanced AMD. However, currently there is not enough evidence to make clear recommendations as to the possible benefits of supplementation with omega-3 fatty acid. Including oily fish in the diet is currently advised for other health reasons and may reduce the risk of developing AMD. Results of ongoing trials are awaited: for example, the AREDS2 trial,[a] which is investigating supplementation with omega-3 long-chain polyunsaturated fatty acids (DHA and EPA).

22.8.5 Light

It is thought that the retina may be particularly vulnerable to oxidative stress because of a combination of exposure to visible light and high oxygen concentrations. Photochemical reactions create problems for cells as the reaction products or intermediaries are often toxic. The action of light on the photoreceptors generates free radicals. These are short-lived molecular fragments that have an unpaired electron in the outer orbital. This unstable structure is highly reactive and toxic. It attacks other molecules, particularly polyunsaturated fatty acids, which are essential components of biological membranes.

The wavelengths of solar ultraviolet radiation that reach the earth's surface (approximately 290–400 nm) are partially absorbed by the cornea and lens. It is largely visible light (wavelength 400–780 nm) that reaches the retina. Animal studies and case reports in humans show that excessive exposure to bright light, from solar or other sources (which may contain wavelengths shorter than 290 nm), can damage the retina. There is also some evidence that intense bright sunlight causes changes in the RPE similar to those seen in early AMD. Whether or not exposure to sunlight or artificial light sources is an important aetiological factor in the development of AMD in human populations is not clear. Light exposure is problematic to study in human populations because the measurement of individual lifetime exposure is very difficult. There have been inconsistent results from a number of

---

[a] http://www.areds2.org; accessed 2/10/2009

cross-sectional and case-control studies, which have used measures of exposure to sunlight such as residential history, time spent outdoors and use of sunglasses. One possibility is that the harmful effects of sunlight may be offset by the protective effects of antioxidants. The EUREYE study provided some evidence to support this hypothesis.[41] People with low levels of antioxidants in the plasma (vitamin C, zeaxanthin, vitamin E) and low dietary levels of zinc had an odds ratio of 1.4 for neovascular AMD for each one standard deviation unit increase in blue light exposure. Associations were also seen for low antioxidant levels and increasing levels of blue light exposure for early AMD. Although on balance the evidence is not conclusive as to the effects of blue light on AMD, some authors have argued that a large-scale clinical trial of blue blocking filters on AMD is indicated.[42]

Melanin is an effective absorber of photons and also acts as a free radical scavenger or sink. The observation that AMD is an uncommon cause of blindness in black people is consistent with a protective effect of ocular melanin. As discussed above, early AMD is, however, common in black people, and it appears to be the late-stage AMD that is less common. A number of studies on individuals have examined features of the hair and iris in an attempt to quantify the amount of pigment in the eye. Inconsistent results have been found and pooled analysis of relevant studies shows little evidence of an association.

22.8.6 Genetic factors

There is now considerable evidence to suggest that genetic factors play a key role in the development of AMD, and it is likely that multiple genes interacting with environmental factors, such as smoking and inflammatory markers, are involved[43] (See Chapter 6, Section 6.4.1).

Twin studies have shown fairly consistent results: there appears to be a higher concordance rate between monozygotic than dizygotic twins in features of the disease. Family-based studies, comparing siblings rather than twins, also provide evidence for a genetic basis for the condition. It has been estimated that siblings of an affected person have nearly a 20-times higher risk of developing the disease than the general population.[44] Segregation analysis of siblings enrolled in the Beaver Dam Eye Study found results consistent with a major gene effect accounting for 62% of the expression of macular degeneration in the right and 59% in the left eye.[45]

The **complement factor H gene (CFH)**, in particular the CFH Y402H polymorphism, has recently been identified as a key genetic risk factor for AMD.[46] CFH helps to regulate the body's response to inflammation by protecting against uncontrolled complement activation. People with CC genotypes are approximately six times more likely to have AMD compared with people with TT genotype. Approximately 60% of AMD might be attributed to this CFH polymorphism. Protective genes have also been identified such as those on either factor B (BF or complement factor B (CFB)) or complement component 2 (C2) genes.[47]

Apolipoprotein E (APOE), which transports lipids and cholesterol in the nervous system, has also been identified as a possible genetic marker of AMD. The ε2 allele has been associated with an increased risk of AMD and an earlier mean age of diagnosis, and the ε4 allele with a modest protective effect. However, several other studies have shown no association between APOE and AMD, although it is unclear why some studies have found an association and others not.[43]

PLEKHA1 and the hypothetical LOC387715 on chromosome 26 have been identified as further possible genes. PLEKHA1 encodes the protein TAPP1 which is involved in lymphocyte activation.[43] Currently it is not clear what function LOC387715 may have; however, it has been observed that there is a strong gene–environment association with smoking.[48]

22.8.7 Alcohol

Alcohol has many effects on the circulation and physiology. In moderate amounts its effects are thought to be beneficial, reducing the risk of coronary heart disease. Excessive consumption, however, has many adverse effects. Pooled analyses suggested that people who are heavy drinkers, that is who drink more than three standard drinks a day, have an increased risk of developing early AMD (pooled OR 1.47, 95% CI 1.10 to 1.95).[49] Data are inconclusive both about the risks of moderate drinking and the risk of late AMD being associated with alcohol consumption.

22.8.8   Oestrogens

Markers of exposure to oestrogen in women, such as age at menarche and menopause and use of hormone replacement therapy, are not consistently associated with AMD. Initial studies suggested a protective effect. The Eye Disease Case-Control study group found that women with neovascular AMD were less likely to have taken postmenopausal oestrogen compared with women without AMD.[50] This was followed by a report from Rotterdam that women with an early surgical menopause had markedly increased risk of AMD.[51] However, subsequent studies, such as the Beaver Dam Eye Study and Blue Mountains Eye Study, found little effect. More recently, the Salisbury Eye Evaluation Study found that women who took hormone replacement therapy were at less risk of large drusen.[52] Inconsistent findings may be a result of the different stages of disease studied, selection bias and other study differences. The Rotterdam Study was the first to observe the association with early menopause, particularly surgical oophorectomy; this may be a chance finding.

One randomized controlled trial has been reported.[53] The Women's Health Initiative clinical trial of hormone therapy randomized women to conjugated equine oestrogens (CEE), CEE with progestin (CEE+P) or placebo. In this trial over 4,000 women aged 65 years and above were evaluated for the presence of AMD after an average of five years' treatment. Overall there was no association between oestrogen supplementation and development of AMD. The group treated with CEE+P had a reduced risk of one early sign (soft drusen) and neovascular disease; however, the study was underpowered to evaluate these associations, and the authors were unable to make a definitive statement regarding these effects.

22.8.9   Cataract and cataract surgery

There is a considerable overlap in suspected risk factors for age-related cataract and AMD, in particular as regards smoking, lack of antioxidant vitamins and exposure to solar radiation. Thus, persons with cataract are thought to have higher risk of AMD. However, this is a potentially difficult area to study as the presence of lens opacities may also mask the detection of retinal changes. The Framingham Study originally suggested an inverse relationship between the two diseases. However, subsequent studies, which have taken into account the quality of the images of the retina, have suggested that lens opacities, particularly of the nuclear type, are associated with an increased risk of AMD.

Clinical observations suggest that cataract surgery increases the rate of progression of AMD. However, an initial review of five observational studies and two non-randomized clinical trials found inconsistent evidence for the hypothesis.[54]

22.9   CONTROL AND TREATMENT STRATEGIES

The main preventive strategy for AMD is to encourage people to stop smoking. Currently there is not enough convincing evidence to recommend other public health measures for the prevention of AMD, although there are many reasons to recommend a diet rich in fruit and vegetables, and regular consumption of oily fish. It is also likely that protecting the eyes from excessive sunlight exposure is a good idea, but there are not enough conclusive studies to promote this as a specific public health measure for AMD prevention.

Antioxidant vitamin and mineral supplements are readily available for purchase without prescription in many countries. The decision as to whether or not to take these supplements is at the discretion of the person with AMD. The following benefits and harms need to be considered. People with moderate or severe disease may delay the progression of their condition if they take antioxidant vitamins and zinc at the levels described in AREDS trial (500 mg vitamin C, 400 IU vitamin E, 15 mg beta-carotene, 80 mg zinc daily). Given that there are few other interventions that offer much in the way of disease prevention or cure, this is an important consideration. Harmful effects associated with long-term vitamin supplementation, particularly in smokers, cannot be ruled out. A healthy diet with a variety of fresh fruit and vegetables will have many benefits and will not do any harm, although it may be difficult to consume as part of a normal diet the recommended levels of antioxidants and zinc.

Until recently, once neovascular AMD had developed, there were few effective treatment options, with direct laser therapy and photodynamic therapy indicated in a limited number of patients. In the last few years, however, a new class of therapies based on the suppression of vascular endothelial growth factor (VEGF) has been introduced, and the use of intra-ocular administration of anti-VEGF agents has changed the paradigm of AMD management.[24] In particular, the anti-VEGF agent, ranibizumab, has been shown to be effective in preventing vision loss and, in many cases, significantly improved vision in eyes with neovascular AMD.[55] Another agent, bevacizumab, which is substantially cheaper, is increasingly used off-label for neovascular AMD treatment in many countries worldwide, and is currently being evaluated in randomized controlled trials.

With the emergence of these new therapies for neovascular AMD, a key issue is the identification, and rapid referral, of people who are at high risk of visual loss from AMD. Age, smoking and family history of AMD are the most consistent risk factors for AMD, knowledge of which might assist physicians to identify people at risk of AMD who might benefit from specialist referral.

22.10 PRIORITIES FOR FUTURE EPIDEMIOLOGICAL RESEARCH

In the last 30 years, there have been major advances in understanding the epidemiology, environmental and genetic risk factors, natural history and treatment of AMD. However, there remain many unanswered questions, which are areas of potential future research.

➤ There is a need for longer-term studies to document more precisely the progression from early to late stages of disease, and to examine 'cohort' effects and temporal trends.

➤ Second, studies should further explore new risk factors including genetic markers and other biomarkers of inflammation and cardiovascular disease. This will refine the aetiology and pathogenesis of AMD, and may lead to new diagnostic and screening tests for high risk groups.

➤ Studies should also seek to determine how major genetic variants for AMD interact with environment factors (for example, light exposure) and lifestyle (for example, smoking and diet) to trigger the development of early AMD or promote the progression from early to late AMD.

➤ There is scope for research in understanding racial/ethnic patterns (for example, why rates of AMD are higher in whites and Chinese and lower in blacks and Hispanics). This may provide further clues to the role of genetic or lifestyle factors (for example, diet) in the development of AMD.

➤ Future studies should include an evaluation of new ocular imaging technologies (for example, high resolution OCT, fundus autofluorescence imaging) to allow better phenotypic classification of both early and late AMD signs. This will improve diagnosis and classification, aid in genetic discovery, and allow more precise data-pooling of different studies around the world.

➤ Finally, whilst there are now some effective treatments for AMD, they have limitations: most are expensive, are only applicable to 10% of people with neovascular disease and are indicated for treatment of late AMD when vision loss is often irreversible. There are also currently no effective treatments for geographic atrophy. Therefore, strategies to identify early modifiable risk factors to prevent the development and progression of AMD remain important public health priorities.

REFERENCES

1. Pascolini D, Mariotti SP, Pokharel GP, *et al.* 2002 global update of available data on visual impairment: a compilation of population-based prevalence studies. *Ophthalmic Epidemiol* 2004; 11:67–115.

2. Klein R, Davis MD, Magli YL, *et al.* The Wisconsin age-related maculopathy grading system. *Ophthalmology* 1991; 98:1128–1134.

3. Age-Related Eye Disease Study Research Group. The Age-Related Eye Disease Study Severity Scale for Age-Related Macular Degeneration: AREDS Report No. 17. *Arch Ophthalmol* 2005; 123:1484–1498.

4. Macular Photocoagulation Study Group. Subfoveal neovascular lesions in age-related macular degeneration. Guidelines for evaluation and treatment in the macular photocoagulation study. *Arch Ophthalmol* 1991; 109:1242–1257.

5. Friedman DS, O'Colmain BJ, Munoz B, *et al.* Prevalence of age-related macular degeneration in the United States. *Arch Ophthalmol* 2004; 122:564–572.

6. Owen CG, Fletcher AE, Donoghue M, *et al.* How big is the burden of visual loss caused by age related macular degeneration in the United Kingdom? *Br J Ophthalmol* 2003; 87:312–317.

7. Evans JR. Risk factors for age-related macular degeneration. *Prog Ret Eye Res* 2001; 20:227–253.

8. Bressler SB, Munoz B, Solomon SD, *et al.* Salisbury Eye Evaluation (SEE) Study Team. Racial differences in the prevalence of age-related macular degeneration: the Salisbury Eye Evaluation (SEE) Project. *Arch Ophthalmol* 2008; 126:241–245.

9. Schachat AP, Hyman L, Leske MC, *et al.* Features of age-related macular degeneration in a black population. The Barbados Eye Study Group. *Arch Ophthalmol* 1995; 113:728–735.

10. Munoz B, Klein R, Rodriguez J, *et al.* Prevalence of age-related macular degeneration in a population-based sample of Hispanic people in Arizona: Proyecto VER. *Arch Ophthalmol* 2005; 123:1575–1580.

11. Klein R, Klein BE, Knudtson MD, *et al.* Fifteen-year cumulative incidence of age-related macular degeneration: the Beaver Dam Eye Study. *Ophthalmology* 2007; 114:253–262.

12. Age-Related Eye Disease Study Research Group. A Simplified Severity Scale for Age-Related Macular Degeneration: AREDS Report No. 18. *Arch Ophthalmol* 2005; 123:1570–1574.

13. Wong TY, Chakravarthy U, Klein R, *et al.* The natural history and prognosis of neovascular age-related macular degeneration: a systematic review of the literature and meta-analysis. *Ophthalmology* 2008; 115:116–126.

14. Sunness JS. The natural history of geographic atrophy, the advanced atrophic form of age-related macular degeneration. *Molecular Vision* 1999; 5:25.

15. Evans J, and Wormald R. Is the incidence of registrable age-related macular degeneration increasing? *Br J Ophthalmol* 1996; 80:9–14.

16. Klein R, Knudtson MD, Lee KE, *et al.* Age-period-cohort effect on the incidence of age-related macular degeneration: the Beaver Dam Eye Study. *Ophthalmology* 2008; 115:1460–1467.

17. Rein DB, Wittenborn JS, Zhang X, *et al.* Vision Health Cost-Effectiveness Study Group. Forecasting age-related macular degeneration through the year 2050: the potential impact of new treatments. *Arch Ophthalmol* 2009; 127:533–540.

18. Wong TY, Loon SC, and Saw SM. The epidemiology of age related eye diseases in Asia. *Br J Ophthalmol* 2006; 90:506–511.

19. Gupta SK, Murthy GVS, Morrison N, *et al.* Prevalence of early and late age-related macular degeneration in a rural population in northern India: the INDEYE feasibility study. *Invest Ophthalmol Vis Sci* 2007; 48:1007–1011.

20. Krishnan T, Ravindran RD, Murthy GV, *et al.* Prevalence of early and late age-related macular degeneration in India: the INDEYE Study. *Invest Ophthalmol Vis Sci* 2010; 51:701–707.

21. Zhou Q, Friedman DS, Lu H, *et al.* The epidemiology of age-related eye diseases in Mainland China. *Ophthalmic Epidemiology* 2007; 14:399–407.

22. Kawasaki R, Yasuda M, Song SJ, *et al.* The prevalence of age-related macular degeneration in Asians: a systematic review and meta-analysis. *Ophthalmology* 2010; 117:921–927.

23. Sun C, Klein R, and Wong TY. Age-related macular degeneration and risk of coronary heart disease and stroke: the Cardiovascular Health Study. *Ophthalmology* 2009; 116:1913–1919.

24. Wong TY. Age-related macular degeneration and cardiovascular disease in the era of anti-vascular endothelial growth factor therapies. *Am J Ophthalmol* 2009; 148:327–329.

25. Hogg RE, Woodside JV, Gilchrist S ECM, *et al.* Cardiovascular disease and hypertension are strong risk factors for choroidal neovascularization. *Ophthalmology* 2008; 115:1046–1052.

26. Klein R, Klein BEK, Tomany SC, *et al.* The association of cardiovascular disease with the long-term incidence of age-related maculopathy: the Beaver Dam Eye Study. *Ophthalmology* 2003; 110: 1273–1280.

27. Cho E, Hung S, Willett WC, *et al.* Prospective study of dietary fat and the risk of age-related macular degeneration. *Am J Clin Nutr* 2001; 73:209–218.

28. Smeeth L, Cook C, Chakravarthy U, *et al.* A case control study of age related macular degeneration and use of statins. *Br J Ophthalmol* 2005; 89: 1171–1175.

29. Peeters A, Magliano DJ, Stevens J, *et al.* Changes in abdominal obesity and age-related macular degeneration: the Atherosclerosis Risk in Communities Study. *Arch Ophthalmol* 2008; 126:1554–1560.

30. Knudtson MD, Klein R, Klein BEK. Physical activity and the 15-year cumulative incidence of age-related macular degeneration: the Beaver Dam Eye Study. *Br J Ophthalmol* 2006; 90: 1461–1463.

31. Cong R, Zhou B, Sun, Q, *et al.* Smoking and the risk of age-related macular degeneration: a meta-analysis. *Ann Epidemiol* 2008; 18:647–656.

32. Thornton J, Edwards R, Mitchell P, *et al.* Smoking and age-related macular degeneration: a review of association. *Eye* 2005; 19:935–944.

33. Shankar A, Mitchell P, Rochtchina E, *et al.* Association between circulating white blood cell count and long-term incidence of age-related macular degeneration: the Blue Mountains Eye Study. *Am J Epidemiol* 2007; 165:375–382.

34. Schaumberg DA, Christen WG, Buring JE, *et al.* High-sensitivity C-reactive protein, other markers of inflammation, and the incidence of macular degeneration in women. *Arch Ophthalmol* 2007; 125:300–305.

35. Seddon JM, Gensler G, Milton RC, *et al.* Association between C-reactive protein and age-related macular degeneration. *JAMA* 2004; 291:704–710.

36. Wang AL, Lukas TJ, Yuan M, *et al.* Changes in retinal pigment epithelium related to cigarette smoke: possible relevance to smoking as a risk factor for age-related macular degeneration. *PLoS One* 2009; 4;e5304.

37. Evans J. Antioxidant supplements to prevent or slow down the progression of AMD: a systematic review and meta-analysis. *Eye* 2008; 22:751–760.

38. Evans JR. Antioxidant vitamin and mineral supplements for slowing the progression of age-related macular degeneration. *Cochrane Db Sys Rev (Online)* 2006; 2:CD000254.

39. Age-Related Eye Disease Study Research Group. A randomized, placebo-controlled, clinical trial of high-dose supplementation with vitamins C and E, beta carotene, and zinc for age-related macular degeneration and vision loss: AREDS report no. 8. *Arch Ophthalmol* 2001; 119:1417–1436.

40. Chong EWT, Kreis AJ, Wong TY, *et al.* Dietary omega-3 fatty acid and fish intake in the primary prevention of age-related macular degeneration: a systematic review and meta-analysis. *Arch Ophthalmol* 2008; 126:826–833.

41. Fletcher AE, Bentham GC, Agnew M, *et al.* Sunlight exposure, antioxidants, and age-related macular degeneration. *Arch Ophthalmol* 2008; 126:1396–1403.

42. Margrain TH, Boulton M, Marshall J, *et al.* Do blue light filters confer protection against age-related macular degeneration? *Prog Ret Eye Res* 2004; 23:523–531.

43. Haddad S, Chen CA, Santangelo SL, *et al.* The genetics of age-related macular degeneration: a review of progress to date. *Surv Ophthalmol* 2006; 51:316–363.

44. Silvestri G, Johnson PB, Hughes AE. Is genetic predisposition an important risk factor in age-related macular degeneration? *Eye* 1994; 8:564–568.

45. Heiba IM, Elston RC, Klein BE, *et al.* Sibling correlations and segregation analysis of age-related maculopathy: the Beaver Dam Eye Study. *Gen Epidemiol* 1994; 11:51–67.

46. Thakkinstian A, Han P, McEvoy M, *et al.* Systematic review and meta-analysis of the association between complementary factor H Y402H polymorphisms and age-related macular degeneration. *Hum Mol Gen* 2006; 15:2784–2790.

47. Patel N, Adewoyin T, and Chong NV. Age-related macular degeneration: a perspective on genetic studies. *Eye* 2007; 22:768–776.

48. Schmidt S, Hauser MA, Scott WK, *et al*. Cigarette smoking strongly modifies the association of LOC387715 and age-related macular degeneration. *Am J Hum Gen* 2006; 78:852–864.

49. Chong EWT, Kreis AJ, Wong TY, *et al*. Alcohol consumption and the risk of age-related macular degeneration: a systematic review and meta-analysis. *Am J Ophthalmol* 2008; 145:707–715.

50. Eye Disease Case-Control Study Group. Risk factors for neovascular age-related macular degeneration. *Arch Ophthalmol* 1992; 110:1701–1708.

51. Vingerling JR, Dielemans I, Witteman JCM, *et al*. Macular degeneration and early menopause: a case-control study. *Br Med J* 1995; 310:1570–1571.

52. Freeman EE, Munoz B, Bressler SB, *et al*. Hormone replacement therapy, reproductive factors, and age-related macular degeneration: the Salisbury Eye Evaluation Project. *Ophthalmic Epidemiol* 2005; 12:37–45.

53. Haan MN, Klein R, Klein BE, *et al*. Hormone therapy and age-related macular degeneration: the Women's Health Initiative Sight Exam Study. *Arch Ophthalmol* 2006; 124:988–992.

54. Bockelbrink A, Roll S, Ruether K, *et al*. Cataract surgery and the development or progression of age-related macular degeneration: a systematic review. *Surv Ophthalmol* 2008; 53:359–367.

55. Vedula SS, Krzystolik MG. Antiangiogenic therapy with anti-vascular endothelial growth factor modalities for neovascular age-related macular degeneration. *Cochrane Db Sys Rev (Online)* 2008; 2:CD005139.

SECTION 4

PREVENTION STRATEGIES

23

From epidemiology to programme

ROBERT LINDFIELD, HANS LIMBURG AND ALLEN FOSTER

23.1	Overview	587	23.6	The planning process	591
23.2	Need for healthcare	587	23.7	Sustainability	593
23.3	The relationship between	588	23.8	Quality of programmes	595
	epidemiological data and planning		23.9	Monitoring and evaluation	596
23.4	Gathering data for planning	590	23.10	Conclusion	598
23.5	Involving the community:	591	23.11	Further reading	599
	Participatory planning			References	599

23.1 OVERVIEW

Epidemiology is defined as the study of the distribution, determinants and control of diseases and injuries in human populations.[1] The study of epidemiology is a rigorous, scientific exploration of a research question. The application of the 'science' of epidemiology provides a detailed understanding of the effect of disease on a particular population.

The majority of this textbook describes the science of epidemiology; this can be broken down into a description of the different approaches to the scientific study of epidemiology and the use of epidemiological data to describe different diseases or populations.

The final two chapters begin to describe the application of the results of epidemiological studies and show how best to use the results of rigorous epidemiological research to change people's lives.

The use of epidemiological data is an important part of planning healthcare programmes. This chapter explores the way that epidemiology can influence planning, and how best to use the results of epidemiological studies for planning.

23.2 NEED FOR HEALTHCARE

23.2.1 Definition of 'need'

There is widespread agreement that planning should be based on the need of the population. A useful definition of 'need' is 'the capacity to benefit'.[2] If the individual or community does not have the capacity to benefit from an intervention or service then it, by definition, does not need the service.

Need is different from demand. Demand is consumer-led and does not necessarily reflect the level of overall need in the population, and demand-driven service provision tends to ignore marginalized or disadvantaged groups in the community whose need may not be appreciated and included in a demand-driven service model.

23.2.2 Using epidemiological data to plan a programme

Epidemiology provides insight into the distribution of a disease using indicators like prevalence and incidence (see Chapter 1), identifies risk factors (causation) and can provide evidence of 'best practice', indicating which intervention is most successful in reducing the prevalence or incidence of a condition.

However, epidemiological studies do not produce all the information necessary to plan and develop a programme.

23.2.3   Assessing the need for healthcare within a population

There are three pieces of information required before a healthcare plan can be developed:

➤ A description of how many people in the population of interest are affected, and how. This requires population-based surveys (see Chapter 3), epidemiological studies and the use of routine data (census, government statistics etc., see Chapter 1) to collect information about prevalence, incidence, degree of severity, or the burden on the health system (number of people treated). This is called a needs assessment or epidemiological needs assessment.

➤ A description of the relevant resources available to the population of interest. The available resources, human, infrastructure, equipment, consumables and financial, are identified using a variety of different methods (information management systems, ad hoc surveys, interviews etc.). It also includes an analysis of the utilization, effectiveness and efficiency of the current services and the possible constraints. This is known as 'situational analysis' or 'corporate needs assessment'.

➤ A description of what should be provided to deal with the condition in the population of interest. This is known as a 'gap analysis' or 'comparative needs assessment'. It uses evidence of best practice, including published studies, as well as evidence from services to similar populations within the same resource considerations, to establish what should be provided.

Once a specific problem has been identified (for example, visual impairment due to cataract) then,

taken together, these three components form a comprehensive approach to identifying healthcare needs, the steps required to address them, and the best way to integrate any new service within the existing set-up. All these activities are essential components of the planning process.

23.3   THE RELATIONSHIP BETWEEN EPIDEMIOLOGICAL DATA AND PLANNING

23.3.1   Planning

Planning is the organizational process of creating and maintaining a plan. It is important to prepare a plan based on the local situation, the available resources and sustainability of activities. Planning can be conducted for an entire country or smaller administrative units (states, provinces or districts). **VISION 2020** suggests planning services for a district of approximately one million people (see Chapter 24). A comprehensive plan will not guarantee success, but lack of such a plan will almost certainly lead to failure. A well-prepared plan demonstrates that the organization knows its area of work and has thought through its development in terms of services, management, quality and finances.

A plan should serve the following three critical functions:

➤ It allows the healthcare provider to clarify, focus, and research its programme's development and prospects.

➤ It provides a considered and logical framework within which a healthcare provider can develop and pursue its strategies over the next three to five years.

➤ It offers a benchmark against which actual performance can be measured and reviewed.

23.3.2   The planning cycle

There are different approaches to healthcare planning with use of different terminologies, but in essence they follow the same process. The processes will be described and the terminology used by the different schools will be indicated.

The planning process is divided into five distinct stages, illustrated in Fig. 23.1.

Where are we now? (Identifying the problem)

The information required to establish the health-care situation, and the need for services, has been described above ('Assessing the need for healthcare within a population'). Eye care needs may vary for different members of the community. It is important to involve all stakeholders in the planning process and particularly the community. This ensures that all relevant groups in the district are included in identifying and describing the problem (see 'Involving the Community', 23.5).

Once the information has been collected, the process of developing the plan is best conducted at a workshop with all stakeholders. Active involvement should be sought from representatives of patient groups, local and international NGOs, representatives of private practitioners, local authorities, related departments and other service providers.

The methodology most commonly used for planning is the 'logical framework approach' (LFA). It follows a logical hierarchy, thereby reducing the risk that certain crucial aspects are missed in the planning.

Where are we going? (Setting priorities, goals, targets)

This is also known as a 'comparative needs assessment'. Data on available resources and current outputs describe the utilization of resources. Combining them with estimates of future need will indicate whether there is sufficient service capacity. This activity is called a 'gap analysis'. When resources are limited, decisions are required as to how best to use the available resources, including money, to meet the future needs.

This allows specific objectives to be established (e.g. shortage of eye surgeons → more eye surgeons trained). Objectives should be stated in a way that will make them measurable. A timeframe should also be included.

All activities, sub-activities and inputs required to achieve each objective should be identified. Creating the list of inputs, required to achieve the objectives, is important in developing the plan.

In countries with resource constraints, it may not be feasible to address all identified problems at once, and objectives have to be prioritized. Usually interventions are selected on the basis of cost-effectiveness, whereby maximum health gain can be achieved with minimal inputs. Aims, objectives and targets must be realistic, keeping in mind the available human, infrastructure, and financial resources.

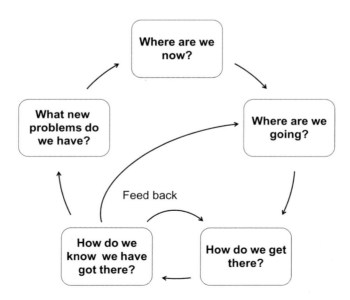

Figure 23.1 *The planning cycle*

Over-ambitious plans often result in activities not being completed, targets not being met and objectives not being achieved. This causes frustration and loss of commitment, and should be avoided. 'If the ideal is not feasible, make what's feasible the ideal'.

How will we get there? (Strategy and approach)

Activities are directed towards the achievement of objectives in the plan. Taken together, the activities are called the 'strategy', i.e. the best way to achieve the objective.

For each activity those responsible, the start and completion time, and the costs are indicated. The people identified should be capable of performing the assigned tasks, tasks are distributed evenly, and particular individuals should not be overloaded with work. Training programmes should be included in the plan. Timescales for delivering any tasks should be defined.

When all objectives, activities and sub-activities have been described, the cost of each individual activity is estimated in terms of money (financial) and person days (human resources). This is a complicated but crucial step in the planning process. Resourcing must be pragmatic and realistic, appropriate for the socio-economic and human resource situation of the area and the country.

How will we know if we are on track and when we arrive? (Monitoring and evaluation)

Monitoring and evaluation of the programme activities and overall programme results are essential. Monitoring provides feedback to assess whether the objectives and targets are realistic, whether strategies chosen are **effective** and **efficient**, and whether the organizational structure is adequate for good management.

Whilst monitoring provides regular feedback on a set of indicators, it does not identify overall success or failure of the project. A more comprehensive approach, namely evaluation, is required to achieve this.

What new problem do we have? (Forward planning)

Planning is a continuously evolving process, with much emphasis on learning (evaluation). Initially, planning may have been based on many assumptions, but during the process, insight and understanding develop, allowing learning and improved planning. Certain objectives may not be achieved using the strategy in the original plan, but with new insight and understanding more effective strategies can be applied in future planning.

23.4 GATHERING DATA FOR PLANNING

The use of relevant data is a critical part of any planning process. The quality and validity of data need to be assessed; for example, if the last census performed in a country was 20 years ago then data from that source will not necessarily be accurate.

23.4.1 Demographic

Demographic data are collected on a regular basis by governments and UN agencies.
Examples (see Chapter 1):

➢ Census data, including predictions of population changes.
➢ Healthcare activity data (in-patient, outpatient, primary care).
➢ Mortality data (from death registrations).
➢ Employment data.
➢ Global data on diseases (e.g. visual loss).
➢ Data from disease registers.

23.4.2 Specific population data

These are data collected as a one-off episode.
Examples (see Chapter 3):

➢ Surveys of diseases, e.g. blindness.
➢ Studies of disease population, including hospital-based studies.

23.4.3 Effectiveness of interventions and services

Evidence-based medicine seeks to define what healthcare interventions or services are effective and safe. Groups like the **Cochrane Collaboration** combine different sources of evidence into a single view on effectiveness (see Chapter 9). A comprehensive literature review (including unpublished data) should be conducted as part of any plan. Where evidence is not available for a particular service, a specific study might be necessary to determine effectiveness. Although studies are expensive and time-consuming, they frequently provide accurate information that is relevant to the local situation. Alternatively, examples of best practice can be sought from other areas, and if possible applied to the correct planning situation.

23.4.4 What is good practice? And how can it be achieved?

Good practice describes activities that are the good way of doing the job in a specific environment. It is efficient in terms of resources and effective in terms of outcome at any particular time. Good practice models can be developed further when new evidence becomes available.

Defining the components of good practice can be difficult. There are certain factors that a model of good practice should fulfil:

➢ Based on the best possible evidence.
➢ Shown to be effective and efficient.
➢ Repeatable (not a combination of atypical unique factors).

For example, good practice for cataract extraction in many low-income settings at the present time is **small incision cataract surgery SICS** (Cochrane reference: http://www.cochrane.org/reviews/en/ab001323.html). The results of SICS are similar to phacoemulsification (SICS is **effective**), it is of lower cost (SICS is **efficient**) and the skills required to perform SICS are transferable and the equipment available (SICS is **repeatable**) whilst being shown to be safe (evidence-based).

23.5 INVOLVING THE COMMUNITY: PARTICIPATORY PLANNING

It is widely recognized that for a healthcare programme to achieve its objectives the community should be involved throughout planning, implementation and evaluation.

Participatory planning (PP) describes the involvement of the community in deciding what services they need, and how best to provide them. There are many benefits arising from participatory planning. These are: the development of a high quality programme; empowerment of local people; learning for local people and programme planners; political commitment and support; and local ownership of the resulting programme making success more likely.

Several tools are available to facilitate participatory planning in communities; these include:

➢ Rapid rural appraisal (RRA): an external facilitator 'listens' to communities, comparing their responses with other available data, observations and recordings.
➢ Participatory rural appraisal (PRA): an external facilitator (the 'humble listener') embeds himself or herself in communities and assists them to formulate ideas, develop local knowledge and implement planning activities.

The World Bank has produced a toolkit to develop a participatory approach. This describes the tools available to aid participation; including PRA, self-esteem, associative strength, resourcefulness, action planning, and responsibility (SARAR), and beneficiary assessment (BA). For more details look under 'Further Reading' (23.11).

23.6 THE PLANNING PROCESS

Planning can be a complicated exercise. In order to ensure that the plan contains all the essential elements such as goal, objectives, outputs and inputs, and that these elements are all measurable by appropriate indicators, the planning process must follow clear guidelines. The methodology most widely used for the planning process is the **logical framework approach (LFA)**.

23.6.1 Logical framework approach (LFA)

LFA is a management tool used in the design, monitoring and evaluation of international development projects. It is also known as goal-oriented project planning (GOPP; ZOPP in German) or objectives-oriented project planning (OOPP). It is widely used by bilateral and multilateral donor organizations and NGOs in their project proposals. It provides a structure for the main elements of a project, highlighting logical linkages between objectives, outcome and inputs.

The output of this process is a four-by-four table (Table 23.1), also called the logframe. An example of a completed logframe for a programme aiming to reduce the prevalence of cataract is shown in Table 23.2.

The four rows are used to describe the different types of events that take place as a project is implemented (*activities, outputs, objectives* and *goal*). The four columns describe the different types of information about the events in each row. The first column gives a *narrative* description of the event. The second column lists one or more *objectively verifiable indicators* of these events taking place. The third column describes the *means of verification* whereby information will be sought, and the fourth column lists the *assumptions*. These are external factors that could possibly influence (positively or negatively) the events described in the narrative column but which cannot be directly controlled by the programme managers. They may include so-called *killer assumptions (major risks)*,

which have major negative consequences for the project. A good project design should be able to substantiate its assumptions, especially those with a high potential to have a negative impact.

There is vertical relationship between the rows which makes it clear why and how the project is undertaken. Moving down the columns and asking 'how' reveals the relationship between goal and purpose, purpose and outputs, outputs and inputs. The same relationship can be described by asking 'why' and going upwards to see how certain inputs will lead to certain outputs, to achieve the logical purpose, and finally to achieve the sector goal of the project.

The horizontal logic in the framework shows what is to be achieved by the project (from right to left) and what is required (from left to right) if it is to be a success. If used properly, LFA provides a practical framework for project design, review and evaluation.

Details of activities and sub-activities are worked out in a second table (Table 23.3), the project matrix. In the matrix, all inputs are divided into activities and further into sub-activities. The columns include the start date, the completion date, those responsible for the activity and the cost and person work days. All activities for each input should be listed in chronological order, thereby demonstrating the inter-dependency.

23.6.2 Project cycle management (PCM)

Whilst LFA is used for the design, planning and management of individual projects, PCM deals with the design, planning and management of many projects within one organization. Most larger organizations with many projects may have

Table 23.1 *Overview of Logframe*

	Description	Indicators	Verification	Comments/Assumptions/Risks
Goal				
Objectives				
Output (Results)				
Input (Activities)				

Table 23.2 *Example of completed logframe*

	Narrative summary	Indicators (objectively verifiable)	Means of verification	Important assumptions
Overall objective (Goal)	Goals/objectives	Measures of goal achievement	Various sources of information, methods used	Goal/purpose linkages
	• Reduce blindness and visual impairment due to cataract	• Prevalence blindness and visual impairment by cataract reduced • CSC increased	• Population-based survey	• Cataract intervention is considered a major health problem
Objectives	Narrative description	End-of-project status	Various sources of information, methods used	Output/purpose linkages
	• Increase number of cataract operations • Improve outcome of cataract operations	• CSR increased from 1,000 to 2,000 • Proportion good outcome (VA > 6/18) > 80%	• MIS on eye care • MIS and Reviews	• Public demand for cataract surgery increased • Eye surgeons monitoring their own outcome
Output (Results)	Narrative description	Magnitude of outputs, planned completion dates	Various sources of information, methods used	Input/output linkages
	• Eye surgeons trained in SICS • OT nurses trained • OTs fully equipped • Outcome monitored in all surgical eye units	• 200 eye surgeons trained in SICS • 350 OT nurses trained • All 100 eye OTs fully equipped • Monitoring systems in place and used	• Reports • Reports • MIS, reports • Reports, MIS	• Eye surgeons willing to monitor
Inputs (Activities)	Narrative description	Types/levels of resources, starting date	Project data, other sources of information	Initial assumptions regarding the causality of the programme
	• Organize SICS training • Train trainers • Supply extra equipment to training institutes • Develop training course for OT nurses • Supply OT equipment • Provide training on outcome monitoring	• Curriculum prepared • Ten trainers trained • Equipment provided • Curriculum prepared • OT equipment supplied • Training given	• Report • Report • Report, MIS • Report • Report • Report, MIS	

MIS = Management information system; OT = Operation theatre; SICS = Small incision cataract surgery; CSC = Cataract surgical coverage; CSR = Cataract surgical rate

certain organizational policies concerning sector approach, target groups and beneficiaries, cooperation with local organizations, accounting, sustainability etc., which apply to all their projects. To ensure that all individual projects meet the standards of the organization, the entire process of identification, formulation, implementation and evaluation of projects has to comply with strict procedures and standards. The entire process is called 'PCM'.

23.7 SUSTAINABILITY

For a healthcare programme to have a lasting impact on the population it should become sustainable.

Table 23.3 *Example of project matrix*

	Activity	Sub-activity	Start date	Completion date	Responsible for implementation	Cost
2	Supply surgical equipment for Small Incision Cataract Surgery (SICS)					
2.1		Calculate total order and specifications	01-01-2010	01-04-10	SICS training committee	
2.2		Invite quotations	01-03-2010	01-07-10	Ministry of Health	200
2.3		Purchase selected equipment	01-06-2010	01-10-10	Medical Stores Department	60,000
2.4		Distribute equipment	01-07-2010	01-12-10	Medical Stores Department	8,500

References to more details on the LFA methodology are provided under Further Reading (23.11)

Planning a programme that is sustainable reduces the risk of collapse once any donor has withdrawn.

A usual definition of sustainability is the ability to continue activities independently, both organizationally and financially, when an external source of oversight or resources is removed. Whilst this definition is useful, it fails to acknowledge other definitions. These include sustaining benefits for intended clients, or maintaining the attention to issues addressed by the programme.[3]

Sustaining the benefits for intended clients is very different from continuing project activities, and the strategies to ensure sustainability will be different depending on which definition is chosen. For example the benefits to clients of a primary eye care clinic might be assured by integrating the clinic into an existing primary health care clinic. It might be necessary for the current project to finish, in order to allow this to happen.[4]

23.7.1 Threats to sustainability

There are two types of threats to sustainability: extrinsic and intrinsic. Extrinsic threats are mostly due to political, economical or environmental factors. Intrinsic threats come from factors within the organization itself, like perceived lack of effectiveness, limited integration, inadequate budget and no community participation or ownership.

The control of intrinsic threats is within the design and planning of the project. These threats can be mitigated or avoided by careful project planning.

23.7.2 Planning sustainable programmes

Steps to ensure sustainability should be considered at every stage of the planning process. Threats to sustainability need to be identified and steps taken to overcome these threats. Programme planning should address each risk to sustainability and develop alternative actions wherever possible.

23.7.3 Cost recovery

Many eye care programmes focus on financial sustainability and establish cost recovery mechanisms that pay for the service. Several models of cost recovery have been developed, for example, for eye care.

23.7.3.1 *Tiered payments*

Patients are charged different amounts depending on their ability to pay. The wealthiest patients receive a 'higher quality hotel service' (air-conditioned rooms, food provided). This subsidises the poorest patients who receive a more basic hotel service (shared rooms, sleeping mats, no food provided) but everyone receives the same surgery and surgical expertise.

23.7.3.2 *Service subsidization*

This is when part of the eye care service subsidizes another part. An example is the development of optical shops. These provide refraction and spectacles for the general public and are run by the hospital, which receives either all or part of any profit. This money is used to subsidize other services which do not have the potential for cost recovery. This example has been shown to work in India.

However, financial self-reliance is only one part of sustainability, and one must also consider human resources, infrastructure and patient demand when planning a sustainable programme.

23.8 QUALITY OF PROGRAMMES

A healthcare programme needs to consider:

➢ The outcome of care (clinical outcome and patient reported outcomes).
➢ The safety of care.
➢ The patient experience of care.

A high quality healthcare programme has excellent outcomes, is safe and the patient experience of care is well received. By definition a high quality programme asks service users for their views and makes changes based on these views.

'Clinical governance' is the term used to describe a systematic approach to maintaining and improving the quality of patient care within a health system.

There are six 'pillars' of clinical governance that assure ongoing quality of healthcare. These are:

1. Education and training — including continuing professional development (an acknowledgement of the need for ongoing training despite the practitioner's experience).

2. Clinical audit — a regular commitment to assess standards through audit.
3. Clinical effectiveness — 'does an intervention work?' This includes 'is it affordable?'
4. Research and development — ensuring that clinical practice is influenced by best available evidence of effectiveness, as well as continuing to encourage enquiry and investigation by each clinician (for example, auditing case notes).
5. Openness — an open and honest culture of care where people are able to report adverse events without fear of reprisal.
6. Risk management — this encompasses risk management for patients, practitioners and the organization. For patients it ensures that 'practitioners do no harm'; for practitioners it means they work in a safe environment. For organizations it means that all practices are high quality (employment, procurement, records).

23.8.1 Quality of eye care

Providing high quality eye care is the responsibility of everyone who works in, or is associated with, an organization. As eye care programmes have begun to evaluate their own effectiveness, the quality of services has become important. This leads to the safety and effectiveness of care being routinely recorded and evaluated as an integral part of service delivery.

23.8.2 Quality of cataract surgery

The simplest measure of clinical effectiveness of cataract surgery is postoperative visual acuity (VA). The WHO benchmark for a high quality cataract service is achievement of a postoperative VA of 6/18 or better with best correction in 90% of patients 6–12 weeks after surgery.

In high-income countries, visual acuity, complication and infection rates, and patient experience are widely accepted as methods for monitoring the quality of cataract surgical services, and most services meet the benchmark set by WHO.

Assessments of visual function (such as VF-14) have also been used in specific settings to measure effectiveness. They measure the perceived impact that cataract surgery has on the patient's visual functioning, and provide a measure of effectiveness. Routine use of current visual function questionnaires is difficult because it requires specialized staff and is time-consuming.

In low-income countries, evidence suggests a marked variation in outcomes after cataract surgery.

Several studies have revealed that poor visual outcomes (VA worse than 6/60 with best correction) are the result in up to 25% of surgeries. Variations in patient-reported outcomes have also been reported.

Poor outcomes can lead to loss of confidence among patients and low utilization of cataract services.

There are four main causes of poor outcome:

> Selection: patient-related risk factors such as other eye diseases affecting VA that were present before surgery.
> Surgery: intra- and peri-operative complications.
> Spectacles: uncorrected postoperative refractive error.
> Sequelae: late complications such as posterior capsule opacification.

It is likely that there is a link between poor patient experience and negative clinical outcomes. For example, poor provision of information about post-discharge care may make poor outcomes more likely.

Inadequate provider–patient interaction is often a key source of dissatisfaction for patients. In a study of over 1,900 patients receiving government healthcare in rural Bangladesh, the politeness of the staff was the most powerful predictor of overall satisfaction with care. Information like this can be used to improve services if staff reflect and act on the results.

To improve the overall quality of the cataract surgical service, the three aspects of quality (outcome of care, safety and patient experience) must be considered in every case. Computer-based tools exist to record clinical outcomes. However, more work is required to develop patient experience questions appropriate for use in low-income settings.

23.9 MONITORING AND EVALUATION

Monitoring is an ongoing process that uses collection of data on specified indicators to provide management with information of progress, achievement of objectives and use of allocated funds, and to inform decision makers.[5]

Management also requires monitoring information to provide feedback reports to stakeholders. Stakeholders want to know whether the project is producing desired results and outcomes, whether it is on target, whether any problems have been encountered, whether these problems can be corrected, how progress is measured, and whether success can be differentiated from failure (evaluation).

Evaluation is an objective assessment of an ongoing or completed project, programme, or policy, including its design, implementation and results. The aim is to determine the relevance and fulfilment of objectives, development efficiency, effectiveness, impact and sustainability. An evaluation should provide information that is credible and useful, enabling the incorporation of lessons learned into the decision-making process of both recipients and donors.

Monitoring and evaluation are distinct yet complementary. Monitoring provides information about where a policy, programme or project is at any given time (and over time) relative to respective targets and outcomes. It is descriptive in intent. Evaluation gives evidence of why targets and outcomes are, or are not, being achieved. It addresses issues of causality.

Monitoring asks: 'Are we doing things right?', whereas evaluation would ask: 'Are we doing the right things?' and 'Are there better ways of achieving the results?'

A **monitoring and evaluation (M&E)** system is a structured approach to collecting and recording project or programme information. This allows a comprehensive analysis of relevant data to either monitor or evaluate the project or programme.

There are two types of M&E systems:

> Implementation-based M&E systems are designed to address compliance — the 'are we doing it?' question. Did we mobilize the needed inputs? Did we undertake and complete the agreed activities? Did we deliver the intended products or services?
> Results-based M&E systems are designed to address the 'so what' question. So what that outputs have been generated? So what that activities have taken place? So what that the outputs from these activities have been counted? A results-based system provides feedback on the actual outcomes and goals of the activities, and can be a powerful tool to demonstrate impact and outcomes to stakeholders and to gain public support.

23.9.1 Developing an M&E system

Any M&E system is likely to fail if there is inadequate local institutional capacity to develop indicators and systems to collect, aggregate, analyze and report performance data; to train managers; and understand what to do with the information once it arrives.

Every M&E system needs four basic elements: ownership, management, maintenance and credibility. Ownership has to come from those at every level who use the system, and demand for performance information at each level needs to be identified. Besides that there needs to be a core group responsible for the management and maintenance of the system. The credibility of the system depends on the validity and reliability of the data and the way the results are presented and used.

The development of an M&E system involves several steps, namely:

> Agreeing on outcomes to monitor and evaluate.
> Selecting key indicators to monitor outcomes.
> Collecting baseline data on indicators (where are we now?).
> Planning for improvement (selecting targets).

M&E should be an ongoing and integral part of any plan from the onset. This will assure high quality in a programme.

Monitoring is important because:

> What gets monitored is more likely to get done.
> If you don't measure results, you can't tell success from failure.
> If you can't see success, you can't reward it.
> If you can't recognize failure, you can't correct it.
> If you can't demonstrate results, you can't win public support.

23.9.2 Indicators

An effective M&E system relies on indicators that report on the key features of the programme. Indicators should be SMART: specific, measurable, achievable, realistic and time-specific.

Other important aspects of monitoring are:

> Collect only indicators that will actually be used for decision-making and discard indicators that are not used.
> Collect data at intervals that your system can cope with. In most countries quarterly reporting of performance data and annual reporting of data on resources will be appropriate. With more advanced systems the frequency of reporting may increase.
> Provide feedback to each unit that provides data for monitoring.
> Educate staff about the benefits of collecting monitoring indicators.
> Don't discard existing monitoring systems before a better system is in place.

With the increased use of computers in healthcare, widespread computer skills of healthcare staff, and expanding internet access, the implementation of M&E systems has become much easier. The analysis of data and generation of reports can now be incorporated in the software of the M&E system, saving much time and reducing the risk of data entry errors.

Each project has activities that achieve objectives or targets, which in turn contribute to an overall goal or aim. The indicators identified in the logframe should reflect the degree of achievement of each of these components.

Indicators

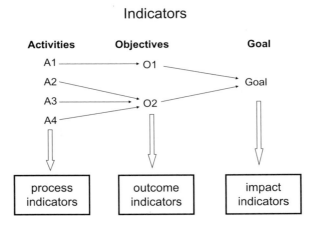

Figure 23.2 *Development of indicators at different levels of a plan*

Figure 23.2 shows that indicators can reflect different levels of the plan; process indicators reflect activities, outcome indicators reflect objectives and impact indicators reflect the goal. Table 23.4 shows a practical example of the different types of indicator applied to a trachoma programme.

23.9.3   Setting the scope of an evaluation

When monitoring indicates change, and questions arise why this occurred, additional information through evaluation may be required. This evaluation can be focused at each stage of the programme, thereby defining its scope, like:

➢ Effectiveness — why have the objectives of the project not been met?
➢ Efficiency — why are the results of the project worth the resources required?
➢ Sustainable — can the activities be continued?
➢ Impact — what are the effects on the final welfare of the target population? (Foreseen and unforeseen, positive or negative?)
➢ Relevance — are the results of the project relevant for the whole country and other countries?

23.9.4   M&E for VISION 2020

Indicators for monitoring VISION 2020 programmes have been defined in a WHO/IAPB workshop in 2003 but no standardized software has been developed to facilitate the implementation of an effective M&E system within countries.[6]

Data from standardized M&E software could be aggregated to monitor VISION 2020 activities at regional or global level.

23.10   CONCLUSION

Epidemiological information is an important part of planning high quality eye care programmes, but

Table 23.4 *Example of indicators for a trachoma programme*

	Trachoma programme	Indicators	
Goal	Elimination of blindness due to trachoma	Prevalence of blindness from trachoma in the population	Impact indicator
Objectives	Reduce trachomatous trichiasis	Proportion of population with TT	Outcome indicators
	Reduce infectious trachoma	Proportion of population with TI	
Activities	Surgery	Number of people with TT operated per month	Process Indicators
	Antibiotics	Community coverage of antibiotics	
	Face hygiene	Number of communities receiving health promotion messages	
	Environmental changes	Proportion of households less than one hour from water source	
		Proportion of households with a functioning latrine	

needs to be complemented by other relevant information. All planning should be based on the healthcare need of the local population. Epidemiological information helps describe the need so that a service can be planned that is relevant to local people.

Tools, such as logframes, exist to allow planning to become a structured step-wise process. Different processes exist that strengthen the planning process, ensuring that it considers sustainability and quality. These include involving local people in developing and planning services relevant to their needs.

Robust monitoring and evaluation of programmes also feed into the planning process, to ensure that objectives are being met, and that lessons learnt are integrated in future plans.

VISION 2020: the Right to Sight is an initiative that provides eye care planners throughout the world with a process and objectives that allow them to use available epidemiological data to plan eye care programmes.

23.11   FURTHER READING

VISION 2020 Toolkit: 'Developing an Action Plan':
- ➢ http://www.who.int/ncd/vision2020_actionplan/contents/frame.htm

Best practice:
- ➢ http://www.cochrane.org

Logical framework approach:
- ➢ http://pdf.usaid.gov/pdf_docs/PNABN963.pdf

- ➢ http://www.norad.no/en/Tools+and+publications/Publications/Publication+Page?key=109408
- ➢ http://www.ausaid.gov.au/ausguide/pdf/ausguideline3.3.pdf

Participatory planning:
- ➢ http://gametlibrary.worldbank.org/FILES/161_Guidelines for participatory planning and evaluation.pdf
- ➢ http://www.uncdf.org/english/local_development/uploads/technical/WP4_ParticipatoryME.pdf

REFERENCES

1. Adapted from Mausner JS, Kramer S. *Mausner & Bahn Epidemiology — An Introductory Text.* Philadelphia: WB Saunders Company; 1985.
2. Stevens A, Gillam S. Needs assessment: from theory to practice. *Br Med J* 1998; 316:1448–1452.
3. Scheirer MA, Hartling G, Hagerman D. Defining sustainability outcomes of health programs: illustrations from an on-line survey. *Eval Prog Plan.* 2008; 31:335–346.
4. Scheirer MA. Is sustainability possible? A review and commentary on empirical studies of program sustainability. *Am J Eval* 2005; 26:320–347.
5. Kusek JZ, Rist RC. *Ten Steps to a Results-Based Monitoring and Evaluation (M&E) System.* The World Bank; 2004.
6. WHO Working Group. *A framework and indicators for monitoring VISION 2020: The Right to Sight: the Global Initiative for the Elimination of Avoidable Blindness.* Geneva: WHO/IAPB; 2003.

24

Global initiative for the elimination of avoidable blindness

ROBERT LINDFIELD, IVO KOCUR, HANS LIMBURG AND ALLEN FOSTER

24.1	What is Vision 2020 — the Right to Sight?	601
24.2	History	601
24.3	Strategy	602
23.4	'I SEE' principles	603
24.5	The structure of Vision 2020	604

24.6	Resources	604
24.7	Implementation	604
24.8	Conclusions	605
24.9	Future research for Vision 2020	606
	References	606

24.1 WHAT IS VISION 2020 — THE RIGHT TO SIGHT?

VISION 2020 is a global initiative to eliminate avoidable blindness. The initiative is a partnership between the World Health Organization (WHO) and the International Agency for Prevention of Blindness (IAPB), which is the umbrella organization for eye care professional groups, the corporate sector and non-governmental organizations (NGOs) involved in eye care.

The primary goal of VISION 2020 is to eliminate avoidable blindness by the year 2020. Long-term goals are to ensure the best possible vision for all people and thereby improve quality of life.

24.2 HISTORY[1]

In the late 1970s the WHO established the Prevention of Blindness Programme (PBL), and at the same time the International Federation of Ophthalmological Societies (IFOS), the World Blind Union and a group of international NGOs formed the IAPB.

Throughout the 1980s a close working relationship developed between WHO/PBL and the NGOs. In 1994 the NGOs and WHO formed a joint taskforce to address the increasing problem of global blindness. With support from the NGOs the World Health Organization convened consultations with experts in the field, and in 1997 this resulted in the publication of 'The Global Initiative to Eliminate Avoidable Blindness'. This document explained the rationale, global strategy and targets for the VISION 2020 initiative.

In 2003 the **World Health Assembly (WHA)** adopted Resolution WHA 56.26, which urged member states to commit their support to VISION 2020, and set up the appropriate structures to define and implement VISION 2020 plans. This resolution was strengthened in 2006 when the

World Health Assembly adopted Resolution 59.25, which reinforced WHA 56.26.

In 2006 the original Global Initiative to Eliminate Avoidable Blindness document was updated with an action plan (VISION 2020 Action Plan: 2006–2011). This recognized that there had been a shift in the causes of preventable blindness, and the challenges faced in tackling them. The Action Plan listed the major activities associated with a VISION 2020 programme, namely, disease control and prevention of visual impairment; human resource development and infrastructure and technology; setting out new objectives for each activity; as well as considering advocacy and resource mobilization.

24.2.1   Priorities for VISION 2020

The priorities for VISION 2020 are based on the facts that approximately 85% of blindness occurs in the poorer communities of the world, and that around 80% of blindness is a result of preventable or treatable conditions (avoidable).[2] If priority is given, at the global level, to improving eye care services for neglected communities, and to targeting causes of avoidable blindness, then, if current trends continue, the number of people affected by blindness should have decreased significantly by 2020.[2]

24.3   STRATEGY

The concept of VISION 2020 is built upon the foundation of community participation, with the four essential components of the VISION 2020 programme being:[3]

➢ Cost-effective disease control interventions.
➢ Human resource development (training and motivation).
➢ Infrastructure development (facilities, appropriate technology/consumables, funds).
➢ Advocacy.

24.3.1   Cost-effective disease control interventions

VISION 2020 initially focused on five 'priority' diseases:

1. Cataract
2. Refractive error
3. Onchocerciasis
4. Childhood blindness
5. Trachoma

However, with the publication of the VISION 2020 Action Plan: 2006–2011,[4] the focus on these five priority diseases has broadened to include important chronic eye diseases; diabetic retinopathy, glaucoma and age-related macular degeneration. The Action Plan recognizes that these diseases are important causes of blindness and visual impairment in many countries, and that effective treatment strategies are becoming more defined and available.

24.3.2   Human resource development

Many governments and non-governmental organizations are emphasizing the importance of human resource development at the primary, secondary and tertiary levels of eye care. This is particularly needed for Sub-Saharan Africa, where, on average, there is only one ophthalmologist per million population, compared with 100 per million in some cities of the Americas and Eastern Europe.

A simple estimate of the requirement for ophthalmologists in a particular place can be established using the **cataract surgical rate (CSR)**. For example, to achieve a CSR of 2,000 in a location would require four ophthalmologists operating on ten cases per week for 50 weeks in each year. To increase the CSR requires either more ophthalmologists (which is the case in many high income countries) or more productivity from each ophthalmologist. Whilst an ophthalmologist's role is far wider than solely operating on cataract, it is one of the critical activities that decreases the prevalence of blindness and is a good marker of the requirement for ophthalmologists.

If the ophthalmologist's expertise is to be used efficiently there is also a need for optometrists and ophthalmic assistants to manage refractive errors, to assist in screening patients for asymptomatic disease, and to perform ophthalmic investigations. Provision of eye care requires more than just clinicians. There is a great need for management skills and a community/public health approach to eye care.

Eye specialists, ophthalmic assistants and managers tend to be hospital-based. They need to be complemented by human resources at the community level, which can identify patients with visual loss, motivate them to present for eye care, and possibly provide first aid for acute red eyes and ocular injuries.

The human resources needed for a VISION 2020 programme are therefore both clinical and non-clinical, and involve all cadres of eye staff as well as the community. It is important that they work together as a team to complement each other's skills and roles in the provision of comprehensive eye care services.

24.3.3   Infrastructure development

The past few years have seen major technological developments in ophthalmological practice in the industrialized world. These developments are often expensive but can improve the quality of eye care offered. Increasingly, these technological developments are being adapted for use in the developing world. High-quality, affordable intraocular lenses and eye sutures are now available. Efforts have been made to produce low-cost spectacles and eye drops. Several companies are involved in the production of affordable ophthalmological equipment and instruments.

A VISION 2020 programme requires the necessary diagnostic, therapeutic and surgical equipment and consumables to manage at least the five priority causes of blindness. This is a minimum requirement. As services develop, equipment for diabetic retinopathy and glaucoma can be added. With limited resources it is important to avoid

wastage on equipment, which is not used, not indicated, or inadequately maintained.

24.3.4   Advocacy

A key part of VISION 2020 is advocacy at global, regional, national and local levels. A core component of the global advocacy programme is World Sight Day, held on the second Thursday of October each year, and focusing on a specific issue related to blindness. Global advocacy has also resulted in the two WHA Resolutions related to prevention of blindness and the development of the Action Plan for the prevention of avoidable blindness and visual impairment adopted by the 62nd WHA.

Lasting change in countries will only occur with government support; therefore, the integral role of WHO and national ministries of health in VISION 2020 is necessary to achieve this change.

24.4   'I SEE' PRINCIPLES

The guiding principles for a VISION 2020 project can be summarized as 'I SEE', standing for Integrated, Sustainable, Equitable and Excellent.

➤ I: Integrated. VISION 2020 activities should be integrated into existing health services. Although certain elements are specialized (e.g. cataract surgery), eye care should not stand alone but wherever possible be integrated into district level health services.
➤ S: Sustainable. Eye care services need to be ongoing and long-term, sustainable both financially and with respect to personnel. This is particularly difficult in Africa and poor areas of Asia, but good models do exist which can be replicated. It is also necessary to acknowledge that we cannot always expect 'self-sustainability', and sometimes people in very poor areas just have to be provided for.
➤ E: Equitable. The eye care service should be available to all sectors of society, not just to those who can afford it, or who live in urban

situations. This again is particularly challenging in Africa because of poor distribution of specialists, poverty, low density of population and difficult terrain.

➢ E: Excellence. Good quality clinical and non-clinical care is essential if people's fears of eye surgery are to be overcome. Just because people cannot pay, they should not be offered poor quality services, either clinical or non-clinical.

24.5   THE STRUCTURE OF VISION 2020[1]

The organogram in Plate 24.1 describes the structure of VISION 2020, and shows the relationship between WHO and IAPB. It also describes the way that VISION 2020 activities are implemented at district or provincial level, directed by National Programmes which, in turn, feed into the WHO/IAPB Regional Offices. At a global level there are advocacy, resource mobilization and programme development activities (Plate 24.1).

24.6   RESOURCES

There are two key resources required for the successful implementation of VISION 2020 — human and financial resources.

24.6.1   Human resources — people's time

The 'human' resource is very important. The world in total has sufficient eye specialists (approximately 150,000), yet at least one third of the world is lacking in trained eye care workers because of poor distribution. As well as clinical training for specialists and eye care workers, there is a need to provide and encourage a public health perspective based upon an understanding of epidemiology.

The implementation of VISION 2020 does not depend on international committees (whose role is priority setting and reviewing activities), but upon individual eye care workers implementing the priorities and strategies of VISION 2020 (eliminating

blindness, maximizing vision and improving quality of life) for the people (community) they serve. The concept of a VISION 2020 movement for eye care is more important than the structure.

24.6.2   Financial resources

Funds are required to improve facilities and infrastructure for eye care, particularly in poor areas of the world. Funds are also required to motivate eye care staff to work in difficult situations. The existing and new funds, be they obtained from government or private sources, need to be used in an effective way. This requires clear priority setting and allocation of the resources based upon community needs rather than professional interests.

24.7   IMPLEMENTATION

24.7.1   District level

At the district level (usually a population of between 100,000 and 2 million), implementation of VISION 2020 involves:

1. Identifying the important preventable and/or treatable causes of blindness and visual loss applying to a particular community. This can be done through a formal survey, rapid assessment, or estimates based on local knowledge and disease patterns.
2. Assessing the available resources:
   a. financial and infrastructural — buildings, beds, equipment, instruments, medicines, spectacles and other consumables; and understanding the running costs and sources of funds — from patient fees, government, or non-governmental sources; and funds for development costs including training and equipment;
   b. clinical and managerial human resources — ophthalmologists, optometrists, ophthalmic assistants, nurses, community health workers; and expertise in leadership and motivation of people; practical management of a programme; and financial accountability.

3. Formulating a plan to strengthen the human resources (technical and managerial), and to improve the infrastructure and facilities needed by the eye care staff to deliver services.

4. Implementing specific disease control interventions integrated into a comprehensive eye care service; for example, if hospital services are improved for the diagnosis and treatment of cataract because this is a priority for VISION 2020, it is likely to also have a positive impact on services for other eye diseases like glaucoma. Similarly the provision of reading spectacles at the community level by ophthalmic assistants may assist in improving case detection for cataract, glaucoma or diabetic retinopathy.

24.7.2 National level

At the national level it is important to develop collaboration and co-ordination between all the relevant stakeholders, including Ministries of Health, ophthalmologists and other eye care professional groups, and local and international nongovernmental eye care providers. A national plan is needed to identify the priorities for action and who will be responsible for each activity. It is advisable to have a small taskforce or executive committee under the Ministry of Health, and made up of the key individuals in national eye care, meeting once every one — three months, and reporting to a larger annual meeting of all involved parties. There is no substitute for one dedicated person to work full-time on the national VISION 2020 programme.

24.7.3 Inter-country/regional level

WHO and IAPB divide the world into six administrative regions, namely, WHO African Region, WHO Region of the Americas, WHO South East Asia Region, WHO European Region, WHO Eastern Mediterranean Region and WHO Western Pacific Region. In each region there is a Chairperson for IAPB and a Regional Working group for VISION 2020. In some regions there is

a specific WHO regional adviser for prevention of blindness. The role of the Regional Group is advocacy and resource mobilization for VISION 2020 in the region, together with offering assistance to countries in developing and implementing their national VISION 2020 plans.

24.7.4 Global level

WHO and IAPB are joint partners of VISION 2020. There are coordinating mechanisms between WHO and the members of IAPB to govern and implement VISION 2020. IAPB tends to focus on global advocacy, resource mobilization and assistance to the regions. WHO sets the technical norms and guidelines for the programme.

24.8 CONCLUSIONS

Epidemiological studies have been used to identify the magnitude and causes of visual impairment, including blindness. Effective interventions for most of the major avoidable causes have been identified and tested. VISION 2020 — the Right to Sight Global Initiative was launched in 1999 as a major global partnership to work towards elimination of avoidable blindness. Two key principles in VISION 2020 are 'partnership' and 'ownership'.

➢ Partnership — the problem of blindness is too great for any one group, be they governments, eye care professionals or non-governmental organizations. There is a need to combine our strengths and work together to plan and implement VISION 2020 if we are to control avoidable blindness.

➢ Ownership — VISION 2020 will only be successful if people 'own' the programme for themselves, be they a national policy maker, a district ophthalmologist or a community health worker identifying cataract patients for surgery.

VISION 2020 is the leading global eye health initiative of concern to all of us, to which epidemiological research contributes essential information.

24.9　FUTURE RESEARCH FOR VISION 2020

Public-health action to prevent blindness and visual impairment needs to be evidence-based and cost-effective. International collaboration in promoting multidimensional and multisectoral research is essential for developing eye care systems that are comprehensive, integrated, equitable, high quality and sustainable. Further research is needed on ways to capitalize on existing evidence. Special emphasis should be placed on evaluating interventions and strategies for early detection and screening of the causes of blindness and visual impairment in different population groups. Epidemiological, behavioural and health-system research should be part of national programmes for eye health and prevention of blindness and visual impairment.

Topics that require further research:

➢ Prevalence and causes of blindness and visual impairment at national and district levels.
➢ Socio-economic determinants, the role of gender, the cost-effectiveness of interventions and identification of high-risk population groups.
➢ The economic cost of blindness and visual impairment and its impact on socio-economic development.
➢ The impact of poverty and other determinants on the gradient of socio-economic disparity in individuals' access to eye care services.
➢ The impact of risk factors such as smoking, unhealthy diet, physical inactivity, ultraviolet radiation and poor hygiene.
➢ The impact of public health policies and strategies on the status of eye health.

REFERENCES

1. IAPB, WHO. VISION 2020: The Right to Sight. [Cited 12th December 2009]. http://www.iapb.org.
2. Resnikoff S, Pascolini D, Etya'ale D, *et al*. Global data on visual impairment in the year 2002. *Bull World Health Organ* 2004; 82:844–851.
3. WHO. *The Global Initiative for Elimination of Avoidable Blindness*. Geneva: WHO; 1997.
4. WHO. *Global Initiative for the Elimination of Avoidable Blindness: action plan 2006–2011*. Geneva: WHO; 2007.

Glossary of acronyms and definitions

AAC acute angle-closure

AAO American Academy of Ophthalmology

AAPOS American Association of Pediatric Ophthalmology and Strabismus

ABCD Trial Appropriate Blood Pressure Control in Diabetes Trial

ABR annual biting rate, in Onchocerciasis

AC accommodation; the reflex thickening of the lens of the eye to bring near objects into focus on the retina

AC angle-closure

AC anterior chamber

ACD anterior chamber depth

ACE angiotensin-converting enzyme

ACG angle-closure glaucoma

AC-IOL anterior chamber intraocular lens

ADDE aqueous tear-deficient dry eye

admixture refers to racial or ethnic outcrossing within a population

ADVS Activities of Daily Vision Scale

AG aphakic glasses

AGIS Advanced Glaucoma Intervention Study

AI adequate intake of vitamin A nutrients to maintain normal status

AIDS acquired immune deficiency syndrome

AK Acanthamoeba keratitis

allele one of several alternative forms of a gene occupying a given locus on a chromosome

amblyopia; a decrease in best corrected visual acuity in an eye which has no obvious pathology in the visual pathway; attributed to 'form vision deprivation', most commonly due to strabismus or unequal refraction in the two eyes (anisometropia) (see Section 8.7.3.1)

AMD age-related macular degeneration (see Section 22.2)

ametropias refractive errors, i.e. myopia, hypermetropia or astigmatism

anisometropia unequal refraction in the two eyes

ANOVA analysis of variance

aphakia (an eye) without a lens

APOC African Programme for Onchocerciasis Control

AP-ROP aggressive posterior ROP

AR attributable risk

Ara-A adenine arabinoside, or vidarabine, an antiviral drug

AREDS Age-Related Eye Disease Study

ARIC Atherosclerosis Risk in Communities Study

ARN acute retinal necrosis syndrome

ARVO Association for Research in Vision and Ophthalmology

AS-OCT anterior segment optical coherence tomography

ASCs antibody-secreting cells

ASCRS American Society of Cataract and Refractive Surgery

association, genetic occurs when risk factors for a disease, including a complex (multifactorial) disease, are represented by genetic factors such as single nucleotide polymorphisms (SNPs) Genetic associations can be investigated by several epidemiological study methods (see Chapter 6)

astigmatism (A) the refractive state of an eye when the outer corneal surface is not spherical because the radii of curvature of two perpendicular meridians are unequal

ATP adenosine triphosphate

ATP annual transmission potential, in onchocerciasis (see Section 18.5.3)

attributable risk (AR) the excess risk of disease in those exposed to the risk factor compared with those not or less exposed (see Chapter 2)

autosomal dominant (AD) a gene capable of expression when carried on only one of a pair of homologous chromosomes (i.e. the heterozygous state)

autosomal recessive (AR) a gene not capable of expression unless the responsible allele is carried by both members of a pair of homologous chromosomes

avoidable blindness blindness which could reasonably be prevented or cured within the limits of resources likely to be made available

AZT zidovudine (azidothymidine) an antiretroviral agent

B-cells (B-lymphocytes) cells involved in antibody-mediated immunity

BDES Beaver Dam Eye Study

bias (general) distortion of an estimate (e.g. prevalence, odds ratio, relative risk, treatment effect) away from the true population value, caused by non-sampling errors; includes **selection bias** and information bias (see Chapter 3), **recall** and **observer bias** (see Chapter 4) and **lead-time bias** and **length bias** (see Chapter 8)

blindness (WHO definition) visual acuity of less than 3/60 (or equivalent) in the better eye with best correction, or visual field in each eye restricted to less than 10° from fixation

blocking (permuted block randomization) a type of restricted randomization procedure in a trial which guarantees that at no time during randomization will there be a large imbalance in size of treatment groups, and that at certain points in the sequence of treatment allocation the treatment groups will be of equal size

BMES Blue Mountains Eye Study; an area to the west of Sydney, Australia

BMI body-mass index [weight (kg) divided by the square of the height (m)]

BTRP bilamellar tarsal rotation procedure; recommended by WHO for surgical correction of trichiasis in trachoma

BUT tear film break-up time: the time from the last blink to the appearance of the first gap in the precorneal tear film, shown up by fluorescein staining

BW birth weight

CANDEES Canada Dry Eye Epidemiology Study

CBD community-based distributor

CBR community-based rehabilitation

CD4 cells cellular differentiation or 'clonal deletion 4' cells, originally called T-helper cells

CD4$^+$ T-lymphocyte a lymphocyte bearing the CD4 receptor complex — a critical component of the immune system

CD8 cells cellular differentiation or 'clonal deletion 8' cells, originally called T-suppressor cells

CDC Centers for Disease Control and Prevention of the United States of America

CDD community-directed distributor

CDHW community-directed health workers

CDK climatic droplet keratopathy

cDNA recombinant deoxyribonucleic acid

CDTI community-directed treatment with ivermectin

CFH complement factor H (applied to a gene and its polymorphisms)

CFR case–fatality ratio (as in measles)

CGMP cyclic guanosine monophosphate

CI confidence interval, as in 95% CI. This indicates a probability of 0.95 that the reported limits contain the true population prevalence (see Chapter 3) or true Odds Ratio (see Chapter 4)

CI also cumulative incidence (see Chapter 2)

CIC conjunctival impression cytology

CIGTS Collaborative Initial Glaucoma Treatment Study

CL contact lens

CLS cluster sampling (see Section 3.4.2)

CLW contact lens wearer

CME cystoid macular edema (oedema)

CMFL community microfilarial load in Onchocerciasis (see Section 18.5.1)

CMI cell-mediated immunity

CMV cytomegalovirus

CNS central nervous system

CNV choroidal neovascularization

CO corneal opacity in trachoma

Cochrane Collaboration an international network of researchers conducting systematic reviews of clinical trials in all medical specialties to improve the evidence base for health intervention. Named in honour of Prof. Archie Cochrane (1908–1988); pioneer epidemiologist at the Welsh National School of Medicine; advocated randomized clinical trials and stressed the importance of demonstrating effectiveness of health interventions

COMET Correction of Myopia Evaluation Trial (USA)

conditional logistic regression see logistic regression

confounding said to exist when all or part of an observed exposure–disease association is attributable to another causal exposure factor (the confounder) (see Section 4.5.2)

CONSORT Consolidated Standards of Reporting Trials; agreed guidelines and checklist for reporting of randomized clinical trials (see Section 7.4)

coverage (of a screening programme) the proportion of the population at risk who are screened in one episode aiming to examine all at risk

Cox proportional hazards regression commonly used for analysis of survival data, allows for changes in the instantaneous incidence rates (hazards) during follow-up, but assumes that the hazard ratios remain constant

CP cerebral palsy

CRS congenital rubella syndrome

CRYO-ROP Cryotherapy for Retinopathy of Prematurity Cooperative Group study, the first multicentre trial of cryotherapy for ROP

CSC cataract surgical coverage: the proportion of patients (or eyes) with 'operable' cataract who have already received surgery

CSR cataract surgical rate: number of operations performed per year per million population

CTL cytotoxic lymphocyte

cumulative incidence the number of new cases of disease occurring in a given time period, divided by the total population at risk

CVFQ Children's Visual Function Questionnaire; a vision-related quality of life instrument developed specifically for children

D dioptre or diopter, a measure of the power of a lens: the reciprocal of the focal length in metres

DCCT Diabetes Control and Complications Trial

DEC diethylcarbamazine citrate

DED dry eye disease

deff (design effect) the actual variance of a parameter estimate in a cluster random sample relative to (divided by) the variance calculated under the assumption of simple random sampling (see Chapter 3)

DEWS International Dry Eye Workshop, 2007

DNA deoxyribonucleic acid

DR diabetic retinopathy

DR 3,4-didehydroretinol

DRS Diabetic Retinopathy Study research group

DRS-HRC Diabetic Retinopathy Study High Risk Characteristics

DZ dizygotic twin; derived from two zygotes, or fertilized ova

EAR Estimated Average Requirement of a nutrient

EB elementary body, infectious particle of Chlamydia

ECCE extracapsular cataract extraction

EDC-CS Eye Disease Case-Control Study

EDE evaporative dry eye

effect modification when the association between the exposure and disease under study varies according to the level of a third factor, such as age; differs from confounding, which is a nuisance effect, distorting the true relationship between the exposure and risk in a particular mix of subjects being studied

effective applied to treatment, intervention or procedure, having the intended effect in a specific population; applied to medicines or treatments in ideal circumstances, as determined by results of randomized clinical trial = efficacious

efficient the results achieved by an intervention or treatment (of known effectiveness) in relation to expenditure of effort, cost and time

EGPS European Glaucoma Prevention Study

ELBW extremely low birth weight, less than 1,000 g

ELISA enzyme-linked immunosorbent assay

EME Established Market Economies (World Bank region)

EMGTS (or EMG study) Early Manifest Glaucoma Treatment Study

emmetropia the refractive state of an unaccommodated eye in which a distant image (more than 6 m away) is focussed on the retina

ENL erythema nodosum leprosum, occuring in type II leprosy reactions

EPESE Study Established Populations for the Epidemiologic Studies of the Elderly Study

EPI WHO Expanded Programme of Immunization of the World Health Organization

epigenetic heritable changes in gene expression that are due not to changes in the DNA sequence itself, but to 'something in addition', such as chemical modification of certain bases or protein factors bound with the DNA

epistasis genetic variance resulting from non-additive effects of alleles at distinct loci (gene–gene interaction, the genotype at one locus affecting the phenotypic expression of the genotype at another locus)

epsem equal probability selection method: a popular type of probability sampling

ERG electroretinogram

ETDRS Early Treatment Diabetic Retinopathy Study

etiologic fraction for a risk factor gives the proportion of all 'cases' (occurring among the population exposed to the risk factor) that is attributable to the exposure (see Chapter 2)

ETROP Early Treatment of Retinopathy of Prematurity Trial

FAO the Food and Agriculture Organization

FAS/D foetal alcohol syndrome/disorder

FDA USA Food and Drug Administration

FES Framingham Eye Study

fluorescein stain a topical stain applied to the cornea which highlights defects in the epithelial cell layer of the cornea

FLV functional low vision

fomites any material, such as bedding or clothing, which can convey disease; an old-fashioned term from Latin, used in connection with trachoma

GA gestational age

GEE generalized estimating equations: statistical procedures for analyzing 'repeated measures' on the same subject in longitudinal studies, and for other 'correlated' or clustered data (e.g. from cluster randomized trials, family studies, cluster sampling surveys, both eyes of same person)

genetic heterogeneity distinct alleles at the same or different loci that give rise independently to the same disease

genotype the genetic constitution of a person or organism

genovars varieties of *C. trachomatis*, differing and identified by gene sequencing of DNA

GLT Glaucoma Laser Trial

GMS Gomori's methenamine silver; stain for identifying fungi

gp120 a surface glycoprotein of the human immunodeficiency virus

GWAS genome-wide association studies

HAART highly active anti-retroviral therapy

HANES USA National Health and Nutrition Examination Study

haplotype a sequence of linked alleles, present in a single chromosome, and transmitted from parent to offspring

Hardy–Weinberg Equilibrium a principle of population genetics which defines a stable frequency of genes and genotypes in a population, assuming random mating

HDL high density lipoproteins

heritability the proportion of population variance in a trait attributable to segregation of a gene or genes

heterozygous (heterozygote) carrying dissimilar alleles of a gene on each of a pair of chromosomes

HHV-8 human herpesvirus 8

HIV human immunodeficiency virus

HLA antigens human-leukocyte-associated antigens, first demonstrated on white blood cells

homozygous (homozygote) having the same allele of a gene on both of a pair of chromosomes

HPLC high pressure liquid chromatography

HPV human papilloma virus

HSV *Herpes simplex* virus; 2 strains HSV1 and HSV2

HTA UK Health Technology Assessment

HTEM harmful traditional eye medicines

hypermetropia or hyperopia (H) a condition where the unaccommodated eye forms the image of a distant object behind the retina

hyphaema accumulation of blood in the anterior chamber of the eye

hypopyon accumulation of pus cells in the anterior chamber of the eye

HZO herpes zoster ophthalmicus

HZV *Herpes zoster* virus, also called VZV

IAPB International Agency for the Prevention of Blindness

IATS Infant Aphakic Treatment Study

ICCE intracapsular cataract extraction

ICD-10 International Statistical Classification of Diseases and Related Health Problems, 10th revision

ICMR Indian Council of Medical Research

ICROP International Classification of Retinopathy of Prematurity

ICT impression cytology with transfer

IDP Ivermectin Distribution Programme

IgA immunoglobulin A

IgE immunoglobulin E

IGF-1 insulin-like growth factor 1

IgG immunoglobulin G

IgM immunoglobulin M

IL interleukin; interleukin-4 (IL-4) and interleukin-10 (IL-10)

IMR infant mortality rate

incidence rate the number of cases that occur in the population per unit of person-time at risk (see Section 2.2.2)

inclusion body the vesicle in which Chlamydia mature within the infected cell

IOL intraocular lens

IOP intraocular pressure

IR incidence rate (incidence density) number of new cases occurring per person-time at risk (e.g. per 1,000 person-years at risk) (see Chapter 2)

IRU immune recovery uveitis

ISGEO International Society for Geographic and Epidemiologic Ophthalmology

IU international unit, e.g. of vitamin A

IVACG International Vitamin A Consultative Group

KAP knowledge, attitudes and practices

Kaplan–Meier method a method of analysis for survival data using exact (or near exact) censoring and failure times, which must be known for all individuals included in the analysis

kappa statistic (k) a measure of the agreement between two observers (inter-observer agreement) which makes allowance for the number of agreements by chance

kD kilodaltons; a unit of relative molecular mass

keratomalacia full thickness necrosis of the cornea ('softening of the cornea')

KIM key informant method

KOH potassium hydroxide; used as a wet mount to detect fungi in a scraping from a corneal ulcer

L3 third-stage (infective) larva of *Onchocerca volvulus*

L4 fourth-stage larva (in human host) of *Onchocerca volvulus*

lagophthalmos (literally 'hare eye'); failure of the eyelids to completely close, so that the globe is visible through the gap between the eyelids on attempted closure; in leprosy, due to damage to temporal or zygomatic branches of facial nerve

LALES Los Angeles Latino Eye Study

LASIK laser *in situ* keratomileusis

LD linkage disequilibrium

LFA logical framework approach, a management tool for planning

LGHS Local Government Health Services

linkage analysis a model explaining the inheritance pattern of phenotypes and genotypes observed in a family pedigree, to examine whether a particular area of the genome is linked to the phenotype

linkage disequilibrium (LD) two alleles at different loci that occur within an individual more often than would be predicted by random chance. Also called allelic association

LOCS Lens Opacity Classification System

locus the position on a chromosome at which the gene for a particular trait resides; the locus may be occupied by any one of the alleles for the gene

LOD expresses the 'log of the odds' scores (Z). They compare the likelihood of obtaining sibship data if two gene loci are indeed linked, with the likelihood of obtaining the same data if there is no linkage (see Section 6.3.4)

log MAR logarithm of the minimal angle of resolution. A design of a visual acuity chart aiming to give consistency of measurement

logistic regression family of regression models for analysis of data where the response (outcome) is not a continuous variable, but is discrete, the usual form being a binary variable (dichotomous outcomes such as 'blind' 'not blind'). **Polytomous logistic regression** is an extension of the method to handle response variables that have three or more categories, e.g. three levels of visual impairment: none, moderate and severe. Conditional logistic regression is a variant of the method applicable in some study designs, e.g. matched case-control studies

LOSOL Longitudinal Study of Ocular Leprosy, a multicentre study of multi-bacillary leprosy running for ten years from 1988

LVA low-vision assistive device, or low-vision aid

LVP-FVQ L V Prasad-Functional Vision Questionnaire; a vision-related quality of life instrument developed at the L V Prasad Institute, India, for children in developing countries

M&E a monitoring and evaluation system

MAC *Mycobacterium avium* complex

Mantel–Haenszel method statistical procedures for analysis of data stratified by levels of a confounder, e.g. to provide estimates for the pooled odds ratio adjusted for confounding effects, when the odds ratios are homogenous across the strata

marker a fragment of DNA in the human genome whose location is known and which can be used to identify loci that may be linked to a disease or trait of interest

masking procedures in a study or trial to keep participants, and often clinic staff and examiners, from knowing the treatment allocation or other facts which might bias their decisions (sometimes called 'blinding')

MB multi-bacillary leprosy (sometimes known as lepromatous)

MDA mass drug administration; drug treatment of whole communities, as may apply in onchocerciasis and trachoma

MDT multi-drug therapy for leprosy (includes dapsone, rifampicin, and clofazamine)

mean a measure of central tendency, calculated as the sum of a set of values divided by the number of values in the set; the arithmetical mean, or average

median a measure of central tendency, which is the middle observation when the observations are arranged in increasing or decreasing order. When the total number of observations (n) is an even number, then the median is taken as the average of the two middle observations

meta-analysis a systematic process for combining the results of a number of well-designed studies into a single quantitative measure

mf(s) microfilaria(e) of *Onchocerca volvulus*

microarray modern genetic technology in which many hundreds or thousands of markers or single nucleotide polymorphisms (SNPs) are arrayed for rapid multiple testing

microsatellite DNA variant resulting from a tandem repetition of a short DNA sequence (usually between two and four nucleotides), often used as a marker

miosis constriction of the pupil

MIS management information system

MMC mitomycin C; antimetabolite

MMPs matrix metalloproteinases — enzymes involved in breakdown of proteins

MMR mumps, measles and rubella immunization

MODY maturity-onset diabetes of the young

MOMP (also called omp1) the major outer membrane protein of chlamydia

MRDR modified relative dose response (see Section 14b.6.1)

MSG monosodium glutamate

mtDNA (multi variable) mitochondrial deoxyribonucleic acid

multivariate (multivariable) regression more than one independent variable in the regression model

MUST Trial the Multicenter Uveitis Steroid Treatment Trial

mydriasis dilation of the pupil

myopia (M) when the un-accommodated eye forms the image of a distant object in front of the retina

MZ monozygotic twin; derived from one zygote, or fertilized ovum

NAATS nucleic acid amplification tests, such as PCR

NCEU Study: Northern California Epidemiology of Uveitis Study

NFL nerve fibre layer of the retina

NGDO non-governmental development organization

NGO non-governmental organization

NHANES National Health and Nutrition Examination Surveys (USA)

NICU newborn intensive care unit

NIH USA National Institutes of Health

NK cells natural-killer cells; part of the 'innate' immune response, e.g. in trachoma

NLES North London Eye Study

NNRTI non-nucleoside reverse transcriptase inhibitor; name of a class of anti-retroviral agents

NNT number needed to treat to prevent the outcome in one person (e.g. in glaucoma, the number of people with ocular hypertension which must be treated to prevent one case of early POAG)

NPCB National Programme for the Control of Blindness (India)

NPV negative predictive value (of a test); the probability of a person being disease-negative if the test is negative (see Section 8.6.1)

NRTI nucleoside reverse transcriptase inhibitor; name of a class of anti-retroviral agents

NSC UK National Screening Committee

NSSDE non-Sjögren syndrome dry eye

NTDs 'Neglected Tropical Diseases'; an initiative for 13 bacterial and worm infections regarded as 'neglected' in comparison with resources available for malaria, tuberculosis and AIDS; includes trachoma, leprosy and onchocerciasis

OAG open-angle glaucoma

OCP the FAO/UNDP/World Bank/WHO Onchocerciasis Control Programme in West Africa

OCT optical coherence tomography

OEPA Onchocerciasis Elimination Programme in the Americas

OHT ocular hypertension

OHTS Ocular Hypertension Treatment Study

ON ophthalmia neonatorum; conjunctivitis in an infant less than 28 days old

ON also optic neuropathies

OR odds ratio; odds of being exposed to the risk factor among the cases, divided by the odds of exposure among non-cases (controls). A measure of association between exposure and disease, sometimes interpreted as relative risk (see Chapter 2 and Section 4.2)

p probability. See also **p-value** (in context of statistical significance)

p also estimated prevalence in a sample

P true prevalence in a population

PAC primary angle-closure

PACG primary angle-closure glaucoma

PACS primary angle-closure suspect

PAR% population attributable risk percentage, gives the proportion of all 'cases' (occurring in a general population) that is attributable to the exposure of interest. Meaningful only when a causal relationship is assumed between a detrimental exposure and the 'case' status (see Chapter 2)

PAS peripheral anterior synechiae

path analysis this involves solving a series of simultaneous structural equations in order to estimate genetic and environmental parameters that best fit observed familial variances and covariances

PB pauci-bacillary leprosy (sometimes known as tuberculoid)

PBD WHO Programme for the Prevention of Blindness and Deafness (replaced WHO-PBL)

PCG primary congenital glaucoma

PC-IOL posterior chamber intraocular lens

PCM project cycle management (see Section 23.6.2)

PCO posterior capsular opacification

PCP *Pneumocystis carinii* pneumonia

PCR polymerase chain reaction

PDR proliferative diabetic retinopathy

PELF Programme for Elimination of Lymphatic Filariasis

PEM protein–energy malnutrition

PFV persistent foetal vasculature

phenocopy a phenotype caused by the environment, which looks the same as the phenotype caused by a genetic disease

phenotype the appearance or other characteristics of an individual resulting from the interaction of its genetic constitution with the environment (the term is something used by geneticists to mean the visible or detectable effect of a gene, the observable properties or make-up of an individual)

PHMB polyhexamethyl biguanide

PHS Physician's Health Study, USA

PI protease inhibitor: name of a class of anti-retroviral agents

PK penetrating keratoplasty, or full-thickness corneal graft

PMMA polymethyl methacrylate

POAG primary open-angle glaucoma

polymorphism ('the ability to exist in different forms'): the situation in which there are multiple allelic forms of a gene maintained in the population, but where their physiological expression is the same

PORNS progressive outer retinal necrosis syndrome

power of a test (or study) is the probability that the test or study will correctly reject the null hypothesis in the presence of a true effect of a given magnitude. Evaluated as 1-b, where b is the probability of a type II error (see Section 7.2.7)

pps probability proportional to size: type of cluster sampling where the probability of selection for each cluster is made proportional to the size of the cluster (see Chapter 3)

PPV positive predictive value (of a test); the probability of a person being disease-positive if the test is positive (see Section 8.6.1)

PR public relations

precision of an estimate: the width of the confidence interval for the estimated value is a measure of precision, and is determined by a) the amount of sampling error, and b) the required level of certainty, i.e. the probability (usually set to 95%) that the confidence interval contains the true population value

presbyopia age-related decline in range of accommodation of the eye

prevalence (P) of a disease in a population is the proportion of individuals who have the disease at a given time

preventive fraction gives the proportion of potential 'cases' prevented by the exposure. It is analogous to PAR% but applies when the exposure is beneficial (see Chapter 2)

probability sampling a method of sampling where the probability of selection is known (specified) for every eligible member of the population (the sampling frame)

proband the first person in a family to be recognized and investigated in a family study

PSC posterior subcapsular cataract

pseudophakia (an eye) with an artificial intraocular lens

PSU primary sampling unit

PUK peripheral ulcerative keratitis

p-value obtained from a statistical significance test: the probability of the observed result (or results even less consistent with the null hypothesis), given that the null hypothesis is true

QA quality assurance, for example of a screening programme

QoL quality of life

quantitative trait a trait (or disease) that can be measured rather than defined as present or absent (e.g. spherical equivalent in refractive error)

RA retinoic acids

RAAB rapid assessment of avoidable blindness

RACSS rapid assessment for cataract surgical services

RAE retinol activity equivalent

RB reticulate body; growing and multiplying phase of Chlamydia

RBP retinol-binding protein

RCT randomized clinical trial

RDA recommended dietary allowance: the daily requirement of vitamin A-containing nutrients

RDR relative dose response (see Section 14b.6.1)

RDS respiratory distress syndrome

RE retinol equivalents

REA rapid epidemiological assessment, in onchocerciasis

recombination in genetics, the crossing-over of chromosomes during meiosis and recombination of the fragments

reliability (of a screening test) the ability of the test to give consistent results when repeated on the same individual

REMO rapid epidemiological mapping of onchocerciasis

RFT 'released from treatment', after completion of course of multidrug therapy for leprosy; regarded as 'cured'

RGC retinal ganglion cell

RNA ribonucleic acid; rRNA = ribosomal RNA; mRNA = messenger RNA

ROC receiver operating characteristic: the ROC curve in the screening context is a plot of sensitivity against 1-specificity of a diagnostic test, for various choices of cut-off points (see Section 8.6.1)

ROL retinol

ROP retinopathy of prematurity

Rose Bengal a dye with an affinity for dead and devitalized epithelial cells, also for mucus, used for assessing the dry eye

RP retinitis pigmentosa

RPE retinal pigment epithelium

RR relative risk, an effect measure; the ratio of two risks, or **risk ratio**, e.g. the risk among the exposed divided by the risk among those not exposed (or less exposed) (see Chapter 2)

SAFE a strategy adopted by WHO for the control of trachoma: surgery, antibiotics, face washing, environmental change

sampling distribution theoretical frequency (probability) distribution of a parameter (e.g. a proportion) that may be obtained from all possible distinct samples of a given size drawn from a defined population (see Chapter 3)

sampling error component of error in estimating a population parameter such as a proportion, arising from random sampling variation, i.e. because of chance differences between the members of the sample and those not included in the sample (see Chapter 3)

sampling frame a complete list of all and only all eligible sampling units (see Chapter 3)

SCBUs special care baby units

Schirmer test a test of tear secretion in which the extent of wetting in mm of a special filter paper 5 mm wide × 32 mm after five minutes is measured

SCORM Cohort Study of Risk Factors in Myopia (Singapore)

SE spherical equivalent of lens to correct astigmatism; expressed as the spherical power plus half of the cylindrical power

SEE Salisbury Eye Evaluation Project (USA)

sensitivity (of a screening test): among the people with a disease, the proportion correctly identified by the test (see Section 8.6.1)

serovars subdivision of *Chlamydia trachomatis* into varieties based on their serology

SES socio-economic status

SICS small incision cataract surgery

SiMES Singapore Malay Eye Study

s.l. sensu lato (in the broad sense), in defining species, e.g. of *Simulium damnosum*

SNP single nucleotide polymorphism; DNA sequence variation resulting from a change in a single nucleotide

specificity (of a screening test): the proportion of persons who are disease-free which the test correctly identifies as disease-free (see Section 8.6.1)

SROL serum retinol

SRR sight restoration rate

SRS simple random sampling (see Section 3.4.1)

s.s. sensu stricto (in the strict sense), in species definition

SSDE Sjögren syndrome dry eye

STD sexually transmitted disease

stratification in cross-sectional studies, the arrangement of the total population into subgroups (strata) of people who share geographical, ethnic or other similarities. Sampling is then applied separately to each stratum (see Section 3.4.5)

SU sampling unit, a defined unit for selection in sampling: may be an individual or some grouping (cluster) of individuals (see Chapter 3)

SUN standardization of uveitis nomenclature

systematic error non-random error in the design, conduct or analysis of a study, producing a spurious (biased) result

TAP Treatment of Age-Related Macular Degeneration with Photodynamic Therapy Study

T-cells (T-lymphocytes) thymus-derived cells involved in cell-mediated immunity

TF follicular trachoma

TFT trifluorothymidine, or trifluridine, an antiviral drug

TI intense inflammatory trachoma

TNF tumour necrosis factor

trichiasis one or more eyelashes rubbing on the globe of the eye, or evidence of epilation

TS scarring of the conjunctiva of the upper lid in trachoma

TT trachomatous trichiasis

type 1 diabetes insulin-dependent diabetes

type I error wrong conclusion drawn from the result of a statistical significance test — rejecting the null hypothesis when it is in fact true. The probability of this type of error is denoted by *alpha*, and is equal to the critical p-value used for the conclusion

type I reaction in leprosy (also known as reversal reaction) thought to result from delayed hypersensitivity (cell-mediated immunity)

type 2 diabetes gradual onset, usually non-insulin-dependent diabetes (occasionally requires insulin if inadequately controlled by diet, exercise and oral medication)

type II error wrong conclusion drawn from the result of a statistical significance test — failing to reject the null hypothesis when it is false. The probability of this type of error is denoted by *beta*, and is equal to 1-power

type II reaction in leprosy (also known as erythema nodosum leprosum or ENL reaction) thought to be an immune complex disease

U5MR under-five mortality rate

UBM ultrasound biomicroscopy

UKPDS United Kingdom Prospective Diabetes Study

UL tolerable upper intake level, the routine daily intake of a nutrient that can be biologically tolerated within a population

UNDP United Nations Development Programme

UNICEF United Nations Children's Fund, known until 1963 as the United Nations International Children's Emergency Fund

UVA ultraviolet within the wavelengths 315–400 nm

UVB ultraviolet within the wavelengths 280–315 nm

UVR ultraviolet radiation

VA visual acuity

VAD vitamin A deficiency

VADD vitamin A deficiency disorders

validity (of a screening test): the ability to differentiate correctly between those who do and those who do not have the disease (see Section 8.6.1)

variance a measure of variation in numeric data; a measure of the spread of a statistical distribution: the average of the squares of the differences between the observations and the mean

VCDR vertical cup–disc ratio

VECAT Vitamin E, Cataract and Age-Related Maculopathy Study

VEGF vascular endothelial growth factor

VEP visually evoked potential

VF-14 an index of visual function based on 14 questions relating to activities of daily life

VI visual impairment

VIP the Melbourne Visual Impairment Project

VISION 2020 The Right to Sight a global initiative to eliminate avoidable blindness by 2020; a partnership between WHO and the International Agency for the Prevention of Blindness (IAPB)

VKC vernal keratoconjunctivitis

VLBW very low birth weight, less than 1,500 g

VRT vision restoration time, after the retina has been exposed to a bright light source

VZV *Varicella zoster* virus, also called HZV

WACS Women's Anti-Oxidant Cardiovascular Study

WARMGS Wisconsin Age-Related Maculopathy Grading System

WESDR Wisconsin Epidemiologic Study of Diabetic Retinopathy

WHA World Health Assembly

WHO World Health Organization

WHO/PBL The Prevention of Blindness Programme of WHO, now PBD

WHS Women's Health Study, USA

X1A conjunctival xerosis (see Table 14b.2)

X1B Bitot's spots (see Table 14b.2)

X2 xerosis of the cornea (see Table 14b.2)

X3A corneal ulceration in vitamin A deficiency, affecting less than one-third of the cornea (see Table 14b.2)

X3B keratomalacia; ulceration and generalized necrosis involving one-third or more of the cornea (see Table 14b.2)

XF xerophthalmic fundus, seen in some cases of vitamin A deficiency (see Table 14b.2)

X-linked transmission a gene carried on sex chromosome X

XN night blindness (see Table 14b.2)

XS corneal scarring in xerophathlmia (vitamin A deficiency) (see Table 14b.2)

yield (of a screening test): the number of persons to be screened to detect one case (see Section 8.6.1)

Index

A

Aboriginal peoples
    climatic droplet keratopathy 441
    pterygium 448
    see also Australasia
Acanthamoeba spp. 409
    classification 410
acanthamoeba keratitis 409–18
    blindness prevalence 410
    diagnosis 413–14
    geographical distribution 410–12
    incidence 410–12
    non-contact lens wearers 410–11, 413
    research priorities 415–16
    risk factors 412–13
        contact lens wear 409, 411, 412
        contaminated water and lens use 412–13
        lens solutions and hygiene practice 413
    treatment
        medical 414–15
        surgical 415
accommodation
    age-related loss *see* presbyopia
    see also refractive errors
aciclovir
    herpes zoster ophthalmicus 526
    viral infectious keratoconjunctivitis 405, 406
acquired immune deficiency syndrome *see* HIV/AIDS
Action in Diabetes and Vascular Disease: Preterax
    and Diamicron Modified Release Controlled
    Evaluation (ADVANCE) trial 556
Action to Control Cardiovascular Risk in Diabetes
    (ACCORD) 556
Activities of Daily Vision Scale (ADVS) 184, 230,
    231
acute haemorrhagic conjunctivitis 404

acute retinal necrosis syndrome (ARN) 531–2
acute retroviral syndrome 521
acyclovir *see* aciclovir
adalimumab 437
adenine arabinoside 405
adenoviral keratoconjunctivitis 403, 404–5
adnexa, opportunistic infections in HIV/AIDS 525–7
adolescents, refractive errors 202
adoption studies 121
Advanced Glaucoma Intervention Study (AGIS)
    259
advocacy 603
Afghanistan, trachoma 465
Africa
    blindness prevalence 12
    climatic droplet keratopathy 441
    glaucoma prevalence 246
        PACG 248
        POAG 247, 249
    microbial keratitis 395
    onchocerciasis 493–4
    Sub-Saharan *see* Sub-Saharan Africa
    see also individual countries
African Programme for Onchocerciasis Control
    (APOC) 488, 499
African-Caribbeans
    cataract 185
    glaucoma 160
        incidence 252
        prevalence 246, 249
    refractive errors 199, 200
    visual impairment 16
    see also Barbados; St Lucia
age distribution
    childhood cataract 332
    climatic droplet keratopathy 442–3

diabetic retinopathy   559–60
dry eye disease   377
ocular disease in leprosy   424–5
POAG   252
presbyopia   216
pterygium   449
refractive errors   206–7
trachoma   468
age-related cataracts see cataracts
Age-Related Eye Disease Study (AREDS)   100, 135,
   187
   AMD   572
   diabetic retinopathy   560
age-related macular degeneration   232, 233,
   571–84
   aetiology and risk factors   576
      alcohol   579–80
      cardiovascular disease   576–7
      cataracts/cataract surgery   580
      diet   578
      genetic factors   579
      inflammation   577
      light   578–9
      oestrogens   580
      smoking   577
   classification   572
   control and treatment strategies   580–1
   definition and diagnosis   571–2
   future research priorities   581
   genetic epidemiology   126–7
   geographical distribution   576
   incidence   73, 574–5
      changes with time   575–6
   prevalence   572–4
      changes with time   575–6
alcohol
   and AMD   579–80
   and diabetic retinopathy risk   560–1
   and dry eye disease   380–1
   see also foetal alcohol syndrome
alemtuzumab   437
allele sharing methods   122–3
allelic variation   118
allergy and dry eye disease   383
allogenic bone marrow transplantation, and dry eye
   disease   383
amblyopia   198, 270, 331
   prevention   165
   screening   163
AMD see age-related macular degeneration
America see North America region; USA
American Academy of Ophthalmology   156

ametropias see refractive errors
amphotericin   400
anaemia of prematurity   358
analysis of variance   120
ANCHOR/Age-Related Macular Degeneration trial
   139
Andhra Pradesh Eye Study   15, 16
   refractive error prevalence   203
angiotensin-converting enzyme (ACE) inhibitors   556
Angola   493, 503
animism   327
aniridia   344–5
anterior chamber
   depth   255–6
   in onchocerciasis   492
anterior segment
   dysgenesis   344
   HIV-related opportunistic infections   525–7
   ocular coherence tomography (AS-OCT)   178,
      244
antiandrogens and dry eye disease   382
antibiotics in trachoma   475–7
antibody secreting cells   462
antidepressants and dry eye disease   382
antihistamines
   and dry eye disease   382
   vernal keratoconjunctivitis   432
antihypertensives and dry eye disease   382
antioxidants
   in AMD   580–1
   and cataract risk   187–8
antiretroviral therapy   522–4
   complications   523–4
   opportunistic infection   523
   see also individual drugs
aphakic glaucoma   345
apolipoprotein E   126, 579
Appropriate Blood Pressure Control in Diabetes
   (ABCD) Trial   557
aqueous tear deficient dry eye   370–1
Argentina
   blindness
      causes   51
      prevalence   35
   cataract   183
ARMS2 and AMD   127
arthritis and dry eye disease   383
Aruba   449
Asia Pacific region
   blindness
      causes   40, 43
      prevalence   23, 31

dry eye disease 375–6
    see also individual countries
Asians
    glaucoma prevalence 246
    see also Asia Pacific region; *and individual countries*
Aspergillus spp. 395
astigmatism 197, 198
    age, gender and ethnic distribution 206
    prevalence
        older adults 202–5
        school age children/adolescents 201, 202
Atherosclerosis Risk in Communities Study 574
atovaquone, ocular toxicity 536
attributable risk 66, 69
audit 595
Australia *see* Australia; New Zealand
Australia
    acanthamoeba keratitis 410–11
    AMD 41, 574, 576
    blindness
        causes 41, 45
        prevalence 26, 34
    climatic droplet keratopathy 441, 443
    diabetic retinopathy 552
    dry eye disease 375
    glaucoma 246, 251–2
    poor vision 229
    pterygium 447–8
    refractive errors 198, 201–4, 206, 212–13
    trachoma 465
avoidable blindness 20–1
    in children 285
    see also Vision 2020 initiative
Axenfeld–Rieger anomaly 344
axial anterior chamber depth test 260
azathioprine 432
azithromycin 475

B
B-cells 430
bacterial keratitis 394
badness-of-fit 120
Baltimore Eye Survey 87
    AMD 574
    cataract 181
    glaucoma 254, 259
Bangladesh
    blindness
        causes 44, 50, 88, 283
        in children 183, 276, 281, 283
        prevalence 34
    cataract outcome 596

leprosy 421–2
microbial keratitis 395
refractive error prevalence 203
vitamin A deficiency 302
Barbados
    AMD 574
    blindness
        causes 16, 19, 20, 45
        prevalence 34
    cataract 179–81, 188
    diabetic retinopathy 552
    glaucoma 40, 41, 245, 249, 251–2
    pterygium 448, 450
    refractive errors 204–6, 208
Barbados Eye Study 84, 90
    AMD 574
    cataract
        blindness and low vision 181
        prevalence 179, 180
    POAG 246, 251
    refractive errors 204, 208
Beaver Dam Eye Study 16, 28, 87–8, 113–14
    AMD 574, 575, 577, 579, 580
    cataract 182
        blindness and low vision 181
        prevalence 179, 180
    diabetic retinopathy 560
    dry eye disease 374, 376, 379
    refractive errors
        incidence/progression 205–6
        prevalence 204
Beijing Eye Study 179
    blindness (cataract-related) 181
    cataract prevalence 179, 180
    refractive error prevalence 203
Benin
    blindness 88
        causes 48
        prevalence 38
    onchocerciasis 493, 498
benzalkonium chloride and dry eye disease 381
beta blockers and dry eye disease 381
β-carotene 293, 296
bevacizumab 360
Bhutan 395, 398
bias 80–2, 114
    lead-time 155–6
    length 156
    risk of 170–1
    screening programmes 155–6
    sources of 89–90
        biased selection 89

faulty coverage 89
   non-response 89–90
Bietti's nodular dystrophy *see* climatic droplet
   keratopathy
bilamellar tarsal–rotation BLTR procedure (BTRP)
   473
biometry 209–10
Bitot's spots 299
blindness
   acanthamoeba keratitis 410
   avoidable *see* avoidable blindness
   cataract
      age-related 182, 184
         prevalence 4, 19, 181
   causes 16–18
      multiple/different 16–17
      nomenclature 16
      numbers for 17–18
      surveys 40–52
      time trends 17
   in children
      causes 281–2, 283
         avoidable 285
         classification 282
         data sources 281–2
         regional variation 282
         time trends 282, 284
      data sources 274–5
      incidence 278–80
      magnitude and causes 269–89
      and mortality rate 273, 277, 278, 280–1
      prevalence 13–14, 273–7
   climatic droplet keratopathy 441
   cortical 535
   data sources 5–6
      blindness registration statistics 5–6
      preliminary data 5
   definition 7–8
   distribution patterns 18–21
      demography 18–19
      geography 19–20
      socio-economic status 20
   glaucoma 4, 19, 248, 249
   global causes 5
   global prevalence 3–60
      by age 18
      by health region 12–13
      surveys 11, 23–39
      time trends 11–12, 14–15
   incidence 15–16
   leprosy 425
   literacy 20

ophthalmia neonatorum 318–19
   WHO categorization 8, 9
   see also data for individual countries and regions
blindness registration 5–6
blocking 136
blood pressure, and diabetic retinopathy risk 556–7
Blue Mountains Eye Study 16, 26, 69, 87–8, 111, 113
   AMD 574, 575, 580
   cataract
      blindness and low vision 181, 233
      prevalence 179, 180
   dry eye disease 375, 376
   glaucoma 254
   pterygium 448
   refractive errors, prevalence 204
body mass index, and myopia 213
Bolivia 217
Botswana
   blindness
      causes 52
      prevalence 38
Brazil
   blindness
      causes 46, 51, 283
      in children 283
      prevalence 36
   leprosy 421–2, 426
   onchocerciasis 495, 501
   pterygium 448
   refractive errors 198, 216–17
   retinitis in HIV/AIDS 532
   ROP 356
   trachoma 465
British Birth Cohort Study 228, 229, 232
British Childhood Visual Impairment Study 278,
   282
Bulgaria
   blindness
      causes 45
      prevalence 35
Burkina Faso
   onchocerciasis 493
   trachoma 465
Burundi, onchocerciasis 491, 493

C
Calabar swellings 503
Cambodia
   blindness
      causes 44
      prevalence 34
   trachoma 465

Cameroon
 blindness
  causes 48, 52
  prevalence 38
 cataract 183
 climatic droplet keratopathy 441
 onchocerciasis 490–3, 503
 trachoma 465
Canada
 acanthamoeba keratitis 411
 blindness
  in children 276, 284
  registration of hereditary disease 6
 dry eye disease 374–5
 glaucoma 250
 low vision 232–3
 see also Labrador
Canada Dry Eye Epidemiology Study (CANDEES)
 374–5
Candida spp. 395
candidate gene association studies 122, 123
Cape Verde Islands
 blindness
  causes 48
  prevalence 39
cardiovascular disease
 and AMD 576–7
 and dry eye disease 383
Caribbean region
 blindness
  causes 41, 45, 51
  in children 283
  prevalence 26, 34–5
 see also African-Caribbeans; *and individual*
  countries
carotenoids 293, 578
 see also vitamin A
case definition 65–6, 97–8
case-control studies 73–4, 95–107
 analysis of 103–4
 case definition 97–8
 definition 95–6
 exposure assessment 102–3
 incident/prevalent cases 98–9
 nested 74, 103
 reporting results 104
 sample size 96–7
 selection of controls 99–102
  matching 101–2
  population controls 100–1
 sources of cases 98
 study hypothesis 96–7
cataract 177–96

 and AMD risk 580
 blindness 182, 184
  prevalence 4, 19, 181
 children 331–40
  aetiology 333–5
   congenital rubella syndrome 334–5
   iatrogenic 335
   idiopathic 335
   metabolic 334
   secondary 335
   syndromic 334
   traumatic 335
  classification 331–2
  clinical trials 337
  future research priorities 337–8
  hereditary 333
  intraocular lenses 337
  molecular genetics 333–4
  prevalence and incidence 332–3
   by gender and age 332
   by geographical distribution 333
   changes with time 333
  prevention 335–6
  surgical management 336–7
 in diabetes mellitus 185, 563
 genetic epidemiology 128
 genetics 189
 impact on quality of life 184
 incidence and prevalence 178–84
  cortical 180
  nuclear 179
  posterior subcapsular 180
 lens opacity types 179, 182
 in leprosy 424
 and low vision 181, 233
 mechanisms 177–8
 medications 188–9
  prevention of cataract formation 188–9
  statins 113
  steroids 188
  topical intra-ocular pressure lowering drugs
   188
 and mortality 189–90
 phenotypes 178
 posterior subcapsular 177, 180
  and myopia 213
 risk factors 184–8
  childbearing 73
  diabetes 185
  oxidative stress/antioxidants 187–8
  radiation exposure 185–7
  smoking 184–5
 subtypes 177–8

surgery
    in children   336–7
    quality of   595–6
    small incision   591
CCR5 antagonists   522
cefotaxime   320
cellular differentiation (CD) markers   461
    CD4   461, 519, 521–2
    CD8   461
cellular immune response   463
Central African Republic
    blindness
        causes   42, 47
        prevalence   37
    onchocerciasis   493, 503
Central Asia region
    blindness
        causes   40, 43, 50
        prevalence   23, 31
Chad
    blindness
        causes   48
        prevalence   38
    climatic droplet keratopathy   441
    onchocerciasis   493
    trachoma   465
χ^2-test   141
children
    astigmatism   201, 202
    cataract   331–40
        aetiology   333–5
            congenital rubella syndrome   334–5
            iatrogenic   335
            idiopathic   335
            metabolic   334
            secondary   335
            syndromic   334
            traumatic   335
        classification   331–2
        clinical trials   337
        future research priorities   337–8
        hereditary   333
        intraocular lenses   337
        molecular genetics   333–4
        prevalence and incidence   332–3
            by gender and age   332
            by geographical distribution   333
            changes with time   333
        prevention   335–6
        surgical management   336–7
    corneal disease   323–30

congenital abnormalities   323–4
corneal dystrophies   324–5
future research needs   329
management   328–9
measles infection   325–7
traditional eye medicines   327–8
glaucoma   341–51
    classification   343
    clinical features   341–2
    primary   342–4
    prognosis   348
    research implications   348–9
    secondary   344–5
    treatment   345–8
        angle surgery   346–7
        drainage implants   348
        trabeculectomy with/without antimetabolites   348
        trabeculotomy–trabeculectomy   347
hyperopia   206
mortality
    blindness   273, 277, 278, 280–1
    measles infection   325–6
    vitamin A deficiency   300–1
myopia
    age, gender and ethnic distribution   206
    incidence/progression   205
    ocular factors   213
    prevalence   199–202
screening programmes   162–4
    amblyopia   163
    pre-school vision tests   163
    refractive error   163–4
vision loss
    causes   281–2, 283
        avoidable   285
        classification   282
        data sources   281–2
        regional variation   282
        time trends   284
    data sources   274–5
    definition and categories   270–3
    epidemiology   270
    functional low vision   284–5
    incidence   278–80
    magnitude   277–8, 280
    and mortality rate   273, 277, 278, 280–1
    prevalence   13–14, 273–7
    self-report   272–3
visual development   270–2

visual function assessment 270–2
  colour vision and contrast sensitivity 272
  distance visual acuity 271–2
  near visual acuity 272
  visual fields 272
vitamin A deficiency *see* vitamin A deficiency in children
Children's Functional Vision Questionnaire (CVFQ) 273
Chile
  blindness
    causes 51
    in children 277, 284
    prevalence 35
China
  blindness
    causes 40, 43, 50
    in children 276–9
    prevalence 23, 31–2
  cataract 181, 185
  childhood cataract 332
  diabetic retinopathy 552
  external eye conditions 318, 423–4, 436, 448
  glaucoma
    incidence 252
    prevalence 246, 249
      PACG 248
      POAG 247
  pterygium 448
  refractive errors and low vision 198, 202, 203, 206–9, 212, 237, 284
  trachoma 464
  see also East Asia region
Chlamydia trachomatis 317–19, 455, 456–8
  detection of 457–8
  developmental cycle 456–7
    elementary body 456
    inclusion body 456
    reticulate body 456
  major outer membrane protein 456–7, 462
  see also trachoma
chloramphenicol ointment 398
cholesterol and dry eye disease 383
choroidal neovascularisation 572
choroidopathy, infectious 533–4
ciclosporin A 432, 437
cidofovir 528, 529
  ocular toxicity 535–6
climatic droplet keratopathy 439–45
  classification 439–40
  control and management 444
  future research priorities 444–5

genetic predisposition 442
geographical distribution 441
grading 440
incidence 442
nomenclature 439
pathology 440–1
prevalence 441
  of blindness 441
risk factors 442–4
  age and gender 442–3
  environmental 442
  ultraviolet radiation 443–4
time trends 442
clinical governance 595
clinical trials 131–45
  data analysis 141–2
    by intention to treat 141
    data and safety monitoring 141–2
    multiple analyses over time 142
    statistical methods 141
    stopping early 142
  diabetic retinopathy 562
  follow-up 139
  future directions 142–3
  glaucoma 258–9
  history 131
  masking 140–1
  objectives 132
  outcome measures 137–9
    primary 137–8
    secondary 138–9
  phase 1 131–2
  phase 2 132
  phase 3 132
  reporting results 142
  sample size 139–40
  study population 134–5
    determination/confirmation of eligibility 135
    eligibility criteria 134–5
    exclusion criteria 135
  treatment assignment 135–7
    by person vs. by eye 135–6
    randomized 136
    timing of 137
  treatments/interventions 132–4
    comparison groups 132–3
    standardization of treatment 133–4
  see also different types of trial
clofazamine, ocular toxicity 536
Clostridium tetani 300
clotrimazole 398, 400
cluster sampling 82, 84–5

eye surveys   86–8
  multi-stage   85
  one-stage   84
  two-stage   84–5
CMV *see* cytomegalovirus retinitis
Cochrane Collaboration   163, 170–1, 591
cohort studies   72–3, 109–16
  alternatives to   115
  description   109–11
  design   111–13
    follow-up   112
    measurement of exposure   111–12
    outcome definition   113
    study population   111
  exposure and disease   113–14
  historical   115
  nested   115
  research priorities   115–16
  strengths   114
  weaknesses   114–15
Cohort Study of Risk Factors of Myopia (SCORM)
  205, 210, 212–13
Collaborative Initial Glaucoma Treatment Study
  (CIGTS)   258
Colombia   495, 501
colour vision assessment   272
community intervention trials   72
community microfilarial load (CMFL)   496
compact segment method   85
comparative needs assessment   588, 589
complement factor H gene   579
complex segregation analysis   120
conditional logistic regression   104
confidence intervals/limits   6, 14, 71, 72, 80
confounders   67, 71, 101, 113
congenital rubella syndrome   333, 334–5
Congo (Republic of Congo, formerly Congo-
  Brazzaville)
  blindness   29, 30, 88
    causes   47
    prevalence   37
conjunctiva
  impression cytology   304
  in onchocerciasis   491
  scarring   471–3
  squamous neoplasia   534–5
  xerosis   299, 303
conjunctival vasculopathy, HIV-related   525
connexins   333
Consolidated Standards of Reporting Trials
  (CONSORT)   142, 143
contact lenses
  and acanthamoeba keratitis   409, 411, 412–13

and dry eye disease   379–80
  and microbial keratitis   397
contraception, as risk factor for diabetic retinopathy
  557–8
contrast sensitivity   230–2
  assessment of   272
Copenhagen City Eye Study   27, 73, 233
corneal disease
  children   323–30
    congenital abnormalities   323–4
    corneal dystrophies   324–5
    future research needs   329
    management   328–9
    measles infection   325–7
    traditional eye medicines   327–8
  onchocerciasis   491–2
  scarring   299–300
    and blindness   19
    in trachoma   459
  ulceration   299
    and measles infection   326
  xerosis   299
corneal elastosis *see* climatic droplet keratopathy
corneal thickness   160–1
Correction of Myopia Evaluation Trial (COMET)
  205, 211
cortical blindness   535
cost recovery   594–5
  service subsidization   595
  tiered payments   594–5
Côte d'Ivoire   493–4
coverage   154
Cox proportional hazards regression   141
cranial nerve palsy   535
craw-craw   487, 492
cross-sectional studies   72, 79–93
  bias and precision   80–2
  probability sampling   82
  sampling schemes   82–9
    cluster sampling   82, 84–5
    design effect   85–6
    simple random sampling   82, 83–4
    stratification   88–9
CRYO-ROP study   359
cryptococcal choroidopathy   534
Cryptococcus neoformans   534
crystallins   333
Cuba
  blindness   26
    causes   51
    prevalence   34
cumulative incidence   7, 67, 68, 113
cyclophosphamide   437

cycloplegia   199
cystoid macular oedema   512
cytomegalovirus retinitis   521
   clinical features   528
   epidemiology and regional variation   527–8
   HIV-related   527–31
   prognosis   531
   and retinal detachment   530–1
   treatment   528–30
      resource-poor settings   537–8
   virology   527
cytotoxic T-cells   461, 463

D
Dahlak Islands   441
data analysis   141–2
   by intention to treat   141
   data and safety monitoring   141–2
   multiple analyses over time   142
   statistical methods   141
   stopping early   142
data gathering   590–1
   demographic data   590
   effectiveness of interventions   591
   population data   590
Democratic Republic of Congo (DRC, formerly Zaire)
   leprosy   421
   onchocerciasis   421, 493, 503
demographic data   18–19, 590
Denmark   73
   blindness
      causes   45
      in children   276
      prevalence   35
   childhood cataract   332
   diabetic retinopathy   552
desiccation   450
design effect   85–6
Diabetes Control and Complications Trial (DCCT)
   75, 555
diabetes mellitus   134
   associated ocular conditions   563
      cataracts   185, 563
      dry eye disease   382–3
      glaucoma   563
   duration of   554–5
   glycaemic control   555–6
   maturity-onset of youth (MODY)   554, 559–60
   type 1   547
      prevalence   552
   type 2   547
      prevalence   552

diabetic retinopathy   547–69
   clinical trials   562
      see also individual trials
   future research priorities   164–5
   genetic factors   561–2
   geographical distribution   551–2
      changes with time   553–4
   incidence   552–3
   and low vision   233
   macular oedema   549, 551
   management   562–3
   non-proliferative   548
   pre-proliferative   548
   prevalence   549–52
      changes with time   553–4
      population-based studies   549–51, 552
      visual impairment   551
   proliferative   548–9
   research priorities   563–4
   risk factors   554–61
      age   559–60
      alcohol   560–1
      blood pressure   556–7
      contraception and pregnancy   557–8
      duration of diabetes   554–5
      ethnicity   558–9
      glycaemic control   555–6
      insulin   558
      kidney disease   561
      lack of exercise   561
      nutrition   560
      obesity   561
      serum lipids   558
      smoking   560
      socio-economic status   561
   screening   156–9
      frequency of   157–8
      population at risk   156
      programme structure   157
      screening test   156–7
   severity levels   550
Diabetic Retinopathy Candesartan Trials (DIRECT)
   study   557
Diabetic Retinopathy Study   131, 562
   High Risk Characteristics (DRS-HRC)   553
Diabetic Retinopathy Vitrectomy Study (DRVS)   562
didanosine, ocular toxicity   536
3,4-didehydroretinol   303
diet
   and AMD   578
   and diabetic retinopathy risk   560
   and dry eye disease   381

diethylcarbamazine 487, 497
different (absolute) measure 69
differential measurement error 103
dioptres 198
dioptric spherical equivalents 198–9
Djibouti 441
DNA 117
  mitochondrial 410
Down's syndrome
  and cataracts 334
  keratoconus 324
doxycycline 504
Doyne honeycomb retinal dystrophy 126
drainage implants in glaucoma 348
dry eye disease 369–90
  age and gender differences 377
  classification 369–71
    aqueous tear deficient dry eye 370–1
    evaporative dry eye 371
  clinical signs 377
  definition 369
  diagnosis 373–4
  future research needs 385
  health-related costs 384
  incidence and natural history 378–9
  pathophysiology 371–3
  prevalence 374–7
    see also individual countries and regions
  quality of life 384
  race and ethnic distribution 377–8
  risk factors 379–83
    environmental 379
    medications and interventions 381–2
    ocular 379–80
    social and dietary 380–1
    systemic diseases 382–3
  therapy 384–5

E
Early Manifest Glaucoma Trial 188, 259
Early Treatment Diabetic Retinopathy Study (ETDRS) 134, 158, 271, 557, 558
Early Treatment of ROP trial (ETROP) 359
East Asia region
  blindness
    causes 40, 44
    prevalence 23, 32
  glaucoma prevalence 246, 250–1
  see also China
Eastern Mediterranean, blindness, prevalence 12
ecological studies 74
Ecuador 501

effect modification 104
Egypt, trachoma 465, 471
elderly persons, screening programmes 164
electroretinogram 138
ELISA 334
emedastine 432
emmetropia 198
endoplasmic reticulum-bound photoreceptor cell-specific factor (ELOVL4) 126
enfuvirtide 522
enteroviral keratoconjunctivitis 403, 404
entropion 471–3
enzyme-linked immunosorbent assay see ELISA
epidermal growth factor 126
epigenetics 125
epilepsy, and onchocerciasis 493
Equatorial Guinea
  blindness
    causes 47
    prevalence 37
  onchocerciasis 493
Eritrea, trachoma 465
erythromycin 319, 320
Eskimo (Inuit)
  climatic droplet keratopathy 438, 439
  glaucoma 250
Established Populations for Epidemiologic Studies of the Elderly (EPESE) 228, 229
Estimated Average Requirement 295
ethambutol, ocular toxicity 536
Ethiopia
  blindness 13, 29
    causes 42, 47, 283
    in children 276, 283
    prevalence 37
  leprosy 421
  onchocerciasis 493–4
  trachoma 465, 469, 471, 474–6
ethnic distribution
  AMD 573
  blindness 19
  diabetic retinopathy 558–9
  dry eye disease 377–8
  inherited disorders 325
  refractive errors 206–7
    see also individual countries/regions
EUREYE Study 579
EURODIAB Controlled Trial of Lisinopril in Insulin-Dependent Diabetes Mellitus (EUCLID) Study 556
Europe
  blindness, prevalence 12, 27

Central 27
    blindness
        causes 41, 45
        prevalence 35
    dry eye disease 376–7
    East 27
    glaucoma
        incidence 251–2
        prevalence
            PACG 248
            POAG 244–7
    West 27
        blindness
            causes 41, 45–6
            prevalence 35
European Glaucoma Prevention Study (EGPS) 160
evaporative dry eye 371
exposure
    assessment 102–3, 111–12
    categorization 112
    and disease 113–14
eye care, quality of 595
Eye Disease Case-Control study 99
eye movement disorders, supranuclear 535
eye worm see Loa loa

F
false negatives 151
false positives 151
famciclovir 406
familial aggregation studies 75, 119
familial clustering 119
faulty coverage bias 89
Faye, Eleanor 227
field trials 72
Fiji
    childhood blindness 276
    trachoma 466
Finland
    blindness
        causes 46
        in children 276
        prevalence 35
        registration 6
    uveitis 511
Fisher, Ronald 118
fisherman's keratitis see climatic droplet keratopathy
flies, in transmission of trachoma 470–1
flubendazole 504
fluorescein angiogram 572
fluorescein staining 375, 377
fluorometholone 432

foetal alcohol syndrome 323
fomivirsen 529
Food and Drug Administration (FDA) 131, 142
forest plot 171–2
form deprivation myopia 211
forward planning 590
foscarnet 406, 528, 529
Framingham Eye Study 15
    diabetic retinopathy 559
    POAG 251
France
    blindness prevalence 35
    childhood cataract 332
    retinitis in HIV/AIDS 532
    uranium workers 111
French Household Survey 229
functional low vision 284–5
fungal keratitis 394–5
Fusarium spp. 395, 397
fusion inhibitors 522

G
Gabon 493, 504
galactosaemia, and cataracts 334
Gambia
    blindness
        causes 48
        prevalence 18, 29, 38, 79, 88
    prevalence surveys 14
    trachoma 458, 462, 465, 470–6
ganciclovir 406, 528, 529
    implants 530
gap analysis 588, 589
gender distribution
    childhood cataract 332
    climatic droplet keratopathy 442–3
    dry eye disease 377
    presbyopia 216
    pterygium 449
    refractive errors 206–7
    trachoma 472
    vernal keratoconjunctivitis 431
gene–environment interaction 127
gene–gene interaction 127
General Practice Research Database (GPRD) 113
generalized estimating equations 104
genetic epidemiology 117–29
    definition 117
    eye diseases 126–8
        AMD 126–7
        cataract 128
        climatic droplet keratopathy 442

glaucoma   127
    refractive error   128
familial aggregation   119
future developments   125, 128
genetic model of inheritance   119–21
history   117–18
shared genes vs. shared environment   119
genetic factors
    AMD   579
    cataract   189
    diabetic retinopathy   561–2
    glaucoma   257–8
    myopia   210–11
    pterygium   449
    vernal keratoconjunctivitis   432
    see also inheritance
genetic heterogeneity   118
genetic mutations   122–5
    allele sharing methods   122–3
    candidate gene association studies   122, 123
    genome-wide association studies   122, 123–5
    linkage analysis   122
genetic studies   75
    glaucoma   257–8
    refractive errors   210
        familial factors   210–11
        molecular genetics   210
genome-wide association studies   122, 123–5
    case selection   124
    control selection   124–5
    functional analysis   125
    quality control   125
    sample size   125
    statistical analysis   125
geographical information systems   105
geography   19–20
    local variations   19–20
    regional variations   20
Germany   27, 100–1, 318
Ghana
    blindness
        causes   48
        in children   276
        prevalence   38
    fungal keratitis   395
    onchocerciasis   493, 498
    prevalence surveys   14, 29
    trachoma   465
    vitamin A deficiency   301, 302
giant papillae   430
glaucoma   241–66
    aphakic   345

blindness   4, 19, 248, 249
in children   341–51
    classification   343
    clinical features   341–2
    primary   341, 342–4
    prognosis   348
    research implications   348–9
    secondary   344–5
    treatment   345–8
        angle surgery   346–7
        drainage implants   348
        trabeculectomy with/without antimetabolites
            348
        trabeculotomy–trabeculectomy   347
classification   243–5
clinical trials   258–9
in diabetes mellitus   563
diagnosis   242–3
functional damage   242
genetic epidemiology   127
genetics   257–8
geographical distribution   248–51
incidence   251–3
infantile   245
and low vision   233
and myopia   213
narrow angle   244
prevalence   17, 245–8
primary angle-closure see primary angle-closure
    glaucoma
primary angle-closure suspect   244
primary open-angle see primary open-angle
    glaucoma
risk factors   253–7
screening programmes   259–61
secondary   245
structural damage   241–2
uveitic   345
Glaucoma Laser Trial   136
glaucomatous optic neuropathy   241–2
Global Burden of Diseases, Injuries and Risk Factors
    Study Group (GBD)   13
Global Initiative for the Elimination of Avoidable
    Blindness   11, 601
glutathione peroxidase   578
glycaemic control in diabetes   555–6
goal-oriented project planning   592
Gomori's methenamine silver   399
gonioscopy   243–4, 260–1
good practice   591
goodness-of-fit   120
gp120   519

Greece 98, 336
Greenland 6, 246, 250, 441
Guatemala
    blindness
        causes 51
        prevalence 27, 35
    cataract 183
    onchocerciasis 495, 501
    vitamin A fortification 309
Guinea
    onchocerciasis 493, 498, 500
    trachoma 465
Guinea-Bissau
    onchocerciasis 493–4
    trachoma 465

H
HAART therapy 522–4, 527–8, 531
Handan Eye Study, refractive error prevalence 203
haplotype 122, 463
Hardy–Weinberg equilibrium 123
Hartmanella spp. 409
health regions 12–13
Health Technology Assessment 159
healthcare need 587–8
    assessment 588
    definition 587
healthcare planning 587–95
    data gathering 590–1
    forward planning 590
    monitoring and evaluation 590, 596–8
    participatory 591
    planning cycle 588–90
    planning process 591–3
        logical framework approach 592
        project cycle management 592–3
    priorities, goals and targets 589–90
    problem identification 589
    programme quality 595–6
    strategy and approach 590
    sustainability 593–5
Herbert's pits 459
heredity 118
heritability 75, 120
Herpes Eye Disease Study Group 406
herpes simplex virus 317
    in HIV 531–2
    keratitis 326, 393
    pterygium 450
    viral keratoconjunctivitis 403, 404
herpes zoster keratitis 393
herpes zoster ophthalmicus 525–6

Herzegovina, blindness 45
heterogeneity 172
heterozygotes 119
Hispanics
    AMD 573
    blindness
        causes 47
        prevalence 36
    diabetic retinopathy 551, 552
    glaucoma
        incidence 252
        prevalence 246
        risk factors 254
    refractive errors 199, 200, 202
    see also Latinos in Los Angeles
historical cohort studies 115
HIV protease 520
HIV retinopathy 524–5
    pathogenesis 525
HIV/AIDS 517–45
    antiretroviral therapy 522–4
    CDC surveillance system 519, 520
    clinical course 521–2
    definition and classification 519
    epidemiology 517–19
    future research priorities 536–8
        monitoring of prevalence/incidence 536–7
        ocular opportunistic complications 538
        treatment of CMV retinitis in resource-poor settings 537–8
    history 517
    ocular complications 524–36
        drug toxicities 535–6
        neuro-ophthalmological lesions 535
        opportunistic infections 525–34
            anterior segment/adnexa 525–7
            posterior segment 527–34
        tumours 534–5
        vascular diseases 524–5
    pathogenesis 519–20
    prevalence 518
    transmission and prevention 520–1
    viral load 521–2
    viral subtypes 520
    WHO staging 520
Home Interview Survey 229
homozygotes 120
Hong Kong
    acanthamoeba keratitis 411, 413
    blindness
        causes 44, 283
        in children 283

prevalence   24, 32
  microbial keratitis   397
  refractive errors   202, 205, 207, 217
Horner–Trantas dots   429
HOX 1.5 gene   324
Human Genome Project   118
human herpesvirus 8 (HHV-8)   534
human immunodeficiency virus see HIV/AIDS
human leukocyte antigens   461
human papillomavirus   534
human resource development   602–3
hypermetropia   198
hyperopia   197, 198
  age, gender and ethnic distribution   206, 207, 208
  and glaucoma risk   254
  molecular genetics   310
  prevalence
    older adults   202–5
    pre-school age children   199–201
    school age children/adolescents   201, 202
hypertension and dry eye disease   383
hypocalcaemia, and cataract   334
hypothesis testing   71

I
'I SEE' principles   603–4
ICD-10   7, 9
Iceland
  AMD   574
  blindness   6
    causes   41, 46
    in children   276
    prevalence   35
  glaucoma   5, 127, 257–8
idoxuridine   405
immune recovery inflammatory syndromes (IRIS)   523
immune recovery phenomena   523
immune recovery uveitis   531
immune system   372
immunization
  measles   326–7
  MMR vaccine   105, 327, 336
  rubella   335–6
immunoglobulin E   430
immunoglobulin G   300, 334
immunoglobulin M   334
impression cytology   304
incidence   7, 15–16, 66, 67–9
  cumulative   67, 68
incidence density see incidence rate

incidence rate   7, 67, 68–9, 113
incidence rate ratio   70–1
  see also relative risk
incident cases   98–9
India
  blindness
    avoidable   21
    causes   40, 44, 50, 283
    in children   276, 277, 283
    prevalence   15, 24–5, 32–3
      surveys   13, 14
      time trends   14, 15
  cataract   183
  diabetic retinopathy   552
  glaucoma prevalence   246, 249
    PACG   248
    POAG   247, 250
  leprosy   421–4, 426
  microbial keratitis   395
  Mooren's ulcer   436, 438
  National Programme for the Control of Blindness   24
  refractive errors   202, 203, 206–8, 212
  trachoma   465
  visual impairment prevalence   15
  vitamin A deficiency   294, 301, 306
  see also South Asia region
Indian Council of Medical Research   24
Indonesia   26
  blindness
    causes   45
    in children   283
    prevalence   34
  dry eye disease   375, 376, 378
  leprosy   421–2
  pterygium   447–8, 450
  vitamin A deficiency   298, 301, 305, 309
Infant Aphakic Treatment Study (IATS)   337
infant mortality rate   354
infantile glaucoma   245
infection
  and AMD   577
  and vitamin A deficiency   300
infectious keratoconjunctivitis   526–7
infliximab   437
information bias   80
infrastructure development   603
inheritance   119–21
  adoption studies   121
  path analysis   121
  segregation analysis   120
  twin and sib-pair studies   121

variance components analysis   120–1
  see also genetic factors
innate immunity   462
institutions for the blind   6
insulin-like growth factor, and ROP   357
integrase inhibitors   522
intention to treat   141
inter-observer variation   154
interleukin-4   461
interleukin-10   461
International Classification of Retinopathy of
  Prematurity (ICROP)
International Council of Ophthalmology   9
International Dry Eye Workshop (DEWS)   369
International Society for Geographic and
  Epidemiologic Ophthalmology (ISGEO)   241
International Statistical Classification of Diseases *see*
  ICD-10
intra-observer variation   154
intraocular lenses in childhood cataract   336, 337
intraocular pressure   159, 160
  in glaucoma   241, 254–5, 341
intravitreous injection   529
iodopsins   293
ionizing radiation and cataract risk   186–7
Iran
  blindness
    causes   46, 283
    in children   276, 283
    prevalence   36
  climatic droplet keratopathy   441
  trachoma   466
Ireland
  blindness
    in children   276
    prevalence   35
  glaucoma   246, 248, 250
  prevalence survey   27, 83, 90
iris damage *see* uveitis
Israel
  childhood blindness   276, 278
  low vision services   234–5
Italy
  blindness
    causes   46
    prevalence   20, 27, 35
  glaucoma   246, 250
itraconazole   400
ivermectin   488, 496, 497–8
  community-directed treatment   499–500

J
Jamaica   246, 335
Japan
  blindness
    causes   40, 43
    prevalence   31
  cataract, radiation   186
  corneal disease   404, 431
  dry eye disease   375–6
  glaucoma prevalence   246
    PACG   248
    POAG   247
  refractive error prevalence   203, 205, 207
Jordan   449
juvenile open-angle glaucoma   344

K
Kaplan–Meier method   141, 574
Kaposi's sarcoma   534
kappa statistic   154
Kenya
  blindness
    causes   52, 183, 283
    in children   283
    prevalence   38
  onchocerciasis   494
  ophthalmia neonatorum   319–20
  trachoma   466
keratinoid corneal degeneration *see* climatic droplet
  keratopathy
keratitis
  acanthamoeba *see* acanthamoeba keratitis
  epithelial   404
  fisherman's *see* climatic droplet keratopathy
  herpes simplex   326, 393, 404
  herpes zoster   393
  microbial *see* microbial keratitis
  neurotrophic   406
  peripheral ulcerative   435
  snowflake/cotton wool   491
keratoconjunctivitis
  infectious   526–7
  sicca *see* dry eye disease
  vernal   429–34
  viral infectious *see* viral infectious
    keratoconjunctivitis
keratoconus   324, 430–1
keratomalacia   299, 302–3, 326
  and measles   301
Key Informant Method (KIM)   276, 281, 283

kidney disease, and diabetic retinopathy risk   561
Klebsiella pneumoniae   300
Korea   413, 425–6
Kuwait   278

L
Labrador
    climatic droplet keratopathy   441–3
    glaucoma   250
    pterygium   448
Labrador keratopathy *see* climatic droplet keratopathy
lacrimal glands   372–3
lagophthalmos   371, 420, 421, 423–4
    global distribution   423
large-vessel vaso-occlusive disease   525
Laser Assisted In Situ Keratomileusis (LASIK)   214,
    371, 380
Latin America
    Andean   27
        blindness
            causes   51
            prevalence   35
        blindness
            in children   279, 283
            prevalence   27, 35
        Central   27
        blindness
            causes   51
            prevalence   35
        glaucoma prevalence
            PACG   248
            POAG   247
        onchocerciasis   493, 495
        Southern   27
        blindness
            causes   51
            prevalence   35
        Tropical   27
        blindness
            causes   41, 46, 51
            prevalence   36
Latinos in Los Angeles
    blindness
        causes   47
        prevalence   37
    cataract   182
    refractive errors, prevalence   204, 209
lead-time bias   155–6
Lebanon
    blindness
        causes   46
        prevalence   36

length bias   156
Lens Opacities Classification System (LOCS III)   98
leprosy   419–28, 533
    blindness prevalence   425
    future trends   426–7
    in HIV/AIDS   533
    multibacillary   419
    ocular   421–5
        cataracts   424
        lagophthalmos   420, 421, 423–4
        leprosy type   421
        multidrug therapy effects   425
        population age   424–5
        uveitis   423, 424
    paucibacillary   419
    prevalence and incidence   421, 422
    prevention and control   425–6
    research needs   427
    systemic disease   419–20
    treatment   420–1
        multidrug therapy   420
levocobastine   432
Liberia   493–4, 498–9
Lighthouse National Survey on Vision Loss   228, 229
lighting levels, and myopia   213
limbal anterior chamber depth (van Herick) test   260
linkage analysis   122
linkage disequilibrium   123
Liwan Eye Study   209
    refractive errors, prevalence   203
lizard skin dermatitis   493
Loa loa   498, 500, 503, 504
LOC387715   579
local variations   19–20
log of odds (LODS) score   122–3
logframe   592–3
logical framework approach   592
logistic regression   104
logMAR   10, 230, 232
logMAR charts   10, 271
Longitudinal Study of Ocular Leprosy (LOSOL)   421,
    425
Los Angeles Latino Eye Study (LALES) *see* Latinos in
    Los Angeles
loss to follow-up   114–15
loteprednol   432
low vision   227–39
    causes   232–3
    definition   7–8, 228
    future research needs   237
    global issues   236–7
    population-based studies   228, 229

prevalence   227–8
  rehabilitation   233–6
    effectiveness of   235–6
    use of low-vision aids   236
  and visual impairment   230–2
    contrast sensitivity   230–2
  see also visual impairment
low-vision assistive devices (LVAs)   234–7
  use of   236
Lowe oculo-cerebro-renal syndrome   333, 343
LOXL1 gene   127, 257–8
LV Prasad–Functional Vision Questionnaire
  (LVP–FVQ)   273
lymphoma   534

M
McNemar's test   141
macular oedema   549, 551
magnitude   7
Malawi
  blindness
    causes   47, 49, 52, 283
    in children   276, 283
    prevalence   37
  onchocerciasis   493–4
  trachoma   466
  vitamin A deficiency   305, 307
Malaysia
  blindness
    causes   45, 283
    in children   276–7, 283
    prevalence   34
  refractive errors   201–2, 206–7, 212
Mali
  blindness
    causes   48
    prevalence   38
  onchocerciasis   493, 500
  trachoma   466
Mantel–Haenszel analysis   103–4
maraviroc   522
masking   140–1
mass drug administration   505
mast cell stabilizers   432
matching   101–2
maturity-onset diabetes of youth (MODY)   554,
  559–60
Mauritania, trachoma   466
maximum likelihood   121
measles   325–7
  case fatality ratios   325
  and corneal ulceration   326

immunization   326–7
  incidence   325
  and keratomalacia   301
  risk factors   325–6
Measles Initiative   327
Mectizan *see* ivermectin
Meibomian glands   373
  dysfunction   371
Meiktila Eye Study   203, 448
melanin   579
Melbourne Visual Impairment Project   87, 90
  cataract, prevalence   179, 180
  dry eye disease   375, 376, 377
  glaucoma   252
  low vision   228, 229, 233
  pterygium   448
  refractive errors, prevalence   204
Mendel, Gregor   118
Mendelian inheritance   118
messenger RNA (mRNA)   463
meta-analysis   171–2
Mexico
  blindness
    causes   51
    prevalence   35
  onchocerciasis   495, 501
  trachoma   466
miconazole   400
microaneurysms   548
microbial keratitis   393–402
  bacterial   394
  clinical features and classification   393–4
  definition   393
  fungal   394–5
  incidence and geographical distribution   396–7
  management   399–400
  prevalence   395–6
  prevention   398–9
  research priorities   400–1
  risk factors   397
microfilaricides   497–8
microtrauma   450
milbemycin B *see* Moxidectin
Millennium Cohort Study   111
mitochondrial DNA   410
mitomycin-C   347
MMR vaccine   105, 327, 336
molluscum contagiosum   526
Mongolia
  blindness
    causes   20, 43
    in children   276, 281

prevalence   31
    climatic droplet keratopathy   441
    glaucoma   246, 249, 256
monitoring and evaluation   590, 596–8
    indicators   597–8
    scope of   598
    system development   597
    Vision 2020 initiative   598
montelukast   432
Mooren's ulcer   435–8
    classification   435–6
    clinical description   435
    definition   435
    geographical distribution   436
    management   437
    mechanisms   436–7
    prevalence   436
    research priorities   437–8
    risk factors   436
Moraxella spp.   394, 395
Morocco
    blindness
        causes   46
        prevalence   36
    trachoma   466
mortality
    age-related cataract   189–90
    and childhood blindness   273, 277, 278, 280–1
    measles infection   325–6
    vitamin A deficiency
        children   300–1
        maternal   301–2
Moxidectin   497, 504
Mozambique
    onchocerciasis   493–4
    trachoma   466
Multi-Ethnic Study of Atherosclerosis   574
Multicenter Uveitis Steroid Treatment (MUST) Trial   135, 512–13, 514
multinomial logistic regression   104
multivariable logistic regression   104
Myanmar (Burma)
    blindness
        causes   45
        in children   283
        prevalence   34
    cataract   183
    leprosy   421
    microbial keratitis   395, 398
    pterygium   448
    refractive error prevalence   203
    trachoma   466

Mycobacterium avium complex (MAC)   533
Mycobacterium leprae   419
    see also leprosy
myocilin   257
myopia   197, 198
    age, gender and ethnic distribution   206, 207, 208
    and body mass index   213
    correction
        LASIK   214
        progressive addition lenses   211, 214
        single vision lenses   211
    definition   199
    form deprivation   211
    genetic factors   210–11
        familial factors   210–11
        molecular genetics   210
    and glaucoma risk   254
    incidence, children   205
    and lighting levels   213
    and near-work   211–12
    ocular factors   213
    outdoor activities protecting against   212–13
    prevalence
        older adults   202–5
        pre-school age children   199–201
        school age children/adolescents   201, 202
        young adults   201–2
    progression, children   205

N
Naeglaeria spp.   409
narrow-angle glaucoma   244
natamycin   399
National Eye Institute Refractive Error Quality of Life Instrument   217
National Health and Nutrition Examination Study (HANES)   208
National Health and Nutrition Examination Surveys (NHANES) III   559, 563
National Institutes of Health (NIH)   131, 142
National Screening Committee   148
native Americans
    blindness, prevalence   28
    diabetic retinopathy   552
natural killer cells   461
Nauru
    diabetic retinopathy   552
    trachoma   466
near-vision impairment   11
near-work, and myopia   211–12
nedocromil sodium   432

negative predictive value 152
neglected tropical diseases (NTDs) 477, 503
Neisseria gonorrhoeae 318
Nepal
    blindness 11
      causes 44
      in children 277, 283, 331
      prevalence 25, 33
    leprosy 421, 424, 426
    microbial keratitis 395–9, 401
    trachoma 41, 466, 475
    vitamin A deficiency 299, 301–2, 304–5, 307
Nepal Blindness Survey 11, 86–7
nerve fibre layer 153, 161
nested case-control studies 74, 103
nested cohort studies 115
Netherlands
    acanthamoeba keratitis 411
    AMD 573–4
    blindness
      causes 45
      prevalence 35
    glaucoma 246
    refractive error prevalence 204
neuro-ophthalmological complications of HIV 535
neurofibromatosis 345
neurotrophic keratitis 406
New Zealand 26, 234, 410–11, 413
new-born intensive care units 354
Newfoundland 6, 442–4
Niger
    onchocerciasis 493, 498–9
    trachoma 466, 477
Nigeria
    avoidable blindness 21–2
    blindness
      causes 20, 48, 52
      incidence 16
      prevalence 16, 39
    cataract 183
    leprosy 421
    Mooren's ulcer 436
    National Blindness and Visual Impairment Survey
      29, 30, 66–7, 72
    onchocerciasis 493, 498–9, 500
    trachoma 466
night blindness 297
nodular band-shaped hyaline keratopathy *see* climatic
    droplet keratopathy
nomenclature 16
non-differential measurement error 103

Non-Governmental Development Organizations
    (NGDOs) 488
non-nucleoside reverse transcriptase inhibitors 522
non-response bias 89–90
non-Sjögren syndrome dry eye (NSSDE) 370
Nordic countries (Scandinavia)
    blindness
      incidence 15
      registration 6, 278, 281, 332
    see also individual countries
North Africa/Middle East region
    blindness
      causes 41, 46, 283
      in children 283
      prevalence 28, 36
    glaucoma prevalence
      PACG 248
      POAG 247
North America region
    blindness
      causes 41–2, 46–7
      prevalence 28, 36–7
    see also Canada; USA
North London Eye Study (NLES) 79, 90
Northern California Epidemiology of Uveitis (NCEU)
    Study 511–12
Norway
    blindness
      in children 276
      registration 6
    glaucoma 246, 248
    leprosy 421
    Oslo Macular Study 574
nucleic acid amplification tests (NAATS) 457
nucleoside reverse transcriptase inhibitors 522
Nurses' Health Study 111, 113, 114
nutrition *see* diet

O

obesity, and diabetic retinopathy risk 561
oblique flashlight test 260
observational studies 72–4, 155
    case-control studies 73–4
    cohort studies 72–3
    cross-sectional studies 72
    limitations of 75–6
    variants of 74–5
      ecological studies 74
      genetic studies 75
      self-controlled case series 74
      space/time cluster studies 74–5

observer bias   103
occurrence   66
Oceania
    blindness
        causes   42, 47, 51
        prevalence   28–9, 37
ocular computerized tomography   161, 549
Ocular Hypertension Treatment Study (OHTS)   160, 188, 254
ocular surface   372
Ocular Surface Disease Index   384
odds ratio   70–1, 95
    and sample size   97
    see also relative risk
oestrogens
    and AMD   580
    and cataract   188–9
    and dry eye disease   382
    and trachoma   472–3
Olmsted County Study
    microbial keratitis   396, 397
    POAG   251
olopatadine   432
omalizumab   432
Oman
    blindness
        causes   46
        in children   276
        prevalence   36
    trachoma   466
omega-3 fatty acids   370, 578
Onchocerca volvulus   18, 487, 488–9
    annual transmission potential   501
    community microfilarial load   496
    control/elimination   497–8
    elimination of transmission   501–2
    life cycle   489
    microfilariae   487, 488
onchocercal papillo-dermatitis   492
onchocerciasis   19, 487–507
    blindness, prevalence   17–18, 19
    clinical features   491–3
        eye disease   491–2
        skin disease   492–3
    management   495–503
        control measures   497–8
        control programmes   498–500
        disease mapping   496–7
        elimination   500–3
    parasite *see Onchocerca volvulus*
    prevalence and geographical distribution   493–5
    research priorities   503–5
        diagnostic tools   504–5

        drug combinations   504
        hypo-endemic zones/transmission zones   504
        ideal treatment frequency   503–4
        mass drug administration   505
        modelling   505
    skin snip surveys   496
    vector   489–91
        control   497
Onchocerciasis Control Programme (OCP)   488, 498–9
Onchocerciasis Elimination Programme in the Americas (OEPA)   488, 501
ophthalmia neonatorum   317–20
    blindness   280, 284, 318–19
    classification   317–18
    clinical features   317–18
    community healthcare management   320
    geographical distribution   319
    incidence   319
    prevalence   318
    prevention   319–20
    research priorities   320
    treatment   320
opportunistic infection   523
opsins   293
optic atrophy, sequential   535
    cause of blindness   43, 52, 283
optic discs   161
optic nerve in onchocerciasis   492
optic neuropathy
    glaucomatous   161, 241–2
    HIV-related   535
    and low vision   233
optical coherence tomography   572
optineurin   257
Orinda Longitudinal Study of Myopia   212
Oslo Macular Study   574
outcome measures   137–9, 155–6
    observational studies   155
    primary   137–8
    randomized trials   155
    secondary   138–9
outcome reporting bias   171
oxidative stress, and cataract risk   187–8

P

PACG *see* primary angle-closure glaucoma
Pacific Islands
    trachoma   466
    see also Oceania; and specific islands
Pakistan
    blindness
        causes   44, 50

prevalence 25, 33–4
    cataract 183
    refractive error prevalence 203
    surveys 13, 25, 79
    trachoma 466
Palestinian Arabs 342
Pan-American Health Organization (PAHO) 488
Panama 336
papilloedema 535
Papua New Guinea
    blindness
        causes 51
        prevalence 28, 37
    cataract 183
    uveitis 511
    vitamin A deficiency 301
Paraguay
    blindness
        causes 51
        prevalence 27, 36
    cataract 183
participatory planning 591
participatory rural appraisal 591
path analysis 121
pedigree studies 75
peripheral anterior synechiae 244
peripheral ulcerative keratitis 435
persistent foetal vasculature 331–2
personal hygiene, and trachoma transmission 470
Peru
    blindness
        causes 51
        prevalence 35
Peters anomaly 344
phenocopies 118
phenotype 117
Philippines
    blindness
        causes 51
        prevalence 34
    cataract 183
    vitamin A fortification 309
photorefractive keratectomy 380
Physicians' Health Study 103, 374
    dry eye disease 376, 382–4
placebos 132–3
PLEKHA1 579
Pneumocystis jirovecii choroidopathy 533
POAG *see* primary open-angle glaucoma
Poland, childhood blindness 283
polyhexamethyl biguanide 414
polymerase chain reaction 412, 458, 489

polymorphism 118
polytomous logistic regression 104
Ponza Island *see* Italy
population 66
population attributable risk percent 70
population controls 100–1
population-based sample surveys 6–10
positive predictive value 151, 152
posterior capsule opacification 337
posterior segment
    HIV-related opportunistic infections 527–34
    in onchocerciasis 492
posterior subcapsular cataracts 177, 180
    and myopia 213
potassium hydroxide 399
povidone–iodine 319–20
pre-school age children
    refractive errors 199–201
    vision screening 163
precision 80–2, 90
pregnancy, as risk factor for diabetic retinopathy 557–8
preliminary data sources 5
presbyopia 197, 215–19
    awareness of 218
    correction
        barriers to 218
        spectacle use 218
    definitions 215–16
    distribution
        age/gender 216
        geographical 216–17
    population-based studies 216
    prevalence 216
        global 11
    prevention/control 219
    public health significance 217–18
    and quality of life 217–18
    research priorities 219
    risk factors 217
prevalence 7, 66–7, 153
    sample size 90–1
prevalence surveys 11
    health regions 12–13
    limitations of 13–14
    methodology 79–88
    time trends 11–12, 14–15
prevalent cases 98–9
primary angle-closure glaucoma (PACG) 244–5
    blindness 249
    diagnostic tests 260–1
    incidence 252–3

prevalence 248
    African/African-derived populations 250
    East Asia region 250–1
prevention of progression 261
risk factors 255–7
screening 260–1
primary open-angle glaucoma (POAG) 110–11, 245
    blindness 249
    future research priorities 165
    genetics 257–8
    incidence 251–2
        age-specific 252
    prevalence 247
        African/African-derived populations 249
        India 250
        South Asia region 250
    risk factors 254–5
    screening 159–62, 259–60
        population at risk 160
        programme structure 162
    screening tests 160
        corneal thickness 160–1
        imaging technologies 161
        intraocular pressure 160
        nerve fibre layer 153, 161
        optic discs 161
        visual field testing 161–2
primary sampling units 85
probability sampling 82
probability-proportional-to-size 84
process measures 151–5
Programme for the Prevention of Blindness and
    Deafness (PBD) 4, 11
progressive addition lenses 211, 214
progressive multifocal leukoencephalopathy 535
progressive outer retinal necrosis syndrome (PORNS)
    532
project cycle management 592–3
proviruses 519
Proyecto VER study 181, 204
pseudogerontoxon 430
pseudohypopyon 492
Pseudomonas spp. 394
Pseudomonas aeruginosa 395
pterygium 447–53
    definition 447
    future research priorities 451–2
    geographical distribution 449
    grading 447
    heredity 449
    management 451
    pathogenesis 451

prevalence and incidence 447–8
    risk factors 449–51
        personal 449
publication bias 171
Puerto Ricans 217

Q
quality assurance 150–1, 158, 595–6
quality of life
    age-related cataract 184
    dry eye disease 384
    presbyopia 217–18

R
radiation exposure and cataract risk 185–7
raltegravir 522
Rand Health Insurance Study 228, 229
random sampling error 80–1
randomized controlled trials 71–2, 132
randomized screening trials 72, 165
ranibizumab 580
Rapid Assessment of Avoidable Blindness (RAAB) 6,
    14, 88
    cataract 182
    India 25
    surveys 49–52
Rapid Assessment of Cataract Surgical Services
    (RACSS) 6, 14, 88
    cataract 182, 183
    India 25
    surveys 49–52
rapid epidemiological assessment 496
rapid epidemiological mapping of onchocerciasis
    (REMO) 496
rapid rural appraisal 591
rate ratio see relative risk
recall bias 102
receiver operative characteristic (ROC) 152
Recommended Dietary Allowance (RDA) 295
refractive errors 197–226
    associated factors 209–13
        anthropometric parameters and dietary changes
            213
        biometry 209–10
        environment 211–13
        genetics 210–11
    and blindness 4
    classification and grading 198–9
    clinical descriptions 198
    distribution
        by age, gender and ethnicity 206–7, 208
        changes with time 208–9

geographical   207–8
future research   214–15
genetic epidemiology   128
and glaucoma risk   254
incidence/progression   205–6
adults   205–6
children   205
presbyopia *see* presbyopia
prevalence   199–205
changes with time   208–9
older adults   202–5
pre-school age children   199–201
school age children/adolescents   201, 202
young adults   201–2
prevention/control   214
public health significance   198
screening in children   163–4
see also individual conditions
refractive surgery and dry eye disease   380
regional variations   20
relative dose response   303
relative humidity and dry eye disease   379
relative risk   66, 69–70, 110
reliability   153
Renin-Angiotensin System Study (RASS)   557
research methods   65–77
case definition   65–6
future directions   76
hypothesis testing   71
incidence   7, 15–16, 66, 67–8
measures of effect   69–71
different (absolute) measure   69
estimation of   71
odds ratio   70–1
population attributable risk percent   71
relative risk   69–70
observational studies   72–4
limitations of   75–6
variants of   74–5
prevalence   7, 66–7
randomized experimental studies   71–2
research synthesis   169–73
future research needs   173
systematic review   170–2
types of   172–3
respiratory distress syndrome   358
retinal detachment in CMV retinitis   530–1
retinal pigment epithelium   297, 571
retinitis
cytomegalovirus *see* cytomegalovirus retinitis
toxoplasmic   532–3
retinitis pigmentosa   118

and low vision   233
retinoic acids   296
retinol activity equivalents   293
retinol, serum   303
retinol-binding protein   296
retinopathy, HIV   524–5
retinopathy of prematurity (ROP)   282, 353–68
aggressive posterior   355–6
blindness risk   354–5
classification/grading systems   355–6
detection and treatment   360–1
digital imaging   361
ophthalmologist-led   360–1
future research   362
and gestational age   354
history and regional variation   353–5
prevalence and incidence   356–7
prevention
primary   357–9
secondary   359–60
tertiary   360
risk factors   354, 357
Reykjavik Eye Study   574, 575
rhodopsin   296–7
ribosomal RNA (rRNA)   458
rifabutin, ocular toxicity   536
rimexolone   432
Risk Factor for Uveal Melanoma Study   100–1
risk management   595
risk ratio *see* relative risk
RNA
messenger (mRNA)   463
ribosomal (rRNA)   458
ROP *see* retinopathy of prematurity
Roscommon Glaucoma Survey   27, 35, 83, 152, 246, 248
Rose Bengal test   372, 377
Rotterdam Eye Study   81, 110–11, 126
AMD   126, 574, 575, 580
glaucoma   246, 250
low vision   233
refractive errors   204
rubella
congenital rubella syndrome   333, 334–5
immunization   335–6
Russia   27, 186
Rwanda
blindness
avoidable   21
causes   52
prevalence   38
cryptococcal meningitis   535

onchocerciasis   493–4

S
SAFE strategy in trachoma   473–8
St Lucia   246, 249
Salisbury Eye Evaluation and Driving Study   111
Salisbury Eye Evaluation Study (SEE)   19, 28, 79, 179
   AMD   573, 580
   blindness
      causes   47
      prevalence   36
   cataract
      blindness and low vision   181
      prevalence   179, 180
   dry eye disease   374, 376, 377
   low vision   228, 229, 232–3
Salnes Eye Study, dry eye disease   376, 377
sample size   139–40
   case-control studies   96–7
   genome-wide association studies   125
   and odds ratio   97
   prevalence estimation   90–1
sample surveys   80
sampling distribution   82
sampling error   80–1
sampling frame   83
sampling interval   83
sampling schemes   82–9
   cluster sampling   82, 84–5
   design effect   85–6
   simple random sampling   82, 83–4
   stratification   88–9
sampling unit   83
Saudi Arabia
   blindness
      causes   46, 283
      in children   283
      prevalence   36
   congenital glaucoma   342
Save Sight America campaign   162
Scandinavia *see* Nordic countries
Schirmer test   372, 377
school age children, refractive errors   201, 202
schools for blind   6
Scotland
   acanthamoeba keratitis   411
   blindness, in children   283
   seasonal allergic rhinoconjunctivitis   431
screening programmes   147–67
   bias   155–6
   children   162–4

amblyopia   163
   pre-school vision tests   163
   refractive error   163–4
definition   147–8
diabetic retinopathy   156–9
elderly persons   164
evaluation of   151–6
   outcome measures   155–6
   process measures   151–5
future research priorities   164–5
glaucoma   259–61
   PACG   260–1
   POAG   159–62, 259–60
justification for   150
primary   147
principles of   148–9
programme planning   150
quality assurance   150–1
secondary   147
setting up   150
target population   150
segregation analysis   120
selection bias   80, 89
self-controlled case series   74
Senegal
   onchocerciasis   493, 500
   trachoma   466
sensitivity   151–2
Serratia spp.   394
serum lipids, as risk factor for diabetic retinopathy   558
serum retinol   303
sexually transmitted diseases   318, 319
sham procedures   132–3
shared environment   119
shared genes   119
Shihpai Eye Study   40
   dry eye disease   376, 377, 378
   refractive error prevalence   203
sibling studies   121
Sierra Leone   29
   blindness
      causes   42, 48
      prevalence   38
   onchocerciasis   493–4, 498
silver nitrate   319
simple random sampling   82, 83–4
Simulium spp. in onchocerciasis   19, 489–91
   annual biting rates   491
Singapore
   blindness
      causes   40, 43

prevalence   31
cataract   246, 249
glaucoma
    incidence   253
    prevalence   179, 180, 253
pterygium   448, 450
refractive error prevalence   199, 200, 202, 203,
    205–9, 211–13
Singapore Malay Eye Study (SiMES)   179
    cataract prevalence   179, 180
    refractive error prevalence   203
single nucleotide polymorphisms   122, 471–3
single vision lenses   211
situational analysis   588
Sjögren syndrome dry eye (SSDE)   370
Slovakia   342
smoking
    and AMD   577
    and cataract risk   184–5
    and diabetic retinopathy risk   560
    and dry eye disease   380–1
    protective effect against pterygium   450
Snow, John   109
socio-economic status   20
    and diabetic retinopathy risk   561
sodium cromoglycate   432
Sorsby fundus dystrophy   126
South Africa
    blindness
        causes   48
        prevalence   29, 38
    children   244, 323
    climatic droplet keratopathy   441
    glaucoma   245, 248, 250
    HIV/AIDS   530
    microbial keratitis   395
    pterygium   448
    refractive error   202, 207, 212
    uveitis   511
South Asia region
    blindness
        causes   41, 44, 50
        prevalence   24, 33–4
    glaucoma prevalence   250
    see also India
South East Asia region
    blindness
        causes   41, 44–5, 50–1
        prevalence   12, 26, 34
    glaucoma prevalence
        PACG   248
        POAG   247

'sowda'   492, 495
space/time cluster studies   74–5
Spain
    blindness prevalence   35
    see also Salnes Eye Study
specificity   151–2
spectacle use
    barriers to   218
    presbyopia   218
Sri Lanka
    blindness
        causes   45
        prevalence   34
standardization of uveitis nomenclature (SUN)   510
Staphylococcus aureus   394
Staphylococcus epidermidis   394
Stargardt disease   126
statistical power   139
steroids, age-related cataract   188
Stevens–Johnson syndrome   536
stigma of blindness   6
stratification   88–9
Streptococcus pneumoniae   300, 394
Streptococcus viridans   394
Sturge–Weber syndrome   345
Sub-Saharan Africa
    blindness
        in children   276, 283
        prevalence   29–30
    Central   29
        blindness
            causes   42, 47
            prevalence   37
    East   29
        blindness
            causes   47, 52
            prevalence   37–8
    Southern   29
        blindness
            causes   42, 47, 48, 52
            prevalence   38
    West   29–30
        blindness
            causes   42, 48, 52
            prevalence   38–9
Sudan
    blindness
        causes   47
        in children   276
        prevalence   38
    onchocerciasis   492–4
    trachoma   467, 471, 478

vitamin A deficiency   301
sunlight *see* ultraviolet radiation
superoxide dismutase   578
Supplemental Treatment of Pre-threshold ROP study
  (STOP-ROP)   360
surgery
      acanthamoeba keratitis   415
      cataract
          in children   336–7
          quality of   595–6
          small incision   591
      glaucoma   346–7
      refractive   380
      trachoma   473–5
sustainable healthcare   593–5
      cost recovery   594–5
      programme planning   594
      threats to   594
Sweden
      acanthamoeba keratitis   410–11
      childhood blindness   280, 283, 319
      childhood cataract   332
      diabetic retinopathy   552
      glaucoma   246, 248, 251, 253
      low vision   236
      optic neuritis   75
      ROP   358
Switzerland
      diabetic retinopathy   552
      vernal keratoconjunctivitis   431
Sydney Myopia Study   210, 212–13
syphilis, ocular   533
systematic review   170–2
systematic sampling   83

T
T-cells   300, 430
      cytotoxic   461, 463
      in trachoma   460–1
T-helper cells   461
T-regulatory cells (Tregs)   461, 463
t-test   141
tacrolimus   432
Taiwan
      blindness
          causes   40, 44
          prevalence   24, 32
      dry eye disease   375, 376, 378
      glaucoma   246, 253
      refractive error prevalence   203
Tajimi Eye Study, refractive error prevalence   203
Tamil Nadu Eye Study, refractive error prevalence   203

Tanzania   29
      blindness
          causes   47, 283
          in children   276, 277, 283
          prevalence   37
      glaucoma   246, 248–9
      leprosy   421
      low vision   229
      onchocerciasis   493–4
      refractive errors   11, 216–18
      trachoma   232, 458, 462, 464, 467–77
      viral infectious keratoconjunctivitis   404
TAPP1   579
tear film   371–2
      break-up time   375, 377
Tear Stability Analysis System (TSAS)   384
tetracycline eye ointment   475
Thailand   21, 249, 448
time trends
      in causes   17
      in prevalence   11–12, 14–15
      see also individual diseases
Timor-Leste
      blindness
          causes   50
          prevalence   34
      cataract   183
      refractive errors   216, 218
TIMP3   126
Togo
      blindness
          causes   19, 48
          prevalence   19, 38
      onchocerciasis   493–4, 498–9
Tonga
      blindness
          causes   47
          prevalence   37
toxic epidermal necrolysis   536
Toxoplasma gondii   532–3
toxoplasmic retinitis, HIV-related   532–3
toxoplasmosis   532–3
trabeculectomy   247–8
trabeculotomy   247
trachoma   455–86
      blindness prevalence   19
      Chlamydia trachomatis   455, 456–8
      classification   459, 460
      clinical signs   459–60
      control and management   473–8
          antibiotics   475–6
          personal hygiene measures   477–8

surgery 473–5
vaccine 478
epidemiology 464–73
follicular 459
fomites 470
future research 478–9
history 455–6
immunopathology 460–4
antibody response 462–3
cellular responses 463
hypersensitivity and chlamydial persistence 463–4
immune response 461–2
innate immunity 462
prevalence 464–9
reinfection 476
risk factors 469–73
flies 470–1
latrines 471
personal 469
personal hygiene 470
scarring and entropion 471–3
water 469–70
trachomatous trichiasis 459
risk factors 471–3
traditional eye medicines, harmful 326, 327–8
transducin 297
traumatic cataract 335
traumatic microbial keratitis 397
trichiasis study 229, 232
trifluorothymidine 405
tuberculosis 533
tumour necrosis factor 471–3
tumours 534
Tunisia
blindness
causes 46
prevalence 36
Turkey
blindness
causes 46, 283
in children 283
prevalence 36
Turkmenistan
blindness 23
causes 50
prevalence 31
cataract 183
twin studies 75, 121, 126, 189
type I errors 139
type II errors 140

U
Uganda
blindness
causes 47, 283
in children 283, 327, 396
prevalence 37
HIV/AIDS 532, 534–5
leprosy 424
onchocerciasis 491, 493–4, 497, 500
presbyopia 216
trachoma 467
UK
acanthamoeba keratitis 411
blindness
causes 45, 283
in children 278, 280, 283, 325
prevalence 35
childhood cataract 332
aphakic glaucoma 345
ophthalmia neonatorum 318
diabetic retinopathy screening programme 157–9
glaucoma 258
low vision 229, 233, 236
refractive errors 212
see also British; Scotland; Wales
ultrasound biomicroscopy 244
ultraviolet radiation
and AMD 578–9
and cataract 185–6
and climatic droplet keratopathy 443–4
and pterygium 449–50
UNICEF 308
United Arab Emirates 319
United Kingdom Prospective Diabetes Study (UKPDS) 555, 556–7
USA
acanthamoeba keratitis 411
causes 283
blindness, prevalence 12, 36–7
cataract
age-related 179, 180, 181
childhood 331–2
climatic droplet keratopathy 441
diabetic retinopathy 552
dry eye disease 374, 376
low vision 228, 233
POAG 246, 251
pterygium 448
refractive error prevalence 200, 202, 204
UVB
and cataract risk 185–6

see also ultraviolet radiation
uveitis   509–16
    classification and grading   509–11
    complications   512–13
    definition   509
    disease associations
        glaucoma   245, 345
        leprosy   423, 424
        onchocerciasis   492
    immune recovery   531
    management   512
    prevalence and incidence   511–12
    research   513–14
    standardization of uveitis nomenclature (SUN)
        510
    syndromes   510
    vision loss attributable to   513

V
vaccines
    herpes simplex   406
    HIV/AIDS   521
    measles   325–6
    rubella (MMR)   105, 335–6, 338
    trachoma   478
Vahlkampfia spp.   409
valaciclovir   406
    cytomegalovirus   528, 529
    herpes zoster ophthalmicus   526
validity   151
Vanuatu
    blindness
        causes   47
        prevalence   37
variance components analysis   120–1
varicella zoster keratoconjunctivitis   403, 404
varicella zoster virus   525
vascular endothelial growth factor (VEGF)
    in AMD   580
    and ROP   357
Venezuela
    blindness
        causes   51
        prevalence   35
    onchocerciasis   495–501
vernal keratoconjunctivitis   429–34
    classification   430–1
    clinical features   429–30
    definition   429
    genetics   432
    geographical distribution   431
    management   432

prevalence   431
    research priorities   432–3
    risk factors   431–2
vertical cup–disc ratio   242
Veteran Administration Diabetes Trial (VADT)   556
VF-14   184
vidarabine   405
Vietnam, trachoma   467
viral infectious keratoconjunctivitis   403–8
    clinical features   403–4
    definition   403
    geographical distribution   305
        changes with time   305
    management   405–6
    prevalence and incidence   404–5
        changes with time   305
    research priorities   407
    risk factors   405
Vision 2020 initiative   79, 269, 588, 601–6
    advocacy   603
    cost-effective interventions   602
    definition   601
    future research   606
    history   601–2
    human resource development   602–3
    'I SEE' principles   603–4
    implementation   604–5
    infrastructure development   603
    monitoring and evaluation   598
    priorities   602
    resources   604
    strategy   602–3
    structure of   604
vision loss *see* blindness
Vision-related Quality of Life Core Measure 1 (VCM1)
    228
visual acuity   7
    children   271–2
    logMAR charts   10, 271
    measurement of   10
    notations for recording   8
visual field testing   161–2
    children   272
Visual Function Questionnaire-25   384
visual impairment
    in children   269–89
    data sources   5–6
    definition   7–8, 10
    diabetic retinopathy   551
    and low vision   230–2
        contrast sensitivity   230–2
    prevalence   4

WHO categorization   8, 9
see also blindness; low vision
vitamin A
   absorption and metabolism   296–7
   dietary sources   293, 295–7
      dietary reference intakes   295
      foods with preformed vitamin A   295
      foods with provitamin A carotenoids   293
   supplementation   301, 302, 307–8
vitamin A deficiency in children   18, 277, 291–316
   biochemical indicators   303–4
   dietary risk factors   377
   epidemiology   302–7
   extent of vitamin A deficiency   304–5
   functional indicators   304
   geographical distribution   294, 305–6
   health consequences   297–302
      infection   300
      morbidity and mortality
         children   300–1
         maternal   301–2
      xerophthalmia   291, 297–300, 302–3
   historical context   292–3
   indicators of   302–4
   prevalence
      periodicity   306
      person-related   306
   prevention   307–10
      dietary improvement   309–10
      food fortification   308–9
      vitamin A supplementation   301, 302, 307–8
vitamins C and E
   in AMD   580–1
   in cataract   187
   in dry eye   370
   in ROP   357
   in vitamin A deficiency   301, 302, 307–8
vitritis   510
   see also uveitis
voriconazole   400

W
Wales, glaucoma in   245–6, 250–2
water, contaminated
   as risk factor for acanthamoeba keratitis   410–13, 415–16
   as risk factor for trachoma   469–70
weighted kappa statistic   154

Wellcome Trust Case Control Consortium (WTCCC) 124
Western Pacific, blindness, prevalence   12
Western Samoa   448
WHO
   Expanded Programme of Immunization (EPI) 326
   HIV staging system   520
WHO/PBL, Global Databank *see* Programme for the Prevention of Blindness and Deafness
Wilcoxon Rank Sum test   141
Wisconsin Age-Related Maculopathy Grading Scheme 572
Wisconsin Epidemiologic Study of Diabetic Retinopathy (WESDR)   68, 549–50
Wolbachia spp.   504
Women's Health Study   374
   dry eye disease   376
World Health Assembly   601
World Health Organization
   Programme for the Prevention of Blindness and Deafness *see* WHO/PBL
   Vision 2020 initiative   79, 269

X
xerophthalmia   291, 297–300, 302–3
   classification   298
   prevalence   298
   treatment and prevention   298
xerophthalmic fundus   303
Xichang Pediatric Refractive Error Study   211

Y
Yemen
   onchocerciasis   492–5
   trachoma   467
yield   153

Z
Zambia
   blindness prevalence   37
   trachoma   467
   vitamin A deficiency   305, 309
zeanthin, in AMD   579
zidovudine   522
zinc
   in AMD   579, 581
   in cataract   187